# Acupuncture, Trigger Points and Musculoskeletal Pain

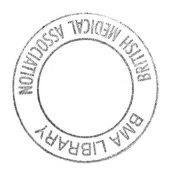

*To Oina, my wife, for her patience and forbearance*
*during the writing of this book.*

The phenomena of pain belong to that borderland between the body and soul about which it is so delightful to speculate from the comfort of an armchair, but which offers such formidable obstacles to scientific inquiry.

J. H. Kellgren (1948)

*Extracts from reviews of the first edition:*

'…I warmly recommend this book to anyone who wants to learn more about this often neglected area of common musculoskeletal pain conditions…'
**Journal of the Royal College of Physicians of London**

'This is a book that should belong to physicians, neurologists, rheumatologists and teachers of medical students…'
**Pain**

*Endorsements of the new edition:*

'Peter Baldry is one of the most respected practitioners of Medical Acupuncture in the UK. This new edition is yet another first-class book, which adeptly combines the theory and practice of treatment of trigger points for musculoskeletal pain. An eminently readable and informative text; this is a *tour du force* and an essential acquisition for those practitioners who want a clear practical guide for the treatment of musculoskeletal pain using trigger point treatment and the scientific understanding that underpins the treatment.'
**Jacqueline Filshie, Consultant in Anaesthesia and Pain Management, Royal Marsden Hospital, London and Surrey; Secretary of the British Medical Acupuncture Society**

'In this fine comprehensive book, Dr Baldry removes much of the mystique from acupuncture as a technique for musculoskeletal pain relief. Using a fully scientific integration of Eastern and Western knowledge, coupled with the relevant literature on clinical effectiveness of acupuncture, he provides an ideal, evidence-based text for the practitioner.

From the beginner to the expert, anyone with an interest in the nature of muscle pain, its pathophysiology and treatment will be informed by this book: the entry-level therapist will gain a better understanding based on sound scientific evidence, while the experienced clinician will be rewarded with a well-written guide to what is significant in everyday clinical practice. Clinicians of several medical specialties (neurologists, orthopaedic surgeons, general practitioners, pain specialists, physiatrists) and other practitioners (acupuncturists, physiotherapists, nurses, occupational therapists) will find this book an indispensable reference in their daily work. For those who wish to implement acupuncture in the clinic, this textbook is an invaluable resource for responsible practice.

In total, this book offers an innovative approach to the diagnosis, understanding and treatment of myofascial trigger point pain using acupuncture that integrates all current concepts of neurophysiology and neuroanatomy principles. Dr Peter Baldry is to be congratulated for conceptualizing, editing and writing such a truly valuable asset for every clinical practice.'
**Dr George Georgoudis, Research Physiotherapist, University of Manchester, UK; Lecturer, Technological Educational Institute of Athens, Department of Physiotherapy, Greece; "Tzanio" General Hospital of Pireaus, Greece**

*For Elsevier Ltd*

*Commissionning Editor:* Karen Morley
*Project Development Manager:* Kerry McGechie
*Project Manager:* Derek Robertson

# Acupuncture, Trigger Points and Musculoskeletal Pain

A scientific approach to acupuncture for use by doctors and physiotherapists in the diagnosis and management of myofascial trigger point pain

THIRD EDITION

**P. E. Baldry** MB BS FRCP

*Emeritus Consultant Physician and Postgraduate Clinical Tutor, Ashford Hospital, North West London, UK*
*Past Chairman, British Medical Acupuncture Society*
*Past President, Acupuncture Association of Chartered Physiotherapists*
*Member of the British and Irish Chapter of the International Association for the Study of Pain*
*Member of the International Myopain Society*

*Foreword by*

**John W. Thompson** PhD MB BS FRCP

*Professor of Pharmacology and Head of Department of Pharmacological Sciences, University of Newcastle upon Tyne*
*Consultant Clinical Pharmacologist and Consultant in Administrative Charge,*
*Pain Relief Clinic, Royal Victoria Infirmary, Newcastle upon Tyne, UK*

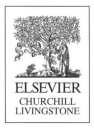

ELSEVIER
CHURCHILL
LIVINGSTONE

EDINBURGH  LONDON  NEW YORK  PHILADELPHIA  SAN FRANCISCO  AND TORONTO  2005

# ELSEVIER
CHURCHILL
LIVINGSTONE

First edition 1989
Second edition 1993
Translated into Japanese 1995
Translated into German 1996
Third edition 2005
    Reprint 2006

ISBN 0 443 06644 2

British Library Cataloguing in Publication Data
A catalogue record for this book is available from the British Library

Library of Congress Cataloguing in Publication Data
A catalogue record for this book is available from the Library of Congress

Notice

Knowledge and best practice in this field are constantly changing. As new
research and experience broaden our knowledge, changes in practice, treatment
and drug therapy may become necessary or appropriate. Readers are advised to
check the most current information provided (i) on procedures featured or (ii) by
the manufacturer of each product to be administered, to verify the recommended
dose or formula, the method and duration of administration, and
contraindications. It is the responsibility of the practitioner, relying on experience
and knowledge of the patient, to make diagnoses, to determine dosages and the
best treatment for each individual patient, and to take all appropriate safety
precautions. To the fullest extent of the law, neither the publisher nor the authors
assumes any liability for any injury and/or damage.

The Publisher

ELSEVIER    your source for books,
            journals and multimedia
            in the health sciences
**www.elsevierhealth.com**

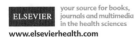
Working together to grow
libraries in developing countries
www.elsevier.com | www.bookaid.org | www.sabre.org
ELSEVIER    BOOK AID    Sabre Foundation
            International

The
publisher's
policy is to use
**paper manufactured
from sustainable forests**

Printed in China

# Contents

# Foreword

*Quod est ante pedes nemo spectat: coeli Scrutantur plagas.* (What is before one's feet no one looks at; they gaze at the regions of heaven.)
Ennius, quoted by Cicero, *De Divinat.*, 2, 13.

This is an important and valuable book that needed to be written. Musculoskeletal or myofascial pain is an all too common and extraordinarily neglected subject of medicine; it is barely mentioned in many textbooks of medicine. In reality it is a ubiquitous condition that causes a great deal of pain and suffering and one which, unfortunately, either slips by unrecognized or is passed off as trivial or untreatable. In this book Dr Peter Baldry has shown how musculoskeletal pain can be simply and effectively treated by acupuncture. But this book is much more than that because it is really three books in one.

The first part presents an interesting historical background to Chinese acupuncture and its spread to the outside world, particularly to the West. The second part deals with the principles of trigger point acupuncture wherein, over the course of six chapters, the reader is presented with a detailed and critical account of the evidence for and the nature of trigger points and the way in which acupuncture can be used to deactivate them. Dr Baldry spares no effort to provide the reader with an up-to-date and accurate account of the neurophysiology of pain and the possible ways in which acupuncture can be used to control it. He also grasps the difficult and important nettle concerning the scientific evaluation of acupuncture. The results of properly controlled experiments and trials demonstrating the efficacy of acupuncture are slowly but surely accumulating and Dr Baldry discusses these critically and points the way to the further rigorous studies that are urgently needed. The third part of the book gives a detailed and splendidly practical account of the many different forms of musculoskeletal pain and the way that these can be treated with acupuncture.

Even for the reader who does not intend to use acupuncture, this book still serves a most valuable purpose by drawing attention to the very large number of common musculoskeletal pain conditions that are all too commonly overlooked. A particularly helpful feature of Dr Baldry's book is the rich admixture of case histories of his own patients, from which the medical reader can learn the correct way to diagnose and subsequently to treat these painful conditions.

There seems little doubt that, through unfamiliarity with this condition, much time and effort are often expended unnecessarily both by the medical profession and by patients seeking the cause and treatment of pain problems that are, in fact, musculoskeletal in origin. Dr Baldry has performed a most valuable service in writing this eminently readable book and I wish it the very considerable success that it richly deserves.

John W. Thompson

# Preface

## The aims of this book

It is because traditional Chinese acupuncture is perforce inextricably bound up with archaic concepts concerning the structure and function of the body that most members of the medical profession in the Western world view it with suspicion and scepticism and assign it, together with various other seemingly esoteric forms of therapy, to what is called alternative or complementary medicine. Moreover, it is evident that attempts during the past 40 years to place Chinese acupuncture on a more rational and scientific basis have done little to dispel this attitude.

My reason for writing this book is to bring to the attention of doctors and physiotherapists a 20th-century-evolved scientific approach to acupuncture for the relief of pain emanating from trigger points in the myofascial pain syndrome and from tender and trigger points in the fibromyalgia syndrome, and to take acupuncture (so far as the alleviation of nociceptive pain of this type is concerned) out of the category of alternative or complementry medicine by describing a method of employing it that has been developed as a result of observations made by physicians during recent years and is now fast becoming incorporated within the framework of present-day orthodox medical practice.

It is because there have been so many advances in our knowledge concerning the pathophysiology, diagnosis and treatment of the myofascial trigger point and fibromyalgia syndromes since the 2nd edition of this book was published, that in this edition four chapters in Part 2 (Principles of Trigger Point Acupuncture) have had to be replaced by entirely new ones. In addition to these changes most of the other chapters in Part 2 and Part 3 (The Practical Application of Trigger Point Acupuncture) have had to be extensively revised.

It is hoped that as a result of reading this book many more anaesthetists, rheumatologists, orthopaedic specialists, general physicians, general practitioners and physiotherapists than at present may not only be led to search for trigger points in their routine clinical investigation of pain, but may also be persuaded to include dry needling at these points in their therapeutic armamentarium.

## Case histories

I offer no apology for having included case histories in this book. They are, of course, by their very nature essentially anecdotal and certainly no inference is meant to be drawn from them concerning the effectiveness of trigger point acupuncture, for any conclusions about that can only come from clinical trials. The sole purpose of including these vignettes is to provide illustrations from everyday clinical practice that serve to highlight certain important principles underlying the diagnosis and management of various painful musculoskeletal disorders.

# Acknowledgements

My very sincere thanks are due to Professor John Thompson for the meticulous manner in which he read the manuscript of this book and then gave me much valuable advice and constructive criticism besides kindly writing a foreword.

I wish to express my gratitude to Dr Alexander Macdonald for it was he who, some years ago, first drew my attention to the aetiological importance of trigger points in the pathogenesis of musculoskeletal pain and introduced me to trigger point acupuncture as a method of alleviating it.

I thank Dr Felix Mann for having initially brought to my notice the close relationship between trigger points and traditional Chinese acupuncture points.

I wish to say how indebted I am to the late Drs Janet Travell and Dr David Simons for the very considerable contribution they made to my knowledge of specific patterns of myofascial trigger point pain referral. It has largely been from studying their descriptions and illustrations of these patterns in various publications referred to later in this book that I am now able to recognize them in my own patients.

I also wish to say how very grateful I am to Dr David Bowsher, for it has been from him in particular that I have learnt so much about what is currently known concerning the mechanisms responsible for the pain-relieving effect of acupuncture.

I have to thank Professors Peter Williams and Roger Warwick, the editors of *Gray's Anatomy* (36th edition 1980) and its publishers Churchill Livingstone for giving me permission to reproduce Figures 12.1, 12.5, 12.9, 12.14, 13.12, 15.1, 15.2, 15.17, 15.23*, 16.8, 16.9, 16.10, 18.1*, 18.6, 18.7*, 18.9*, 18.11*, 20.1, 20.2, 20.5*, 20.6. The illustrations from *Gray's Anatomy* marked with an asterisk originally appeared in *Quain's Anatomy* 11th edition.

Finally, I have to thank the following: Dr J. H. Kellgren and the editor of *Clinical Science* for permission to publish Figures 4.1 and 4.2; Dr Kellgren and the editor of the *British Medical Journal* for permission to publish Figure 4.3; Dr Howard Fields and McGraw Hill, New York for permission to reproduce Figures 6.1, 6.2, 6.3 and 7.3 from *Pain* 1987; Dr David Bowsher and the editor of *Acupuncture in Medicine – The Journal of the British Medical Acupuncture Society* for permission to reproduce Figures 6.5 and 9.1; Dr David Simons and Haworth Press for permission to reproduce Figure 7.2; Dr Alexander Macdonald and George Allen & Unwin, London for permission to reproduce Figures 7.4 and 7.5 from *Acupuncture – from Ancient Art to Modern Medicine* 1982; Mr R. J. D'Souza for providing me with Figure 7.6; Professor Yunus and Lea & Febiger, Philadelphia for permission to reproduce Figure 7.7; Dr J. Park and the editor of *Acupuncture in Medicine* for permission to reproduce Figure 11.1; Dr David Simons and Churchill Livingstone, Edinburgh for permission to reproduce Figure 16.6 from *Textbook of Pain* (Wall P., Melzack R., eds) 2nd edition 1989; Professor R. W. Porter and Churchill Livingstone, Edinburgh for permission to reproduce Figures 17.2 and 17.3 from *The Lumbar Spine and Back Pain* (Jason M. I. V., ed) 3rd edition 1987.

P.E.B. (p.baldry@ukonline.co.uk)

# Introduction to the third edition

For reasons to be explained later in this book, the early 1970s saw the dawn of an era when people in the Western world began taking an increasing interest in the ancient oriental mode of therapy known as acupuncture, with lay practitioners of it leading the public to believe that it has such wide ranging healing properties as to be an effective alternative to orthodox medicine in the treatment of a large number of diseases.

There is clearly no justification for such extravagant claims and it has to be said that, at the onset of this era, the medical profession in Europe and America viewed this form of therapy with considerable suspicion and continued to do so for so long as explanations as to how it might work remained inextricably bound up with abstruse concepts formulated by the Chinese 3000 years previously. This reluctance to believe in these long-established but somewhat esoteric hypotheses was, of course, because they had been conceived at a time when ideas concerning the structure and function of the body together with those concerning the nature of disease belonged more to the realms of fantasy than fact, and for this reason it was difficult to reconcile them with the principles upon which the present-day Western system of medical practice is based.

During the latter part of the 20th century, however, there has been a considerable increase in knowledge concerning the neurophysiology of pain and because of this there is now a scientific explanation for acupuncture's ability to alleviate pain. It has become apparent that this technique, which involves the use of dry needles (*acus* (Latin),

needle) for the purpose of stimulating peripheral nerve endings, achieves its pain-relieving effect by virtue of its ability to evoke activity in pain-modulating mechanisms present in the peripheral and central nervous systems.

In the light of this discovery and a number of others the public in general and the medical profession in particular have had to revise their attitudes towards acupuncture.

Furthermore, when the House of Lords select committee in science and technology (2000) took a close look at various types of treatment at present included within the ambit of complementary/alternative medicine, it divided them into three groups and placed acupuncture in the one containing therapeutic procedures deemed to be the most organized and regulated.

The committee, in addition, considered that the research bases of these procedures are of sufficiently high standards to allow them to be used within the UK's National Health Service.

Prior to the publication of this report the British Medical Acupuncture Society (1997) had published a discussion paper entitled 'Acupuncture's Place Within Mainstream Medicine'. In this it was stated:

'...Medical acupuncture practice depends on three important principles: an orthodox Western diagnosis needs to be made for every patient; acupuncture should be integrated with conventional medicine; and it must be appreciated that the traditional Chinese view of acupuncture is being replaced in many areas by an approach based on modern physiology and neuroanatomy. ...'

In accordance with the above, in 2000 The Royal College of Physicians of London set up a subcommittee to assist with the present task of bringing acupuncture and a strictly selected number of other hitherto somewhat pejoratively called complementary or alternative therapeutic procedures within the framework of orthodox medical practice.

Lewith et al (2003), moreover, during the course of discussing the current status of certain therapeutic procedures in the *Journal of the Royal College of Physicians of London*, including acupuncture, made the following two apposite comments concerning the latter: (1) 'needling trigger points is particularly effective in the treatment of pain'; (2) 'acupuncture is currently used in at least 84% of pain clinics in the UK…'

A paucity of suitably funded research has been the principle hindrance to getting certain therapeutic procedures including acupuncture integrated within the fabric of conventional medical practice. This has prompted Lesley Rees, Director of Education at the Royal College of Physicians of London and Andrew Weil, Professor of Medicine at the University of Arizona (Rees & Weil 2001), to emphasize the need for the NHS research and development directorate and the Medical Research Council to now help correct this unfortunate state of affairs.

The purpose of this book is to discuss the scientific aspects of acupuncture in general and trigger point acupuncture in particular and to show how this latter type of therapy can readily be used by doctors and physiotherapists in the treatment of the myofascial pain and fibromyalgia syndromes.

For those trained in the Western system of medicine there are obvious advantages in using this particular method rather than the traditional Chinese one, but clearly these advantages cannot be fully appreciated without knowing something about the latter. This book is, therefore, divided into three parts with Part 1 containing a brief account of traditional Chinese acupuncture. It also gives reasons as to why doctors in Europe on first learning about this type of treatment in the 17th century rejected it, and describes how certain 19th-century European and American doctors, having put on one side what they considered to be unacceptable Chinese concepts concerning this mode of therapy, devised a method of practising it principally for the relief of musculoskeletal pain that may be considered to be a forerunner of the somewhat more sophisticated one developed in recent years and described in this book. It is also pointed out that, although physicians who advocated the use of acupuncture in the Western world during the last century wrote enthusiastically about it, it was never widely practised by their contemporaries, mainly it would seem because at that time there was no satisfactory explanation as to the manner in which it might work.

In Part 2 attention is drawn to fundamental laboratory investigations into the phenomenon of referred pain from musculoskeletal structures carried out by J. H. Kellgren at University College Hospital, London, in the late 1930s. In addition it is explained how these investigations prompted many physicians during the 1940s, in particular the late Janet Travell in America, to study the clinical manifestations of this particular type of pain, and how, as a result of this, she came to recognize the importance of what she termed trigger points as being the source of pain in many commonly occurring musculoskeletal disorders.

It is also shown how once it had been discovered that it is possible to alleviate such pain by injecting trigger points with a local anaesthetic or with one or other of a variety of different irritant substances, it was found that this could be accomplished even more simply, as well as more safely and equally effectively, by means of the carrying out of needle-evoked nerve stimulation at trigger point sites.

Part 2 also contains a brief account of advances in knowledge concerning the neurophysiology of pain during the 1960s and 1970s and describes the various pain-modulating mechanisms now considered to be brought into action when acupuncture is carried out. In addition, it includes a discussion of some of the difficulties so far encountered in scientifically evaluating the pain-relieving efficacy of this particular type of therapy and in determining its place relative to other forms of treatment in the alleviation of musculoskeletal pain.

Part 3 is devoted to the practical applications of trigger point acupuncture.

# References

British Medical Acupuncture Society 1997 Acupuncture's place within mainstream medicine. Acupuncture in Medicine 15(2): 104–107

House of Lords Select Committee on Science and Technology 2000 6th report, Session 1999–2000. Complementary and alternative medicine. Stationary Office, London

Lewith G T, Breen A, Filshie J, Fisher P et al 2003 Complementary medicine: evidence base, competence to practice and regulation. Clinical Medicine (Journal of the Royal College of Physicians of London) 3(3): 235–240

Rees L, Weil A 2001 Integrated medicine. British Medical Journal 322: 119–120

# PART 1

# Acupuncture – a historical review

# Chapter 1

# Traditional Chinese acupuncture

The Chinese first carried out acupuncture, that seemingly strange practice whereby needles are inserted into people for therapeutic purposes, at least 3000 years ago. News of this, however, did not reach the Western world until about 300 years ago when European medical officers employed by the Dutch East Indies Trading Company in and around Java saw it being used there by the Japanese, and when at about the same time Jesuit missionaries came across it whilst endeavouring to convert the Chinese to Christianity.

From their writings it is clear that both these groups found the concepts upon which the Chinese based their curious practice difficult to comprehend, due to the fact that these appeared to be completely at variance with what Europeans by that time had come to know about the anatomy and physiology of the human body. And it has been this inability to reconcile the theoretical concepts put forward by the Chinese in support of acupuncture with those upon which modern scientific medicine is based that has for so long been the cause of such little interest being taken in it in the Western world. During the past 30 years, however, attitudes towards acupuncture in the West have been changing since research into the mechanisms of pain has provided a certain amount of insight as to how possibly it achieves its effect on pain. These, as might be expected, are entirely different from those originally put forward by the Chinese.

The prime purpose of this book is to describe a recently developed method of practising acupuncture in which dry needles are inserted into the tissues overlying what have come to be known as trigger points as a means of alleviating musculoskeletal pain. Before turning to this, however, it is necessary to give a brief account of the discovery and development of the traditional practice of Chinese acupuncture as it is only by having a proper understanding of this that the merits of the trigger point approach to acupuncture can be fully appreciated. For an explanation as to how the Chinese came to discover the therapeutic properties of acupuncture in the first place it is helpful to turn to an early Chinese medical book entitled *Huang Ti Nei Ching* and known in the English-speaking world as *The Yellow Emperor's Manual of Corporeal Medicine*. This is a most unusual textbook of medicine as it is written in the form of a dialogue between the Emperor Huang Ti and his minister Chhi-Po. It is a work which incorporates much concerning the philosophical thoughts of the ancient Chinese, their religious beliefs with particular reference to Taoism, their observations concerning the workings of the universe in general, and the application of all this to their practice of medicine.

The Western world is much indebted to the American scholar, Ilza Veith, who, in February 1945 at the Institute of the History of Medicine at Johns Hopkins University, undertook the extremely difficult task of translating this important treatise into English. This translation together with her own invaluable introductory analysis of the work was first published in 1949. Also, for those who wish to read a detailed account of how the Chinese practice of acupuncture has gradually evolved over the centuries, there is much of considerable interest in *Celestial Lancets*, an erudite study of the subject written by the two distinguished Cambridge historians, Lu Gwei-Djen and Joseph Needham (1980).

It is by no means certain that Huang Ti ever lived, with the general consensus of opinion being that he is a legendary figure, but nevertheless he is to this day worshipped as the father of Chinese medicine. It is very difficult to determine with any degree of accuracy the date the *Nei Ching* first appeared, but it seems likely that Part I, the *Su Wên* (Questions and Answers), originated in the 2nd century BC and that Part II *Chen Ching* (Needle Manual) first appeared in the 1st century BC. However, not only was the latter re-named the *Ling Shu* (Vital Axis) in about AD 762, but both parts have been repeatedly revised with the addition

each time of extensive commentaries by a variety of different people. This prompted Ilza Veith to say:

> It is obvious that any work that has undergone the fate of the *Yellow Emperor's Canon of Internal Medicine* contains but little of its authentic original text; it is also clear that its various commentators have frequently obscured rather than elucidated its meaning. It seems impossible to determine now how much of the original text remains; especially since in former times it was difficult to distinguish text from commentary.

Nevertheless, in spite of all these difficulties it is generally agreed that from a study of this work it is possible to gain a clear idea as to how the practice of acupuncture had developed in China by the 2nd century BC.

Acupuncture and a related form of heat therapy and counter irritation known as moxibustion almost certainly had their origins long before this, as may be seen from recently discovered medical manuscripts written on sheets of silk in the tomb of the son of the Lord of Tai, a young man who died in 168 BC. As Lu Gwei-Djen & Joseph Needham point out 'the style and contents of the texts is similar to that of the *Nei Ching* but more archaic, so that they present a picture of Chinese medical thought during the two or three centuries preceding the compilation of that great classic'.

It is interesting to observe that these manuscripts, whilst certainly referring to the practice of acupuncture with needles made of stone, discuss moxibustion in even greater detail and there are reasons for believing that that technique may have been introduced even longer ago than acupuncture itself.

## MOXIBUSTION

This is a process by which heat is applied to the body by the burning of Artemisia leaves that have been dried to a tinder. This Artemisia tinder has come to be known in the West as moxa – a word of Japanese derivation (*mogusa*, herb for burning) because it was from Japan that the Western world first heard about this technique in the 17th century.

The classical method of performing moxibustion is to make the tinder into a cone and apply it to the skin at points identical to those used for acupuncture. Sometimes it is used as a counter irritant by being allowed to blister and scar the skin. At other times it is used as a milder form of heat treatment, by applying it to the skin with a layer of vegetable material interposed between this and the cone in order to protect the former from damage. Yet another method is to combine moxibustion with acupuncture by placing a piece of moxa on top of a needle inserted into the body, and igniting it, when the heat from the moxa is conducted down the needle to the surrounding tissues.

## ACUPUNCTURE

The concepts which prompted the ancient Chinese to use acupuncture for therapeutic purposes were complex and to the modern Western mind difficult to comprehend. They were intricately bound up with their views concerning all aspects of the living world, including in particular their belief in the existence of two cosmic regulators known as Yin and Yang.

The supremacy of power and influence accorded to these two forces in the creation of the world is well illustrated by the following quotations from the *Nei Ching*.

> The principle of Yin and Yang is the basis of the entire universe. It is the principle of everything in creation. It brings about the transformation to parenthood; it is the root and source of life and death …
>
> Heaven was created by an accumulation of Yang; the Earth was created by an accumulation of Yin.
>
> The ways of Yin and Yang are to the left and to the right. Water and fire are the symbols of Yin and Yang. Yin and Yang are the source of power and the beginning of everything in creation.
>
> Yang ascends to Heaven; Yin descends to Earth. Hence the universe (Heaven and Earth) represents motion and rest, controlled by the wisdom of nature. Nature grants the power to beget and to grow, to harvest and to store, to finish and to begin anew.

Further, the Chinese considered that, following the creation of the world, Yin and Yang continued to exert a considerable influence, and that indeed the preservation of order in all natural phenomena, both celestial and terrestrial, was dependent on the maintenance of a correct balance between them. It should be noted in this connection that neither of these two opposing forces were ever envisaged as existing in pure form but rather that each contained a modicum of the other. And moreover, there was the belief that all events, both in nature and in the human body, were influenced by a constantly changing relationship between them.

Yin and Yang were thus said to be ubiquitous essential components of all things, with in some cases Yang being predominant and in others Yin. In the universe for example, phenomena such as the sun, heaven, day, fire, heat and light were all considered to be predominantly Yang in nature, whereas their opposites, the moon, earth, night, water, cold and darkness were considered to be predominantly Yin. The individual structures of the body were also thought to have either Yang or Yin qualities. For example, five hollow viscera – the stomach, small intestine, large intestine, bladder and gall bladder – were said to be Yang organs because lying near to the surface on opening the body they get exposed to light. In contrast, five solid viscera – the heart, lungs, kidneys, spleen and liver – were said to be Yin organs due to their being in the dark recesses of the body.

The conclusion reached by the Chinese that five organs had Yang and five had Yin characteristics was apparently not a fortuitous one but seemingly because five was considered to be a dominant number in their conception of the universe. This stemmed from their fundamental belief in the theory of the five elements, which stated that Yin and Yang consist of five elements, namely water, fire, metal, wood and earth, and that man and, indeed, all natural phenomena are products of an interaction between these two opposing forces.

The theory of the five elements was extremely complicated and there is little to be gained by going into it in detail except to say, in view of its relevance to the traditional practice of Chinese acupuncture, that in its application to the organs of the body the *Nei Ching* teaches that:

> The heart is connected with the pulse and rules over the kidneys. The lungs are connected with the skin and rule over the heart. The liver is connected with the muscles and rules over the lungs.

The spleen is connected with the flesh and rules over the lungs. The kidneys are connected with the bones and rule over the spleen.

With this background it is now possible to see how these various considerations concerning Yin and Yang came to be applied to matters concerning the maintenance of health and the development of disease. It was considered that in order to be healthy these two opposing forces have to be in a correct state of balance (crasis) and that it is when this is not so that disease occurs (dyscrasia).

Further, it was considered that this health-giving balance between Yin and Yang only exists when a special form of energy, known as chhi, flows freely through a system of tracts. And, as a corollary to this, that disease develops when a collection of 'evil air' in one or other of the tracts obstructs the flow of chhi through it as this leads to an imbalance between Yin and Yang. It was in attempting to dispel this 'evil air' or wind that the Chinese were first led to insert needles into these tracts, and then from this, over the course of centuries, to develop a somewhat complex system of therapy now known to the Western world as acupuncture (from the Latin *acus*, a needle; and *punctura*, a prick).

As it is only possible to understand how the Chinese developed their system of acupuncture by having some knowledge of their original, somewhat primitive ideas concerning the anatomy and physiology of the body, these will now be discussed.

The knowledge of anatomy and physiology possessed by the Chinese when they first started to practise acupuncture was obviously both scanty and inaccurate. It is, therefore, surprising to find that from an early date and certainly by the time the *Su WÊn* was compiled in the 2nd century BC they had with considerable perspicacity come to realize that blood circulates continuously around the body. For in this manuscript Chhi-Po says:

> The flow (of blood) … runs on and on, and never stops; a ceaseless movement in an annular circuit.

Chhi-Po is here showing remarkable intuition especially when it is remembered that it was another 1700 years before the Western world came round to this view. This tardy realization of the true state of affairs in the West was of course because Galen, that remarkably influential early Greek physician, had categorically stated that the movement of blood in the vessels of the body is by means of a tidal ebb and flow. This remained the official view for centuries and anyone who dared to question it was considered a blasphemous heretic. Indeed, it was not until 1628 that William Harvey with considerable courage published his proof that blood moves around the body in a continuous circle in his *Exercitatio Anatomica de Motu Cordis et Sanguinis in Animalibus*.

The ancient Chinese admittedly had no scientific evidence to support their belief in the circulation of the blood but because of their inherent conviction that the workings of the body are a microcosmic representation of those to be found in the macrocosm or universe itself, they may have come to this conclusion from observing the meteorological water-cycle that occurs in nature.

It should be noted that the Chinese at an early date not only correctly concluded that blood circulates around the body but also that this is effected by a pumping action of the heart, for in the *Su WÊn* it says 'the heart presides over the circulation of the blood and juices and the paths in which they travel'. Moreover, they were quick to appreciate that the action of the heart is reflected in movements of the pulse felt at the wrist, and were able to measure the pulse rate by using an instrument capable of measuring time by a regulated flow of water, an apparatus similar to that used by the ancient Greeks for timing speeches in their law courts and called by them a clepsydra.

The ancient Chinese also with much ingenuity attempted to estimate the time it takes for blood to circulate around the body and to assist with this calculation measured the approximate total length of the great blood vessels. Although their conclusion that the circulation time is 28.8 minutes was about 60 times too slow, modern methods having now shown it to be only 30 seconds, it was nevertheless a praiseworthy effort, especially when it is remembered that even William Harvey several hundred years later got the calculation wrong!

The Chinese whilst realizing that blood circulates around the body in specially designed vessels also believed, as did the ancient Greeks, that there is a separate substance very difficult to define in modern terms but which could perhaps best be described as a vital force or special form of energy, that also circulates around the body.

The Greeks referred to it as pneuma and considered it to be present with the blood in arteries. The Chinese called a substance of similar nature chhi, with part of it having Yang properties and the other part Yin properties. Following the appearance of the *Ling Shu* in about 762 AD it has always been said that the Yin chhi circulates around the body in the blood vessels, whilst the Yang chhi travels outside them in a completely separate system of channels or tracts.

This system of tracts, which anatomically is not demonstrable, has nevertheless always been very real to the Chinese who from the beginning believed it to consist of an intricate network of main channels, connecting channels and tributaries similar to the rivers, tributaries and canals which together make up the waterways of the earth. The idea is to be found clearly expressed in a book entitled the *Kuan Tzu* written about the late 4th century BC where it says 'one can say water is the blood and the chhi of the earth, because it flows and penetrates everywhere in the same manner as the circulation ... in the tract and blood vessel systems'.

A belief in the existence of such tracts was vital to the Chinese in developing their practice of acupuncture and it is because of the essential part these channels play in this that they are specifically known as acu-tracts. Nonetheless, it must be emphasized that it is the lack of any tangible proof of their existence that has been one of the main reasons why the Western world has viewed the traditional Chinese method of practising acupuncture with such considerable suspicion since first hearing about it 300 years ago.

The Chinese have always visualized and described these tracts in a three-dimensional form and considered them to be at variable depths along their individual courses. Clear descriptions of this are given in their writings, although their illustrations merely give the impression that the tracts run in a relatively straight line along the surface of the body. It should be noted that modern Western writers often refer to the Chinese acutracts as meridians but this is better avoided because as Lu Gwei-Djen & Joseph Needham in the *Celestial Lancets* point out 'the analogy with astronomical hour-circles or terrestrial longitude is so far-fetched that we do not adopt the term'.

The Chinese described 12 main acu-tracts corresponding in number with the months of the year with each one being considered to have a connection with and taking its name from an organ of the body. However, as already stated, the Chinese were of the opinion that there were only ten principal organs, five with Yin characteristics and five with Yang characteristics. Therefore, in order that the 12 tracts could be linked with 12 organs they found it necessary to include the pericardium amongst the Yin organs, and to invent a structure with no known equivalent in modern anatomy, which they called the san chiao (triple warmer) and included this amongst the Yang organs.

It is of interest to note that because the brain was considered to be nothing more than some form of storage organ it was not included amongst the principal organs. The *Nei Ching* in fact states that it is the liver that 'is the dwelling place of the soul or spiritual part of man that ascends to heaven'.

Those who pioneered the development of acupuncture in ancient China believed that acu-tracts for most of their course are situated in the depths of the body's tissues, but that at certain points, now known in the West as acu-points, they come to lie immediately under the skin surface where needles can readily be inserted into them.

It will be remembered that, according to traditional Chinese teaching, the purpose of inserting needles into acu-points in disease is to release noxious air or 'wind' (malignant chhi) that impedes the free flow of chhi in acu-tracts and thereby disturbs the balance between Yin and Yang.

It is possible to gain some idea as to how the Chinese have always thought about acu-points by studying the various names they use to describe them in their writings. One of the commonest of these being chhi hsüeh – hsüeh being a word meaning a hole or minute cavity or crevice; in the *Su Wên*, chhi hsüeh are described as pores or interstices in the flesh that are connected to the naturally occurring Yin and Yang forms of chhi in the acu-tract and blood vessel systems. It is also said that these 'holes' in the flesh are open to invasion by malignant chhi from outside the body but that if and when this onslaught occurs it is readily repelled by acupuncture!

The *Nei Ching* in several places says that there are 365 acu-points. A figure no doubt arrived at because of its symbolic association with the number of degrees in the celestial circle, the number of days in the year and the number of bones in the human body. This, however, was only the number of points supposed to be present in theory, as even in the *Nei Ching* itself only 160 points actually receive names, and with the passage of time even fewer have remained in regular use.

The Chinese have given each of their acupoints a specific name and just as they have named acu-tracts after various rivers so they have incorporated into the names of acu-points references to such parts of nature's waterway system as tanks, pools and reservoirs. Also, during the course of time, acu-points along the length of each tract have been individually numbered, and, as every tract bears the name of the organ to which it is supposed to be linked, it necessarily follows that each point may be identified by reference to the name of the tract along which it is situated and its number on this tract. For example, the point on the gall bladder tract situated half-way between the neck and the tip of the shoulder at the highest point of the shoulder girdle has been named by the Chinese Jianjing but is more commonly referred to as Gall Bladder 21 (GB 21); the point situated between the head of the fibula and the upper end of the tibia called by the Chinese Zusanli is more usually known as Stomach 36 (St 36); and the point just above the web between the first and second toes known as Taichong is more often referred to as Liver 3 (Liv 3).

In the recently developed Western type of approach to acupuncture to be described in this book, acu-tracts and their alleged links with internal organs are not of themselves of any practical importance. However, because most of the trigger points employed in this Western form of acupuncture have been found to have a close spatial correlation with many of the traditional Chinese acu-points, some of the latter will be referred to in the text as a matter of interest.

In traditional Chinese acupuncture it is from an examination of the pulse that disease is mainly diagnosed. The *Nei Ching* contains a clear account of how, from a detailed study of the pulse at the wrist, it is possible to establish the nature of a disease, its location in the body and where best to insert needles to combat it.

The reason why the Chinese have placed such importance on examining the pulse is because they have always considered that it is at that site that the Yin chhi in the blood vessels and the Yang chhi in the tracts converge, and the pulse in some of their writings is referred to as *The Great Meeting Place*.

In the *Nan Ching* – The Manual of Explanations of Eighty-one Difficult Points in the Nei Ching – a work that first appeared some time around the 1st century AD it says:

> The Yin chhi runs within the blood vessels, while the Yang chhi travels outside them (in the tracts). The Yin chhi circulates endlessly, never coming to a stop (save at death). After fifty revolutions the two chhi meet again and this is called a 'great meeting'. The Yin and Yang chhi go along with each other in close relation, travelling in circular paths which have no end. So one can see how the Yin and Yang mutually follow one another.

The Chinese method of examining the pulse consists of placing three fingers along the length of the radial artery at both wrists and by first applying superficial pressure to these points and then deep pressure 12 separate observations can be made. From this it is said to be possible to ascertain the state of chhi in the 12 main tracts, and when disease is present, to tell which organ is affected and into which tract needles have to be inserted.

Chinese sphygmology is therefore basically complicated and has been made even more complex over the centuries by the laying down of rules as to when the examination might most profitably be carried out, including the taking into account of certain astrological considerations in determining the best day for it. Next, the right time of day has to be selected for according to the *Nei Ching* the examination must be done very early in the morning 'when the breath of Yin has not yet begun to stir and when the breath of Yang has not yet begun to diffuse, when food and drink have not yet been taken, when the twelve main vessels are not yet abundant, … when vigour and energy are not yet exerted'.

It is clear that the technique of pulse diagnosis must always have been extremely difficult to master and yet it would seem that those who devised the procedure must have achieved some measure of agreement as to the significance of the various nuances that they considered they could detect at the wrist. Nevertheless, their diagnostic interpretation of these was of necessity expressed in nosological terms quite irreconcilable with those based on our present-day knowledge of pathology, and, therefore, it is surprising to find that certain Western-trained doctors even to this day still try to base their practice of acupuncture on this archaic approach to diagnosis, and are quite unwilling to accept that such an anachronistic procedure should long ago have been relegated to the realms of history.

As the practice of acupuncture has of necessity always depended on the insertion of needles into the body it is of considerable interest to discover how primitive Asiatic man found objects of sufficient tensile strength and sharpness for this purpose.

Thorns of various plants, slivers of bamboo, and needles fashioned from bone have always been available. Bone needles have in fact been found in recent years in tombs from the neolithic age, and by the 6th century, which is about the date of the oldest existing reference to acupuncture, it would have been technically possible to make needles from bronze, copper, tin, silver and even gold. And certainly gold needles have recently been discovered in the tomb of the Han Prince, Liu-ShÊng (113 BC). It is therefore somewhat surprising to find that seemingly needles in the early days of acupuncture were commonly made of stone, for in *Huang Ti Nei Ching* (2nd century BC), Chhi-Po says:

> In the present age it is necessary to bring forward powerful drugs to combat internal illnesses, and to use acupuncture with sharp stone needles and moxa to control the external ones.

Also, in manuscripts written on silk before this and found in the tomb of the son of the Lord of Tai, there are two separate specific references to the use of stone needles.

It seems difficult to conceive how needles made of stone could have been sharpened sufficiently to penetrate the tissues of the body, but, of the various mineral substances available in those far off days, it has been suggested that the following might have been employed: flint, mica, asbestos and jade. However, there is no confirmatory evidence that any of these were utilized and the exact nature of

the type of stone originally used still remains a matter for conjecture. The only certainty is that as iron and steel did not become available to the Chinese until the 5th century BC and as the practice of acupuncture was started long before this, it necessarily follows that materials other than iron must have initially been employed.

It is impossible in this brief review to mention all the various stages in the development of this technique over the centuries. Reference will however be made to the *Chen Chiu Chia I Ching* as this is the oldest existing book entirely devoted to acupuncture and moxibustion. It was written soon after the Chinese Empire became re-unified in AD 265 by one Huang Fu-mi who apparently became interested in medicine partly because his mother was paralysed and partly because he himself suffered from rheumatism! In this book Huang Fu-mi for the first time groups the various acu-points under the names of the various tracts to which they belong and, after numbering them, gives a detailed description of their positions and how to locate them. Further, he names specific acu-points recommended in the treatment of various illnesses and gives much advice as to how he considers acupuncture should best be practised. This is, therefore, an outstanding book in the history of acupuncture and one which was to exert a great influence on the practice of this technique throughout the East.

Mention must be made of the eminent physician Sun Ssu-mo (AD 581–673) as it was he who introduced the so-called module system for determining the exact position of acu-points on people's bodies irrespective of their various sizes by taking measurements using relative or modular inches. He defined a modular inch as being the distance between the upper ends of the distal and middle interphalangeal folds when a person flexes the middle finger; and recommended that measurements should be made by using strips of bamboo, paper, or straw, cut to the length of a person's individual modular inch.

Sun Ssu-mo was also the author of two outstanding books on acupuncture and moxibustion and was the first to draw attention to the importance of inserting needles into exquisitely tender points, particularly, he said, in treating low back pain. He called these ah-shih (oh-yes!) points, from the expletive often uttered by the patient when pressure is applied over them! This is of particular interest as he was clearly practising what is known now as trigger point acupuncture, and which having been rediscovered in recent years is described in Parts 2 and 3 of this book.

The Imperial Medical College, with a departmental professor of acupuncture, lecturers, and demonstrators, had been founded by AD 618, and by AD 629 a similar college of medicine had been established in each province.

From AD 1027 the teaching of acupuncture at these institutions was carried out with the help of life-size bronze figures of the human body. The walls of these figures had holes punched in them at the sites of all the known acu-points. The figures with their holes filled with water and covered by wax were then used for examining medical students in acupuncture. This was done by making the students insert needles into sites on these figures where they considered acupoints points might exist, and if, on attempting this, no water poured out they failed their examination!

The Chinese have always had a deep conviction that the workings of the body are intimately linked with those of nature in general, and that various cyclical events external to the body have an important influence over matters of health and disease. Further, that for the successful eradication of disease by acupuncture it is necessary to perform the latter at a propitious time and one that can only be determined by taking into consideration the interrelationship of these various external factors. It is, therefore, not surprising to find that the *Nei Ching* clearly states that in order to discover the right time for both the application of acupuncture and moxibustion the physician must first establish the position of the sun, the moon, other planets, and the stars in addition to taking into account the season of the year and the prevailing weather conditions!

The following is a quotation from Chapter 26 of that book:

> Therefore one should act in accordance with the weather and the seasons in order to have blood and breath thoroughly adjusted and harmonized – and consequently – when the weather is cold, one should not apply acupuncture. But when the days are warm there should not be any hesitation. …

In an earlier part of the same book there is a statement that when acupuncture is applied for an excess of Yang it has a draining effect, and when for a deficit of Yin it supplements vigour. Later on in the same chapter it states:

> At the time of the new moon one should not drain, and when the moon is full one should not supplement. When the moon is empty to the rim one cannot heal diseases, hence one should consult the weather and the seasons and adjust the treatment to them.

This concept that cyclical events have an important controlling influence over matters of health and disease was still further developed with the introduction of the wu-yün liu-chhi system (the cyclical motions of the five elements and the six chhi) in AD 1099, and of the tzu-wu liu-chu system (noon and midnight differences in the following of the chhi) in about the middle of the 12th century.

These are complex systems the details of which will not be entered into. Suffice it to say that the first was based on the conviction that external cyclical, astronomical, meteorological, and climatic factors influence the workings of the body and that from a study of these the occurrence of disease and particularly epidemics of it may be predicted. And that the second was based on the idea that there are internal cyclical changes occurring inside the body and that these have to be taken into account when deciding upon ideal times for performing acupuncture and moxibustion. It is of great interest that such ideas concerning circadian rhythms in the body were put forward so long ago considering that it is only in very recent years that proof has been obtained of the existence of internal biological clocks.

From this brief review it may be seen that the Chinese did not discover the therapeutic effects of acupuncture as a result of some astute clinical observation nor alternatively were they inspired to use it by the logical development of some well-founded hypothesis. On the contrary, it would seem that it was very much by luck that they stumbled upon this valuable form of therapy because their original reasons for using it have subsequently been shown to be entirely fallacious. And further, to a very large extent they succeeded in obscuring the merits of this therapy by grafting upon it a somewhat esoteric set of rules for its application. The manner in which all this prevented acupuncture from becoming readily accepted in the Western world during the past 300 years will be discussed in detail in the next two chapters but before this it is necessary to say something about its changing fortunes in China itself.

From the time that acupuncture was first used in China it remained in the ascendance in that part of the world until reaching its zenith at about the end of the 16th century. From then onwards during the Ch'ing dynasty (1644–1911), when China was under Manchu rule, the practice of it went into a gradual decline. This initially was mainly because the Confucian religion practised by the Manchu people was associated with much prudishness so that the baring of the body, as clearly is so often necessary with treatment by acupuncture, was considered to be immoral. And also because the religion discouraged the inserting of needles into a person's body for fear that this might damage that which was considered to be sacred by virtue of it having been bestowed on that individual by loving parents. Another important reason was that from the 17th century onwards missionaries from Europe, with initially these mainly being Portuguese Jesuits, in bringing the Christian religion to China, also brought with them the Western form of medical practice, and this over the next 300 years profoundly influenced the type of medicine practised in the Far East with the practice of acupuncture gradually being displaced.

Events moved so quickly that when Hsü Ling Thai, an eminent Chinese physician and medical historian, wrote about the history of Chinese medicine in 1757, he had to report that by that time acupuncture had become somewhat of a lost art with few experts left to teach it to medical students.

During the 19th century its status declined still further, with the Ch'ing emperors in 1822 ordering that it should no longer be taught at the Imperial Medical College. From then on an increasing number of colleges were opened by medical missionaries for the express purpose of teaching Chinese students Western medicine, until finally this ancient form of treatment reached its nadir in 1929 when the Chinese authorities officially outlawed the practice of it in that country.

It has to be remembered, however, that what has been said only really applied to a minority of the population because China has always been a land of the rich and poor, of the rulers and the oppressed, and whilst Western medicine increasingly displaced traditional Chinese medicine in the wealthy coastal cities the rural peasants that inhabited most of the country continued to depend on traditional forms of treatment including acupuncture, and increasingly, what health care system was available to them became more and more chaotic due to years of Japanese occupation, civil war, and lack of doctors trained in this type of medicine.

The Chinese communist victory in the so-called War of Liberation in 1949, however, changed all this with Mao Tse Tung being determined to improve the health service for the poor by ensuring that more doctors became trained in traditional Chinese medicine; and by ensuring that the practice of this form of medicine and Western medicine became closely integrated with both being taught in the medical colleges.

Following the Great Proletariat Cultural Revolution during the years 1966–69 there was even further emphasis placed on the importance of traditional Chinese medicine including acupuncture with the result that most hospitals offered both forms of treatment to their patients. It is therefore not surprising that when President Nixon and his entourage visited China in 1972, with acupuncture by then having been fully restored to its former prestigious position, its use in the treatment of disease and in particular as an anaesthetic was demonstrated to them with considerable pride. And it was because his personal physician was so impressed with what he saw that, on returning to America, he generated a wave of enthusiasm for it in the Western world that advances in knowledge concerning the neurophysiology of pain since that time have helped to sustain.

# References

Lu Gwei-Djen, Needham J 1980 Celestial lancets. A history and rationale of acupuncture and moxa. Cambridge University Press, Cambridge

Veith I 1949 Huang Ti Nei Ching Su Wen The Yellow Emperor's classic of internal medicine. University of California Press, Berkeley

## Recommended further reading

Kaptchuk T J 1983 Chinese medicine: the Web that has no weaver. Hutchinson, London

Macdonald A 1982 Acupuncture from ancient art to modern medicine. George Allen & Unwin, London

Ma Ran-Wen 2000 Acupuncture: its place in the history of Chinese medicine. Acupuncture in Medicine 18(2): 88–98

Porkert M 1974 The theoretical foundations of Chinese medicine. MIT Press, Cambridge, Massachusetts

# Chapter 2

# How news of acupuncture and moxibustion spread from China to the outside world

The Chinese had practised acupuncture and moxibustion for several centuries before news of it reached the outside world. The first people to hear about it were the Koreans and then not until about the beginning of the 6th century AD. It was not long after that, however, that both Chinese and Korean missionaries introduced it to Japan during the course of converting the people of that country to Buddhism.

The Western world, on the other hand, did not learn about these oriental practices until the 17th century when Jesuit missionaries, whilst attempting to convert the Chinese to Christianity, saw them being used in Canton, and when European doctors employed by the Dutch East Indian Company in and around Java saw them being used by the Japanese in that part of the world. Willem ten Rhijne (1647–1700), a physician born in the Dutch town of Deventer, and who received his medical education at Leyden University, must be given the credit for being the first person to give the Western world a relatively detailed, if unfortunately a somewhat misleading, account of the Chinese practice of acupuncture and moxibustion.

His opportunity to see orientals practising these techniques came when, soon after qualifying as a doctor, he joined the Dutch East India Company in 1673 and was sent to Java. During the latter part of his life there he was to become the director of the Leprosarium but as a young man he had no sooner arrived than he was ordered to go to the island of Deshima in Nagasaki Bay. It was during the 2 years he was stationed there that he first saw the techniques of Chinese acupuncture and moxibustion being practised by the Japanese, and managed to acquire four illustrations depicting acupuncture points lying along channels. He not unnaturally assumed that the latter must be blood vessels, but found the matter confusing as the directions in which they appeared to run in no way conformed with those taken by any anatomical structures with which he was familiar. He was nevertheless very much impressed with the therapeutic effects of these two techniques and was therefore determined to learn more about them and in particular to get someone to explain the drawings to him. This however was not to prove easy because as he later said in his book on the subject:

> The zealous Japanese are quite reluctant to share, especially with foreigners, the mysteries of their art which they conceal like most sacred treasures in their book cases.

It would seem, however, that the Japanese on the other hand had no such inhibitions when it came to them wanting to know all about Western medicine for, on the orders of the Governor of Nagasaki, a Chinese-speaking Japanese physician, Zoko Iwanga, was sent to see ten Rhijne in order to question him closely about the way in which medicine was practised in Europe. Ten Rhijne however seemed to take all this in good part for when writing about it later he refers to the various questions put to him as nothing but 'bothersome trifles, to be sure', and moreover in return for the information he gave Iwanga he managed to persuade the latter to attempt to explain to him the drawings in his possession. Unfortunately as ten Rhijne later pointed out in his book, in order for him to understand Iwanga's explanations of the notes attached to the drawings it necessitated one interpreter having to translate the Chinese into Japanese and then another interpreter, whose command of the Dutch language was limited, having to translate the Japanese into Dutch. It therefore follows that the information ten Rhijne received was of necessity inaccurate and yet he himself then had to do his best to translate this into Latin, which was the universal language in the Western world at that time.

In spite of these difficulties there is no doubt that ten Rhijne convinced himself that he had sufficient understanding as to how the Japanese practised acupuncture for him to write an essay on it

which he included with essays on other subjects in his book *Dissertatio de Arthritide; Mantissa Schematica; de Acupunctura …*, written some time after he had left Nagasaki on 27 October 1676 and returned to Java, and which was published simultaneously in London, The Hague, and in Leipzig in 1683.

In the introduction to this essay on acupuncture, in which he also included comments on moxibustion, he gave reasons why the Chinese and Japanese preferred these two particular forms of therapy to the therapeutic form of bleeding (phlebotomy; venesection) that was so widely practised in Europe in his time, by saying:

> Burning and acupuncture are the two primary operations among the Chinese and Japanese who employ them to be free from every pain. If these two people (especially the Japanese) were deprived of the two techniques, their sick would be in a pitiful state without hope of cure or alleviation. Both nations detest phlebotomy because, in their judgement, venesection emits both healthy and diseased blood, and thereby shortens life. They have, accordingly, attempted to rid unhealthy blood of impurities by moxibustion; and to rid it of winds, the cause of all pain, with moxibustion and acupuncture.

It is interesting to learn from him that in Japan at that time therapy was mainly carried out by technicians working under the direction of medical practitioners, but as ten Rhijne said, 'For difficult illnesses the physicians themselves administer the needle.'

These technicians called by the Chinese Xinkieu, and by the Japanese Farritatte, must have had a fair degree of independence and clinical freedom for they had their own establishments with each of the latter having a distinctive sign outside it in the form of a wooden statue with acupuncture and moxibustion points marked in different colours, an eye-catching device, similar to the multicoloured striped pole often seen outside a barber's shop in the Western world representing the splint for which the barber-surgeon in former times bound the arms of his patients during the process of blood-letting.

From ten Rhijne's account it would seem that the needles used by the Japanese in the 17th century were made of gold, or occasionally of silver, which is somewhat surprising considering that steel must have been readily available to them. The main indication for their use according to him was for the release of 'winds' for as he says:

> The Japanese employ acupuncture especially for pain of the belly, stomach and head caused by winds … They perforate those parts in order to permit the confined wind to exit.

In an attempt to explain this further, he adds the following somewhat homely simile: 'in the same way, sausages, when they threaten to explode in a heated pan, are pierced to allow the expanding wind to go out'.

It would seem therefore that although the Chinese originally employed acupuncture for the purpose of clearing collections of 'wind' in acutracts (p. 7) in due course both they and the Japanese came to use it for the relief of abdominal pain brought about by the entrapment of a quite different type of 'wind' in the intestinal tract.

It is of particular interest in this respect that the only case history ten Rhijne includes in his book is of a Japanese soldier with some abdominal pain. The soldier believing this to be due to 'wind' produced as a result of drinking an excessive amount of water, is reported to have carried out his own treatment by inserting an acupuncture needle into his abdomen. Ten Rhijne was obviously present when he did this for he says:

> … lying on his back, he drove the needle into the left side of his abdomen above the pylorus at four different locations … while he tapped the needle with a hammer (since his skin was rather tough) he held his breath. When the needle had been driven in about the width of a finger, he rotated its twisting-handle … Relieved of the pain and cured by this procedure, he regained his health.

Ten Rhijne whilst watching this demonstration of auto-acupuncture must have cast his mind back to his youth for by a strange coincidence the title of his dissertation for his doctorate in medicine was *De dolore intestinorum e flatu* … ! In his essay he also gives a long list of other disorders that the Japanese in those days were treating with acupuncture including conditions such as headaches, rheumatic pains, and arthritis that people all over the world are still using it for. The one notably bizarre and

certainly very hazardous use for it at that time was in the field of obstetrics with the acupuncturist being advised to 'puncture the womb of a pregnant woman when the foetus moves excessively before the appropriate time for birth and causes the mother such severe pains that she frequently is in danger of death; puncture the foetus itself with a long and sharp needle, so as to terrify it and make it cease its abnormal movement fraught with danger for the mother'!

It is very unfortunate considering that ten Rhijne was sufficiently impressed with the practical value of acupuncture to feel that he wanted to pass on his knowledge of the subject to the Western world by writing an essay on it, that this should have proved to be a totally inaccurate account, due to his failure to understand that the Chinese believed in the existence of a system of channels (now referred to in the West as acutracts or meridians) completely separate from and yet closely associated with blood vessels. His knowledge of anatomy was extensive for at one stage in his life he taught the subject and therefore in all fairness there was no reason why it should have ever crossed his mind that the acutracts depicted in the illustrations he acquired could be anything but structures already well known to him from dissecting the human body. As a result he repeatedly refers to them as arteries, and to confuse the matter even more insists that the Chinese and Japanese use the terms artery, vein, and nerve interchangeably and so in some places he even refers to them as veins and in others as nerves.

His belief that these tracts were arteries is also readily understandable when it is remembered how much importance the Chinese placed on their long-held beliefs concerning the circulation of the blood in developing their practice of acupuncture. This is clearly expressed by ten Rhijne when he said:

> Although Chinese physicians (who are the fore-runners from whom Japanese physicians borrowed these systems of healing) are ignorant in anatomy, nonetheless they have perhaps devoted more effort over many centuries to learning and teaching with very great care the circulation of the blood, than have European physicians, individually or as a group. They base the foundation of their entire medicine upon the rules of the circulation, as if the rules were oracles of Apollo at Delphi.

He then goes on to point out how, 'among the Chinese the masters employ hydraulic machines to demonstrate the circulation of the blood to their disciples who have earned the title of physician; in the absence of such machines the masters assist understanding with clear figures'. It is obvious that ten Rhijne was under the impression that the drawings he possessed were examples of such figures.

Another reason for his confusing acu-tracts with arteries was that he knew that the Chinese place considerable emphasis on the examination of the pulse in making a diagnosis before undertaking acupuncture or moxibustion. In referring to the latter for instance he says:

> … wherever pain has set in, burn; burn however in the location in which the arteries beat most strongly. For in that place the seat of the pain is lodged, where harmful winds inordinately move the blood. After prior examination of the pulse of the arteries, place the burning tow on the location marked with its own sign.

And in another place he says:

> … wherever pain has lodged, burn. To which I add, when it is necessary puncture, puncture and burn where the arteries beat strongest. What the patient can detect by the sensation of pain the physician can detect by feeling the pulses in the affected part.

At the same time he is clearly aware that if the channels depicted in his illustrations and which he describes in the text of his book are arteries then they are a very inaccurate anatomical representation of the course known to be taken by such vessels. And it would seem that, fearing that for this reason alone authorities in the Western world might reject out of hand the whole system of acupuncture and moxibustion, he finds it necessary to apologize for the apparent ineptness of those who drew the illustrations by saying:

> In many instances, a person especially skillful at the art of anatomy will belittle the lines and the precise points of insertion, and will censure the awkward presentation of the short notes on the diagrams, when these should be more closely identified with walls of the blood vessels. But we must not on this account casually abandon our

confidence in experiments undertaken by the very great number of superb and polished intellects of antiquity. Chinese physicians prefer to cast the blame for a mistake upon their own ignorance, rather than diminish in the slightest the authority of and trust in antiquity …

Although the account of acupuncture in ten Rhijne's book was the first detailed one to appear in the Western world, a passing reference to the subject had already been made in a book written by Jacob de Bondt (1598–1631) who as surgeon-general to the Dutch East India Company in Java had also seen the technique being used in that part of the world. This book, *Historia Naturalis et Medica Indiae Orientalis*, published in 1658, is in the main an account of the natural history of animals and plants found in the East, but it contains a paragraph about acupuncture.

When ten Rhijne quotes this paragraph in his own book he cannot refrain from putting in parentheses his own critical comments thus causing de Bondt's description of acupuncture to read as follows:

> The results with acupuncture in Japan which I will relate even surpass miracles [without undermining belief in their authenticity]. For chronic pains of the head [and moreover for recent ones, especially those arising from winds], for obstruction of the liver and spleen, and also for pleurisy [and for other ailments, as is here made clear] they bore through [and they perforate] with a stylus [he should have said, with a needle] made of silver or bronze [more correctly, from gold] and not much thicker than ordinary lyre strings. The stylus [here the good author is quite in error] should be driven slowly and gently through the above mentioned vitals so as to emerge from another part.

One book that presumably ten Rhijne did not read, but which could have been a help to him in understanding something about acu-tracts, was written anonymously but almost certainly by a French Jesuit missionary working in Canton. This work was based on a translation of a 1st-century manual, the *Mo chüeh* (Sphygmological Instructions). This book printed at Grenoble in 1671 clearly refers to acu-tracts although admittedly there is very little detail about them or about the Chinese system of pulse-diagnosis in spite of its title *Les*

*Secrets de la Médecine des Chinois, consistant en la parfaite Connoissance du Pouls, envoyez de la Chine par un Francois, Homme de grand mérite.*

It is more surprising that ten Rhijne did not learn about the belief of Chinese physicians in a system of channels or acu-tracts separate from the anatomically demonstrable circulatory system from the German Andreas Cleyer as they were together as medical officers in the service of the Dutch East India Company on Java. And Cleyer edited a book giving clear references to acu-tracts that was published in 1682, the year before ten Rhijne's book appeared.

Cleyer attributes several parts of this book *Specimen Médicinae Sinicae, sive Opuscula Medica ad mentem Sinesium* to an 'eruditus Europaeus' living in Canton. The possibility therefore exists that this was none other than the anonymous author of the book *Les Secrets de la Médecine des Chinois, consistant en la parfaite Connoissance du Pouls, envoyez de la Chine par un Francois, Homme de grand mérite* that appeared in 1671. Like the latter, Cleyer's book also includes translations from the *Mo chüeh* (Sphygmological Instructions) but is far more informative with a lengthy discussion of the various types of pulse found in health and disease; there are also no less than 30 drawings depicting the course of acu-tracts. In addition there are numerous references to acu-tracts, or viae (ways) as they are called in the text but unfortunately, as might be expected, the author is quite unable to explain how the Chinese believed that circulatory disturbances in these invisible tracts could be diagnosed from observations on the pulse.

Nevertheless, the book certainly aroused the interest of Sir John Floyer (1649–1734) who included an abridged and paraphrased form of it in his famous two-volume work, *The Physician's Pulse-Watch or an Essay to Explain the Old Art of Feeling the Pulse, and to improve it by the help of a Pulse-Watch*, the first volume of which was published in 1707 and the second in 1710.

Floyer's pulse-watch was a portable instrument that he carried in a box, it having been made under his direction by a Mr Samuel Watson, a watchmaker in Long Acre, London. Its great virtue was that it ran for 60 seconds, and with it he studied the effects of a variety of different factors on the pulse rate including food, drink, tobacco, anxiety and fevers. He implored all young physicians to use the instrument 'to discern all those dangerous exorbitances which are caused by an irregular diet, violent passions, and a slothful life'.

His reference to Cleyer's observations on Chinese medicine comes in the first part of the second volume under the title of *An Essay to make a new Sphygmologia, by accommodating the Chinese and European observations about the Pulse into one System*. As may be gathered from the title this only discusses the Chinese method of pulse diagnosis and there is no mention of acupuncture in it. It would seem in fact that Floyer had no interest in the latter believing that the Chinese in the main treated most diseases pharmaceutically after having diagnosed them in the first place by means of observations on the pulse. Curiously enough he was not all that wrong because unbeknown to him, at the time his book was being written, acupuncture in China was going through one of its periodic phases of being out of fashion.

In spite of Floyer's enthusiasm for Chinese sphygmology his contemporaries failed to show any real interest in it, or for that matter in the practice of acupuncture itself. This perhaps is surprising considering that in the early part of the 17th century William Harvey dramatically changed long-held ideas in the Western world concerning the physiology of the circulatory system when in 1628 he published his famous book *Exercitatio Anatomica de Motu Cordis et Sanguinis in Animalibus*. In this he was at last able to refute the hitherto seemingly inviolable but erroneous teaching of Galen concerning the structure of the heart and the manner in which he had insisted that blood ebbs and flows in the vessels. Harvey proved by means of carefully conducted experiments what the Chinese had surmised centuries before that blood flows around the body in a continuous circle.

As might be expected, in view of the manner in which Galen's views had been revered for so many centuries, there was initially considerable opposition to Harvey's revolutionary discovery, but, based as it was on such sound evidence, its gradual acceptance over the course of years became inevitable.

Considering that the system of sphygmology devised by the Chinese and their practice of acupuncture were both firmly founded on the principle that blood circulates around the body one might therefore have thought that in the climate of opinion prevailing in the West towards the end of the 17th century that more interest might have been shown in them. Yet when the book *Clavis Medica ad Chinarum Doctrinam de Pulsibus*, which basically was yet another translation of the *Mo chüeh*, written by Michael Boym (1612–1659) a Polish Jesuit missionary in China, was published in 1686, it prompted Pierre Bayle in reviewing it that year in *Nouvelles de la République des Lettres* to say:

> The Reverend Father expounds to us the Chinese system of medicine very clearly, and it is easy to see from what he says that the physicians of China are rather clever men. True, their theories and principles are not the clearest in the world, but if we had got hold of them under the reign of the philosophy of Aristotle, we should have admired them very much, and we should have found them at least as plausible and well based as our own. Unfortunately, they have reached us in Europe just at a time when the mechanick Principles invented, or revived, by our Modern Virtuosi have given us a great distaste for the 'faculties' of Galen, and for the calidum naturalis and the humidum radicale too, the great foundations of the Medicine of the Chinese no less than that of the Peripateticks.

It should be noted that the Galenic-Aristotelian calidum naturalis or 'innate heat' was widely considered in the 17th century to correspond to the Chinese yang whilst the Galenic-Aristotelian humidum radicale or 'primigenial moisture' was considered to correspond to the Chinese yin.

It may therefore be seen from the sentiments expressed by Bayle that what really deterred most physicians in the Western world from taking any particular interest, either in the Chinese method of pulse-diagnosis, or in acupuncture itself, on first learning about them in the 17th century, at a time when they had only recently come to terms with Harvey's new and enlightened approach to anatomy and physiology after centuries of slavish adherence to Galenic dogma, was that the curiously esoteric and nebulous concepts including yin, yang, chhi and invisible acu-tracts upon which these Chinese practices seemed to be based, were all too reminiscent of some of the bizarre Graeco-Roman beliefs from which they had just been liberated.

Most European physicians also showed little or no enthusiasm for the Chinese practice of applying heat to the skin by burning moxa on it, when they first heard of this in the 17th century, in spite of the fact that at that time they were still firm believers in blistering their patients with strong irritants, and burning them with boiling oil and red hot irons! One person, however, who did advocate its use was Hermann Buschof, a Dutch Reformed Minister and a friend of ten Rhijne when they worked together in Java. He wrote a laudatory account of its use in gout and other arthritic conditions in a book published in 1674 entitled *Het Podagra* … Another protagonist was Sir William Temple the eminent 17th-century diplomat who wrote appreciatively about it in an essay 'The cure of Gout by Moxa' in his *Miscellanea* published in 1693, after having received this form of treatment for a painful attack of this affliction during an international conference at Nijmegen in 1677. Conversely the eminent physician Thomas Sydenham (1624–1689), when writing about gout some time earlier, had referred disparagingly to the use of moxa in its treatment.

The most comprehensive account of moxibustion to reach the West, however, was that written by the German physician Englebert Kaempfer (1651–1716). Kaempfer, who was brought up in Germany at a time when it had recently been devastated by the ravages of the Thirty Years War (1618–1648), decided after qualifying as a doctor that rather than continue to live there he would prefer to seek work abroad. He therefore joined the United East India Company and became yet another of the surgeons to work at the Dutch trading station on the island of Deshima in Nagasaki Bay.

His observations on Japanese medical practice in that part of the world led him to write two essays, one 'Acupuncture, a Japanese Cure for Colic', and the other 'Moxa, a Chinese and Japanese Substance for Cautery', which appeared together with a large number of essays on other subjects in his *Amoenitatum Exoticarum Politico-Physico-Medicarum Fasciculi V* … published in 1712.

The essay on acupuncture is of limited value because as may be seen from the title it confines itself to the use of this technique in one condition only, namely the relief of cramp-like pains occurring in association with a severe type of diarrhoea that was endemic in that part of the world at the time and known to the Japanese as senki. There is a detailed account of how needles should be inserted in this condition but all reference to acu-tracts is avoided, and it does not really add anything to that which had by that time already been written on the subject.

The essay on moxibustion, however, is far more wide ranging. His description of the sites at which he saw a moxa cautery applied, and the reasons for doing this make fascinating reading, as may be seen from the following quotation:

> Considering the places cauterised, you would think the unexpected successes illusory. For example to facilitate birth, the tip of the small toe on the left foot; to prevent conception or to promote sterility, the navel; to relieve toothache, the adducting muscle of the thumb on the same side as the aching tooth.

The latter is a clear reference to the classical Chinese acupuncture and moxa point Ho-Ku, stimulation of which to this day is widely recognized as having a powerful analgesic effect.

From what has been said it will be clear that much information concerning acupuncture and moxibustion reached Europe during the 17th century but only limited use was made of these techniques either during that century or the following one because physicians in the Western world were completely mystified as to how these particular forms of therapy achieve their effects. One of the few men to think deeply about this matter was Gerhard van Swieten, the famous Dutch physician, who concluded that any beneficial effects that they may have must be for reasons entirely different from those that had been put forward by the Chinese, for as he said in 1755:

> The acupuncture of the Japanese and the cautery of various parts of the body with (Chinese) moxa

seems to stimulate the nerves and thereby to alleviate pains and cramps in quite different parts of the body in a most wonderful way. It would be an extraordinarily useful enterprise if someone would take the trouble to note and investigate the marvellous communion which the nerves have with one another, and at what points certain nerves lie which when stimulated can calm the pain at distant sites. The physicians of Asia, who knew no (modern) anatomy, have by long practical experience identified such points.

It was of course another 200 years before research into the neurophysiology of pain provided objective evidence in support of van Swieten's hypothesis.

It is now necessary to consider the attitudes of doctors, both in Europe and America, to acupuncture during the 19th century as this was a period when a few of the more courageous of them, in spite of not being able to accept the traditional theories upon which the Chinese based their practice of it, decided to explore empirically its clinical applications. And having convinced themselves of its merits in alleviating musculoskeletal pain, they attempted to popularize its use for this purpose. They were, however, to find their efforts thwarted by entrenched conservatism. Members of the medical profession at that time showed a strangely inconsistent attitude whereby they were more than willing to prescribe potentially toxic substances of uncertain efficacy whilst being quite unwilling to try out the relatively harmless procedure of inserting needles into people, presumably because they could not bring themselves to believe that anything so simple could have the effects claimed for it – an attitude of mind, regretfully, still adopted by some in the late 20th century!

## References

Bowers J Z 1966 Englebert Kaempfer; Physician, explorer, scholar and author. Journal of the History of Medicine and Allied Sciences 21: 237–259

Bowers J Z, Carrubba R W 1970 The doctoral thesis of Englebert Kaempfer on tropical diseases, oriental medicine and exotic natural phenomena. Journal of the History of Medicine and Allied Sciences 25: 270–310

Carrubba R W, Bowers J Z 1974 The Western world's first detailed treatise on acupuncture: Willem ten Rhijne's De Acupunctura. Journal of the History of Medicine and Allied Sciences 29: 391–397

Floyer Sir John 1707 The physician's pulse watch: or, an essay to explain the old art of feeling the pulse, and to improve it by the help of a pulse-watch. London

Harvey William 1628 Exercitatio anatomica de motu cordis et sanguinis in animalibus. London – an anatomical disquisition on the motion of the heart and blood in animals. Translated by Robert Willis, Barnes, Surrey, England 1847. In: Willius F A, Keys T E (eds) Classics of cardiology, Vol 1. Dover Publications, New York, 1961

Lu Gwei-Djen, Needham J 1980 Celestial lancets. A history and rationale of acupuncture and moxa. Cambridge University Press, Cambridge

# Chapter 3

# The practice of acupuncture in the Western world during the 19th century

There is good evidence to show that acupuncture came to be widely practised by the medical profession in Europe during the first half of the 19th century.

Its protagonists, however, turned their backs on the complexities of the traditional Chinese approach to the subject and, in a determined effort to shed it of all its mysticism, ignored the acu-tract system and refused to attempt to use the oriental system of pulse-diagnosis. They confined themselves for the most part to the treatment of painful conditions and the method adopted was simply a straightforward insertion of needles into painful areas, similar to the ah shih hsüeh type of acupuncture practised by Sun Ssu-mo in China in the 7th century (see Ch. 1). Both of these forms of acupuncture 'in loco dolenti', as Lu GweiDjen & Needham (1980) so aptly call it, were clearly the forerunners of the more sophisticated type of trigger point acupuncture recently developed in the Western world and described in detail later in this book.

The circumstances leading to this renewal of interest were not the same in every country. In Germany the somewhat unlikely source of inspiration was a letter published in 1806 by the playwright, August Von Kotzebue in his magazine *The Candid Observer (Funny and Serious)*. This letter ostensibly from his son travelling in Japan gave a somewhat satirical account of the way acupuncture was being practised there. This might have attracted no more than passing interest if it had not been for the fact that it caught the eye of some unknown physician who wrote a long rejoinder urging that the subject be treated with more seriousness. In spite of this it was some time before the clinical application of the technique became widely adopted but in 1828 some important papers appeared, including one by Bernstein and another by Lohmayer, reporting good results with this form of treatment in the alleviation of rheumatic pain.

In France, interest in acupuncture was reawakened in a far more direct manner. When Isaac Titsingh, a surgeon attached to the Dutch East India Company at Deshima, eventually returned to Europe, he brought with him among the memorabilia of his travels, an ebony case containing needles and moxa tinder; and also a teaching-aid in the form of a cardboard doll with acu-points and tracts painted on it that had been presented to him by a Japanese Imperial Physician. His friends in Europe showed considerable interest in these items, but what was to prove to be of even greater importance was his translation of an 18th-century Japanese treatise on acupuncture, for when this came to the attention of the Parisian physician Sarlandière he was so intrigued with it that he began to practise acupuncture himself and persuaded several other physicians in Paris to do likewise. Included among these were Berlioz, the father of the composer, who in 1816 wrote the first book on the subject in France, and Cloquet & Dantu who reported their results of treating patients with this technique in an article *Observations sur less Effets Thérapeutiques de l' Acupuncture* in Bayle's *Bibliothèque de Thérapeutique* published in 1828.

Sarlandière himself was the first to apply electric currents to implanted needles, and his book giving an account of this was published in 1825. This will no doubt surprise anyone who might have thought that electroacupuncture is a recent invention.

From their reports it is clear that these Parisian physicians were using acupuncture in the treatment of many different disorders but that their best results, as might be expected, were in the relief of musculoskeletal pain and migraine.

In Italy the first book to be published on the practice of acupuncture was that of Bozetti in 1820, but the one that was to become best known was that of Antonio Carraro published in 1825. Also of particular interest were two books, the first appearing in 1834 and the second in 1837, in which da Camin describes how following the example of Sarlandière

he employed electroacupuncture and used Leyden jars as the source of electricity.

In England the medical practitioner who did most to interest his colleagues in the clinical application of acupuncture by writing two books on the subject was J. M. Churchill. The first, entitled *A Treatise on Acupuncturation, being a Description of a Surgical Operation originally peculiar to the Japanese and Chinese, and by them denominated Zin-King, now introduced into European Practice, with Directions for its Performance and Cases illustrating its Success*, was published in 1821, and the second consisting of a number of case histories was published in 1828. His treatise on acupuncturation, a modest volume of only 86 pages, was dedicated to the famous surgeon Astley Cooper as follows:

> To Astley Cooper Esq. the steady friend and patron of humble merit the author respectfully inscribes this little treatise. Less from presumption of its deserving his approbation than as a mark of respect for splendid achievements and of gratitude towards a great master.

Churchill said it was his friend Mr Scott of Westminster, the first person as far as he knew to perform acupuncture in England, who initially drew his attention to the subject by demonstrating to him several successfully treated cases, and it was this which led him to study the technique himself.

From reading Churchill's books it is obvious that he restricted himself to treating cases of what he called 'rheumatalgia', and judging from the case histories this was invariably of short duration. This no doubt accounts for his uniformly excellent results and clearly because of this he considered it only necessary to present a limited number of cases for as he said:

> I would certainly add many others to the list but to minds open to conviction and truth no stronger impression would be made by multiplying examples, whilst the sceptical would not be persuaded though one rose from the dead!

He admits that he did not know how acupuncture works stating:

> I have by no means made up my mind as to the nature of its action and rather than venture into speculations which may be received as doubtful

by some and visionary by others I prefer to preserve a profound silence.

Such honesty has to be admired particularly as he clearly recognizes that his self-confessed ignorance concerning its action could seriously undermine his efforts to popularize the technique for he says '… if on the other hand, a rational theory, built on sound logical reasons, be the only evidence to which any value can be attached, then will my efforts have been unavailing and fruitless'. Such fears, however, proved groundless because his book undoubtedly aroused much interest with it, not only being translated into German in 1824 and into French in 1825, but it also inspired many of his English colleagues to take an interest in the subject. One such person was Mr Wansborough of Fulham, who writing in the *Lancet* in 1826 says:

> As respects the modus operandi I have proceeded in every case according to the recommendation of Mr Churchill in his useful little work on acupuncturation to which I beg the readers of the Lancet to consult for further information on the subject.

In his paper he describes how by the use of acupuncture he alleviated the pain of various musculoskeletal disorders in eight patients. He says the latter were all so impressed with the result as to pronounce them as being magical!

He, like Churchill, was unwilling to commit himself as to how inserting needles into the body could have a therapeutic effect, but he clearly thought that the Chinese were wrong in believing that it was due to noxious air being released from the tissues for he says:

> I shall not hazard a hypothesis of the modus operandi of acupuncturation but at the same time I am free to confess myself sceptical on the creed, that its effects are produced by the escape of air from the cellular membranes through the punctures made by needles.

He then proceeds to give three cogent reasons for his incredulity:

> 1. The very form of the needle is a barrier to the escape of air; 2. the cure is often performed before the needles are withdrawn; and 3. the cure is often performed by causing acute pain in the act of introducing them.

His first observation, being self-explanatory, needs no further comment; his second may sound farfetched to anyone who has not practised acupuncture but on occasions it is surprising how rapidly pain is relieved in response to needle stimulation; and his third is in line with the currently held view that for acupuncture to be successful in the relief of chronic pain the needling itself has to be such as to produce a brief intensely painful stimulus (see Ch. 8).

Another person whose interest in acupuncture was aroused by Churchill was John Elliotson, a physician who was originally on the staff at St Thomas's Hospital, London but who later became Professor of Medicine at University College Hospital. Elliotson writing in the *Medico-Chirurgical Transactions* in 1827 stated that the use of acupuncture both in his private practice and at St Thomas's Hospital over several years had led him to agree with Mr Churchill that it was mainly of value in the 'rheumatism of the fleshy parts', which he also in places referred to as 'rheumatalgia'.

In view of Elliotson's high standing as a teacher in a leading medical school it was unfortunate that his enthusiastic support for animal magnetism, a form of hypnosis introduced by Mesmer, caused him to suffer professional opprobrium, as this in turn served to undermine any influence he might otherwise have had in furthering the cause of acupuncture.

It is clear that in 19th-century Britain any interest that may have been shown in acupuncture both by the medical profession and the general public was intermittent, as may be seen from the following contribution to the subject by Dr T Ogier Ward of Kensington, in the *British Medical Journal* on 28th August 1858:

> … acupuncture is a remedy that seems to have its floods and ebbs in public estimation; for we see it much belauded in medical meetings every ten years or so, even to its recommendation in neuralgia of the heart, and then it again sinks into neglect or oblivion. And it is not unlikely that its disuse may be occasioned partly by fear of the pain, and partly by the difficulty the patient finds to believe so trifling an operation can produce such powerful effects. Its use is not as frequent as it deserves and now that we know

the rationale of its operation I venture to bring forward a few cases in illustration of its remedial powers in order that others may be induced to give it a more extensive trial, and thus ascertain its true value in the treatment of neuralgia or rheumatic pains.

There then follows six case reports describing how muscle pain in various parts of the body including the shoulder, lower back and thigh was alleviated by inserting needles into the areas where the pain was most intensely felt. Acupuncture may not have been widely adopted by the British medical profession during the 19th century but there is evidence to show that at least one large provincial general hospital in this country favoured its use in the alleviation of musculoskeletal pain. T. Pridgin Teale, Surgeon to the General Infirmary at Leeds, writing in the *Lancet* in 1871, states:

> In the present essay it is my wish to record some facts concerning a method of treatment of great antiquity which seems in a great measure to have dropped out of use, or at any rate to be at the present day but little employed or even known in many parts of the United Kingdom. It has however been for years a favourite traditional practice at the Leeds Infirmary.

He then goes on to say 'when it does succeed the relief it gives is almost instantaneous, generally permanent, and often in cases which for weeks or months have run the gauntlet of other treatments without benefit'.

He then proceeds to describe five cases including two with pain and restricted movement of the shoulder joint, one with pain around the coccyx following labour, one with persistent pain around the os calcis, and one with long-standing pain around the wrist following trauma. He expresses the opinion that cases suitable for acupuncture include trauma to muscle, stretching or tearing of muscle or tendon, and disuse pain. Certainly, even by today's standards, this is a reasonably comprehensive list of 'surgical' indications.

It is interesting to note that Teale, from observing the area of redness that so frequently arises in the skin around the site where an acupuncture needle has been inserted, was misled into thinking that acupuncture must work by producing some form of temporary congestion.

Another surgeon to write about the use of acupuncture in hospital practice at Leeds was Simeon Snell. Snell writing in the *Medical Times and Gazette* in 1880 at a time when he was ophthalmic surgeon to the Sheffield General Hospital says:

> At the Leeds Infirmary the use of it is almost traditional. It was there that I both saw it employed, practised it myself and witnessed the remarkable benefits frequently resulting.

He then proceeds to describe five cases of pain with limitation of movement of the shoulder joint he had treated successfully at Leeds.

Presumably when he became an ophthalmic surgeon at Sheffield he had little opportunity to use the technique but one can be sure that he encouraged others to do so. And certainly he was more enlightened than Teale in his view as to how it works believing 'it may act as a stimulant to the nerve twigs'.

News concerning the manner in which acupuncture was being practised in Europe from the beginning of the 19th century quickly reached America. American physicians, however, at that time viewed this form of therapy with considerable suspicion and were reluctant to make use of it. An anonymous reviewer in admitting this, when reviewing Churchill's *Treatise on Acupuncturation* in the *Medical Repository* in 1822, was forced to say:

> … but we have probably been mistaken. Acupuncture is likely to become, employed with discrimination and directed with skill, a valuable resource.

In spite of these words of encouragement, and also that during the 1820s American medical journals published a number of European reports on the subject, the only physicians in the whole of that great continent who seemed to take any interest in it were a few in Philadelphia, with one of the most enthusiastic of these, as Cassedy (1974) has pointed out, being Franklin Bache.

Franklin Bache was the assistant physician at the Philadelphia State Penitentiary and in 1825 he decided to try the effects of acupuncture on prisoners suffering from various painful disorders, which as he said, when reporting his results a year later (Bache 1826), 'may be arranged into the four general heads of muscular rheumatism, chronic pains, neuralgia, and ophthalmia'. In his report in which he reviewed the results of the effects of acupuncture on 29 people, most of whom were convicts, he concluded that the treatment had much to offer in removing and mitigating pain, and that it was 'a proper remedy in almost all diseases, whose prominent symptom is pain'.

One cannot help but feel that if only more notice had been taken of this wise dictum that interest in acupuncture in 19th-century America might have become more widespread, but, unfortunately, certain other Philadelphian physicians decided to direct their energies to exploring its use in conditions of a far more dubious nature.

These included E. J. Coxe, D. T. Coxe, and Samuel Jackson, who having heard reports from Europe about it being possible to revive drowned kittens by inserting needles into their hearts, decided to investigate whether the same procedure had anything to offer in resuscitating drowned people! And finding, as might be expected, that it had not, they clearly became disillusioned with the therapeutic properties of acupuncture in general, for as Edward Coxe (1826) in reporting the results of their experiment remarked:

> Whatever others may think of the possibility of resuscitating drowned persons by acupuncture, I can only say that I should think myself highly culpable, if, called to a case of asphyxia, I were to waste time, every moment of which is precious, in endeavouring to resuscitate by a means which I sincerely believe to be good for nothing.

This in my opinion is a very good example as to how acupuncture can so readily be brought into disrepute when it is not employed in a selective and discerning manner, and should serve as an object lesson to all those currently engaged in investigating the clinical applications of acupuncture. Despite this adverse report the cause of acupuncture in America received a boost when in 1833 the editors of the *Medical Magazine* reprinted a paper that John Elliotson, the physician at St Thomas's Hospital, London, had originally contributed to the *Cyclopaedia of Practical Medicine*. Also, in 1836 the editors of the prestigious and widely read *Boston Medical and Surgical Journal* reprinted an article that

had appeared shortly before in the *Southern Medical and Surgical Journal*. In this paper, William M. Lee of South Carolina reported how he had used acupuncture for 6 years in the treatment of rheumatism and concluded that this method of treatment was 'entitled to far more attention than it has yet received in the United States'.

Such a view, however, does not seem to have been widely shared, for there continued to be a paucity of literature on acupuncture in America at that time with the only further outstanding contribution being that of Robley Dunglison, another Philadelphian physician. This took the form of an eight-page account of the subject in a compendium of his entitled *New Remedies*, and published in 1839. The same article was reproduced in subsequent editions of the book up to the last one which appeared in 1856, but in spite of this any interest that there may have been in this type of treatment was gradually fading leaving Samuel Gross in his book *A System of Surgery*, published in 1859 to state:

> Its advantages have been much overrated and the practice … has fallen into disrepute.

This certainly may have been true so far as America was concerned but up in Canada none other than the famous physician Sir William Osler was using it in the late 19th and early 20th centuries, for in the eighth edition of his book *The Principles and Practice of Medicine* published in 1912 at the time when he was Regius Professor of Medicine at Oxford University he wrote:

> For lumbago, acupuncture is, in acute cases, the most efficient treatment. Needles of from three to four inches in length (ordinary bonnet needles, sterilised, will do) are thrust into the lumbar muscles at the seat of pain, and withdrawn after five or ten minutes. In many instances the relief of pain is immediate, and I can corroborate the statements of Ringer, who taught me this practice, as to its extraordinary and prompt effect in many instances.

He had clearly been in the habit of using the technique for many years because Harvey Cushing (1925) in his book *The Life of Sir William Osler* refers to an unfortunate experience the great man had when he was a physician at the Montreal General Hospital.

It would seem that early in Osler's career at that hospital a certain Peter Redpath, a wealthy Montreal sugar refiner and member of the hospital's board, having suffered from intractable lumbago for some time, had high hopes that the newly appointed physician might be able to cure him.

Arrangements were therefore made for him to consult Osler in his office at the hospital and it is recounted that Redpath, having arrived exhausted from the effort of mounting the stairs, did not take kindly to being treated with acupuncture, for Cushing reports that:

> … at each jab the old gentleman is said to have rapped out a string of oaths, and in the end got up and hobbled out, no better of his pain, this to Osler's great distress, for he had expected to give him immediate relief which as he said 'meant a million for McGill'.

It should be noted that, unlike the Chinese who have always attached much importance to manipulating needles such as twirling them between thumb and finger, once they have been inserted into the body, most 19th-century European exponents of acupuncture were content merely to insert their needles and then to leave them without touching them again for a short period of time. The actual time varied considerably and ranged from Mr Wansbrough of Fulham leaving them in situ for from 20 seconds to 4 minutes, and Mr Pridgin Teale leaving them on average for about 1 minute; up to Mr Churchill who advised leaving them for about 5–6 minutes, and Sir William Osler who recommended that they remain for 5–10 minutes.

This was of considerable practical interest during the resurgence of interest in acupuncture in the latter part of the 20th century, as many people, including myself, for reasons to be explained in Chapter 8, favoured the technique whereby needles, having been inserted, were left in position without any form of manipulation. However, it is also now realized that it is wrong to stipulate any particular period of time for which they should be left, as this varies widely from a few seconds to 10 minutes according to a patient's individual central nervous system's speed of reaction to peripheral nerve stimulation with dry needles.

It is also worth stressing once again that none of these physicians put needles into traditional Chinese acupuncture points but so far as musculoskeletal disorders were concerned, which very sensibly is what in the main they used it for, they simply inserted them into the painful areas. However, it is now realized that musculoskeletal pain does not necessarily originate at the site where it is felt, but is referred there via the central nervous system from some focus of neural hyperactivity – now known as a trigger point – that is often situated some distance away. Therefore, rather than inserting a needle into the area where pain is felt, the pain is more likely to be relieved if the needle is inserted into the tissues overlying the trigger point for the purpose of stimulating Adelta nerve fibres in its vicinity.

This is the fundamental principle upon which the recently developed Western approach to trigger point acupuncture is based, and the manner in which it was discovered will now be explained.

## References

Anon 1822 Review of James Churchill's treatise on acupuncturation. Medical Repository (New Series) 7: 441–449

Bache F 1826 Cases illustrative of the remedial effects of acupuncturation. North American Medical and Surgical Journal 1: 311–321

Berlioz L V J 1816 Mémoires sur les maladies chroniques, les évacuations sanguines et l'acupuncture, 2 vols. Croullebois, Paris

Bozetti S 1820 Memoria sull'agopuntura. Milan

Carraro A 1825 Saggio sull'agopuntura. Udine

Cassedy J H 1974 Early use of acupuncture in the United States. Bulletin of the New York Academy of Medicine 50 (8): 892–896

Churchill J M 1821 A treatise on acupuncturation being a description of a surgical operation originally peculiar to the Japanese and Chinese, and by them denominated zin-king, now introduced into European practice, with directions for its performance, and cases illustrating its success. Simpkins & Marshall, London (German trans 1824, French trans 1825)

Churchill J M 1828 Cases illustrative of the immediate effects of acupuncturation in rheumatism, lumbago, sciatica, anomalous muscular diseases and in dropsy of the cellular tissue, selected from various sources and intended as an appendix to the author's treatise on the subject. Callow & Wilson, London

Cloquet J, Dantu T M 1828 Observations sur les effects thérapeutiques de l'acupuncture. In: Bayle A L J (ed) Bibliotheque de Thérapeutique, vol 1, p. 436

Coxe E J 1826 Observations on asphyxia from drowning. North American Medical and Surgical Journal 2: 292–293

Cushing H 1925 The life of Sir William Osler. Clarendon Press, Oxford

da Camin F S 1834 Sulla agopuntura, con alcuni cenni sulla puntura elettrica. Antonelli, Venice

da Camin F S 1837 Dell'agopuntura e della galvano-puntura. Osservazioni, Venice

Dunglison R 1839 Acupuncture. In: New remedies. Waldie, Philadelphia, pp. 23–30

Elliotson J 1827 The use of the sulphate of copper in chronic diarrhoea together with an essay on acupuncture. Medicochirurgical transactions 13, part 2: 451–467

Elliotson J 1833 Acupuncture. Medical Magazine 1: 309–314

Gross S D 1859 A system of surgery, vol 1. Blanchard and Lea, Philadelphia, pp. 575–576

Lee W M 1836 Acupuncture as a remedy for rheumatism. Southern Medical and Surgical Journal 1: 129–133

Lu Gwei-Djen, Needham J 1980 Celestial lancets. Cambridge University Press, Cambridge, p. 295

Osler Sir William 1912 The principles and practice of medicine, 8th edn. Appleton, New York, p. 1131

Sarlandière le Chevalier J B 1825 Mémoires sur l'electropuncture … Private publication, Paris Snell S 1880 Remarks on acupuncture. Medical Times and Gazette 1: 661–662

Teale T Pridgin 1871 Clinical essays no. III. On the relief of pain and muscular disability by acupuncture. Lancet 1: 567–568

Wansborough D 1826 Acupuncturation. Lancet 10: 846–848

Ward T Ogier 1858 On acupuncture. British Medical Journal (Aug 28): 728–729

# PART 2

# Principles of trigger point acupuncture

# Chapter 4

# Some basic observations leading to its development

## INTRODUCTION

The traditional practice of Chinese acupuncture having become officially recognized once again in China during the 1950s, and it having since then been increasingly used by some doctors, and to an even greater extent by non-medically qualified practitioners in the West, there are at present many acupuncturists throughout the world who claim it is beneficial in the treatment of a wide variety of disorders. It is, however, only in the alleviation of pain, and in particular musculoskeletal pain, that there is any scientific basis to its use. And, even when used within these strictly defined limits, the traditional Chinese approach to this form of therapy has serious drawbacks.

The principal disadvantage is that, for most practitioners of traditional Chinese acupuncture, needles have to be inserted somewhat arbitrarily in accordance with the numerous lists of points that are recommended for use in the treatment of various rather ill-defined clinical conditions in every standard textbook on the subject. Moreover, before a person is able to use these lists, recipes, or prescriptions, as they are sometimes called, it is first necessary to memorize the course taken by the various Chinese acu-tracts, and the exact anatomical position on them of the various acu-points. It can only be assumed that these traditional guides to point selection owe their origin to the time-honoured, but highly contentious, Chinese method of pulse-diagnosis, and for this reason alone they are unlikely to be acceptable to most doctors trained in 20th-century scientific Western medicine.

However, fortunately for those who wish to avoid this somewhat empirically determined and impersonal method of point selection and prefer to employ one based on a carefully conducted clinical examination of each individual patient, there is now a trigger point approach to acupuncture. This recently developed Western approach to acupuncture has as its main application the alleviation of pain that is referred to some part of the body from a focus or foci of neural hyperactivity in one or other of the structures that together form the musculoskeletal system. In order to explain the principles upon which it is based, it is first necessary to review the outstanding pioneer research into referred pain carried out by J. H. Kellgren at University College Hospital Medical School in the late 1930s.

## THE REFERRAL OF MUSCULOSKELETAL PAIN – SOME EARLY OBSERVATIONS

It was Sir Thomas Lewis, the director of the clinical research department at University College Hospital who, because of his particular interest in the subject of pain in general, prompted Kellgren to carry out clinical observations on the referral of musculoskeletal pain.

Lewis in his paper *Suggestions Relating to the Study of Somatic Pain* published in February 1938 states:

> As an experimental method of producing muscle pain the injection of a minute quantity of a salt solution is the most satisfactory … In these observations I have noted that muscle pain is referred to a distance. Thus pain arising from the lower part of the triceps is often referred down the inner side of the forearm to the little finger, from the trapezius it is usually referred to the occiput. I have been fortunate in interesting Dr Kellgren in this matter. In a long series of very careful researches carried out in my laboratory he has formulated some very striking principles underlying the reference of pain from muscle – principles which appear to have an important practical bearing.

Kellgren, in his paper *Observations on Referred Pain Arising from Muscle*, published later the same year, states that in taking on the task set him by Sir Thomas Lewis he was aware that the latter's

experimental findings had already received support from the clinical observations made by several physicians, who, from 1925 onwards, had noted that certain painful conditions of the extremities are associated with tender areas in the muscles of the limb girdles and because of this had suggested the possibility that in such cases pain arising in muscle may be of the referred type.

In his experiments that he carried out on himself and healthy volunteers working in the same laboratory, he first anaesthetized the skin and then injected small amounts (0.1–0.3 cc) of hypertonic (6%) saline into various muscles; and then carefully observed the distribution of pain. For example, in studies involving the gluteus medius muscle the skin of the buttock was first anaesthetized with Novocain at three sites. Then intramuscular needles were inserted through these anaesthetized areas until they impinged upon the gluteal fascia. An injection of hypertonic saline into this fascia produced localized pain. The needles were then advanced into the muscle itself and a further injection into this produced a diffuse pain felt at some distance from the injection site in the lower part of the buttock, the back of the thigh, and on occasions as far down as the knee (Fig. 4.1). Injections into the fascia enveloping the tibialis anticus (anterior) muscle and into the muscle itself produced similar findings (Fig. 4.2).

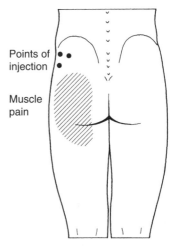

Points of injection

Muscle pain

**Figure 4.1**    The distribution of diffuse referred pain (hatched area) produced by injecting 6% saline into three points in the gluteus medius muscle. (Reproduced with permission of J. H. Kellgren from *Clinical Science*, vol. 3. pp 175–190 © 1938 The Biochemical Society, London.)

Kellgren also points out in this paper that an injection of saline into muscle produces pain at some distance from the point stimulated and that, in certain cases, the maximal pain is not experienced in muscle itself but in other structures. From his experimental work he was able to show, for example, that when an injection is given into the occipital muscle, pain is felt diffusely as a headache; when into the masseter muscle, it is felt in the mouth as toothache; when into the infraspinatus muscle, it is felt at the tip of the shoulder; when into the vastus intermedius, it is felt around the knee joint; when into the peroneus longus, it is felt at the ankle joint; and when into the multifidus muscle opposite the first and second lumbar vertebrae, it is felt in the scrotum.

His finding that referred pain from a focus of irritation in a muscle may be felt in such structures as joints, teeth, or the testicles is, of course, of considerable importance, and one which has constantly to be borne in mind in everyday clinical practice.

From these observations he decided that the distribution of referred pain, induced artificially in normal people, by injecting hypertonic saline into muscle broadly follows a spinal segmental pattern

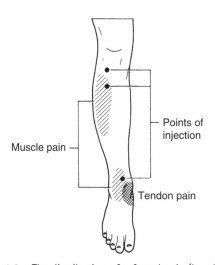

**Figure 4.2** The distribution of referred pain (hatched area) from injecting 6% saline into points in the tibialis anterior muscle. Also, the pattern of locally referred pain (stippled area) from injecting saline into the tendon of this muscle at the ankle. (Reproduced with permission of J. H. Kellgren from *Clinical Science*, vol. 3, pp 175–190 © 1938 The Biochemical Society, London.)

but that it does not correspond with the sensory segmental patterns of the skin.

Kellgren did not confine himself to laboratory experiments but applied knowledge gained from these to clinical medicine. And his paper, *A Preliminary Account of Referred Pains Arising from Muscle*, published in 1938, is of the greatest possible interest because, unbeknown to him, from his study of a number of cases of what he calls 'fibrositis' or 'myalgia' he laid down certain principles upon which the practice of modern Western acupuncture is now based. As his observations are therefore of such fundamental importance, part of his paper will be quoted in full:

During the last year I have made an extensive investigation of the character and distribution of muscular pain produced experimentally in normal subjects … Briefly I find that pain arising from muscle is always diffuse and is often referred, with a distribution which follows a spinal segmental pattern; and that this referred pain is associated with referred tenderness of the deep structures.

A number of cases of 'fibrositis' or 'myalgia' have been investigated from this point of view. The distribution of pain was noted as accurately as possible, and experience of the distribution of pain provoked from normal muscles guided me to the muscles from which spontaneous pain might have arisen. Such muscles almost always presented tender spots on palpation. Pressure on these spots sometimes reproduced the patient's pain; but a method more often successful was the injection of sterile saline into the tender muscle. The injection of Novocain may also reproduce the pain momentarily.

The search for the source of trouble by defining areas of tenderness is often confused by the patients calling attention to areas of referred tenderness. But referred tenderness is rarely conspicuous, and I have found it a useful guide to consider tenderness to be referred unless the patient winces under the palpation of a given spot. When these acutely tender spots were not too extensive they were infiltrated with 1% Novocain … This infiltration often produced relief of the symptoms and signs, and sometimes abolished them completely.

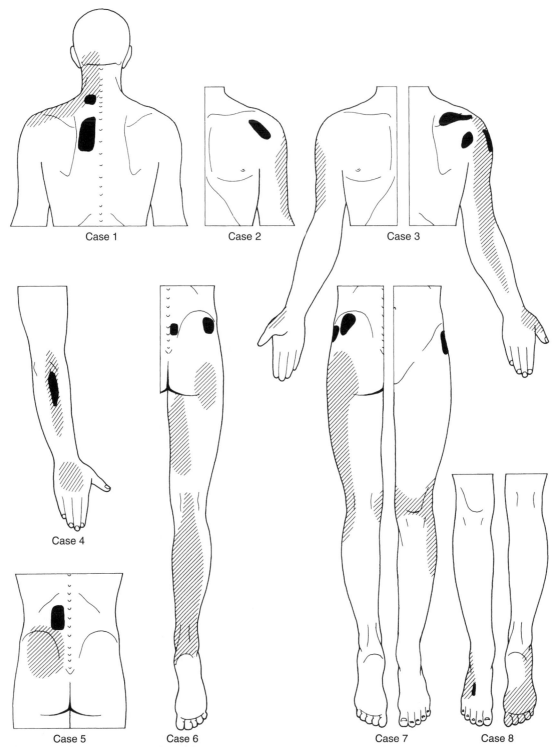

**Figure 4.3** The distribution of pain (hatched area) and tender spots (black) in eight cases in which the pain was abolished by injecting Novocain into the tender spots. (Reproduced with permission of J. H. Kellgren from the *British Medical Journal*, 1938.)

It should be noted from this that Kellgren made a clear distinction between certain 'spots' in muscle so exquisitely tender that palpation of them makes the patient wince; and diffuse rather ill-defined areas of referred pain which on palpation are only slightly tender. Also, that he realized that such 'spots' as he called them, or trigger points as they are now termed, are the cause of this referred pain with it being possible to alleviate the latter by de-activating these acutely tender 'spots' or trigger points by infiltrating them with Novocain (Fig. 4.3).

Kellgren (1939) also investigated referred pain arising from experimentally-induced irritant foci in interspinous ligaments, tendons, joints and the periosteum. Two others who also made a valuable contribution to our understanding of skeletal pain were Verne Inman, an anatomist, and John Saunders, an orthopaedic surgeon working at the University of California Medical School. In their paper, *Referred Pain from Skeletal Structures*, published in 1944, they describe how they studied experimentally induced pain in healthy volunteers by artificially stimulating periosteum, ligaments and tendons by mechanically traumatizing them either by scratching them with the point of a needle, or by drilling them with a special type of wire; and, secondly, by chemically stimulating them by injecting into them either normal isotonic Ringer's solution, or a weak solution of formic acid or hypertonic saline.

From these experiments they conclude:

> Stimulation of the periosteum or the tendinous attachments of ligaments and tendons is accompanied by an extensive radiation of the pain, which, if sufficiently intense, radiates for considerable distances … so constant is the direction and locality to which the pain radiates that it has been found possible to chart and map out the extent of the areas to which the pain radiates, and an attempt has been made to relate them to areas of segmental innervation.

It should be noted that they refer to these areas of segmental innervation in the case of skeletal structures as sclerotomes in order to distinguish them from myotomes or dermatomes.

In this paper they also state that for several years they had been making detailed clinical observations on the radiation of pain from pathological disorders affecting bony and ligamentous structures. And they had found that in every case the type of pain was similar to that produced experimentally and that, like the latter, its radiation to distant areas had a distinctive pattern but one which could not be accounted for by reference to the distribution of peripheral nerves.

## The anatomical distribution of referred musculoskeletal pain

It has to be admitted that there is much confusion concerning the anatomical distribution of referred pain in disorders of the musculoskeletal system. It will be remembered that Kellgren concluded that pain referred from skeletal muscle usually follows spinal segmental patterns but that this is not dermatomal, and that he also noted many exceptions when pain extended over several segments.

Travell & Bigelow (1946) also concluded from clinical observations on patients with referred pain from skeletal muscle that it does not follow a simple segmental pattern for, as they say, 'the reference from a single site may comprise fragments of several "segmental pain areas" without including any one entirely, or may take in a whole "segmental area," skip the adjacent one and reappear distally'.

Hockaday & Whitty (1967) in attempting to clarify the situation studied referred sensations produced by injecting 6% saline into interspinous ligaments in 28 normal subjects, and concluded that the:

> … site of reference for a given site of stimulus was constant and replicable in the individual, but was not always confined to the segment of innervation in which the injection was given. Site of reference within a group of subjects varied widely and could not be interpreted as segmental or having a fixed anatomical substrate.

It is difficult, however, to be certain as to how much credence should be placed on conclusions drawn from any of the experiments carried out over the past 50 years in which hypertonic saline has been injected into various musculoskeletal structures in an attempt to map out the distribution of referred pain for as Wyke (1987) says, in discussing these during the course of considering various aspects of spinal ligamentous pain:

> Although such saline solutions provide a very effective chemical irritant for connective tissue nociceptive receptors, it must be emphasised here that because of the diffuse distribution of this receptor system through the vertebral connective tissues, and because of the widespread intersegmental linkages between their afferent nerve fibres, attempts to use such a procedure as a means of delineating a supposed segmental nociceptive innervation of the spinal tissues are clearly fallacious, especially as it is impossible (even with the introduction of radio-opaque material into the injected solution) to be certain just how much of the diffuse nociceptive afferent system is being stimulated by any given volume of hypertonic saline.

The situation, therefore, is far from straightforward and Travell & Simons (1983) after years of extensively studying referred pain in patients with disorders of the musculoskeletal system have been forced somewhat negatively to conclude that referred pain of this type 'does not follow a simple segmental pattern. Neither does it follow familiar neurological patterns, nor the known patterns for referred pain of visceral origin'.

## The relevance of these discoveries to the development of trigger point acupuncture

Kellgren's discovery that it is possible to alleviate referred musculoskeletal pain by injecting a local anaesthetic into what he called tender points has proved to be an important therapeutic advance. The relevance of this to the recent development of trigger point acupuncture might however at first sight seem to be somewhat obscure until it is explained that there are now sound neurophysiology grounds for believing that it is more rational as well as being simpler, safer and just as effective to alleviate this type of pain by stimulating with dry needles, nerve endings in the superficial tissues directly overlying these intramuscularly situated tender points, or what, for reasons to be explained in the next chapter, are now called trigger points.

## References

Hockaday J M, Whitty C W M 1967 Patterns of referred pain in the normal subject. Brain 90: 481–496

Inman V T, Saunders J B de C M 1944 Referred pain from skeletal structures. Journal of Nervous and Mental Diseases 99: 660–667

Kellgren J H 1938 Observations on referred pain arising from muscle. Clinical Science 3: 175–190

Kellgren J H 1938 A preliminary account of referred pains arising from muscle. British Medical Journal 1: 325–327

Kellgren J H 1939 On the distribution of pain arising from deep somatic structures with charts of segmental pain areas. Clinical Science 4: 35–46

Lewis Sir Thomas 1938 Suggestions relating to the study of somatic pain. British Medical Journal 1: 321–325

Travell J, Bigelow N H 1946 Referred somatic pain does not follow a simple 'segmental' pattern. Federation Proceedings 5: 106

Travell J, Simons D G 1983 Myofascial pain and dysfunction. The trigger point manual. Williams and Wilkins, Baltimore

Wyke B 1987 The neurology of low back pain. In: Jayson M I V (ed) The lumbar spine and back pain, 3rd edn. Churchill Livingstone, Edinburgh, p. 78

# Chapter 5

# Evolution of knowledge concerning muscle pain syndromes for which it is employed

## INTRODUCTION

Trigger point (TrP) acupuncture is mainly employed for the alleviation of pain arising from points of maximum tenderness in the muscles of patients suffering from what is now known as the myofascial trigger point pain syndrome (MTrPPS).

Acupuncture of a similar type, together with other forms of treatment, may also be used to relieve the pain that affects those suffering from what is presently termed fibromyalgia syndrome (FS).

The purpose of this chapter is to show how our current concepts concerning these two syndromes have gradually evolved.

## NOSOLOGICAL OBFUSCATION

Before MTrPPS and FS were recognized to be separate disorders, over the past 200 years they were known collectively by a variety of different names. The original term was rheumatism, which was first introduced by Guillaume de Baillou in the latter part of the 16th century. Unfortunately, as Ruhmann (1940) has pointed out in his introduction to an English translation of De Baillou's book *Liber de Rheumatismo*, de Baillou used the term rheumatism not only when describing clinical manifestations of muscular rheumatism, but also when writing about what has since become known as acute rheumatic fever.

Thomas Sydenham then added to this terminological confusion when in his *Observationes Medicae* published in 1676 he included a chapter entitled 'Rheumatism' that dealt only with the characteristic migratory type of arthropathy seen in acute rheumatic fever. This confusion was further compounded when, in 1810, Wells called the carditis that develops in this febrile disorder rheumatism of the heart (Baldry 1971). Fortunately, Jean Bouillau helped to clarify the situation when in 1840 he made a clear distinction between the arthropathy and carditis of acute rheumatic fever and muscular rheumatism (Reynolds 1983).

By that time two British physicians, Balfour (1815) and Scudamore (1827) had put forward the idea that the pain of muscular rheumatism occurs as the result of inflammation developing in the fibrous connective tissue in muscle. This concept differed from the one held by 19th-century German and Scandinavian physicians who believed that the pain develops as the result of an inflammatory process in the muscle itself. Nevertheless, it was one that was to persist throughout England and France for the rest of that century and in 1904 caused Sir William Gowers to recommend that the disorder hitherto known as muscular rheumatism should be called fibrositis.

Gowers did this during the course of a lecture on lumbago at what was then called the National Hospital for the Paralysed and Epileptic (National Hospital for Nervous Diseases, London). The arguments he put forward in support of his proposition were, in retrospect, distinctly specious, but nevertheless they led him to conclude: 'We are thus compelled to regard lumbago in particular, and muscular rheumatism in general, as a form of inflammation of the fibrous tissues of the muscles … (and thus) … we may conveniently follow the analogy of "cellulitis" and term it "fibrositis." '

Ralph Stockman, the then Professor of Medicine at Glasgow University, seemed to provide him with the pathological confirmation he required when, on examining microscopically some nodules removed from the muscles of patients affected by this disorder, he reported the presence of 'inflammatory hyperplasia … confined to white fibrous tissue' (Stockman 1904).

Although Stockman's findings have never subsequently been confirmed, their publication at that particular time helped to ensure that Gowers' term fibrositis became widely adopted. Any diagnostic specificity Gowers may have hoped to confer upon this term, however, was soon removed when in 1915 Llewellyn, a physician at the Royal Mineral Water Hospital in Bath, and Jones, a surgeon in that city, published a book entitled *Fibrositis*. In this they included under the term fibrositis a variety of disorders including gout and rheumatoid arthritis. Since that time, the term has been used in such an imprecise manner as to make it virtually meaningless.

A search for a more suitable term for what was originally called muscular rheumatism has therefore continued, and some of the synonyms employed during this century include nodular fibromyositis (Telling 1911), myofascitis (Albee 1927), myofibrositis (Murray 1929), neurofibrositis (Clayton & Livingstone 1930), idiopathic myalgia (Gutstein-Good 1940), rheumatic myalgias (Good 1941) and even myodysneuria (Gutstein 1955).

Simons (1975, 1976) and Reynolds (1983), in their wide-ranging historical reviews of the subject, have shown that, in addition to this longstanding terminological confusion, there has also been much disagreement over the years concerning the diagnostic significance of the nodules, palpable bands and tender points found in this disorder.

## NODULES AND PALPABLE BANDS

The Edinburgh physician William Balfour (1816), as a result of massaging muscles to relieve the pain of muscular rheumatism, was one of the first to report the presence of nodules in this disorder. However, it was not until the middle of the 19th century, when the Dutch physician Johan Mezger placed massage on a sound scientific basis (Haberling 1932), and this 'hands-on' technique then became widely adopted for the treatment of muscular rheumatism, that nodules and the elongated cord-like structures now known as palpable bands, which are found in this disorder, became generally recognized.

It was Mezger's Swedish and German students who were particularly influential in disseminating knowledge about these structures. In 1876, the Swedish physician Uno Helleday wrote extensively about nodules occurring in what he called chronic myitis (Helleday 1876). Following this, the German physician Strauss (1898) distinguished between nodules – which he described as being small, tender, apple-sized structures – and palpable bands – which he described as being painful, pencil-sized to little finger-sized elongated structures. The identification of these structures requires more than a cursory examination and, as Müller (1912) pointed out, the main reasons why so many doctors fail to identify them is because it requires a skilled technique, one that he considered difficult to learn but that could be made easier by the application of a lubricant to the skin.

He also thought that the reason why his contemporaries tended to deny the existence of nodules and palpable bands was because they did not bother to look for them conscientiously, unlike masseurs who, according to him, had no difficulty in detecting them from palpating muscles systematically and then treating them appropriately. A similar state of affairs prevails today, with physiotherapists being far more practised in the art of palpating muscles than many doctors.

## Nodules

By the beginning of this century doctors in Britain were being taught to regard the presence of nodules as essential for the diagnosis of what was then called fibrositis. However, it soon became apparent that not only are nodules not always present in the disorder, but also they can occasionally be present in people with no history of it. It is because of their somewhat enigmatic and elusive nature, and because of their distinctly nebulous morphology (Ch. 7), that over the course of this century their diagnostic significance has increasingly come to be questioned. Despite this, there is no doubt that when nodules are specifically sought they are frequently found in the lumbar region in patients with chronic low-back pain, and also, though less frequently, in the neck and shoulder girdle of those affected by persistent musculoskeletal pain at that site. Moreover, the insertion of dry needles into these nodules helps to relieve this pain (Ch. 8).

## Palpable bands

Unlike nodules which only develop in muscles in the lumbar and cervical regions, palpable bands are liable to develop in any muscle of the body. Like nodules, however, they are only discovered if conscientiously and skilfully looked for. When these elongated bands are carefully palpated they are found to contain one or more focal points of exquisite tenderness, now known as TrPs, but which Kellgren and others before him called tender points.

### Tender points

Balfour (1824a,b) not only found tender nodules in patients with muscular rheumatism, but also observed that, separate from these, there are focal points of tenderness in the muscles. However, the first person to write at length about these was the French physician François Valleix.

Valleix, in his *Treatise on Neuralgia* published in 1841 described a disorder characterized by pain of a shooting nature and the finding of painful points (*points douloureux*) on palpation of the tissues. He realized that the pain emanated from these points for he states:

> If, in the intervals of the shooting pains, one asks (a patient with neuralgia) what is the seat of the pain, he replies by designating limited points … It is with the aid of pressure … that one discovers the extent of the painful points. …

Some of the pain syndromes he described would clearly be included in a present-day classification of neuralgias but others, such as what he termed femoropopliteal neuralgia, would not. Furthermore, 7 years later he somewhat confused the situation by calling muscular rheumatism a form of neuralgia (Valleix 1848). With reference to this he states:

> I conclude that pain, capital symptom of neuralgia expresses itself … in different ways. If it remains concentrated in the nerves one finds characteristic, isolated, painful points; this is *neuralgia in the proper sense*. If the pain spreads into the muscles … this is *muscular rheumatism* … an obvious muscular rheumatism can transform itself into a true neuralgia. …

Despite his belief that neuralgia can turn itself into muscular rheumatism and vice versa, he must be given credit for recognizing that the pain in muscular rheumatism emanates primarily from focal points of neural hyperactivity, and also that it travels some distance from its source. He was wrong, however, in believing that this is because it is 'propagated along neighbouring nerves'.

Since then many other European physicians have erroneously subscribed to Valleix's idea that rheumatic pain spreads along the course of peripheral nerves, but they have differed in their views as to how this might occur. Stockman's (1904) explanation was that 'a branch of a nerve may be pressed upon by a nodule, or may even pass through it, hence the pain often radiates over a wide area perhaps far from a nodule'. Others believed that it occurred as a result of pressure on a nerve when a muscle goes into spasm. A third hypothesis, and one which was widely held well into the 20th century, was that it is due to rheumatic inflammation of connective tissue in or around nerves, and it was for this reason that the terms neurofibrositis and perineuritis were introduced (Gowers 1904, Llewellyn & Jones 1915, Clayton & Livingstone 1930).

Those who put forward such ideas seem to have been oblivious of the fact that the British physician Thomas Inman, as long ago as 1858, had shrewdly noted that the radiation of pain in muscular rheumatism 'is independent entirely of the course of nerves'. They also seem to have ignored the observations made by the German physician Cornelius, who at the beginning of this century noted that 'this radiation often enough absolutely does not keep to the individual nerve trunks' and is bound 'to no anatomical law' (Cornelius 1903).

Cornelius not only confirmed Inman's observation that the radiation of pain is not along the course of peripheral nerves and, therefore, cannot be due to compression of these structures, but went further than this by showing that pressure on tender points in muscles evokes this type of pain and that the latter must therefore emanate from these points. He clearly realized that the reason why these points are tender is because they are sites where nerve endings are in a state of hyperactivity and for this reason he called them nerve points (*nervenpunkte*). He also stated that he thought this neural hyperactivity occurred as a result of external factors such as changes of temperature, alterations in weather conditions, physical exertion and emotional upsets, or, alternatively, because of 'heightened excitability' of the nervous system occurring as the result of such influences as heredity, intemperance and illness in general.

He was, therefore, beginning to formulate ideas concerning the pathogenesis of muscular rheumatism, which were very much in line with the modern view that the pain develops as a result of nerve endings at tender points (or what today are more often called TrPs) becoming sensitized for one or other of a variety of different reasons. In the light of all this, it may be seen that Valleix may not have been so far off the mark as at first sight might be thought when he called muscular rheumatism a type of neuralgia. There is also no doubt that Sir William Osler (1909), with his customary perspicacity, must have had Valleix and Cornelius in mind when, in writing about what he called muscular rheumatism or myalgia in his famous textbook of medicine, he said:

> It is by no means certain that the muscular tissues are the seat of the disease. Many writers claim, perhaps correctly, that it is a neuralgia of the sensory nerves of the muscles.

Early 20th-century physicians, however, had difficulty in explaining why pain occurring as the result of the sensitisation of nerve endings at tender points should be felt some distance away from them. Cornelius (1903) stated it was due to 'reflex mechanisms' but did not enlarge much on the nature of these. Nobody else seems to have been able to take the matter much further until 1952, when Neufeld attributed the heterotopic nature of rheumatic pain to cortical misinterpretation of sensation. It was, however, the 3rd decade of the 20th century that was particularly notable for studies concerning the clinical aspects of rheumatic heterotopic pain.

Hunter (1933) described cases in which there was referral of pain from tender points in the muscles of the abdominal wall. Edeiken & Wolferth (1936) described how, in some patients with coronary thrombosis who had developed pain in the shoulder during the course of strict bed rest, pressure on tender points in muscles over the left scapula caused the spontaneously occurring shoulder pain to be reproduced. Then, in 1938 there were no less than three important contributions to the subject.

One of these was Kellgren's experimental and clinical observations concerning the referral of pain from tender points, which were of such considerable importance, both from a diagnostic and therapeutic point of view, that they have already been considered at some length in Chapter 4. A second was that of the Czechoslovakian physician Reichart, who was one of the first to describe and illustrate diagramatically specific patterns of radiating pains from tender points in muscles. The third came from a Polish physician, Gutstein, following his arrival in England as a political refugee.

Gutstein, unlike Kellgren, who in 1938 published his clinical observations in the British Medical Journal, published his findings that year in the less widely read British Journal of Physical Medicine, and that is possibly one of the reasons why it did not receive the attention it deserved. Nevertheless, in an attempt to get the medical profession to take notice of what he had to say about musculoskeletal pain, he wrote a number of papers on the subject over the next 10 years. Confusingly, however, during the course of this he changed his name three times and even more confusingly kept giving the musculoskeletal pain disorder he was discussing a different name. Thus, in 1938 and again in 1940, under the name of M Gutstein, he wrote about what he called muscular or common rheumatism. In 1940 under the name of Gutstein-Good he called the disorder idiopathic myalgia. Then, a year later, by which time he had changed his name yet again to Good, he wrote about rheumatic myalgias! In 1950 he called it fibrositis, and in 1951 non-articular rheumatism. To add to the confusion, there was at about the same time an R. R. Gutstein (1955) calling this disorder myodysneuria!

Despite all this, Good made the valuable observation that pressure applied to tender points, or what he called myalgic spots in a muscle or tendon, gives rise to both local and referred pain, and he must be given the credit for being the first person to stress that the patterns of pain referral from tender points in individual muscles are the same in everyone; these patterns he illustrated in well-executed drawings. In a similar manner to Kellgren he alleviated this type of pain by injecting a local anaesthetic into these tender points.

Sadly, the medical profession in Britain largely ignored Kellgren's and Good's valuable observations. One reason for this was that by the 1950s many of its leading rheumatologists had come to the conclusion that fibrositis, or non-articular rheumatism as it was by that time more commonly called, is not an organic disorder and that a more appropriate name for it is psychogenic rheumatism. They were led to believe this because of doubts concerning the significance of its physical signs, the absence of any characteristic histological appearances and the lack of any specific laboratory tests for it. Typical of this view was the one expressed by Ellman & Shaw (1950) who, during the course of discussing patients with this disorder stated:

> From the striking disparity between the gross nature of their symptoms and the poverty of the physical findings … it seems clear that the nature of this often very prolonged incapacity is psychiatric in the majority of cases … the patient aches in his limbs because in fact he aches in his mind.

Another reason was that by the 1950s specialists in the field of physical medicine were of the opinion that there is no such disorder as muscular rheumatism and that the pain, said to be associated with it, occurs as the result of disorders in the vertebral column with, in particular, degenerative discs impinging upon nerve roots (Cyriax 1948, de Blecourt 1954, Christie 1958).

Fortunately, there were physicians in other parts of the world who were sufficiently perspicacious to recognize the merits of Kellgren's observations. One of these was Michael Kelly in Australia. Kelly not only adopted Kellgren's methods of diagnosing and relieving referred pain from tender points in muscles but recorded his clinical observations in a series of valuable papers published over a period of 21 years from 1941 onwards. References to the majority of these are to be found in his last paper (Kelly 1962).

## MYOFASCIAL TRIGGER POINT PAIN SYNDROME

The physician, however, who from the 1940s onwards has done the most to further the subject is Janet Travell (Fig. 5.1). She first began to take an interest in it after reading how Edeiken & Wolferth (1936) had been able to reproduce spontaneously occurring shoulder pain by applying pressure to tender points in muscles around the scapula, and then reading about observations made both by Kellgren and by the American orthopaedic surgeon Steindler (1940).

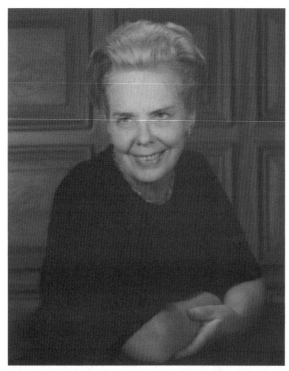

**Figure 5.1** Janet Travell. (With permission from Virginia P. Wilson, USA.)

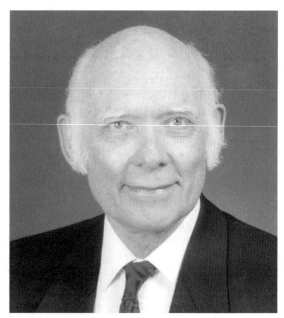

**Figure 5.2** David Simons.

It was Steindler who, during the course of reporting how he was able to relieve 'sciatica' by injecting Novocain into tender points in muscles in the lumbar and gluteal regions, first called these points trigger points (TrPs). It was, however, Travell who brought this term into general use when, in the early 1950s, she introduced the adjective myofascial and began to refer to myofascial TrPs and to describe the pain coming from these as myofascial pain. She adopted the term myofascial as a result of observing, whilst doing an infraspinatus muscle biopsy, that the pain pattern evoked by stretching or pinching the fascia enveloping the muscle is similar to that when the same is done to the muscle itself. Following this, she realized that each muscle in the body has its own specific pattern of myofascial TrP pain referral and she introduced the term myofascial pain syndromes – a term that has since been generally accepted.

By 1951, Travell & Rinzler had had sufficient experience in recognizing these patterns of pain referral to enable them to give a detailed description of a large number of them at that year's meeting of the American Medical Association. In the following year they published an account of them in a classic contribution to the subject, 'The Myofascial Genesis of Pain', which is particularly notable for the clarity of its illustrations (Travell & Rinzler 1952). Thirty-one years later, Travell and her colleague David Simons (Fig. 5.2) had gained such considerable experience in the diagnosis and management of the myofascial pain syndromes that they were able to produce the first authoritative textbook on the subject (Travell & Simons 1983).

## FIBROMYALGIA SYNDROME

In 1965 Smythe, a rheumatologist, and Moldofsky, a psychiatrist in Toronto, Canada, began to take a fresh look at so-called fibrositis and investigated electroencephalographically sleep disturbances in patients suffering from this disorder (Moldofsky et al 1975, Moldofsky 1986, Smythe 1986). They found that the rapid 8–10 c/s alpha rhythm normally found in rapid eye movement (REM) sleep intrudes into the usual slow 1–2 c/s delta rhythm of non-REM stage IV deep sleep. It is for this reason that 60–90% of patients with fibromyalgia complain of a non-restorative sleep that causes them to wake feeling tired and with generalized muscle stiffness (Goldenberg 1987).

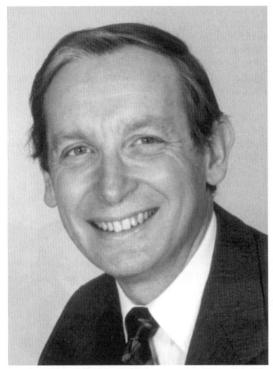

**Figure 5.3**    Harvey Moldofsky.

It was this renewed interest in fibrositis that eventually led to the recognition of a syndrome characterized by persistent generalized muscle pain, non-restorative sleep, early morning stiffness, marked fatigue, and multiple tender points scattered over the body at certain specific sites.

When Smythe & Moldofsky (1977) (Fig. 5.3) first drew attention to this syndrome they somewhat confusingly referred to it as the 'fibrositis' syndrome, but, for the same reason that made this term unacceptable earlier in this century, it was soon abandoned and in 1981 it was re-named the fibromyalgia syndrome (Yunus et al 1981). This term has since been officially included in the World Health Organization's 10th revision of its International Classification of Diseases, where it has been given the number M79.0 (Consensus document on fibromyalgia) (WHO 1993). Before discussing present knowledge concerning the pathophysiology of MPS and FS it will be first necessary in the next chapter to consider the various pain-arousing and pain-suppressing mechanisms present in the peripheral and central nervous systems.

# References

Albee F H 1927 Myofascitis. A pathological explanation of many apparently dissimilar conditions. American Journal of Surgery 3: 523–533

Baldry P E 1971 The battle against heart disease. University Press, Cambridge

Balfour 1815 Observations on the pathology and cure of rheumatism. Edinburgh Medical and Surgical Journal 11: 168–187

Balfour 1816 Observations with cases illustrative of new simple and expeditious mode of curing rheumatism and sprains. … Adam Black, Edinburgh

Balfour 1824a Illustrations of the efficacy of compression and percussion in the cure of rheumatism and sprains. The London Medical and Physical Journal 51: 446–462

Balfour 1824b Illustrations of the efficacy of compression and percussion in the cure of rheumatism and sprains. The London Medical and Physical Journal 52: 104–115, 200–208, 284–291

Christie B G 1958 Discussion on non-articular rheumatism. Proceedings of the Royal Society of Medicine 51: 251–255

Clayton E G, Livingstone J L 1930 Fibrositis. Lancet 1: 1420–1423

Cornelius A 1903 Narben und Nerven. Deutsche Militärärztlische Zeitschrift 32: 657–673

Cyriax J 1948 Fibrositis. British Medical Journal 2: 251–255

de Blecourt J J 1954 Screening of the population for rheumatic diseases. Annals of Rheumatic Diseases 13: 338–340

Edeiken J, Wolferth C C 1936 Persistent pain in the shoulder region following myocardial infarction. American Journal of Medical Science 191: 201–210

Ellman P, Shaw D 1950 The chronic 'rheumatic' and his pains. Psychosomatic aspects of chronic non-articular rheumatism. Annals of Rheumatic Diseases 9: 341–357

Goldenberg D L 1987 Fibromyalgia syndrome. An emerging but controversial condition. Journal of the American Medical Association 257 (20): 2782–2787

Good M G 1941 Rheumatic myalgias. Practitioner 146: 167–174

Good M G 1950 The role of skeletal muscle in the pathogenesis of diseases. Acta Medica Scandinavica 138: 285–292

Good M G 1951 Objective diagnosis and curability of nonarticular rheumatism. British Journal of Physical Medicine and Industrial Hygiene 14: 1–7

Gowers W R 1904 Lumbago: Its lessons and analogues. British Medical Journal 1: 117–121

Gutstein M 1938 Diagnosis and treatment of muscular rheumatism. British Journal of Physical Medicine 1: 302–321

Gutstein M 1940 Common rheumatism and physiotherapy. British Journal of Physical Medicine 3: 46–50

Gutstein R R 1955 A review of myodysneuria (fibrositis). American Practitioner 6: 570–577

Gutstein-Good M 1940 Idiopathic myalgia simulating visceral and other diseases. Lancet 2: 326–328

Haberling W 1932 Johan Georg Mezger of Amsterdam. The founder of scientific massage (translated by Emilie Recht). Medical Life 39: 190–207

Helleday U 1876 Nordiskt medicinskt arkiv 6 and 8 Nr 8. P A Norstedtosöner, Stockholm

Hunter C 1933 Myalgia of the abdominal wall. Canadian Medical Association Journal 28: 157–161

Inman T 1858 Remarks on myalgia or muscular pain. British Medical Journal 407–408, 866–868

Kelly M 1962 Local injections for rheumatism. Medical Journal of Australia 1: 45–50

Llewellyn L J, Jones A B 1915 Fibrositis. Rebman, New York

Moldofsky H 1986 Sleep and musculoskeletal pain. The American Journal of Medicine 81(suppl 3A): 85–89

Moldofsky H, Scarisbrick P, England R, Smythe H 1975 Musculoskeletal symptoms and non-rem sleep disturbance in patients with fibrositis syndrome and healthy subjects. Psychosomatic Medicine 371: 341–351

Müller A 1912 Untersuchungsbefund am rheumatisch erkranten muskel. Zeitschift Klinische Medizin 74: 34–73

Murray G R 1929 Myofibrositis as a simulator of other maladies. Lancet 1: 113–116

Neufeld I 1952 Pathogenetic concepts of 'fibrositis' – fibropathic syndromes. Archives of Physical Medicine 33: 363–369

Osler W 1909 The principles and practice of medicine, 7th edn. S. Appleton & Co, New York, p 396

Reichart A 1938 Reflexschmerzen auf grund von myogelosen. Deutsch Medizinische Wochenshrift 64: 823–824

Reynolds M D 1983 The development of the concept of fibrositis. The Journal of the History of Medical and Allied Sciences 38: 5–35

Ruhmann W 1940 The earliest book on rheumatism. The British Journal of Rheumatism II (3): 140–162 (This paper includes an original translation of de Baillou's *Liber de Rheumatismo* which, originally written in medieval Latin, was first published by a descendant M J Thevart in 1736, i.e. 120 years after the author's death.)

Scudamore C 1827 A treatise on the nature and cure of rheumatism. Longman, London, p. 11

Simons D G 1975 Muscle pain syndromes – Part I. American Journal of Physical Medicine 54: 289–311

Simons D G 1976 Muscle pain syndromes – Part II. American Journal of Physical Medicine 55: 15–42

Smythe H 1986 Tender points: evolution of concepts of the fibrositis/fibromyalgia syndrome. The American Journal of Medicine 81 (suppl 3A): 2–6

Smythe H A, Moldofsky H 1977 Two contributions to understanding of the 'fibrositis' syndrome. Bulletin of Rheumatic Diseases 28: 928–931

Steindler A 1940 The interpretation of sciatic radiation and the syndrome of low-back pain. Journal of Bone and Joint Surgery 22: 28–34

Stockman R 1904 The causes, pathology and treatment of chronic rheumatism. Edinburgh Medical Journal 15: 107–116, 223–225

Strauss H 1898 Über die sogenannte 'rheumatische muskelschwiele'. Klinische Wochenshrift 35: 89–91, 121–123

Sydenham Thomas 1676 Observationes medicae. The works of Thomas Sydenham translated by R G Latham in 1848. Sydenham Society, London

Telling W H 1911 Nodular fibromyositis, an everyday affliction, and its identity with so-called muscular rheumatism. Lancet 1: 154–158

Travell J, Rinzler S H 1952 The myofascial genesis of pain. Postgraduate Medicine 11: 425–434

Travell J, Simons D G 1983 Myofascial pain and dysfunction. The trigger point manual. Williams and Wilkins, Baltimore

Valleix F 1841 Traité des Neuralgies; ou, affections douloureuses des nerfs. Ballière, Paris.

Valleix F 1848 Études sur le rhumatisme musculaire, et en particulier sur son diagnostic et sur son traitement. Bulletin général de thérapeutique médicale et chirurgicale 35: 296–307

WHO 1993 Consensus Document on Fibromyalgia: the Copenhagen Declaration 1993. Journal of Musculoskeletal Pain 1(3/4): 295–312

Yunus M, Masi A T, Calabro J J, Miller K A, Feigenbaum S L 1981 Primary fibromyalgia (fibrositis) clinical study of 50 patients with matched controls. Seminars in Arthritis and Rheumatism 11: 151–171

# Chapter **6**

# Neurophysiology of pain

## INTRODUCTION

This brief and therefore somewhat superficial account of the neurophysiology of pain is simply to provide a certain amount of insight into its complexities. Its purpose is to serve as a basis for discussing in subsequent chapters the various physiological mechanisms that are involved in the development of pain in the myofascial pain and fibromyalgia syndromes and the alleviation of this by means of stimulating peripheral nerve endings with dry needles.

As space does not permit the neurophysiology of pain to be considered at length, anyone interested to learn more about this fascinating subject is recommended to read an extremely lucid account of it in Melzack & Wall's book *The Challenge of Pain* (1988) or an even more detailed presentation of its various aspects by a number of authorities in their *Textbook of Pain* (Wall & Melzack 1999).

Modern concepts concerning the transmission of noxious impulses from the periphery to the cortex and how the sensation of pain may be modulated by various physiochemical mechanisms in the central nervous system have been profoundly influenced by the gate-control theory first put forward by Melzack & Wall (1965). Although this theory, as might be expected, has had to be revised over the years in the light of further knowledge, it, nevertheless, remains a remarkably useful hypothesis and as Liebskind & Paul (1977), when discussing reasons for the current interest in pain research, have said:

> Probably the most important was the appearance in 1965 of the gate control theory of pain by

Melzack & Wall. This theory, like none before it, has proved enormously heuristic. It continues to inspire basic research and clinical applications.

It will, therefore, be necessary to consider this particular theory at some length but, in order fully to understand its ingenuity and implications, it is first necessary to say something about the nature of pain, and the parts of the central nervous system in which pain-modulating mechanisms are to be found.

## THE NATURE OF PAIN

Pain is not a simple, straightforward sensory experience, in the manner of, for example, seeing or hearing, since it has both emotional and physical components. The definition of pain put forward by the International Association for the Study of Pain is that it is 'an unpleasant sensory and emotional experience associated with actual or potential tissue damage, or described in terms of such damage' (Merskey 1979).

As Hannington-Kiff (1974) points out, pain has three main components: physical, emotional and rational. The physical component is determined by the responsiveness of an individual's nociceptive system to a given stimulus; the rational component is derived from an objective interpretation of pain in the cerebral cortex; the emotional component is determined by the responsiveness of an individual's limbic system to any particular noxious stimulus.

It, therefore, follows that for a given noxious stimulus the intensity with which pain is felt varies from person to person, and with regard to this a distinction has to be made between an individual's pain threshold and pain tolerance. The pain threshold is the least stimulus intensity at which a subject perceives pain and, contrary to popular belief, this is much the same in everyone (Thompson 1984a). As Wyke (1979) has pointed out, it is an all too common misconception:

> ... that measuring pain thresholds tells one something about the mechanisms that influence the intensity of a patient's experience of pain. On the contrary, of course, what one should assess in this regard is not a patient's pain threshold but his pain tolerance, because what brings patients to

doctors to seek relief is not the occurrence of some minor pain of which they are just aware when their pain threshold is reached (we have this every day of our lives) but is when the limit of their individual pain tolerance is reached.

This, of course, is of considerable practical importance when attempting to assess pain and the effect of any particular form of treatment on it, for it is not changes in pain threshold that have to be measured but rather changes in pain tolerance.

Pain tolerance clearly depends on a person's emotional response to a noxious stimulus. It is very interesting with respect to this to note that the 17th-century Dutch philosopher Benedict Spinoza (1632–1677) referred to pain as 'a localized form of sorrow'.

It therefore follows that throughout a person's life the intensity with which pain is felt depends on his or her psychological make-up, cultural background, parental influence and ethnic origin (Zborowski 1952, Bond 1979). The manner in which perception of, and reaction to, noxious stimuli is influenced by past experiences has been demonstrated in ingenious experiments carried out on various animals, including dogs (Melzack & Scott 1957, Melzack 1969) and monkeys (Lichstein & Sackett 1971).

The reaction to pain at any specific time is also dependent on an individual's current mood, with anxiety or depression intensifying it. The experience of pain also depends upon the prevailing circumstances so that, for example, a severe wound sustained in the heat of battle may hardly be noticed, whereas a similar injury incurred in a less stressful environment may be the cause of severe pain (Beecher 1959). Conversely, the intensity with which pain is felt is diminished by distraction of attention. It is for this reason that some people find background music helpful whilst undergoing some painful experience such as at the dentist (Gardner & Licklider 1959). This is also why chronic pain sufferers find that their pain is far less intrusive if the mind is occupied by carrying out an absorbing task (Wynn Parry 1980).

## TYPES OF PAIN

Pain is of three types. Very occasionaly it is solely due to a disorder of the mind (psychogenic pain).

Not infrequently it arises as a result of damage to either the peripheral or central nervous system (neuropathic pain). Most commonly it develops because of the primary activation and sensitisation of nociceptors in either the skin, a muscle or a viscus (nociceptive pain).

As will be discussed in Chapter 7, the pain present in the myofascial pain and fibromyalgia syndromes is nociceptive. For that reason pain of this particular type will be discussed at some length.

## NOCICEPTIVE PAIN

Our understanding of the psychological and physical components of nociceptive pain has been greatly advanced by recent detailed studies showing that the behavioural and physiological response to it is dependent on a number of facilitatory and inhibitory modulating mechanisms in various parts of the central nervous system. The structures that are of particular importance in this complex process are sensory receptors, their associated afferent nerve fibres, the dorsal horns, ascending and descending tracts in the neuraxis, the reticular formation in the midbrain and medulla, the thalamus, the limbic system and the cerebral cortex. Each of these will be considered in turn.

### Sensory receptors in the skin

**A-delta nociceptors** These nociceptors are connected to the spinal cord's dorsal horns via medium diameter (1–5 μm) myelinated A-delta nerve fibres with a conduction velocity of 12–30 m/s (25–70 mph).

These A-delta nociceptors are activated by any noxious mechanical stimulus such as that delivered by a sharp pointed instrument or needle and for this reason are also known as high-threshold mechanonociceptors. Approximately 20–50% of them, in addition, respond to suddenly applied heat in the noxious range of from 45° upwards and, because of this, are known as mechanothermal nociceptors.

A-delta myelinated nociceptors are found mainly in and just under the skin and, as will be discussed in Chapters 9 and 10, it is these receptors which are stimulated when carrying out the acupuncture procedure known as superficial dry needling.

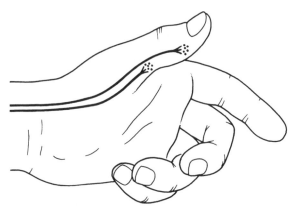

**Figure 6.1**  The multipunctate receptive field of an A-delta nociceptor. Reproduced with permission from Howard Field's *Pain*. McGraw-Hill 1987.

The receptive field of a high-threshold mechanonociceptor in the skin (Fig. 6.1) consists of a number of sensitive spots about 1 mm in diameter grouped together in a cluster covering on average a total area of 5 mm$^2$ (Georgopoulos 1974).

**C-polymodal nociceptors**  C-polymodal nociceptors, are connected to the spinal cord's dorsal horns via small diameter (0.25–1.5 μm) unmyelinated C afferent nerve fibres. The conduction velocity rate of these is only 0.5–2 m/s (1–4.5 mph). These receptors are termed polymodal because under experimental conditions it is possible to activate them by applying either a mechanical, thermal or chemical stimulus (Fig. 6.2). However, it is somewhat of a misnomer as, clinically, such activation is invariably only produced by chemicals released as a result of tissue damage.

The receptive field of C-polymodal nociceptors is usually a single area rather than a cluster of spots as in the case of A-delta nociceptors.

### Low-threshold mechanoreceptors in the skin

Low threshold mechanoreceptors in the skin are connected to the spinal cord's dorsal horns via large diameter A-beta myelinated nerve fibres with a diameter of 5–15 μm and the relatively fast conduction velocity of 30–70 m/s (70–155 mph).

They are stimulated physiologically when the skin is stretched or lightly touched and also when its hairs are bent.

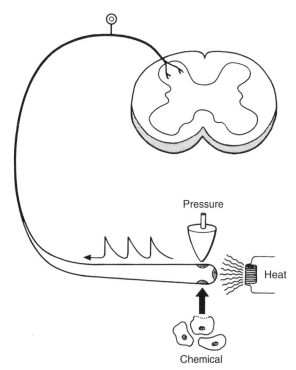

**Figure 6.2** Sensitivity range of the C-polymodal nociceptor. Its terminals are sensitive to direct heat or mechanical distortion, and to chemicals released from damaged cells. Reproduced with permission from Howard Field's *Pain*. McGraw-Hill 1987.

## Sensory receptors in muscle

Lloyd (1943) divided muscle sensory afferents into the following groups:

**Groups IA, IB and II** Group IA and Group IB, which have a diameter of 15–20 μm and transmission velocity of 70–120 m/s (155–270 mph), together with Group II, which have a diameter of 3–6 μm and a transmission velocity of 15–30 m/s (35–70 mph), have a proprioceptive function and are attached to annulospiral muscle spindles, Golgi tendon organs and flower spray muscle spindles respectively (Thompson 1994). Their role is to transmit to the brain information about changes in the length of muscle fibres and the rate at which this takes place.

**Group III and Group IV sensory afferents** Many of a muscle's Group III sensory afferents and all of its Group IV ones have free nerve endings that terminate in arterioles' adventitia and it is

presumably because of this that they are so markedly sensitive to chemical stimuli and particularly to those accompanying disturbances of the microcirculation (Mense 2001, p. 31).

Group III small diameter (2–5 μm) myelinated fibres with a conduction velocity of 12–30 m/s (25–70 mph) are divided (Mense 2001, p. 42) into those that have contraction sensitive receptors (23%), those that have nociceptive receptors (33%) and those that have low-threshold mechanosensitive receptors (44%).

Group IV unmyelinated fibres with an even smaller diameter (0.4–1.2 μm) and a conduction velocity of 0.5–2 m/s (1–4.5 mph) are divided (Mense 2001, p. 42) into those that have low-threshold mechanosensitive receptors (19%), those that have contraction sensitive receptors (19%) and the vast majority of them that have nociceptive receptors (43%).

## Muscle nociceptors

**Group III nociceptors** It has for long been known that pain may be produced by the low-intensity stimulus provided by squeezing a muscle between the fingers and thumb (Lewis 1942). And it was Paintal (1960) who, from experiments on cats, came to the conclusion that this pressure-evoked pain develops when those sensory afferents in this group with nociceptive terminals (33%) are stimulated.

**Group IV nociceptors** It has been shown in animal experiments that the 43% of sensory afferents in this group that have terminal nociceptors are not responsive to a low-intensity stimulus such as that provided by weakly applied pressure or stretching within the physiological range, but are responsive to high-intensity noxious ones such as those that cause myofascial trigger points (TrPs) to become active (see Ch. 7).

## First and second pain (Fig. 6.3)

Stimulation of A-delta nociceptors gives rise to an immediate, sharp, relatively brief pricking sensation – the so-called first or fast pain. This sensation serves to provide a warning of impending tissue damage and is accompanied by reflex withdrawal

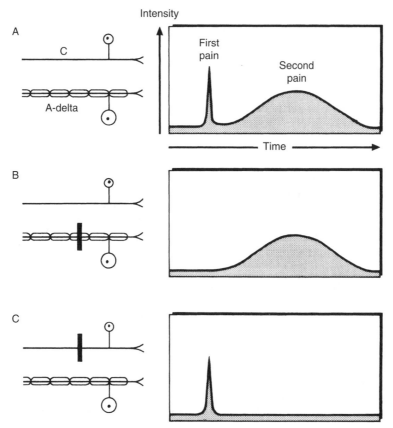

**Figure 6.3** A. First pain – produced by stimulation of A–delta afferent nerve fibres. Second pain – produced by stimulation of C afferent nerve fibres. B. First pain suppressed by the selective application of pressure to the A–delta fibres C. Second pain suppressed by selectively blocking, with low concentrations of local anaesthetic, the C afferent fibres. (Reproduced with permission from Howard Field's *Pain*. McGraw-Hill 1987.)

movements designed to avoid or minimize such damage.

Stimulation of C-polymodal nociceptors in the skin or Group IV nociceptors in muscle leads to the development of pain that, because its onset is delayed beyond the first few seconds, is known as 'second' or 'slow' pain. It is because pain of this type tends to persist for some time that it almost invariably requires treatment.

### Activation of C (skin) and Group IV (muscle) unmyelinated sensory afferent nociceptors

The effect of subjecting skin or muscle to a high-intensity noxious stimulus is to activate C or Group IV nociceptors respectively and to cause them to become pain-producing.

The mechanisms responsible for this activation are twofold, one being electrical and the other chemical.

Firstly, the noxious stimulus by deforming a nociceptive sensory afferent nerve ending opens ion channels present in its membrane with, as a consequence, the development of an ion flux across this membrane and a resultant depolarization of it. The difference in membrane potential between the stimulated depolarized nerve ending and the afferent fibre then causes a current to develop that depolarizes the latter and by so doing elicits a propagated action potential in it.

Secondly, the noxious stimulus brings about the release of the neuropeptides Substance P and calcitonin gene-related peptide stored in vesicles in nociceptive sensory afferents' nerve endings.

Both of these have a vasodilatory effect and cause an increase in vascular permeability with, as a consequence, the development of oedema and the liberation of algesic vasoneuroactive substances (Sicuteri 1967) from the blood. These include bradykinin from plasma proteins, serotinin (5-hydroxytryptamine) from platelets, potassium ions from plasma and other tissues, and histamine from mast cells.

### Sensitisation of C (skin) and Group IV (muscle) unmyelinated sensory afferent nociceptors

Bradykinin not only activates nociceptors but also increases the synthesis and release of prostaglandins, particularly prostaglandin E2, from damaged tissue cells (Jose et al 1981). This has a powerful sensitising effect on nociceptors with a lowering of their pain threshold so as to make them responsive not only to high-intensity noxious stimuli, but also to low-intensity ones. One of the consequences of this is the development of a zone of primary hyperalgesia at the injury site.

### The dorsal horn

**Laminae** It was the Swedish anatomist, Bror Rexed (1952), who established that the cells of the spinal cord are arranged in layers or laminae. There are six laminae in the dorsal (Lamina I–VI); three in the ventral horn (Lamina VII–IX) and an additional column of cells clustered around the central canal known as Lamina X (Fig. 6.4).

At the outer part of the dorsal horn there is a clear zone visible to the naked eye and it was because of this appearance that the Italian anatomist Luigi Rolando (1773–1831) in 1824 named it the substantia gelatinosa. Some neurophysiologists (Wall 1990) state that the substantia gelatinosa includes both Lamina I and II, whilst others (Bowsher 1990, Fields 1987, p. 44) call Lamina II the substantia gelatinosa and Lamina I the marginal zone.

The thin unmyelinated C nociceptive afferents terminate mainly in Laminae I and II where their axon terminals secrete either Substance P or vasoactive intestinal polypeptide (VIP) according to whether they arise from somatic structures or visceral ones respectively (Thompson 1988).

The medium-sized myelinated A-delta nociceptive afferents terminate chiefly in Laminae I, II and V.

In contrast to this, most of the large diameter myelinated A-beta low-threshold mechanoreceptive afferent fibres, on entering the spinal cord, pass directly up the dorsal column to end in the medulla oblongata's gracile and cuneate nuclei. Axons from these nuclei then form the medial lemniscus and this, after decussating in the medulla, terminates principally in the ventrobasal thalamus. However, what is of particular importance, as far as the pain modulating effect of A-beta afferent activity is concerned, is that the medial lemniscus is connected, via the anterior pretectal nucleus, to the periaqueductal grey area in the midbrain at the upper end of the opioid peptide mediated serotinergic descending inhibitory system (see p. 61).

Therefore, as a result of these connections, A-beta afferent activity is enabled to block the C afferent input to the spinal cord by promoting activity in this descending system (Bowsher 1991). In addition, Todd & Mackenzie (1989) have shown that large diameter A-beta nerve fibres, on entering the spinal cord, give off branches which make contact with gamma-aminobutyric acid mediated interneurons (GABA-ergic interneurons) in Lamina II. These also exert an inhibitory effect on the C afferent input to the cord.

It therefore follows that high-frequency, low-intensity transcutaneous nerve stimulation (TENS), which exerts its pain modulating effect by recruiting A-beta nerve fibres (Ch. 9), achieves this effect partly by these fibres, when stimulated, evoking activity in the opioid peptide-mediated descending inhibitory system, and partly by them evoking activity in dorsal horn GABA-ergic interneurons (Fig. 6.5).

**Dorsal horn transmission cells** The neurons in the dorsal horn responsible for transmitting sensory afferent information to the brain are of three main types – low-threshold mechanoreceptor cells, nociceptive-specific cells, and wide dynamic range cells.

Low-threshold mechanoreceptor cells, found chiefly in Laminae III and IV, transmit to the brain information received via large diameter low-threshold A-beta afferents that have become

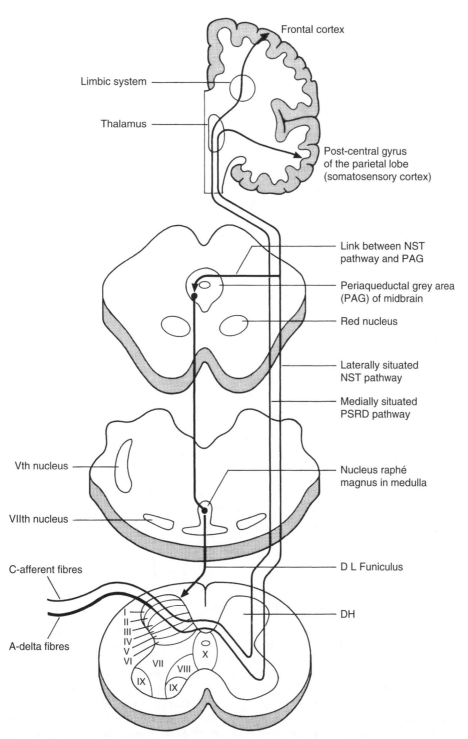

**Figure 6.4**   Diagramatic representation of the course taken by the two ascending 'pain' pathways – the neospinothalamic (NST) pathway carrying A-delta 'pin prick' information, and the paleo-spino-reticulo-diencephalic pathway carrying C 'tissue damage' information. It also shows the descending inhibitory pathway – the dorsolateral funiculus (DLF) which links the periaqueductal grey area (PAG) and the nucleus raphé magnus (NRM) with the dorsal horn (DH).

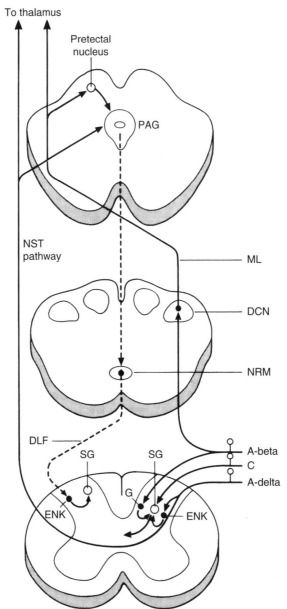

**Figure 6.5** Tissue damage nociceptive information reaches the substantia gelatinosa (SG) vis C afferent fibres. The onward transmission of this information is inhibited by enkephalinergic interneurons (ENK) which are activated via A-delta 'pin prick' fibres as they enter the cord and via serotinergic inhibitory fibres that descend in the dorsolateral funiculus (DLF) from the nucleus raphé magnus (NRM) in the medulla and periaqueductal grey area (PAG) in the midbrain (the descending inhibitory system). The descending inhibitory system is brought into action either via collaterals which link the neospinothalamic 'A-delta pin prick' ascending pathway (NST) with the PAG: or via collaterals which form a link between the PAG and the medial leminiscus (ML), which arises from dorsal column nuclei (DCN) connected to A-beta fibres in the dorsal column. The onward transmission of tissue damage nociceptive information in C afferent fibres is also inhibited by inhibitory GABA-ergic interneurons (G) which are activated by the A-beta fibres that enter the substantia gelatinosa.

(Based on Dr David Bowsher's diagram in the Journal of the British Medical Acupuncture Society (1991). Reproduced with permission).

activated by some innocuous stimulus such as light touch to the skin.

Nociceptive-specific cells, principally present in Lamina I but also to a lesser extent in Lamina IV and V (Christensen & Perl 1970), as their name implies, are only excited by nociceptive primary afferents. Somewhat paradoxically, a study by Mayer et al (1975) suggests that interpretation of pain is related more closely to activity in wide dynamic range cells than it is to that in nociceptive-specific ones.

Wide dynamic range cells, which are present in all laminae but are mainly concentrated in Lamina V and to a lesser extent in Lamina I, transmit to higher centres information received via A-beta, A-delta and C afferents. The message they pass on to the higher centres therefore varies according to whether the peripherally applied stimulus is innocuous or noxious. It thus follows that the sensation ultimately experienced may be one of touch, or the brief localized pricking type of 'first' pain, or the persistent wide-spread aching type of 'second' pain.

The wide-dynamic range cells that receive small diameter afferents from the heart and abdominal organs also receive low-threshold afferents from the skin (Cervero 1983). Melzack & Wall (1988, p. 173) suggest that this may be the reason why pain from a pathological lesion in some internal structure may appear to be coming from the surface of the body and why in such circumstances the skin is liable to be tender.

It needs to be understood that none of these transmission cells possess physiological specificity, as they are capable of changing from one to another depending on the excitability of the spinal cord. For example, animal experiments have shown that, under light barbiturate anaesthesia, nociceptive-specific cells become wide dynamic range ones (Collins & Ren 1987) and that under deeper anaesthesia the latter become nociceptive specific (Dickhaus et al 1985).

**Dorsal horn inhibitory interneurons**  In Laminae I and II there are interneurones that contain inhibitory neurotransmitters such as enkephalin and gamma-aminobutyric acid (Todd et al 1992).

**Dorsal horn neuroplasticity**  From animal experiments it is clear that the effect of prolonged or repetitious high-intensity stimulation of nociceptors is to bring about a progressive build-up of excitability in dorsal horn-situated nociceptive transmission neurons (wind-up) and the eventual sensitisation of them (central sensitisation).

Central sensitisation develops when these neurons' N-methyl-D-aspartate (NMDA) receptors become activated. This is brought about as a result of the co-release of excitatory amino acids (glutamate and aspartate) and neuropeptides (SP and calcitonin gene-related peptide). The NMDA receptor channel is normally blocked by a magnesium 'plug'. The effect of activating these transmission neurons is to remove this 'plug' and by so doing allow an influx of calcium ions into them. This in itself gives rise to considerable cell hyperexcitability. It also leads to the expression of oncogenes such as c-fos which brings about long-term changes in the responsiveness of these neurons; to the production of nitrous oxide which is now believed to contribute to the maintenance of pain; and to the activation of a number of secondary messengers including inositol triphosphate and diacylglycerol that further increase the excitability of the cells (Coderre et al 1993).

The effects of this central sensitisation are to increase the receptive fields of these dorsal horn nociceptive neurons; to bring about the development of large diameter A-beta sensory afferent-mediated hyperalgesia and allodynia; and to cause the nociceptive pain to persist (Cousins & Power 1999; Doubell et al 1999).

As will be discussed in Chapter 7 there are grounds for believing that central sensitisation not infrequently takes place in the myofascial pain syndrome and invariably does so in the fibromyalgia syndrome.

## Ascending pathways

The long-held belief that nociceptive information is transmitted centripetally via a single contralateral spinothalamic tract had to be revised in the 1950s when it was shown that the transmission is through a number of pathways each of which has its own conduction velocity and termination in the brain (Kerr et al 1955).

It is now recognized that these pathways have developed over the course of time as part of an evolutionary process (Melzack & Wall 1988, p. 125) and that their relative importance varies from one species to another (Willis 1989).

Two major ascending systems have been identified, one phylogenetically much older than the other. The principal pathway in the newer of the two systems is the neospinothalamic pathway and the main one in the earlier developed system is the paleo-spino-reticulo-diencephalic pathway (Bowsher 1987).

## The neospinothalamic pathway (Fig. 6.4)

The neospinothalamic pathway arises from the dorsal horn's Laminae I and V, where the majority of the small myelinated A-delta nociceptive fibres terminate. It ascends in the contralateral anterolateral tract to reach the ventrobasal nucleus in the lateral part of the thalamus, and from there it projects to the somatosensory cortex in the postcentral gyrus. This topographically organized lateral pathway subserves the sensory-discriminative process responsible for the localization and identification of a noxious stimulus (Melzack & Casey 1968) and for determining when such a stimulus reaches the pain threshold.

## The paleo-spino-reticulo-diencephalic pathway (Fig. 6.4)

This pathway, which Melzack & Casey (1968) call the paramedian pathway, arises from the dorsal horn's Laminae VII and VIII and to a lesser extent from Lamina V. As this pathway carries information ultimately interpreted as 'second' or 'slow' pain that is conveyed to the dorsal horn by C afferent fibres, and as these terminate in neurons in Laminae I and II, it follows that electrical impulses from these neurons have to pass through several internuncial relays before reaching Laminae V, VII and VIII. From the dorsal horn, it ascends in the contralateral anterolateral tract alongside the neospinothalamic pathway until it reaches the base of the brain where it separates from this by passing medially into the brainstem's reticular tissue. From there, C afferent nociceptive information is projected to the cerebral cortex via

the medially situated intralaminar nuclei of the thalamus.

## Brainstem's reticular formation

The reticular formation that ramifies throughout the medulla and midbrain is so-called because its dense mass of neurons with overlapping and intertwining dendrites give it a net-like appearance.

As Casey (1980) has pointed out, it is because neurons in the reticular formation have bifurcating axons that project downwards to the spinal cord and upwards to the thalamus and hypothalamus that this structure is so extremely well adapted to playing a major integrating role in pain experience and behaviour.

Its links with the motor neurons of muscle spindles enable it to bring about alterations in muscle tone. With respect to this, it is because people who are psychologically tense have an overactive reticular system that they tend to hold certain groups of their muscles persistently taut (Nathan 1982). When this happens, pain is liable to develop in these muscles as a result of TrPs in them becoming activated (see Ch. 7). As Mense (1990) has succinctly put it, 'skeletal muscle is a tool for expressing emotional state in higher mammals and, thus, psychogenic changes of muscle tone may become a source of pain'.

The reticular formation contains several nuclei that make important contributions to the experience of pain and the behavioural activities associated with this. One of these is the nucleus reticularis gigantocellularis situated in the medulla. This nucleus, which receives a large input from the paramedian pathway and that has an upwards projection to the intralaminar part of the thalamus, contains neurons whose discharge in response to a noxious stimulus, as Casey has shown in a series of experiments on cats, sets off aversive escape behaviour (Casey 1971a, b; Casey et al 1974). In addition, serotonin-containing cells in this nucleus and the adjacent nucleus raphe magnus, together with neurons in the periaqueductal grey area of the midbrain from which they receive an excitatory input, form the upper part of the opioid peptide mediated descending inhibitory system that is of such considerable importance in the control of pain.

Most of the fibres in the paramedian pathway terminate at the reticular formation but some continue upwards to the medially situated intralaminar nuclei of the thalamus. There are also separate ascending projections from the reticular formation that reach both these thalamic nuclei and the hypothalamus. It is because of this link between the reticular formation and the hypothalamus that so-called second or slow C afferent tissue damage type pain has autonomic concomitants.

From the intralaminar nuclei of the thalamus there are projections to a number of structures clustered around the thalamus that collectively form the limbic system, as well as projections to other parts of the brain including, in particular, the frontal lobe.

## The limbic system

The limbic system consists of a group of structures clustered around the thalamus. These include the hypothalamus; the hippocampus (Greek, *sea horse*); the amygdala (Latin, *almond*); and the cingulum bundle connecting the hippocampus with the frontal cortex.

There is evidence that the limbic structures control the motivational or behavioural responses to pain together with the emotional response to it or what may be called its affective dimension. With respect to the latter, it is the extent to which the limbic system becomes activated in response to any given noxious stimulus that determines how much any particular individual suffers from it – in other words, the degree to which it hurts that person. It is therefore activity in the limbic system that governs a person's pain tolerance.

## The frontal cortex

As mentioned when discussing the nature of pain, this physico-emotional experience is considerably influenced by cognitive activities such as memories of past experiences, mood and prevailing circumstances. By virtue of the frontal cortex having a two-way communication system not only with all sensory cortical areas but also with the limbic and reticular structures, it controls both of these cognitive activities as well as the paramedian system's motivational-affective ones (Melzack & Casey 1968).

Knowledge as to exactly where in the brain noxious information transmitted to it is processed, with the development of pain as a consequence, has been considerably advanced by recent studies employing positron emission tomography to measure the regional blood flow to various parts of the brain and functional magnetic resonance to measure changes in blood oxygenation (Bushnell et al 2002, Ingvar & Hsieh 1999).

From these studies, which have been carried out both in humans and animals, it is apparent that when noxious information is transmitted to the brain a number of cortical and subcortical regions are activated. These include the primary and secondary somatosensory cortices (S1 & S2), the anterior cingualate cortex (ACC) and the insular cortex (IC ).

That so many regions are activated is a measure of the complexity of the processes involved in pain perception, and a reflection of the fact that pain has three separate components: a sensory, discriminative one that provides information concerning the type of sensation experienced (e.g. aching, burning or stabbing) and the part of the body from which it is arising; an affective (emotional), motivational (behavioural ) one; and an autonomic one that is responsible for such responses to pain as tachycardia, elevation of the blood pressure and sweating.

From studies carried out both on animals and humans it is now evident that the S1 & S2 cortices are the principal regions involved in the process. It is also evident that ACC activity determines behavioural, emotional and autonomic responses, and that IC has a role in associating the immediate affective response to a pain experience with memories of the suffering caused by a previous similar one.

In the past, extensive resections of the frontal lobes were performed as a last resort for intractable pain. Patients who underwent this, because the sensory component of pain subserved by the somatosensory cortex was still present, remained aware of the pain and often said it was as intense as before, but they were no longer worried about it and no longer needed medication for it. The effect of a lobotomy, therefore, was to reduce the motivational-affective and aversive dimensions of the pain experience. As Freeman & Watts (1950) remarked, 'Prefrontal lobotomy changes the attitude of the individual towards his pain, but does not alter the perception of pain.'

## ADVANCES IN KNOWLEDGE DURING THE 1950s AND 1960s

There were several important advances concerning the neurophysiology of pain during the 1950s and 1960s. The Swedish anatomist, Bror Rexed (1952), established that the cells of the spinal cord are arranged in layers or laminae; Hagbarth & Kerr (1954) found evidence of a descending inhibitory system; and Kerr et al (1955) established that there are a number of ascending pathways related to pain. In addition, Noordenbos (1959) furthered the theory first put forward by Head in 1920 that a rapidly conducting afferent fibre system inhibits transmission in a more slowly conducting one by establishing that the fast system is made up of large diameter myelinated fibres and the slow one by small diameter unmyelinated ones. In referring to the interaction between these two systems, he pithily commented; 'stated in the most simple terms, this interaction could be described as fast blocks slow'.

This comment, as Wall (1990) has recently admitted, profoundly influenced Melzack's and his thinking when eventually they came to formulate their gate-control theory. Also influential was the fact that Wall (1960), by a series of ingenious recordings from single dorsal horn cells, was able to confirm Noordenbos's observations concerning this interaction, and was able to show that it is strongly influenced by descending inhibitory systems first identified by Melzack et al 1958.

## THE GATE-CONTROL THEORY

It was thus in the light of knowledge acquired by a number of different workers during the 1950s that Melzack & Wall in 1965 developed their now famous theory that in each dorsal horn of the spinal cord there is a 'gate-like mechanism which inhibits or facilitates the flow of afferent impulses into the spinal cord'. The theory, as originally propounded, stated that the opening or closing of the 'gate' is dependent on the relative activity in the large diameter (A-beta) and small diameter fibres (A-delta and C), with activity in the large diameter fibres tending to close the 'gate', and activity in the small diameter fibres tending to open it. Also, an essential part of the theory ever since the time it was first put forward is that the position of the 'gate' is in addition influenced by the brain's descending inhibitory system.

## Substantia gelatinosa

From the start, Melzack & Wall envisaged the gate as being situated in the substantia gelatinosa where, as they said, inhibitory interneurons are to be found in Lamina II. They also premised that the interaction between the large and small diameter fibres influences activity both in these interneurons and in the dorsal horn transmission cells (T cells). It was thought and subsequently confirmed that the large-diameter myelinated afferents excite the inhibitory interneurons, and that the effect of this is to presynaptically reduce the input to the T cells and thereby to inhibit pain. They further postulated that activity in small diameter unmyelinated fibres, by inhibiting activity in the inhibitory interneurons, facilitates the flow of noxious impulses to the T cells and by so doing enhances pain.

By the time that Melzack & Wall introduced their theory, there was already good evidence to support their belief that it is the substantia gelatinosa (i.e. Laminae I & II) that acts as the 'gate'. Szentagothai (1964) and Wall (1964) had shown that it receives axons directly and indirectly from large and small diameter fibres, that it has connections with cells in deeper laminae and, that its cells connect with one another and are connected to similar cells at distant sites – on the ipsilateral side by means of Lissauer's tract and on the opposite side by means of fibres that cross the cord.

Although it remains reasonable to assume that it is the substantia gelatinosa that acts as the spinal gating mechanism, Melzack & Wall (1982, p. 236) have found it necessary to emphasize that there is still no absolute proof of this. They also posed the question rhetorically, 'If the substantia gelatinosa is a gate control, why is it so complex?', and answered this by saying that it would be wrong to consider that this structure is only concerned with the modulation of nociceptive impulses, but rather that it has to monitor all forms of incoming information and that it is likely to have 'to control and emphasize different aspects of the arriving messages with the emphasis changing from moment to moment'.

There can be no doubt, therefore, that the substantia gelatinosa has the properties of a complex computer and, the greater the detail in which its structure and function are studied, the more intricate the mechanisms contained in it are found to be. There is now experimental evidence to show that the cells that make up this structure, together with those in the underlying laminae, are somatotopically organized (Melzack & Wall 1982, p. 237) in the same way as cells in the dorsal column-medial lemniscus system (Millar & Basbaum 1975) and cells in midbrain structures (Soper & Melzack 1982).

It is also now known that the afferent nociceptive input into the substantia gelatinosa is influenced by several descending inhibitory systems linking cortical and brain-stem structures with the dorsal horn via the dorsolateral funiculus.

It is obvious from the number of peptides found in the substantia gelatinosa in recent years, that its function must be extremely complicated. It is now known that nerve terminals at this site contain at least five peptides, these being vasoactive intestinal peptide, somatostatin, angiotensin, cholecystokinin and SP (Jessell 1982). Endogenous opioids are to be found in the dorsal horn of the spinal cord in the same areas as small diameter primary pain afferents containing SP neurons and opiate receptors (Clement-Jones 1983). Now that it is known that morphine inhibits the release of SP – a primary afferent nociceptor transmitter – it has been proposed that, in addition to the opioid-mediated descending inhibitory system, opioid-containing interneurons presynaptically control the afferent nociceptive input (Jessell & Iversen 1977). Such a hypothesis would certainly provide a neurochemical basis for the 'gate' theory of pain control.

There are thus strong arguments in support of Melzack & Wall's original idea that the substantia gelatinosa acts as a complex 'gating' mechanism that modulates input signals to the spinal cord by means of decreasing their effect on other highly specialized transmission cells (T cells), the function of which is to pass on these messages to various centres in the brain. For a more detailed account of the evidence in support of the substantia gelatinosa's role as a controlling 'gate', reference should be made to Wall's (1980a, b; 1989) comprehensive reviews of the subject.

## Revision of the gate–control theory

Advances in knowledge since 1965 have inevitably led to the theory being revised. For example, Melzack & Wall soon came to the conclusion that there are excitatory as well as inhibitory interneurons in the substantia gelatinosa and that inhibition not only occurs presynaptically, as originally thought, but also takes place postsynaptically.

Furthermore, when the gate-control theory was first put forward, it was considered that the flow of centripetal impulses into the dorsal horn, and from it up to the brain, was influenced partly by descending inhibitory mechanisms and partly by the relative activity in small diameter and large diameter afferent nerve fibres, and that it was always the net result of these various facilitatory and inhibitory effects that controlled the activation of T cells. When Wall, however, re-examined the theory in 1978, he pointed out that the situation was not as straightforward as might have appeared at first, and that large diameter fibre activity is, in certain circumstances, capable of firing T cells, so that the inputs from large and small fibres may at times summate with each other. He also admitted that their original ideas concerning the inhibitory effects of large diameter fibres was much influenced by Noordenbos (1959) who, having shown that in post-herpetic neuralgia there is a loss of large myelinated fibres, generalized from this observation by proposing that pain in general is due to a loss of inhibition normally provided by large fibres. As Wall (1978) then goes on to say, 'We now know that loss of large fibres is not necessarily followed by pain. In Friedreich's ataxia there is just such a preferential large-fibre defect without pain' … (and) 'the polyneuropathy of renal failure in adults is not associated with complaints of pain although there is preferential destruction of large fibres.' He then cites many other examples to show that 'any attempt to correlate the remaining fibre diameter spectrum with the symptomatology of neuropathies is no longer possible'.

This notwithstanding, it would seem that when the central nervous system is intact and unaffected by disease, the balance between the large and small diameter fibres in determining the output of T cells remains an acceptable hypothesis. The theory has also been subjected to criticism by others for neglecting the known facts about stimulus specificity of nerve fibres that have emerged since Von Frey first developed his theory about this in the closing years of the last century (Nathan 1976).

For all these various reasons and others, including advances in knowledge concerning the relative functions of A-delta and C nerve fibres (to be discussed later), Melzack & Wall have had to subject their theory to certain modifications (Wall 1978, Melzack & Wall 1982, p. 260; 1988, pp. 165–193). Nevertheless, it remains remarkably useful and has been considerably enriched by subsequent biochemical discoveries. Much, however, remains to be explained. For example, the descending control system has turned out to be not one system but a number of systems involving a complexity of chemical substances yet to be unravelled. And when enkephalin-containing terminals and opiate receptor-bearing axons were discovered, it was assumed that they must make contact but, surprisingly, this apparently is not so (Hunt et al 1980).

Despite all this, 20 years after Melzack & Wall first put forward their gate-control theory, Verrill (1990) reviewed its influence on current ideas concerning pain modulation and was led to conclude that:

> … despite continuing controversy over details, the fundamental concept underlying the gate theory has survived in a modified and stronger state accommodating and harmonizing with rather than supplanting specificity and pattern theories. It has stimulated multidisciplinary activity, opened minds and benefited patients.

### The relevance of the gate–control system to the 1st and 2nd phases of nociceptive pain

As stated earlier, when some deep-seated structure such as muscle is damaged, the resultant inflammatory reaction leads to the release of chemical substances which sensitize A-delta and C afferents. The outcome of this is that two types of pain develop one after the other. Initially there is a sharp, well-defined sensation – the first pain – brought on as a result of activity in the A-delta afferent nerve fibres. The pain during this first phase is only of brief duration and is followed by a less well-defined and more prolonged second pain, which develops as a result of activity in C afferent nerve fibres. Melzack & Wall (1988, pp. 165–193) have now pointed out that the gate-control pain modulating mechanisms only operate during the 1st phase and that the prolongation of the pain during the 2nd phase is due to C afferent fibres, where they terminate intraspinally, liberating a variety of peptides including substance P, cholecystokinin, neurokinins, vasoactive intestinal peptide and others, giving rise to immediate neuronal excitation in the dorsal horn followed by a slow-onset, prolonged facilitation.

It should be noted with respect to this that the peptide content of unmyelinated sensory afferents is not the same in every type of tissue. The peptide make-up of Group IV fibres in muscle, for example, is very different from that of C fibres in the skin. That is why Group IV afferents, unlike C afferents, produce prolonged facilitation.

## ADVANCES IN KNOWLEDGE DURING THE 1970s AND 1980s

### Opiate receptors

During the 1970s, biochemists and pharmacologists were becoming increasingly convinced that the reason why morphine was such a powerful analgesic was because there were highly specialized chemical receptors in the central nervous system to which this substance could readily attach itself. In 1973, Solomon Snyder of the Johns Hopkins School of Medicine, Baltimore, and Candice Pert of the U.S. National Institute of Mental Health discovered, during the course of basic research on drug addiction, that there are clusters of cells in certain parts of the brain, including the brain stem nuclei, the thalamus and hypothalamus, which serve as opiate receptors (Pert & Snyder 1973). A number of cells in the dorsal horn were then also found to have the same function (Atweh & Kuhar 1977). The finding of opiate receptors in the midbrain perhaps was not so surprising as it had already been shown that an injection of only a small amount of morphine into the area has a considerable analgesic effect. However, of particular interest was the discovery that there are also cells with the same function in the substantia gelatinosa of the dorsal horn and that a local injection of a small amount of morphine into this structure (laminae I and II) has a markedly inhibitory effect on the response of lamina V transmission cells to afferent nociceptive stimuli (Duggan et al 1976); this lent considerable support to the idea that the substantia gelatinosa has an important pain-modulating function. It is now known that there are at least three distinct types of opioid receptors termed mu, kappa and delta (Paterson et al 1983).

The distribution of opiate receptors in the central nervous system is of considerable interest. There are numerous ones in the paramedian system's intralaminar (medial) thalamic nuclei, reticular formation and limbic structures. In contrast, however, there are only a few in the neospinothalamic system's ventrobasal thalamus and postcentral gyrus. This explains why a microinjection of morphine into structures in the paramedian system has a powerful analgesic effect but not when injected into the ventrobasal thalamus. It also explains why morphine suppresses so-called second or 'slow' tissue damage type of pain but not the so-called first or 'rapid' type of pain produced, for example, by a pinprick.

In the dorsal horn there are large numbers of opiate receptors situated postsynaptically on neuronal membranes. There are also some situated presynaptically on the intraspinal part of C afferent nerve fibres, but at present the biological significance of these remains unknown (Fields & Basbaum 1989).

It is because of a particularly high concentration of opiate receptors in the substantia gelatinosa, that a micro-injection of morphine into this structure has a marked pain-suppressing effect. It is also why lumbar intrathecal injections of opiates produce profound analgesia in animals (Yaksh & Rudy 1976) and man (Wang et al 1979).

There is a high concentration of opiate receptors in the corpus striatum, where their function is unknown. They are also extremely numerous in

the brain stem's respiratory centre, thus explaining why morphine is such a powerful respiratory depressant.

During the 1990s it was also established that opiate receptors are present on the peripheral terminals of sensory afferents (Stein et al 1990, Coggeshall et al 1997).

## Opioid peptides

Once these opiate receptors had been located, it was argued that nature was hardly likely to have provided animals, including man, with them for the sole purpose of having somewhere for opium and its derivatives to latch on to should they happen to be introduced into the body. It was far more likely that they are there because morphine-like substances (opioid substances) are produced endogenously.

A search for physiologically occurring morphine-like substances was therefore instituted. Many scientists took part in this, including Snyder and his colleagues at Baltimore; Terenius & Wahlstrom in Uppsala; and Hughes et al in Aberdeen.

The big breakthrough occurred in 1975 when Hughes et al in the Unit for Research on Addictive Drugs at Aberdeen University in collaboration with a research team at Reckitt & Colman isolated a substance from the brains of pigs that appeared to act like morphine and that latched onto opiate receptors in the brain. They named it enkephalin ('in the head'). It was a major discovery, and Lewin (1976) showed considerable prescience by commenting in the *New Scientist*:

> With the structure of enkephalin now at hand ... we are now poised for an exciting breakthrough in the complete understanding of opiate analgesia, addiction and tolerance. Probably the most intriguing aspect of all this is the inescapable implication of the existence of an unexpected chemical transmitter system in the brain, a system which may have something to do with dampening pain, but almost certainly has more general effects also.

Enkephalin having been isolated, Linda Fothergil at Aberdeen and Barry Morgan at Reckitt & Colman attempted to analyze its structure and soon established that it was a peptide, but came up against certain technical difficulties in establishing the exact sequence of its amino acids. Therefore they enlisted the help of a spectroscopist, Howard Morris at the Imperial College, London. Morris was able to show that in fact there are two enkephalin polypeptides – leucine (leu) and methionine (met) enkephalin – but for a time the chemical source from which these substances are made in the body remained a mystery.

By a strange chance, about the time that Morris was considering this, he attended a lecture at Imperial College given by Derek Smythe of the National Institute for Medical Research on beta-lipotrophin, a 91 amino acid peptide that had been isolated from the pituitary glands of sheep 10 years previously (Li et al 1965). Smythe showed a series of slides illustrating its chemical structure and as Morris sat there looking at these, he suddenly saw to his amazement the amino acid sequence of met enkephalin hidden away in the 61–65 position of the betalipotrophin structure. It subsequently became apparent, however, that met and leu enkephalin are derived by enzyme cleavage not from this substance but from the precursor proenkephalin A. Since the discovery of the enkephalins, opioid bioactivity has been found in various beta-lipotrophin fragments with the most potent of these being one in the 61–91 position known as beta-endorphin (Fig. 6.6).

It is now known that beta-endorphin, together with beta-lipotrophin and ACTH (corticotrophin) are all derived by enzyme cleavage from a large precursor pro-opiomelancortin, but that of these three polypeptides only beta-endorphin has known analgesic activity, and also that ACTH acts as a physiological antagonist of this (Smock & Fields 1980).

Recently, two other opioid peptides with N-terminals identical to that of leuenkephalin have been isolated. These are dynorphin, a 17 amino

acid peptide (Goldstein et al 1979), and the decapeptide alpha-neoendorphin (Weber et al 1981), both of which are cleaved from yet another precursor proenkephalin B (prodynorphin).

These various substances are sometimes referred to collectively as the endorphins (endogenous morphine-like substances) but, as may be seen, there are three distinct families of these peptides – the enkephalins, the dynorphins and the endorphins – and therefore it is better simply to call them opioid peptides (Thompson 1984b).

## Distribution of endogenous opioid peptides

Studies using radioimmunoassays and immunohistochemical techniques have demonstrated high levels of enkaphalins and dynorphins in the limbic structures, the periaqueductal grey, the nucleus raphe magnus and the substantia gelatinosa of the dorsal horn. From these sites, opioid peptides spill over into the cerebrospinal fluid. In addition, opioid peptides are released from the anterior pituitary and adrenal medulla into the plasma.

By means of radioimmunoassays and gel filtration techniques, it has been possible to demonstrate the presence of beta-endorphin and metenkephalin in human plasma (Clement-Jones 1983). Beta-endorphin is found there in association with beta-lipotrophin and ACTH with all three showing the same pattern of circadian secretion from the anterior pituitary (Shanks et al 1981). Plasma metenkephalin levels, however, show no relationship to those of the other peptides just mentioned during circadian studies and corticosteroid suppression tests. It is not derived from the pituitary, as levels are detectable in subjects with pan-hypopituitarism (Clement-Jones & Besser 1983) but released from the adrenal gland into the circulation (Clement-Jones et al 1980). It is also derived from the gut, sympathetic ganglia and peripheral autonomic neurons (Smith et al 1981).

**Figure 6.6** Schematic representation of the 91 amino acid peptide beta-lipotrophin and other peptides structurally related to it.

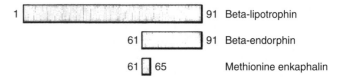

Endogenous opioid peptides have also been found to be present in macrophages, monocytes and lymphocytes present in inflamed tissues (Przewlocki et al 1992, Stein et al 1990). Schafer et al (1996) have shown that the liberation of these opioids is induced by corticotrophin-releasing hormone.

When opioid peptides were first discovered, it was assumed that any structure containing them must have a pain-modulating function. It is clear, however, that this is not so because there is, for example, a very high concentration of them in the basal ganglia where their function has yet to be explained (Bowsher 1987). They are also present in vagal nuclei in the medulla where they presumably contribute to various reflexes such as those associated with the control of coughing.

## Descending pain inhibitory systems

During the 1970s, exciting discoveries were made concerning the biochemistry of the descending inhibitory system, although it was observations made in the 1950s, firstly by Hagbarth & Kerr (1954) and then by Melzack et al (1958) – with their unexpected discovery in experiments on cats that damage to the central tegmental tract in the midbrain markedly enhances pain in these animals – that set the stage for these discoveries.

It was because of their observations that David Reynolds, a young psychologist at the University of Windsor, Ontario, decided to investigate whether, by electrically stimulating this central tegmental-lateral periaqueductal grey area, it might be possible to increase the effects of any inhibitory system that might be present there to such an extent as to bring about pain suppression. In 1969 he was able to report that such stimulation did, in fact, produce such a profound degree of analgesia that it was possible to carry out surgical operations on conscious rats without any other form of anaesthesia, and later he reported being able to control pain by this method during operations on higher species of animals.

Unfortunately, although Reynolds' observations were of the utmost importance, regrettably they were viewed with considerable scepticism and largely ignored. It was not until Mayer, Liebeskind and their colleagues (Mayer et al 1971), with no knowledge of Reynolds' contributions to the subject, independently carried out similar experiments on rats, that any notice was taken of the remarkable phenomenon, now generally referred to as stimulation-produced analgesia.

### Stimulation-produced analgesia

It has been found possible to produce analgesia by electrically stimulating one or other of several sites, but the most consistently effective manner of doing this is to place electrodes either on the periaqueductal grey area in the midbrain or on the nucleus raphé magnus in the medulla (Liebskind & Paul 1977).

Although stimulation-produced analgesia was first demonstrated in experimental animals, it was quickly shown to have considerable therapeutic value in relieving humans of persistent severe pain. In fact, man has been shown to obtain more lasting analgesia using this method than do many types of animals (Adams 1976, Hosobuchi et al 1977).

Electrical stimulation of the brain stem for the purpose of suppressing pain had not been in use for long before it was discovered that its analgesic effect could be abolished by the morphine-antagonist naloxone (Akil et al 1976) and that the injection of a small amount of morphine directly into the periaqueductal grey area produces analgesia (Herz et al 1970, Mayer & Price 1976, Mayer & Watkins 1981). It was therefore concluded that the morphine must act by activating neurons in the descending inhibitory system situated in the brain stem, and it raised the possibility that stimulation-produced analgesia might also occur as a result of the release of endogenous opioids (Basbaum et al 1976). Melzack & Melinkoff's observation (1974), that the analgesic effect of electrically stimulating the brain stem is enhanced by carrying this out for several minutes before a painful stimulus is administered, provided support for this idea.

### Opioid peptide-mediated descending inhibitory system

It is now realized that there are several descending inhibitory systems, but the one about which most is known and the one that is mainly brought into action when acupuncture is employed for the relief of nociceptive pain is opioid peptide-mediated.

**Periaqueductal grey**  This opioid peptide-mediated descending inhibitory system (OPMDIS) has its origin in the midbrain's periaqueductal grey (PAG).

The PAG is divided into two components: a dorsolateral one that projects to the pons and ventrolateral medulla (both of these are involved in autonomic control) and a ventrolateral one that, together with the adjacent nucleus cuneiformis (NC), forms the upper part of the OPMDIS with descending projections from these to structures in the rostral ventromedial medulla (Cameron et al 1995).

**Rostral ventromedial medulla**  The rostral ventromedial medulla (RVM) includes the midline situated nucleus raphe-magnus (NRM) and the adjacent reticular formation in the vicinity of the nucleus reticularis gigantocellularis.

Confirmation that the RVM is an important relay station in the OPMDIS comes from the discovery that electrical stimulation of or a microinjection of an opioid peptide into it has an inhibitory effect on dorsal horn neuronal responses to noxious stimuli (Fields et al 1991).

**Dorsolateral funiculus**  From the RVM axons project down the dorsolateral funiculus (DLF) and terminate on nociceptive neurons in the dorsal horn. Proof of this was obtained when it was shown that neither opiate – induced nor stimulation – produced analgesia occurs when this tract is cut (Basbaum et al 1977).

**Spinal terminals**  The spinal terminals of these descending axons are mainly to be found in Laminae I, II, & V (Basbaum et al 1978) the laminae to which nociceptive sensory afferents mainly project (Willis & Coggeshall 1991).

*Serotonin (5-hydroxy tryptamine)*  There are reasons to believe that serotonin is the main transmitting agent in the OPMDIS (Basbaum & Fields 1978). These include the discovery that electrical stimulation of the RVM causes this substance to be released into the cerebrospinal fluid and the analgesia produced by this type of stimulus is reduced by its antagonists (Yaksh & Wilson 1979, Barbaro et al 1985). Also the analgesia produced by a microinjection of morphine into the PAG is partially blocked by intrathecally administered methysergide a non-selective serotonin antagonist (Yaksh

1979). Finally, para-chlorophenylalanine, a serotonin inhibitor, suppresses analgesia brought about either by electrical stimulation of the PAG or the NRM, and by the microinjection of morphine into either of these structures (Anderson & Proudfit 1981).

With respect to all this it should be noted that Thompson (1984a) believes that the pain-suppressing effect of certain trycyclic antidepressants is probably because of their ability to enhance transmission down this descending pathway by blocking the re-uptake of serotonin.

**Rostral projections to the periaqueductal grey**
There are downward projections to the PAG from the medial prefrontal and insular cortex (Bandler & Shipley 1994). Also, from the hypothalamus; the electrical stimulation of or opioid microinjection into which has an analgesic effect (Manning et al 1994). There are also projections from various other structures, including the amygdala, the almond shaped nucleus at the front of the temporal lobe (Gray & Magnuson 1992), the nucleus cuneiformis, the postmedullary reticular formation, and the bluish-grey coloured locus coeruleus in the floor of the fourth ventricle (Herbert & Saper 1992).

**Caudal projections to the periaqueductal grey**
Nociceptive neurons in the dorsal horn's Laminae I & V project caudally to the PAG and the adjacent nucleus cuneiformis via the neospinothalamic tract, as this not only conveys A-delta nociceptive-generated information to the somato-sensory parietal cortex, but also has a collateral at the midbrain level that connects with these two structures (Fig. 6.5).

It is because of this collateral that needle stimulation of A-delta nerve fibres is able to bring the OPMDIS into action when acupuncture is being used to alleviate nociceptive pain.

The OPMDIS is also brought into action, as stated earlier in this chapter, when A-beta nerve stimulation, such as, for example, by means of high-frequency low intensity TENS, sets up activity in the dorsal column-medial leminiscus ascending pathway as this also has a projection to the PAG.

**Anti–opioid peptide effect of cholecystokinin octapeptide**  Cholecystokinin octapeptide is an endogenous opioid antagonist found to be present in the spinal cord (Yaksh et al 1982). It is also liable to be released into the RVM where it has an antagonistic effect on the antinociceptive action of endogenous opioids at that site (Crawley & Corwin 1994).

## Opioid peptide-mediated pain modulating mechanisms in the dorsal horn

The enkephalinergic inhibitory interneurons situated on the border of Laminae I and II of the dorsal horn not only block C afferent transmission as a result of A-delta afferent activity causing the descending inhibitory system to come into action in the manner just described. These interneurons also do this because A-delta nerve fibres make direct intraspinal contact with them in the dorsal horn (Fig. 6.5). In addition, enkephalinergic interneurons present on the terminals of C afferent fibres exert a presynaptic inhibitory effect (Bowsher 1990). It therefore follows that the acupuncture technique of stimulating A-delta nerve fibres with dry needles relieves C-afferent-transmitted tissue damage-type pain as a result of this kind of stimulus evoking activity in opioid peptide mediated pain modulating mechanisms situated at both supraspinal and spinal levels.

These two endogenous pain control mechanisms collectively constitute what Fields & Basbaum (1989) refer to as the opioid-mediated-analgesia system (OMAS).

**The physiological activation of the opioid–mediated–analgesia system**  When opiate receptors and their opioid peptides were found to be present in the central nervous system it was assumed, because the administration of naturally occurring opium and its derivatives has long been known to have an analgesic effect, that the body's own opioid peptides must be capable of modulating pain. Support for this idea came from finding that a microinjection of morphine either into certain midline nuclei in the brain stem or into the substantia gelatinosa produces analgesia (Herz et al 1970), and from the fact that the administration of high doses of beta-endorphin into the cerebrospinal fluid (Oyama et al 1980) and the intravenous injection of an enkephalin analogue (Calimlim et al 1982) has an analgesic effect.

Although it is now accepted that opioid peptides exert their analgesic effect both at supraspinal and spinal levels, the question that has to be addressed is: under what circumstances is this OMAS activated?

It was thought that, because naloxone is an opiate receptor antagonist with a particular affinity for $\mu$ receptors, that observations on the effects of this substance on pain produced by various means might throw some light on the matter. Unfortunately, the results of experiments designed to study the effects of naloxone on pain in man have proved to be bewilderingly conflicting. As Woolf & Wall (1983) point out, 'each positive result is matched by negative ones', and they go on to say:

> … the hodge-podge of conflicting results cannot be explained by the use of inadequate doses since many of the negative studies used higher doses than the positive ones. It is obvious that there must be an uncontrolled naloxone-reversible variable unrelated to pain in these studies, which may well be the degree of the subjects' stress.

Now this would seem to be the nub of the matter – that both noxious inputs and stress activate the OMAS. Whilst there is no doubt that a noxious input brought about by stimulating A-delta afferent nerve fibres, with, for example, acupuncture needles, may activate the system, so also may this be achieved either by environmental or surgical stress (Gracely et al 1983).

Many experiments have been conducted by Lewis et al (1980, 1981, 1982) on stress-produced analgesia in rats. The rats were stressed by having electric currents applied to their feet. Lewis and his colleagues found that what determines whether or not the analgesia produced by this type of shock is naloxone reversible, and therefore opioid peptide mediated or not, depends on its duration. Thus the analgesia produced by foot shock applied for 30 minutes is naloxone reversible, whereas that produced by foot shock applied for 3 minutes is not.

It is important to note that it was only when stress, such as that produced in these experiments on rats with an electric shock, is applied for a relatively long period that the OMAS is activated, because Levine et al (1979) have similarly shown, with respect to noxious stimuli, that this analgesia producing system also only operates when such a stimulus is of long duration. They demonstrated this by showing that naloxone has little or no effect on relatively brief, experimentally produced pain but markedly increases the intensity of any protracted pain such as that which may be experienced following a dental operation.

In summary, therefore, it has now been established that the OMAS is physiologically activated either by a prolonged, intense, noxious stimulus or some form of prolonged stress. A briefly applied noxious or stressful stimulus is also capable of producing analgesia. However, the question that has been asked is whether they do so by activating some less well-understood, non-opioid-mediated system, because as will be discussed in Chapter 10, the possibility that different analgesia-producing systems are activated according to whether the noxious stimulus is strong or weak is of considerable relevance when it comes to considering whether or not the pain suppressing mechanisms involved with either prolonged or brief stimulation with acupuncture needles are different.

Finally, it has to be said that the exact manner in which endogenous opioid peptides achieve their analgesic effect is not known. It is particularly confusing that electrical stimulation, which presumably has an excitatory action, and an opiate microinjection, which presumably has an inhibitory action, both produce analgesia when applied to certain midline brain stem nuclei. Fields & Basbaum (1989) suggest that this is because 'the opioid peptides may act by inhibiting inhibitory interneurons, thus disinhibiting the output neurons in these analgesia-producing regions'.

### Non-opioid peptide-mediated descending systems

For many years now the morphine antagonist naloxone has been used to investigate brain stem stimulation-analgesia, the action of opiates introduced into the central nervous system and the role of endogenous opioid peptides in suppressing pain.

As long ago as 1965, Lasagna showed that naloxone seemed to increase pain when administered to experimental subjects already experiencing some level of clinical pain. A more recent double-blind clinical study of postoperative dental pain (Levine et al 1978) has demonstrated that compared with a placebo, naloxone considerably increased the intensity of pain.

However, it was not long before contradictory reports started to appear, with Lindblom & Tegner (1979) even questioning whether the endogenous opioids are active in suppressing chronic pain as the administration of naloxone in their patients did not make the pain worse. Also, Dennis et al (1980) found that the adminstration of naloxone does not impair the analgesia produced by midbrain stimulation in rats suffering pain produced by injecting formalin subcutaneously.

Furthermore, as will be discussed again in Chapter 10, despite the fact that there have been many reports of acupuncture-induced analgesia being suppressed by naloxone, Chapman et al (1980) was unable to confirm this in a trial designed to study the effects of acupuncture on experimentally induced dental pain.

It is now accepted that one of the reasons for these conflicting reports must be that there are several descending control systems and that, whereas one of these is opioid peptide mediated, others must be mediated by various other transmitters. Most of these have yet to be discovered and their transmitters identified. However, it is now known that one such system has its origin in the dorsolateral pons where noradrenalin-containing cells project into the spinal cord (Melzack & Wall 1988, p. 141).

**Noradrenergic descending inhibitory system**
Noradrenergic axons, which mainly arise in the locus coeruleus in the pons, descend down the spinal cord to bring about direct inhibition of dorsal-horn-situated nociceptive neurons.

This system, like the OPMDIS, has projections to it from the prefrontal cortex and arcuate nucleus of the hypothalamus.

In addition, stimulation of A-delta nerves such as happens when the skin is penetrated by an acupuncture needle also brings this system into action because the neospinothalamic tract up which A-delta nociceptive information is conveyed has a collateral projection to the locus coeruleus (Craig 1992).

It therefore follows that another reason for the contradictory evidence concerning these various descending inhibitory pain-modulating mechanisms is the likelihood that in some of the experiments more than one of these systems is active at any given time (Watkins & Mayer 1982).

**Diffuse noxious inhibitory controls**   Lebars et al (1979) identified a powerful pain suppressing system that they have called diffuse noxious inhibitory controls (DNIC). The upper part of this system is the subnucleus reticularis in the caudal medulla (Villanueva et al 1988, 1990). From there, projections descend down the dorsolateral funiculus to dorsal horns where they have an opioidergic effect on wide dynamic range transmission neurons (Bernard et al 1990).

The importance of the DNIC system with respect to acupuncture is that Bing et al (1991) have shown that it is brought into action when needle stimulation of A-delta nerves is carried out anywhere on the body surface.

## THE DISTINCTION BETWEEN NOCICEPTIVE AND NEUROPATHIC PAIN

The tissue-damage type of nociceptive pain described earlier in this chapter occurring as a result of the activation and sensitisation of either C-polymodal nociceptors in skin or Group IV nociceptors in muscle has to be distinguished from the neuropathic type of pain that develops as a result of malfunction of either the peripheral or central nervous system.

One reason for this so far as acupuncture is concerned is that neuropathic pain is very much less responsive than nociceptive pain is to this form of therapy that acts by evoking activity in endogenous opioid-peptide-mediated pain modulating mechanisms. This is hardly surprising considering that neuropathic pain is extremely resistant to the effects of opioids (Portenoy et al 1990).

Therefore, before considering the use of acupuncture (or for that matter any other form of therapy) for the alleviation of persistent pain, it is essential to establish whether it is of a nociceptive or neuropathic type.

With certain types of pain, such as, for example, post-herpetic neuralgia, trigeminal neuralgia and central pain from spinal cord or brain stem damage, there is usually no difficulty in recognizing it to be of a neuropathic type. However, when pain develops during the course of some neurological disorder such as a stroke, multiple sclerosis, or subacute combined degeneration, whilst it may be neuropathic, it should not automatically be assumed

to be so, as, not infrequently, myofascial TrP nociceptive pain develops in such disorders as the result of the overloading of weakened muscles. Similarly, with post-herpetic neuralgia, because this neuropathic type of pain is difficult to alleviate it may cause a patient to tense muscles in the vicinity of the affected area and, as a consequence, acupuncture-responsive nociceptive TrP pain may develop as a secondary event.

Cancer is another commonly occurring disorder where pain may be either nociceptive or neuropathic and it is necessary to take this into consideration when deciding how best to alleviate it (Banning et al 1991), including whether or not to attempt to do this with acupuncture (Filshie 1990).

Furthermore, it has to be remembered that myofascial TrP nociceptive pain and neuropathic pain may be present concomitantly. This may happen when an active TrP causes the muscle containing it to become shortened with, as a consequence, the compression of underlying nerve roots (see Ch. 7). And, conversely, it may happen when cervical or lumbar nerve root compression, for reasons to be discussed in Chapter 7, causes TrP activity to develop.

In order to differentiate between nociceptive and neuropathic pain it is essential to pay close attention to the patient's description of the pain and to carry out a carefully conducted clinical examination.

Nociceptive pain of myofascial origin takes the form of a widespread dull aching sensation with tenderness of the tissues in the affected area and systematic examination revealing the presence of well-demarcated exquisitely tender TrPs some distance from it.

In contrast to this, neuropathic pain occurring as a result of peripheral nerve injury or dysfunction is commonly described as being of a burning nature or taking the form of shooting electrical sensations that, though not necessarily painful, are extremely distressing.

In addition, there is characteristically a latent interval between the time that the neural damage occurs and the onset of the pain. The intensity of the pain usually increases gradually to reach its maximum some weeks or months after onset. During this time, the skin becomes markedly hypersensitive so that it only requires a slight breeze or the rubbing of clothes to bring on an episode of pain (allodynia).

With neuropathic pain occurring as a result of nerve injury or dysfunction, there is inevitably some activation of nociceptors but the reason why this type of pain differs from that which is entirely nociceptive must be that the structural damage, as pointed out by Fields (1987, p. 216), causes 'disruption of the sensory apparatus so that a normal pattern of neural activity is no longer transmitted to the perceptual centers'. Melzack & Wall (1988, p. 118), with reference to this, state:

> ... the presence of peripheral nerve damage is signalled rapidly by nerve impulses and slowly by chemical transport. The long-term end result is that central cells whose input has been cut in the periphery increase their excitability and expand their receptive fields ... The duty of sensory cells is to receive information. When cut off from the source of their information, the cells react by increasing their excitability to such an extent that they begin to fire both spontaneously and to distant inappropriate inputs.

From experiments with the C nerve inactivator capsaicin, it has been shown that it is due to damage to C fibres that the prolonged central effects develop (Melzack & Wall 1988, p. 181). It is this central cell hyperexcitability which is responsible for various sensory abnormalities detectable on clinical examination.

When the skin over an area of the body affected by neuropathic pain and over a non-painful area (preferably the contralateral mirror image region) are in turn gently brushed with strands of cotton wool the sensation produced over the affected area is abnormally intense (hyperaesthesia). It may also be unpleasant (dysaesthesia) or even painful (allodynia). The noxious sensation produced by sticking a pin into the skin overlying an area affected by this type of pain is also far more intense than when such a stimulus is applied to skin in a non-painful area (hyperalgesia).

In addition, with neuropathic pain the phenomena of summation, spatial spread, and after discharge are often present. When the skin over an area affected by neuropathic pain is repeatedly pricked with a pin for 30 seconds or more the perceived intensity grows with successive stimuli (summation); this unpleasant sensation may also spread beyond the area stimulated (spatial spread); also, it may persist after the stimulation has been discontinued (after discharge).

## THE EMOTIONAL ASPECTS OF PAIN

Finally, it is necessary to examine the emotional aspects of pain and to discuss what influence these may have on the assessment and treatment of chronic pain. Pain is a complex physico-emotional experience with its emotional component largely determining how much suffering it causes. It is, therefore, not surprising that in describing pain, no matter whether it is nociceptive, neuropathic or entirely of emotional origin, patients are liable to include not only adjectives like aching, tingling or burning to describe its sensory qualities, but also adjectives like depressing, horrible or excruciating to convey the suffering caused by it.

Melzack & Torgerson (1971), in recognizing that there are three main categories of pain experience – sensory, affective and evaluative – drew up the McGill Pain Questionnaire and this, together with a subsequently introduced shortened version (Melzack 1987) has been shown to be of considerable value in the assessment of pain. It is, however, because all types of pain experience have an emotional component that it must never be assumed that pain is due to some primary psychological disturbance simply because a patient uses a predominance of affective terms to describe it.

Pain may very occasionally be a hallucinatory sensation experienced by schizophrenics. It may also be a manifestation of conversion hysteria or hypochondriasis. It therefore has to be admitted that there is such an entity as psychogenic pain (Feinmann 1990) but there are good grounds for believing that this is relatively rare and that affective disorders such as anxiety or depression are mostly the result of chronic pain rather than the cause of it.

The relationship of emotional factors to chronic pain can be assessed by giving patients with it specially designed standardized questionnaires such as the Minnesota Multiphasic Personality Inventory (MMPI). Sternbach et al (1973) used this inventory to compare the relative significance of psychological symptoms occurring in patients with acute (i.e. less than 6 months' duration) and chronic low-back pain. They found that although those with the shorter history of pain had elevated scores on the scales for depression, anxiety, hysteria and hypochondriasis, the scores were significantly higher in those with chronic pain. The MMPI was also used by Sternbach & Timmermans (1975) in their study of 113 patients with low-back pain of at least 6 months' duration. An assessment was made before and after either surgery followed by rehabilitation or rehabilitation only. From this assessment it was found that there was a significant decrease in the hysteria, depression, anxiety and hypochondriasis scales following successful alleviation of the pain.

Observations such as these confirm that chronic pain is usually the cause rather than the result of neurotic symptoms and Melzack & Wall (1988, p. 32) in discussing this conclude:

> It is evident from studies such as these that it is unreasonable to ascribe chronic pain to neurotic symptoms. The patients with the thick hospital charts are all too often prey to the physicians' innuendos that they are neurotic and that their neuroses are the cause of the pain. Whilst psychological processes contribute to pain, they are only part of the activity in a complex nervous system. All too often, the diagnosis of neurosis as the cause of pain hides our ignorance of many aspects of pain mechanisms.

The error of failing to recognize pain as being organic in origin and considering it to be entirely psychological most commonly occurs in my experience when myofascial TrP activity causes pain to persist long after all clinical evidence of tissue damage has disappeared (Ch. 7). This error, of course, is particularly likely to be made when the pain has led to the development of appreciable anxiety or depression or both. The reason why this mistake is so frequently made is clearly because of a widespread failure amongst health professionals to search for myofascial TrPs when attempting to find a cause for persistent pain.

It is as a result of this that many injustices are committed concerning the cause of protracted pain in accident compensation cases. Accidents

undoubtedly give rise to much psychological distress (Muse 1985, 1986) but this does not mean that post-accident pain that does not respond readily to some of the more conventional methods of treating organic pain is necessarily psychological in origin and in some way associated with an unconscious or even at times a conscious desire for compensation.

Such an assumption is all too prevalent and in the past has led experienced physicians such as Henry Miller (1961, 1966) to believe that once compensation is awarded, persistent post-accident pain invariably starts to improve. That this is not so has been demonstrated by Mendleson (1982, 1984) who, from a study of accident compensation cases in Australia, concludes that 'patients are not cured by the verdict', and that, in general, the pain remains as intense after the financial settlement as before. This is confirmed by Melzack et al (1985) who, in commenting both on Mendelson's findings and their own psychological studies of accident compensation cases, states:

> ... the phrase 'compensation neurosis' is an unwarranted, biased diagnosis. Not only are the disability and pain not cured by the verdict but compensation patients do not exaggerate their pain or show evidence of neurosis or other psychopathological symptoms greater than those seen in pain patients without compensation.

From serving on medical appeal tribunals that deal with people seeking compensation for post-accident disablement, it has become evident to me that of those who seek financial assistance because of persistent pain only relatively few are malingerers. This observation is in keeping with that of Leavitt & Sweet (1986) in their study of the frequency of malingering amongst patients with low-back pain.

What, however, has become apparent to me is that a disturbingly large number of these claimants are allowed to suffer from the myofascial pain syndrome for unnecessarily long periods of time simply because the dictum laid down by Livingston as long ago as 1943 is so frequently ignored. He said that in every case of persistent pain following trauma it is essential to search for TrPs. It was because Crue & Pinskey (1984) did not do this that they failed to find a nociceptive peripheral input in a group of patients with chronic back pain; introduced the totally inept diagnostic term 'chronic intractable benign pain'; and made the unwarranted assumption that such pain is a central phenomenon – a polite way of saying 'it is all in the mind!' As Rosonoff et al (1989) have now shown, in 96–100% of patients with chronic low-back or neck pain of the type studied by Crue & Pinskey, the pain emanates from myofascial TrPs.

Finally, it is necessary to reiterate that whilst anxiety is rarely the cause of pain, persistent pain is commonly associated with the development of anxiety. When this happens, the anxiety causes muscles to be held in a state of tension and with musculoskeletal pain this results in an increase in TrP activity with a consequent exacerbation of the pain (Craig 1989). In all such cases it is not sufficient simply to deactivate the TrPs but it is also necessary to reduce the anxiety. My personal preference is to employ hypnotherapy (Orne & Dinges 1989, Hilgard & Hilgard 1994) and to teach the patient how to practise autohypnosis on a regular daily basis.

# References

Adams J E 1976 Naloxone reversal of analgesia produced by brain stimulation in the human. Pain 2: 161–166

Akil H, Mayer D J, Liebeskind J C 1976 Antagonism of stimulation produced analgesia by naloxone, a narcotic antagonist. Science 191: 961–962

Anderson E G, Proudfit H K 1981 The functional role of the bulbospinal serotonergic system. In: Jacobs B L, Gelperin A (eds) Serotonin neurotransmission and behaviour. M.I.T. Press, Cambridge, Massachusetts, pp. 307–338

Atweh S F, Kuhar M J 1977 Autodiographic localization of opiate receptors in rat brain 1. Spinal cord and lower medulla. Brain Research 22: 471–493

Bandler R, Shipley MT 1994 Columnar organization in the midbrain periaqueductal gray: Modules for emotional expression? Trends in Neuroscience 17: 379–389

Banning A, Sjøugren P, Henreksen H 1991 Pain causes in 200 patients referred to a multidisciplinary cancer pain clinic. Pain 45: 45–48

Barbaro NM, Hammond DL, Fields HL 1985 Effects of intrathecally administered methysergide and yohimbine on microstimulation – produced antinociception in the rat. Brain Research 343: 223–229

Basbaum A I, Fields H L 1978 Endogenous pain control mechanisms: review and hypothesis. Annals of Neurology 4: 451–462

Basbaum AI, Clanton CH, Fields HL 1976 Opiate and stimulus-produced analgesia: functional anatomy of a medullospinal pathway. Proceedings of the National Academy of Sciences USA 73: 4685–4688

Basbaum AI, Clanton CH, Fields HL 1978 Three bulbospinal pathways from the rostral medulla of the cat: an autioradiographic study of pain modulating systems. Journal of Comparative Neurology 178: 209–224

Basbaum A I, Marley J J E, O'Keefe J, Clanton C H 1977 Reversal of morphine and stimulus-produced analgesia by subtotal spinal cord lesions. Pain 3: 43–56

Beecher H K 1959 Measurements of subjective responses. Oxford University Press, Oxford

Bernard JF, Villaneuva L, Carroue J, Le Bars D 1990 Efferent projections from the sub-nucleus reticularis dorsalis (SRD) : A *Phaseolus vulgaris* leucoagglutinin study in the rat Neuroscience Letters 116: 257–262

Bing Z, Villanueva L, Le Bars D 1991 Acupuncture-evoked responses of subnucleus reticularis dorsal neurons in the rat medulla. Neuroscience 44: 693–703

Bond M R 1979 Pain. Its nature, analysis and treatment. Churchill Livingstone, Edinburgh

Bowsher D 1987 Mechanisms of pain in man. ICI Pharmaceuticals Division

Bowsher D 1990 Physiology and pathophysiology of pain. Journal of the British Medical Acupuncture Society 7: 17–20

Bowsher D 1991 The physiology of stimulation-produced analgesia. Journal of the British Medical Acupuncture Society IX(2): 58–62

Bushnell MC, Villemure C, Strigo I, Duncan GH, 2002 Imaging pain in the brain: The role of the cerebral cortex in pain perception and modulation. Journal of Musculoskeletal Pain 10(1/2): 59–72

Calimlim J F, Wardell W M, Sriwatanakue K et al 1982 Analgesic effect of parenteral metkephamid acetate in treatment of postoperative pain. Lancet 1: 1374–1375

Cameron AA, Kahn IA, Westlund KN, Willis WD 1995 The efferent projections of the periaqueductal gray in the rat: a *Phaseolus vulgaris* – leucoagglutinin study. 11 Descending projections. Journal of Comparative Neurology 351: 585–601

Casey K L 1971a Somatsensory responses of bulboreticular units in awake cat: relation to escape-producing stimuli. Science 173: 77–80

Casey K L 1971b Responses of bulboreticular units to somatic stimuli eliciting escape behavior in the cat. International Journal of Neuroscience 2: 15–28

Casey K L 1980 Reticular formation and pain: towards a unifying concept. In: Bonical J J (ed) Pain. Raven Press, New York, pp. 93–105

Casey K L, Keene J J, Morrow T 1974 Bulboreticular and medial thalamic unit activity in relation to aversive behavior and pain. In: Bonica J J (ed) Pain, Advances in neurology. Raven Press, New York, Vol. 4, pp. 197–205

Cervero F 1983 Somatic and visceral inputs to the thoracic spinal cord of the cat. Journal of Physiology 337: 51–67

Chapman C R, Colpitts Y M, Benedetti C, Kitaeff R, Gehrig J D 1980 Evoked potential assessment of acupuncture analgesia: attempted reversal with naloxone. Pain 9: 183–197

Christensen B N, Perl E R 1970 Spinal neurons specifically excited by noxious or thermal stimuli: marginal zone of the dorsal horn. Journal of Neurophysiology 33: 293–307

Clement-Jones V 1983 Role of the endorphins in neurology. Practitioner 227: 487–495

Clement-Jones V, Besser G M 1983 Clinical perspectives in opioid peptides. British Medical Bulletin 39(1): 95–100

Clement-Jones V, Lowry P J, Rees L H et al 1980 Metenkaphalin circulates in human plasma. Nature 283: 295–297

Coderre T J, Katz J, Vaccarino A L, Melzack R 1993 Contribution of central neuroplasticity to pathological pain : review of clinical and experimental evidence. Pain 52: 259–285

Coggeshall R E, Lekan HA, Doubell T P, Allchorne A , Woolf C J 1997 Central changes in primary afferent fibers following peripheral nerve lesions. Neuroscience 77: 1115–1122

Collins J G, Ren K 1987 WDR response profiles of spinal dorsal horn neurons may be unmasked by barbiturate anesthesia. Pain: 28: 369–378

Cousins M, Power I 1999 Acute and postoperative pain. In: Wall PD, Melzack R (eds) Textbook of pain, 4th edn. Churchill Livingstone, Edinburgh, pp. 447–491

Craig AD 1992 Spinal and trigeminal lamina 1 input to the locus coeruleus anterogradely labeled with *Phaseolus vulgaris* leucoagglutinin (PHA-L) in the cat and the monkey. Brain Research 584: 325–328

Craig K D 1989 Emotional aspects of pain. In: Wall P D, Melzack R (eds) Textbook of pain, 2nd edn. Churchill Livingstone, Edinburgh, pp. 220–230

Crawley JN, Corwin RL 1994 Biological actions of cholecystokinin. Peptides 15: 731–755

Crue B L, Pinskey J J 1984 An approach to chronic pain of non-malignant origin. Postgraduate Medical Journal 60: 858–864

Dennis S G, Choinière M, Melzack R 1980 Stimulation-produced analgesia in rats: assessment by two pain tests and correlation with self-stimulation. Experimental Neurology 68: 295–309

Dickhaus H, Pauser G, Zimmerman M 1985 Tonic descending inhibition affects intensity coding of nociceptive responses in spinal dorsal horn neurones in the cat. Pain 23: 145–158

Doubell T P, Mannion R J, Woolf C J 1999 The dorsal horn: state – dependent sensory processing, plasticity and the generation of pain. In: Wall P D, Melzack R (eds) Textbook of pain, 4th edn. Churchill Livingstone, Edinburgh, pp. 165–181

Duggan A W, Hall J G, Headley P M 1976 Morphine, enkephalin and the substantia gelatinosa. Nature 264: 456–458

Feinmann C 1990 Psychogenic regional pain. British Journal of Hospital Medicine 43: 123–127

Fields H L 1987 Pain. McGraw-Hill, New York, pp. 31, 35, 44, 216, 82–94

Fields H L, Basbaum A I 1989 Endogenous pain control mechanisms. In: Wall P D, Melzack R (eds) Textbook of pain, 2nd edn. Churchill Livingstone, Edinburgh, pp. 206–220

Fields HL, Heinricher MM, Mason P 1991 Neurotransmitters in nociceptive modulatory circuits. Annual Review of Neuroscience 14: 219–245

Filshie 1990 Acupuncture for malignant pain. Journal of the British Medical Acupuncture Society 8: 38–39

Freeman W, Watts J W 1950 Psychosurgery in the treatment of mental disorders and intractable pain. C C Thomas, Springfield, Illinois, USA

Gardner W J, Licklider J C R 1959 Auditory analgesia in dental operations. Journal of the American Dental Association 59: 1144–1149

Georgopoulos A P 1974 Functional properties of primary afferent units probably related to pain mechanisms in primate glabrous skin. Journal of Neurophysiology 39: 71–83

Goldstein A, Tachibana S, Lowney L I, Hunkapiller M, Hood L 1979 Dynorphin (1–13) an extraordinarily potent opioid peptide. Proceedings of the National Academy of Sciences of the United States of America 76: 6666–6670

Graceley R H, Dubner R, Wolskee P J, Dector W R 1983 Placebo and naloxone can alter post-surgical pain by separate mechanisms. Nature 306: 264–265

Gray TS, Magnuson DJ, 1992 Peptide immunoreactive neurons in the amygdala and the bed of the stria terminalis project to the midbrain central gray in the rat. Peptides 13: 451–460

Hagbarth K E, Kerr D I B 1954 Central influences on spinal afferent conduction. Journal of Neurophysiology 17: 295–307

Hannington-Kiff J F 1974 Pain relief. Heinemann Medical, London

Herbert H, Saper CB 1992 Organization of medullary adrenergic and noradrenergic projections to the periaqueductal gray matter in the rat. Journal of Comparitive Neurology 315: 34–52

Herz A, Albus K, Metys J, Schubert P, Teschemacher H 1970 On the sites for the anti-nociceptive action of morphine and fentanyl. Neuropharmacology 9: 539–551

Hilgard ER, Hilgard JR 1994 Hypnosis in the relief of pain. Brunner/Mazel, New York

Hosobuchi Y, Adams J E, Linchitz R 1977 Pain relief by electrical stimulation of the central gray matter in humans and its reversal by naloxone. Science 177: 183–186

Hughes J, Smith T W, Kosterlitz H W, Fothergill L A, Morgan B A, Morris H R 1975 Identification of two related pentapeptides from the brain with potent opiate agonist activity. Nature 258: 577–579

Hunt S P, Kelly J S, Emson P C 1980 The electron microscope localization of methionine enkephalin within the superficial layers of the spinal cord. Neuroscience 5, 1871–1890

Ingvar M, Hsieh J-C 1999 The image of pain. In: Wall PD, Melzack R (eds) Textbook of pain, 4th edn. Churchill Livingstone, Edinburgh, pp. 215–233

Jessell T W 1982 Neurotransmitters and CNS disease – Pain. Lancet 2: 1084–1087

Jessell T W, Iversen L L 1977 Opiate analgesics inhibit substance P release from rat spinal trigeminal nucleus. Nature 268: 549–551

Jose P J, Page D A, Wolstenholme B E et al 1981 Bradykinin – stimulated prostaglandin E2 production of endothelial cells and its modulation by antiinflammatory compounds. Inflammation 5: 363–378

Kerr D I B, Haughen F P, Melzack R 1955 Responses evoked in the brain stem by tooth stimulation. American Journal of Physiology 183: 253–258

Lasagna L 1965 Drug interaction in the field of analgesic drugs. Proceedings of the Royal Society of Medicine 58: 978–983

Leavitt F, Sweet J J 1986 Characteristics and frequency of malingering among patients with low back pain. Pain 25: 357–364

Lebars D, Dickenson AH, Besson J-M 1979 Diffuse noxious inhibitory controls (DNIC). 1-Effects on dorsal horn convergent neurones in the rat; 11 – Lack of effect on non-convergent neurones, supraspinal involvement and theoretical implications. Pain 6: 283–327

Levine J D, Gordon N C, Jones R T, Fields H L 1978 The narcotic antagonist naloxone enhances clinical pain. Nature 272: 826–827

Levine J D, Gordon N C, Fields H L 1979 Naloxone dose dependently produces analgesia and hyperalgesia in postoperative pain. Nature 278: 740–741

Lewin R 1976 The brain's own opiate. New Scientist 69: 13

Lewis T 1942 Pain. Macmillan, New York

Lewis J W, Cannon J T, Liebeskind J E 1980 Opioid and non-opioid mechanisms of stress analgesia. Science 208: 623–625

Lewis J W, Sherman J E, Liebeskind J C 1981 Opioid and non-opioid stress analgesia: assessment of tolerance and cross tolerance with morphine. Journal of Neuroscience 1: 358–363

Lewis J W, Tordoff M G, Sherman J E, Liebeskind J C 1982 Adrenal medullary enkephalin-like peptides may mediate opioid stress analgesia. Science: 217: 557–559

Li C H, Barnafi L, Chrétien M, Chung D 1965 Isolation and amino-acid sequences of beta-LPA from sheep pituitary glands. Nature 208: 1093–1094

Lichstein L, Sackett G P 1971 Reactions by differentially raised rhesus monkeys to noxious stimulation. Developmental Psychobiology 4: 339–352

Liebeskind J C, Paul L A 1977 Psychological and physiological mechanisms of pain. American Review of Psychology 28: 41–60

Lindblom U, Tegner R 1979 Are the endorphins active in clinical pain states? Narcotic antagonism in chronic pain patients. Pain 7: 65–68

Livingston W K 1943 Pain mechanisms. Macmillan, New York

Lloyd DPC 1943 Neuron patterns controlling transmission of ipsilateral hind limb reflexes in cat. Journal of Neurophysiology 6: 293–315

Manning BH, Morgan MJ, Franklin KBJ 1994 Morphine analgesia in the formalin test: evidence for forebrain and midbrain sites of action. Neuroscience 63 : 289–294

Mayer D J, Price D D 1976 Central nervous system mechanisms of analgesia. Pain 2: 379–404

Mayer D J, Price D D, Becker D P 1975 Neurophysiological characterization of the anterolateral spinal cord neurons contributing to pain in man. Pain 1: 51–58

Mayer D J, Watkins L R 1981 The role of endorphins in endogenous pain control systems. In: Emrich H M (ed) Modern problems in pharmopsychiatry: The role of endorphins in neuropsychiatry. S Karger, Basel

Mayer D J, Wolfle T H, Akil H, Carder B, Liebeskind J C 1971 Analgesia from electrical stimulation in the brainstem of the rat. Science 174: 1351–1354

Melzack R 1969 The role of early experience in emotional arousal. Annals of New York Academy of Science 159: 721–730

Melzack R 1987 The short-term McGill Pain Questionnaire. Pain 30: 191–197

Melzack R, Casey K L 1968 Sensory, motivational, and central control determinants of pain: a new conceptual model. In: Kenshalo D (ed) The skin senses. C C Thomas, Springfield, Illinois, pp. 423–443

Melzack R, Katz J, Jeans M E 1985 The role of compensation in chronic pain. Analysis using a new method of scoring the McGill Pain Questionnaire. Pain 23: 101–112

Melzack R, Melinkoff D F 1974 Analgesia produced by brain stimulation: evidence of a prolonged onset period. Experimental Neurology 43: 369–374

Melzack R, Scott T H 1957 The effects of early experience on the response to pain. Journal of Comparative Physiology and Psychology 50: 155–161

Melzack R, Stotler W A, Livingston W K 1958 Effects of discrete brainstem lesions in cats on perception of noxious stimulation. Journal of Neurophysiology 21: 353–367

Melzack R, Torgenson W S 1971 On the language of pain. Anesthesiology 34, 50–59

Melzack R, Wall P D 1965 Pain mechanisms. A new theory. Science 150: 971–979

Melzack R, Wall P D 1982 The challenge of pain. Penguin, Harmondsworth, Middlesex, pp. 236, 237, 260

Melzack R, Wall P D 1988 The challenge of pain, 2nd edn. Penguin, Harmondsworth, Middlesex, pp. 32, 56, 118, 125, 141, 165–193, 173, 181

Mendelson G 1982 Not 'cured by a verdict': effect of legal settlement on compensation claimants. Medical Journal of Australia 2: 132–134

Mendleson G 1984 Compensation, Pain Complaints and Psychological Disturbance. Pain 20: 169–177

Mense S 1990 Physiology of nociception in muscles. In: Fricton J R, Awad E (eds) Advances in pain research and therapy, Vol 17. Raven Press, New York

Mense S 1997 Pathophysiologic basis of muscle pain syndromes. An update. Physical Medicine and Rehabilitation Clinics of North America 8(1): 23–52

Mense S 2001 Local pain in muscle. In: Mense S, Simons D (eds) Muscle pain, understanding its nature diagnosis and treatment. Lippincott, Williams & Wilkins, pp. 31, 42

Merskey H 1979 Pain terms: a list with definitions and notes on usage. Recommended by the IASP sub-committee on taxonomy. Pain 6: 249–252

Millar J, Basbaum A I 1975 Topography of the projection of the body surface of the cat to cuneate and gracile nuclei. Experimental Neurology 49: 281–290

Miller H 1961 Accident neurosis. British Medical Journal 1: 919–925

Miller H 1966 Accident neurosis. Proceedings of the Medico-Legal Society, Victoria 10: 71–82

Muse M 1985 Stress-related, post-traumatic chronic pain syndrome: criteria for diagnosis and preliminary report on prevalence. Pain 23: 295–300

Muse M 1986 Stress-related post-traumatic chronic pain syndrome: behavioral treatment approach. Pain 25: 389–394

Nathan P W 1976 The gate-control theory of pain. A critical review. Brain 99: 123–158

Nathan P 1982 The nervous system, 2nd edn. Oxford University Press, Oxford, pp. 104–113

Noordenbos W 1959 Pain. Elsevier, Amsterdam

Orne M T, Dinges D F 1989 Hypnosis. In: Wall P D, Melzack R (eds) Textbook of pain, 2nd edn. Churchill Livingstone, Edinburgh, pp. 1021–1031

Oyama T, Jin T, Yamaya R 1980 Profound analgesic effects of beta-endorphin in man. Lancet 1: 122–124

Paintal AS 1960 Functional analysis of Group III afferent fibres of mammalian muscles. Journal of Physiology 152: 250–270

Paterson S J, Robson L E, Kosterlitz H W 1983 Classification of opioid receptors. British Medical Bulletin 39: 31–36

Pert C D, Snyder S H 1973 Opiate receptor: demonstration in nervous tissue. Science 179: 1011–1014

Portenoy R K, Foley K M, Inturrisi C E 1990 The nature of opioid responsiveness and its implications for neuropathic pain: new hypotheses derived from studies of opioid infusions. Pain 43: 273–286

Przewlocki R, Hassan AHS, Lason W, Epplen C, Herz A, Stein C 1992 Gene expression and localization of opioid peptides in immune cells of inflamed tissue: functional role in antinociception. Neuroscience 48: 491–500

Rexed B 1952 The cytoarchitectonic organization of the spinal cord in the cat. Journal of Comparative Neurology 96: 415–495

Reynolds D V 1969 Surgery in the cat during electrical analgesia induced by focal brain stimulation. Science 164: 444–445

Rosonoff H L, Fishbain D A, Goldberg M, Santana R, Rosonoff R S 1989 Physical findings in patients with chronic intractable benign pain of the neck and/or back. Pain 37: 279–287

Schafer M, Mousa SA, Zhang Q, Carter L, Stein C 1996 Expression of corticotrophin – releasing factor in inflamed tissue is required for intrinsic peripheral opioid analgesia. Proceedings of the National Academy of Sciences USA 93: 6096–6100

Shanks M F, Clement-Jones V, Linsell C J et al 1981 A study of 24 hour profiles of plasma mentenkaphalin in man. Brain Research 212: 403–409

Sicuteri F 1967 Vasoneuroactive substances and their implication in vascular pain. In: Friedman AP (ed) Research and clinical studies in headache, Vol 1. Karger, New York, pp. 6–45

Smith R, Grossman A, Gaillard R et al 1981 Studies on circulating metenkephalin and beta-endorphin: normal subjects and patients with renal and adrenal disease. Clinical Endocrinology 15: 291–300

Smock T, Fields H L 1980 ACTH (1–24) blocks opiate-induced analgesia in the rat. Brain Research 212: 202–206

Soper W Y, Melzack R 1982 Stimulation-produced analgesia. Evidence for somatotopic organization in the midbrain. Brain Research 251: 301–311

Stein C, Hassan AHS, Przewlocki R, Gramsch C, Peter K, Herz A 1990 Opioids from immunocytes interact with receptors on sensory nerves to inhibit nociception in inflammation. Proceedings of the National Academy of Sciences USA 87: 5935–5939

Sternbach R A, Timmermans G 1975 Personality changes associated with reduction of pain. Pain 1: 177–181

Sternbach R A, Wolf S R, Murphy R W, Akeson W H 1973 Traits of pain patients: the low-back 'loser'. Psychosomatics 14: 226–229

Szentagothai J 1964 Neuronal and synaptic arrangement in the substantia gelatinosa rolandi. Journal of Comparative Neurology 122: 219–239

Thompson J W 1984a Pain mechanisms and principles of management. In: Evans J, Grimley, Laird F I (eds). Advanced geriatric medicine 4. Pitman, London

Thompson J W 1984b Opioid peptides. British Medical Journal 288 (6413): 259–260

Thompson J W 1988 Acupuncture or TENS for pain relief? Scientific and clinical comparisons. New Zealand Journal of Acupuncture. August 21–33

Thompson J W 1994 Acupuncture: current ideas on mechanisms of action. Summary from lecture to meeting of Pain Society. April 14th–16th, UMIST, Manchester

Todd A J, MacKenzie J 1989 GABA – immunoreactive neurons in the dorsal horn of the rat spinal cord. Neuroscience 32: 799–806

Todd AJ, Spike RC, Johnston HM 1992 Immunohistochemical evidence that met-enkephalin and GABA co-exist in some neurons in rat dorsal horn. Brain Research 584: 149–156

Verrill P 1990 Does the gate theory of pain supplant all others? British Journal of Hospital Medicine. 43: 325

Villaneuva L, Bouhassira D, Bing Z, Le Bars D 1988 Convergence of heterotopic nociceptive information on to subnucleus reticularis dorsalis neurons in the rat medulla. Journal of Neurophysiology 60: 980–1009

Villaneuva L, Cliffer KD, Sorkin LS, Le Bars D, Willis WD 1990 Convergence of heterotopic nociceptive information on to neurons of caudal medullary reticular formation in monkey (Macaca *fascicularis*). Journal of Neurophysiology 63: 1118–1127

Wall P D 1960 Cord cells responding to touch, damage and temperature of skin. Journal of Neurophysiology 23: 197–210

Wall P D 1964 Presynaptic control of impulses at the first central synapse in the cutaneous pathway. In: Physiology of spinal neurons. Progress in Brain Research 12. Elsevier, Amsterdam, pp. 92–118

Wall P D 1978 The gate-control theory of pain mechanisms. A re-examination and a re-statement. Brain 101: 1–18

Wall P D 1980a The role of substantia gelatinosa as a gate control. In: Bonica J J (ed) Pain. Raven Press, New York, pp. 205–231

Wall P D 1980b The substantia gelatinosa. A gate control mechanism set across a sensory pathway. Trends in Neurosciences (Sept): 221–224

Wall P D 1989 The dorsal horn. In: Wall P D, Melzack R (eds) Textbook of pain, 2nd edn, Ch. 5. Churchill Livingstone, Edinburgh

Wall P D 1990 Obituary – William Noordenbos (1910–1990) Pain 42: 265–267

Wall P D, Melzack R (eds) 1999 Textbook of pain, 4th edn. Churchill Livingstone, Edinburgh

Wang J K, Nauss L A, Thomas J E 1979 Pain relief by intrathecally applied morphine in man. Anesthesiology 50: 149–151

Watkins L R, Mayer D J 1982 Organization of endogenous opiate and non-opiate pain control systems. Science 216: 1185–1192

Weber E, Roth K A, Barchas J 1981 Colocalisation of alphaneo-endorphin and dynorphin immunoreactivity in hypothalamic neurons. Biochemical and Biophysical Research Communications 103: 951–958

Willis W D 1989 The origin and destination of pathways involved in pain transmission. In: Wall P, Melzack R (eds) Textbook of pain, 2nd edn. Churchill Livingstone, Edinburgh

Willis W D, Coggeshall R E 1991 Sensory mechanisms of the spinal cord, 2nd edn. Plenum press, New York, p. 575

Woolf C J, Wall P D 1983 Endogenous opioid peptides and pain mechanisms: a complex relationship. Nature 306: 739–740

Wyke B 1979 Neurological mechanisms in the experience of pain. Acupuncture and Electro-therapeutics Research 4: 27–35

Wynn Parry C B 1980 Pain in avulsion lesions of the brachial plexus. Pain 9: 41–53

Yaksh T L 1979 Direct evidence that spinal serotonin and noradrenaline terminals mediate the spinal antinociceptive effects of morphine in the periaqueductal grey. Brain Research 160: 180–185

Yaksh T L, Abay EO, Go VLW 1982 Studies on the location and release of cholecystokinin and vasoactive intestinal peptide in the rat and cat spinal cord. Brain Research 242: 279–290

Yaksh T L, Rudy T A 1976 Analgesia mediated by a direct spinal action of narcotics. Science 192: 1357–1358

Yaksh T L, Wilson PR 1979 Spinal serotonin system mediates antinociception. Journal of Pharmacology and Experimental Therapeutics 208: 446–453

Zborowski M 1952 Cultural components in responses to pain. Journal of Social Issues 8: 16–30

Chapter **7**

# Myofascial trigger point pain and fibromyalgia syndromes

## CHAPTER CONTENTS

## INTRODUCTION

In this chapter there will firstly be an account of current knowledge concerning what is widely known as the myofascial pain syndrome, or what will be called here the myofascial trigger point (MTrP) pain syndrome, in order to draw attention to the all-important source of the pain and the one to which treatment with acupuncture has to be directed.

This will be followed by a review of what is presently known about the fibromyalgia syndrome (FS) because, although due to the complexity of this disorder its treatment perforce has to include the employment of a wide variety of pharmacological agents and physical forms of therapy, acupuncture is becoming increasingly often included amongst these.

## MYOFASCIAL TrP PAIN SYNDROME

Nociceptor activity at MTrP sites is one of the commonest causes for musculoskeletal pain developing (Travell 1976). And yet despite the appearance of numerous wide ranging reviews of the MTrP pain syndrome in recent years, including those by Baldry (2001), Gerwin (1994), Hong (1999), Hong & Simons (1998), Mense (1990, 1993 a, b; 1997, 2001), Mense et al (2001), Rachlin (1994), Simons (1996, 1999), Simons et al (1999) and Travell & Simons (1992), the importance of searching for MTrPs when investigating the cause of pain of uncertain origin is still not sufficiently well recognized.

In an attempt to redress this unfortunate state of affairs, the incidence, pathophysiology, clinical characteristics and criteria for the diagnosis of the

MTrP pain syndrome will be discussed at some length.

## Incidence

There have been no large epidemiological studies but as McCain (1994) states, 'anecdotal evidence from expert examiners suggest that MTrP pain syndrome is a very common condition, particularly in industry, where it is a frequent cause of disability after trauma'. Confirmation that the incidence of this syndrome is high also comes from Fricton et al's (1985) finding that 54.6% of a large group of patients with chronic head and neck pain had pain emanating from MTrPs; from Skootsky et al's (1989) finding that 85% of patients presenting with low-back pain to a general internal medicine practice had MTrPs as the source of their pain; and from Schiffman et al (1990), who in an epidemiological study of orofacial pain in young adult females, found that in 50% of them the pain emanated from MTrPs.

MTrP pain mainly affects adults but children may also develop it (Aftimos 1989, Bates & Grunwaldt 1958, Fine 1987). Unlike the fibromyalgia syndrome, in which over four-fifths of patients are females (Yunus 1989) the incidence of the MTrP pain syndrome is about the same in both sexes.

## Pathophysiology of myofascial TrPs

### Myofascial TrP sites

The principal TrPs in a muscle are located at its centre (central TrPs) in the motor endplate zone. This zone is where the motor nerve on entering a muscle divides into a number of branches with each of these, as Salpeter (1987) has shown, having a terminal claw-like motor endplate embedded in the surface of a muscle fibre (Fig. 7.1). When a centrally placed MTrP becomes active the muscle fibre containing it becomes so markedly contracted as to form a taut band and then because of the tension in this, an enthesopathy may develop at the fibre's lateral attachments with, as a consequence, the production of TrP activity at these sites (attachment TrPs).

### Structures present at a MTrP site

Each MTrP contains a neurovascular bundle. This contains a motor axon with branching motor nerve endings that have terminal motor endplates with juxtapositional contraction knots. In addition, the bundle contains nociceptive and proprioceptive sensory afferents; also, blood vessels with closely related sympathetic fibres (Fig. 7.1).

### Physiological contraction of a muscle fibre

When, as a result of alpha-motor neuronal activity in the spinal cord's anterior horn, a nerve action potential enters the central part of a muscle fibre, acetylcholine becomes liberated from the motor endplate's synaptic clefts and causes the muscle fibre to contract.

### Development of contraction knots at MTrP sites

When a MTrP develops pain-producing activity, the release of an appreciable amount of calcitonin gene-related peptide from its activated and sensitized nociceptor sensory afferents causes an excessive amount of acetycholine to be liberated from

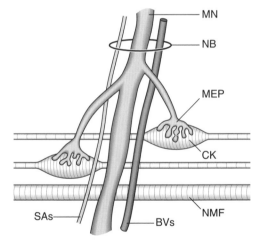

**Figure 7.1** Diagramatic representation of part of a myofascial trigger point showing two motor endplates (MEPs) and juxtapositional contraction knots (CKs); also a neurovascular bundle (NB) containing motor nerves (MNs), nociceptive and proprioceptive sensory afferents (SAs) and blood vessels (BVs) with closely associated sympathetic fibres. Note: in normal muscle fibre (NMF) the sarcomeres are of equal length. In a muscle fibre containing a contraction knot there is a shortening of the sarcomeres at that site and compensatory lengthening of them on either side.

dysfunctional motor endplates so that the muscle fibres into which these are embedded then become so markedly contracted as to form contraction knots. These were first identified by Simons & Stolov (1976) when during the course of palpating muscles in dogs they identified points of tenderness with characteristics similar to those of human MTrPs. On examining longitudinal sections of biopsy material taken from these sites under the microscope they found that the muscle fibres contained fusiform swellings (contraction knots). They also observed that each of them was located in close proximity to a motor endplate and was approximately about the same length as it. They concluded that a knot of this type is a segment of muscle fibre which has become abnormally thickened as a result of its sarcomeres having become considerably shortened; and that the reason why the sarcomeres on either side of it are considerably thinner is because of compensatory stretching (Fig. 7.1).

## Electrical activity at myofascial TrP sites

Knowledge concerning motor endplate activity at MTrP sites has recently been considerably advanced by electromyographic (EMG) studies. The first to examine a MTrP's electrical activity were Weeks & Travell (1957), who recorded a series of high-frequency spike-shaped discharges with an amplitude of approximately 1000 μV and a duration of 1–3 m/s from MTrP sites in the trapezius muscle. The next to turn their attention to this were Hubbard & Berkoff (1993) who, from working with a monopolar EMG needle, recorded similar high-amplitude spike activity of about 100–700 μV and a continuous low amplitude potential of about 50 μV at active TrP sites in the trapezius muscle. They decided that:

> ... the activity is not localised enough to be generated in an endplate, nor does it have the expected location or waveform morphology for end plate activity. We theorize that TrP EMG activity is generated from sympathetically stimulated intrafusal muscle fibre contractions...

A theory that led them to conclude that:

> ... a MTrP is located in the muscle spindle as the intrafusal fibres of this are sympathetically innervated ...

It has to be said, however, that EMG studies carried out both in the middle of the 20th century and again more recently have not provided support for this. Jones et al (1955), using an iron deposition technique to confirm the position of their needle, recorded an electrical activity of 50–700 μV when they inserted it into muscle at a site which histologically was shown to have iron deposited around a number of small nerve endings. And, although this wave pattern was similar to the one Hubbard & Berkoff believed arose in a muscle spindle, they were unable to identify such a structure within the vicinity of their recording needle. Furthermore, their observations that denervation abolished the electrical activity, that the insertion of the needle into the site gave rise to acute pain and also led to the development of brief muscle twitches (see local twitch response p. 86) all strongly suggest, as Gerwin (1994) has pointed out, that the plexus of motor nerves into which their needle was inserted was at a MTrP site.

More recent evidence that a MTrP is not located at a muscle spindle but rather in the vicinity of branches of a muscle's motor nerve and their terminal motor endplates comes from studies carried out by Simons et al (1995a,b,c,d) who, in the carrying out of these, employed a fivefold higher amplification and a tenfold increase in sweep speed for their recordings than had been previously used (Simons et al 1999).

With this technique (Fig. 7.2), they recorded from active MTrP sites intermittent high-amplitude biphasic spike potentials (100–600 μV) similar to those recorded firstly by Weeks & Travell and then by Hubbard & Berkoff. They also drew special attention to having in addition to this recorded spontaneous electrical activity (SEA) made up of constantly present continuous low-amplitude noise-like action potentials (10–50 μv).

It is now clear from studies carried out by Heuser & Miledi (1971) and others that this SEA found at a MTrP site corresponds to an abnormal pattern of motor endplate electrical activity brought about by an excessive release of acetylcholine (Hong 1999).

Support for the belief that MTrPs are not located in muscle spindles but in motor endplate zones also comes from the finding made by Cheshire et al (1994) that it is possible to abolish the pain

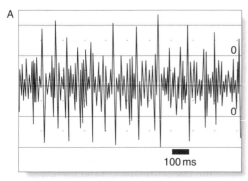 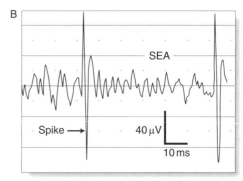

**Figure 7.2**   Spontaneous electrical activity (SEA) and spike characteristic of an active locus in a human trigger point. Both records are of essentially the same activity; the difference is in the recording speed. A, slow speed which presents a one-second record that shows the general pattern of activity, but little detail. B, recording at 10 times faster speed (0.1 s record) that shows the noise-like spontaneous activity of low amplitude and two superimposed, intermittent, sharp, initially negative spikes of high amplitude. Amplification is less for the slow record. Reproduced from Simons 1996, with permission.

emanating from a MTrP by injecting the botulinum A toxin into it as the effect of this substance is to block the release of acetylcholine from motor nerve terminals.

## A MTrP's GroupIV nociceptors

For reasons stated in Chapter 6, there are grounds for believing that the pain that develops when MTrPs become active does so as a result of the activation and sensitisation of Group IV nociceptors.

### Activation of a MTrP's Group IV nociceptors

As discussed at some length in Chapter 6, this is brought about in two ways. Firstly, by a high-intensity noxious stimulus transiently deforming Group IV sensory afferent nerve endings and by so doing causing electrical changes to take place that culminate in the development of propagated action potentials in them. Secondly, by this type of stimulus releasing from vesicles in these nerve endings the neuropeptides Substance P (SP) and calcitonin gene-related peptide that, by having a vasodilatory effect and giving rise to an increase in vascular permeability, cause oedema to develop and algesic vasoneuroactive substances such as bradykinin, serotonin, potassium ions and histamine to be liberated (Sicuteri 1967).

With respect to this, however, it is of interest to note that the nociceptive sensory afferents in

muscle contain much less SP and calcitonin gene-related peptide than their counterparts in the skin (McMahon et al 1989).

It has been suggested that the teleological reason for this may be because these neuropeptides cause the tissues to become oedematous and if this was allowed to become excessive in skeletal muscle, encased as it is in unyielding fascia, it would be liable to become ischaemic or even necrotic (McMahon et al 1984).

### Sensitisation of a MTrP's Group IV nociceptors

As also discussed in Chapter 6, bradykinin not only activates nociceptors but also sensitizes them with, as a consequence, a lowering of their threshold so as to make them responsive not only to high-intensity noxious stimuli, but also to low-intensity mildly noxious or innocuous ones (Mense 1993b). In addition, it has the effect of releasing prostaglandins of the E type (particularly E2) from damaged tissue cells (Jose et al 1981). And these in turn have a powerful nociceptor sensitizing effect.

It is this sensitisation of its nociceptors that makes a MTrP so exquisitely tender that when firm pressure is applied to the tissues overlying it the patient involuntarily carries out a reflex flexion withdrawal movement – the 'jump' sign (Kraft et al 1968) and may, on occasions, utter an expletive – the 'shout ' sign. It is this latter vocal reaction that led the 5th century Chinese physician Sun Ssu-Mo to call these points of maximal tenderness in muscle ah shih (oh yes it hurts) points (Lu & Needham 1980).

## Factors responsible for development of MTrP nociceptor activity

### Trauma

The usual reason for MTrP nociceptor activity developing is the subjection of muscle to the high-intensity stimulation provided by trauma. This may be brought about either by a direct injury to a muscle or by the sudden or repeated overloading of it. Alternatively, it may develop when a muscle is subjected to repeated episodes of microtrauma, such as occurs with a repetitive strain injury (see Ch. 15).

### Anxiety

Not uncommonly a patient who, because of anxiety, holds a group of muscles in a persistently contracted state develops MTrP activity in them. One suggested reason for this happening is because of sympathetic nerve overactivity (McNulty et al 1994). Another possibility is that it is brought about as a result of psychologically determined stimulation of brain-stem structures. This is because neurons in the brain stem's reticular tissue have axons that project upwards to the thalamus and hypothalamus, and axons that project downwards to the spinal cord's alpha motor neurons. These, in turn, have connections with MTrP's motor endplates.

### Radiculopathic compression of motor nerves

Chu (1995, 1997), during the course of carrying out electromyographic studies in patients with persistent back pain, has observed that when this occurs as a result of spinal nerve root entrapment, such as from spondylosis or disc prolapse in the cervical or lumbar region, it may be followed by pain arising as a result of the secondary development of TrP activity in the paraspinal muscles. With reference to this Simons et al (1999) state that 'there is much clinical evidence that compression of motor nerves can activate and perpetuate the primary TrP dysfunction at the motor endplate'.

### Muscle wasting

TrP activity may develop in muscles that have become weakened and overloaded such as a result of malignant disease or various neurological disorders. Examples of the latter include poliomyelitis, motor neurone disease and strokes.

With respect to strokes, TrP nociceptive pain may develop during the recovery stage when weakened muscles become overloaded during attempts to restore movements to them. It may also arise in conjunction with glenohumeral joint capsulitis pain in cases where following a stroke the joint has not been kept adequately mobilized.

This TrP-evoked nociceptive pain of a dull aching character, because it is liable to radiate down a limb affected by a stroke has to be distinguished from post-stroke neuropathic pain that arises as a result of damage to the central nervous system (central pain). This, however, is not usually difficult as the latter often takes the form of a severe burning, similar to that experienced when a hand is plunged into ice cold water. Alternatively, it may be either a lacerating, shooting, squeezing or throbbing type of sensation.

### Muscle ischaemia

TrP activity may arise in muscles that have become ischaemic because of arterial obstruction sufficient to cause the development of intermittent claudication (see Ch. 18). It may also develop in muscles that have become ischaemic as a result of neurological disease – induced spasticity (Mense 1993b).

### Visceral pain referral

Pain arising as a result of visceral disease is frequently referred to both skin and muscles. When this happens TrPs in muscles situated in this zone of pain referral are liable to become active with the production of superimposed MTrP pain.

There are grounds for believing that the underlying reasons for this happening (Gerwin 2002, Giamberardino et al 2002) are because the dorsal horn neurons activated by a sensory afferent input from visceral nociceptors also have a similar input from muscle nociceptors. And because the central sensitisation brought about as a result of the sensory afferent barrage sustained by these convergent viscero-somatic dorsal horn neurons results in an expansion in the number and size of their receptive fields (see Ch. 6).

An example of when this may happen is TrP activity developing in anterior chest muscles following the referral to them of coronary heart disease pain. Another is TrP activity developing in abdominal muscles following the referral of pain to them from a peptic ulcer.

### Other causes

TrPs may also become active when the muscles containing them are exposed to adverse environmental conditions such as damp, draughts, excessive cold or extreme heat (Melzack & Wall 1988).

## Primary, secondary and satellite active MTrPs

An active MTrP is one whose nociceptors have become sufficiently activated and sensitized for pain to be referred from it to a site some distance away (zone of pain referral). Active MTrPs are of three types – primary, secondary and satellite.

### Primary MTrPs

These are TrPs whose nociceptor activity in a muscle or a group of muscles is primarily responsible for the development of the MTrP pain syndrome.

### Secondary MTrPs

These are TrPs that develop activity in the initially affected muscle or group of muscles' synergists or antagonists. They develop activity in the synergists when these become overloaded as a result of compensating for the weakened primarily affected muscles and in the antagonists when these become overloaded as a result of combating the tension in and shortening of the primarily affected ones.

### Satellite MTrPs

These are TrPs that become active when the muscle in which they are present is situated in a primarily affected muscle's zone of TrP pain referral. Pain from these satellite TrPs is then referred to an even

yet more distant site. For example, it is not uncommon for a TrP in the lower part of the posterior chest wall to refer pain to the buttock and for pain from satellite TrPs in the gluteal muscles to then be referred down the leg.

### Latent MTrPs

A latent MTrP is one whose nociceptors have become activated and sensitised but not enough to cause pain to develop. Nevertheless, the nociceptor sensitisation makes it sufficiently tender for a 'jump' and 'shout' reaction (see p. 85) to be elicited when firm pressure is applied to the overlying tissues. It, therefore, follows that latent TrPs are liable to be found when examining the muscles of pain-free people. Sola & Kuitert (1955), during the course of examining 200 fit young people in the American Air Force (100 males, age range 17–27 years; and 100 females, age range 18–35 years) found latent TrPs to be present in 45 of the males and 54 of the females.

## The natural history of MTrP pain

MTrP pain may disappear spontaneously once the inflammatory reaction responsible for releasing nociceptor activating and sensitizing substances has resolved.

Not infrequently, however, the pain persists long after tissue healing has taken place. This is liable to cause much diagnostic confusion as all too often it is erroneously concluded that this prolongation of the symptom for months or even years in the absence of physical signs of tissue damage cannot possibly be organic and that the person complaining of it must be neurotic. This may lead to the person concerned being unnecessarily referred for psychiatric assessment.

Alternatively, it may mistakenly be assumed that the pain is being consciously or unconsciously allowed to persist in an attempt by the person concerned to gain financially from it. The case outlined below typifies this.

A man (27 years of age), whilst at work, fell from a ladder on to his back. This caused considerable bruising and pain in the lower lumbar and sacral regions. Radiographs of the spine showed no evidence of a fracture and all signs of soft-tissue damage fairly quickly disappeared. The pain, however, persisted and when 6 months later it continued to be disabling despite intensive physiotherapy an orthopaedic surgeon expressed the opinion in his report that this might be due to the patient subconsciously exaggerating his symptoms in the hope of claiming industrial compensation. Nothing, however, could have been further from the truth for the patient, frustrated by his poor response to physiotherapy, asked his general practitioner if he thought acupuncture might be helpful and as a consequence was referred to me for assessment.

On examination, several TrPs were found to be present in muscles on both sides of the lower back. The pain from these was alleviated after they had been deactivated with dry needles on four occasions at weekly intervals. He was then only too glad to get back to work with no thought of trying to claim compensation.

## Mechanisms responsible for MTrP pain's persistence

As it is not certain why MTrP pain tends to persist long after all evidence of soft-tissue damage has disappeared it is only possible to hypothesize about this (Mense 1990).

The four mechanisms that have to be considered are (1) the development of dorsal horn neuronal plasticity; (2) the development of self-perpetuating ischaemic changes at MTrP sites; (3) the development of self-perpetuating activity in motor efferents; and (4) the development of such activity in sympathetic efferents. Each of these will be considered in turn.

### Spinal dorsal horn neuroplasticity

As stated in Chapter 6 the sensory afferent barrage set up when nociceptors become activated and sensitized eventually causes dorsal horn transmission neurons to develop the neuroplastic changes known as central sensitisation. It, therefore, follows that when MTrP nociceptors have been subjected to prolonged high-intensity stimulation this central sensitisation must inevitably develop and one of its effects is to cause the pain that emanates from them to persist (Mense 1993b).

### Development of self-perpetuating ischaemic changes at MTrP sites

When the MTrP nociceptor-sensitizing substances bradykinin and prostaglandins are released into the tissues as a result of trauma-induced inflammation, they give rise to the development of both vasodilatation and increased vascular permeability. The effect of this is to cause oedema to develop with compression of veins and resultant tissue ischaemia. As a consequence of this a vicious circle is liable to be created because the ischaemia then leads to the release of still more MTrP nociceptor-sensitizing chemical substances.

### Self-perpetuating circuits between a MTrP and the spinal cord motor efferent activity (Fig. 7.3, lower drawing)

Fields (1987) has postulated that the sensory afferent input to the spinal cord from activated and sensitized MTrP nociceptors projects not only to dorsal horn nociceptive neurons but also to ventral horn-situated motor neurons with, as a result, the setting up of motor efferent activity. And it was thought by him that this in turn may cause the muscle containing the TrP to go into sufficient spasm to make it ischaemic with, as a consequence, the release of still more MTrP nociceptor activating substances and the development of a self-perpetuating circuit.

It requires, however, a very considerable amount of spasm to render a muscle ischaemic and the more likely explanation is that it is the effect of this motor efferent activity on a MTrP's dysfunctional motor endplates that leads to the perpetuation of its nociceptor activity.

### Sympathetic efferent activity (Fig. 7.3, top drawing)

Livingston (1943) was the first to put forward the hypothesis that a self-perpetuating circuit of this type may also be set up by the development of efferent activity in the sympathetic nervous system. He did this in an attempt to explain the persistence of pain in his patients with the sympathetic disorder currently called the complex regional pain syndrome-type 1 (RSD). With some of them the disorder was of a primary type and

**Figure 7.3** Livingston's vicious circle. *Top*: A stimulus delivered at S activates a primary afferent nociceptor that, in turn, activates the sympathetic preganglionic neuron in the intermediolateral column (IML). The preganglionic neuron activates the noradrenergic postganglionic neuron in the sympathetic ganglion (SG), which sensitizes, and can activate, primary afferent nociceptors (H) which, feed back to the spinal cord, maintaining the pain. *Bottom*: Nociceptive input may also set in motion another nociceptive input by activating motoneurons that cause muscle spasm. Prolonged muscle spasm activates muscle nociceptors which feed back to the spinal cord to sustain the spasm.

In both situations, the original noxious stimulus sets in motion a spreading and potentially self-sustaining process. In some cases the precipitating noxious input may be trivial and short lasting. In such cases, blocking the spasm or interruption of the reflex loops may provide long-lasting relief. Reproduced with permission from Howard Fields' *Pain*, McGraw Hill 1987.

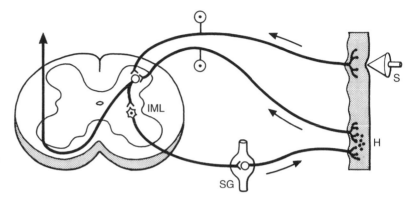

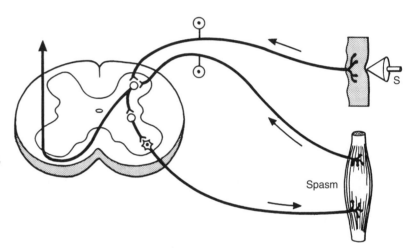

with others there was concomitant MTrP activity (see Ch 8).

His theory was that a MTrP's nociceptive sensory afferent input to the spinal cord, on reaching it, is in some cases liable to activate sympathetic preganglionic neurons in the intermediolateral column situated between the dorsal and ventral horns. And that this, in turn, causes noradrenergic postganglionic neurons in the sympathetic chain to become activated with, as a consequence, the release of noradrenaline (norepinephrine), which then helps to maintain MTrP nociceptor activity. This hypothesis has since received support from in vitro experimental rat muscle receptor studies carried out by Kieschke et al (1988).

All this notwithstanding, it has to be said that often there is no clinically obvious muscle spasm

or sympathetic involvement to account for the long-term persistence of MTrP activity. The following case is a good example of this.

A 65-year-old woman was referred to me with a pain in the lateral chest wall that had been present for 31 years! On examination there was no evidence of sympathetic involvement and no muscle spasm. There were, however, three well-defined TrPs in the serratus anterior muscle and despite the exceptionally long history it only required the deactivation of these by means of dry needling on three occasions for the pain to disappear. She stated that the pain had developed as a result of trauma to the chest wall incurred when 31 years previously she fell off her bicycle. She complained to doctors on many occasions about the pain but it was not until she eventually had to consult a physician about her heart that the TrP origin of this long-standing pain in the lateral chest wall was recognized.

## MTrP pain referral

Lewis (1942) was one of the first to point out that pain that develops as a result of the application of a noxious stimulus to the skin is accurately located by the brain, but that pain that develops as a result of trauma to muscle is perceived as arising some distance away from the affected site.

It was also about that time, as discussed in Chapter 4, that John Kellgren was able to demonstrate that pain emanating from what would now be called a MTrP, is referred to a site some distance from it (zone of pain referral). And that not only is the MTrP itself exquisitely tender, but that there is also a certain amount of tenderness of the healthy tissues in the zone of pain referral.

Since then many hypotheses have been put forward to explain MTrP pain referral, but despite considerable progress having been made in our understanding of the neurophysiology of pain, the reason for it happening is still not certain. The theories that have been advanced include convergence–facilitation, convergence–projection and central sensitisation.

### Convergence–facilitation and convergence–projection theories

These two theories, the first put forward by Mackenzie (1909) and the second by Ruch (1949) to explain the referral of visceral pain, may also apply to the referral of muscle pain. This is because of the extensive convergence of sensory afferent inputs to the dorsal horn, with neurons to which muscle afferents project, also processing noxious information generated in nociceptors in other tissues, including viscera.

The assumption underlying these two theories with respect to the referral of MTrP pain is that this takes place because information transmitted centripetally from these dorsal horn-situated convergent neurons is not sufficiently specific for the brain to be able to distinguish between inputs to the spinal cord from various sources. The validity

of this supposition, however, has to be questioned in view of people usually having little or no difficulty in determining whether a pain is arising from either skin, muscle or a viscus.

### Central sensitisation

Animal experiments carried out by Mense (1990, 1994) have shown that dorsal horn neurons with sensory afferent inputs from nociceptors in a muscle are capable of changing both the size and number of their receptive fields in response to the application of a noxious stimulus to the muscle. Mense (2001), therefore, suggests that the referral of MTrP pain may be due to the neuroplastic changes that develop in dorsal horn neurons in the phenomenon known as central sensitisation with, as part of this process, enlargement and increased sensitivity of dormant nociceptive neurons' receptive fields and a concomitant opening up of previously silent synaptic connections.

### Specific patterns of MTrP pain referral

It has for long been known that pain referred from MTrPs does not follow a segmental or nerve root distribution pattern (Travell & Bigelow 1946). It is no doubt because of this that the majority of clinicians, when presented with pain of MTrP origin, fail to recognize it as being of organic origin (Bonica 1957). Yet, as discussed in Chapter 5, it was at least 50 years ago that Good in Britain, Kelly in Australia and Travell & her colleagues in America, all showed in numerous profusely illustrated reports, that each individual muscle in the body has its own specific pattern of TrP pain referral.

Admittedly, the clinical picture becomes somewhat confused when, as so often happens, there is a composite pain pattern due to more than one muscle being affected. However, knowledge of all the various individual patterns, each of which has to be learnt separately, reduces the chances of overlooking the myofascial origin of such pain and gives much needed guidance as to which muscles in particular should be examined in order to find the TrPs responsible for it.

With respect to this, it should be noted that, although MTrPs are exquisitely tender to touch, somewhat surprisingly, patients themselves are nearly always totally unaware of their presence and, therefore, cannot be of any assistance when a search for them is being made. It also has to be remembered that pain from any one TrP is often felt a considerable distance away from it. For example, TrP activity in the levator scapulae muscle gives rise to pain that is felt not only at the base of the neck and down along the inner border of the scapula but it may also extend upwards towards the occiput, downwards along the inner side of the arm and occasionally around the chest wall. It is because a knowledge of the various specific patterns of MTrP pain referral is therefore so essential that, during the course of this book, each one will be described in detail.

### Directions in which MTrP pain is referred

Simons (1993) has estimated that in 48% of muscles MTrP pain is referred in a downwards direction; in 17% it is referred both locally and downwards; in 10% it is confined to the region around the MTrP; in 20% it is in an upwards and downwards direction; and in only 5% is it in an upwards direction alone.

**MTrP pain pathways and their relationship to those taken by Chinese acu-tracts**    When, during the 17th century, news reached the Western world that the Chinese believed in the existence of structures now known in the West as acu-tracts, channels or meridians and had precisely defined the various courses taken by them, they were immediately dismissed as figments of their imagination, as it was impossible to demonstrate their presence anatomically. However, when one comes to study the paths taken by pain referred from MTrPs it is remarkable how often these coincide with those of Chinese acu-tracts.

Macdonald (1982) describes how he persuaded 52 consecutive patients with chronic musculoskeletal pain seen in his practice, to draw maps of their pain on diagrams of the human body. Somewhat to his surprise, he found that 85% of them drew thin lines linking one area of pain with another. And even more surprisingly he found that 96% of these thin lines corresponded with that of the course taken by one or another of the acu-tracts (meridians) described by the ancient Chinese.

One of his patient's response to needle stimulation was particularly remarkable insomuch as

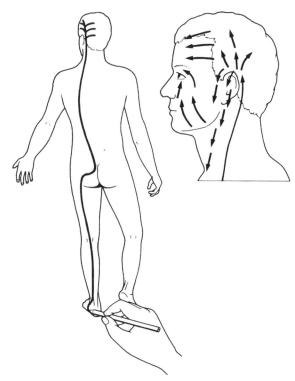

**Figure 7.4**    The pattern of sensation drawn by a patient on an outline of the body following the insertion of a needle into his heel. Reproduced with permission from Alexander Macdonald's *Acupuncture from Ancient Art to Modern Medicine*, 1982.

that whenever a needle was inserted into him he had a feeling of 'warm water' flowing from it; and, although the patient had no previous knowledge of Chinese acupuncture, when needles were inserted into various parts of his body, the paths taken by this 'water' coincided with those taken by meridians. Figure 7.4 shows the drawing the patient made of the path taken by it flowing up his leg and back from a needle inserted into the heel and by comparing it with Figure 7. 5 it will be seen that this is identical with that taken by the traditional Chinese 'urinary bladder' meridian.

### Needle-evoked sensations

As will also be discussed in Chapter 10, from the time that the Chinese first began to practise acupuncture they have described various sensations that may be elicited as a result of inserting a needle into an acupuncture point. These are

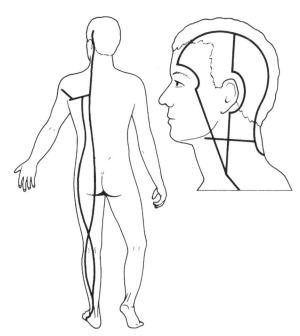

**Figure 7.5**   Composite drawing of the urinary bladder meridians taken from several traditional Chinese sources. It will be seen that the course taken is much the same as the pattern of sensation drawn by the patient in Figure 7.1. Reproduced with permission from Alexander Macdonald's *Acupuncture from Ancient Art to Modern Medicine*, 1982.

collectively known as tê-chhi (sometimes in Western literature spelt de-qi). They include numbness, distension, aching, heaviness and soreness. In most cases a sensation of this type remains confined to the site where the needle is inserted, but occasionally it radiates some distance from it and in rare instances it travels along the entire course taken by a traditional Chinese acu-tract. When this happens it is known as propagated sensation along a channel (PSC).

The Cooperative Group of Investigation of PSC (1980) in China studied the distribution of these needle sensations in 64 228 patients and found that these were localized in the majority of them. However, about 20% of the patients described sensations that radiated for short distances and about 0.4% of them had sensations propagated along a channel.

The Research Group of Acupuncture Anaesthesia at the Institute of Medicine and Pharmacology in the Fujian Province of China reported

in 1986 that mechanically compressing, cooling, or locally anaesthetizing the soft tissues at some site along the course of a PSC blocked its spread. Such an observation is somewhat surprising for it tends to support what is now generally accepted to be the untenable belief that acupuncture tracts or what in the West have come to be known as meridians are anatomical structures.

It would seem far more likely, as Becker et al (1976) have pointed out, that such channels and the propagated sensations along them owe their existence to some as yet unidentified electrical activity in the central nervous system.

In support of this are observations made by Xue (1986), which led him to believe that PSC occurs as a result of activity in the parietal cortex. He came to this conclusion from descriptions of pain referral given to him by patients with a variety of different neurosurgical disorders. One of the most striking of these was that of a below-knee amputee who described propagation of sensation from a point on his stump not only upwards along the surface of it but also downwards into his phantom limb. It is, possible therefore, that the ancient Chinese evolved their ideas concerning acu-tracts or channels from similarly observing the pathways taken by pain arising both spontaneously and in response to needle stimulation.

## Diagnosis of MTrP pain syndrome

As there are no laboratory tests or routine imaging techniques currently available to assist with confirming the presence of this syndrome its diagnosis can only be made by means of a carefully taken case history and the skilled elicitation of a number of characteristic physical signs.

### Symptoms

**Pain**   The nociceptive type of pain which arises as a result of MTrP activity in the MtrP pain syndrome typically takes the form of a widespread dull ache exacerbated by the carrying out of certain movements. This is in contrast to the burning or electric shock-like sensations experienced by patients with neuropathic pain.

The syndrome is usually confined to one region of the body but in some cases it affects several regions concomitantly with the pain then being generalized in the same way as it invariably is in patients with fibromyalgia.

**Restricted movements** A muscle containing one or more active MTrPs becomes shortened and because of both this and the nociceptive pain, movements are liable to be restricted. This restriction may either be a symptom complained of by the patient, or a physical sign elicited on examination.

**Muscle weakness** TrP activity in muscles is liable to weaken them with, as a consequence, difficulty in the carrying out of certain movements.

**Sleep disturbance** Sleep is liable to be disturbed when the posture adopted for this causes pressure to be applied to active MTrPs with, as a consequence, exacerbation of the pain. This sleep disturbance, however, is never as severe or as disabling as that experienced by patients with fibromyalgia.

**Sympathetically–mediated symptoms** As there are sympathetic fibres at a MTrP site (see Fig. 7.1), it is hardly surprising that MTrP activity is not infrequently associated with the development of sympathetically-mediated symptoms. These include the pilomotor changes of goose flesh and localized sweating, with each of these appearing either spontaneously or when pressure is applied to the tissues overlying an active MTrP. The one, however, which often proves to be the most troublesome is intense coldness of the distal part of a limb as is shown by the following case.

A female (35 years of age), who had been complaining of persistent intense coldness of the right foot for 3 years, was referred to a vascular surgeon for an opinion as to whether a sympathectomy might be helpful. No operation was advised but shortly after, as she had been complaining of pain around the right hip for the same period of time, she informed her doctor that she would like to try the effects of acupuncture and so was sent to see me.

On examination, she had exquisitely tender TrPs at the insertion of muscles into the greater trochanter and also along the tensor fasciae latae. And once these had been deactivated by means of the carrying out of superficial dry needling (see Ch. 10) on a few occasions she not only lost her pain but in addition the right foot, subjectively, became as warm as the left one.

*Physical signs*

**The search for MTrPs** The locating of active MTrPs is clearly the most important part of the clinical examination. The technique required for carrying this out, however, requires much skill and practice. It is therefore unfortunate that medical students are still not being taught how to do this because as discussed in Chapter 4, it was before World War II that John Kellgren, by carefully designed experiments and shrewd clinical observations, made fundamental contributions to our understanding of the importance of TrPs as a common source of pain. The failure of most clinical teachers to recognize this is shown by there still being little or no mention of the MTrP pain syndrome in any of the standard undergraduate textbooks.

One reason why so little attention is paid to this disorder is because muscle pain in general is still all too frequently erroneously considered to be no more than a self-limiting minor disability of no particular importance. The result of this attitude is that whenever persistent and severe pain affects the musculoskeletal system, the muscles themselves are given no more than a perfunctory examination, whilst skeletal structures such as the joints, bones and intervertebral discs are subjected to close scrutiny with particular attention paid to changes detected either radiographically or in some cases by magnetic resonance imaging.

The potential danger of this is that should some irrelevant abnormality be discovered during the course of carrying out investigations such as these it may be accorded undue significance. Alternatively, should none be found then the pain is liable to be considered to be of little or no consequence. Furthermore, if, in spite of reassurance that nothing serious has been found, the patient has the temerity to continue to complain about the pain, there is always the risk that it will be assumed to be of psychological origin without the possibility of its emanation from MTrPs ever having even been considered. The following case history exemplifies this.

A secretary (42 years of age), who had complained of persistent low-back pain for 2 years, was referred to an orthopaedic surgeon who, in view of radiographs of the lumbar spine and sacro-iliac joints showing no significant abnormality, informed her that there was nothing serious to worry about and gave no specific therapeutic advice. As the pain continued to be disabling she was next referred to a gynaecologist who decided to carry out a dilatation and curettage. No abnormality was found but 10 days post-operatively she had a pulmonary infarct!

Her general practitioner then finding that she had marital problems decided that the low-back pain must be associated with these and referred her to a psychiatrist. The latter, however, to his credit came to the conclusion that her disability was physical in origin. This led the patient to ask whether acupuncture might be of help and she was referred to me for an opinion about this.

On examination of the back several MTrPs were located, and after these had been deactivated by means of the superficial dry needling technique described in Chapter 10 on five occasions at weekly intervals she lost her long-standing pain.

Another mistake often made is to assume that pain that radiates down a limb must be due to nerve root entrapment even when there are no objective neurological signs to support this diagnosis and when the possibility that it might have been referred from MTrPs has not even been taken into consideration.

It therefore cannot be stressed too strongly that in the investigation of pain of uncertain origin a search for MTrPs is mandatory. Guidance as to which muscles are likely to contain these is obtained by paying careful attention to the distribution of the pain and by observing which movements of the body are restricted. Each muscle under suspicion should then be placed slightly on the stretch and systematically palpated with the tips of the fingers drawn firmly across it in a manner similar to that employed when kneading dough. The necessity for employing firm pressure has to be emphasized because, otherwise, TrPs are liable to be overlooked. When this type of flat palpation is carried out over a normal muscle it causes no discomfort. In the vicinity of a TrP it is slightly uncomfortable. And over a TrP itself, because this is a site where nociceptors are in a state of activation and sensitisation, the tenderness is so great as to cause the patient to carry out an involuntary flexion withdrawal reflex (the 'jump'

sign) and in some cases to utter an expletive (the 'shout' sign).

It is my personal preference when searching for TrPs, which by definition are points of maximum tenderness, to employ the flat palpation technique just described for all muscles. Some authorities advocate the use of pincer palpation for those muscles that can readily be squeezed between the thumb and fingers. However, this, in my view, cannot be recommended, as even a healthy muscle is extremely tender when compressed in this manner (Lewis 1942).

**Pain reproduction**   The application of pressure to an active MTrP for about 10–15 seconds results in the patient's spontaneously occurring pain being reproduced. As Gerwin (1999), however, has pointed out the reliability of this test depends on whether or not the patient is able to provide relevant information concerning what is felt. Another difficulty, as Hong et al (1996) have said, is that pain may be referred from a latent MTrP should it be subjected to particularly strong pressure.

**Palpable taut bands**   A MTrP that is no more than a few millimetres in diameter is often to be found at the centre of a palpable taut band several centimetres in length.

There is much controversy as to what causes bands of this type to develop, particularly as they have been found to be present not only in muscles of patients with the MTrP pain syndrome, but also in muscles of seemingly healthy people (Wolfe et al 1992, Njoo &Van der Does 1994).

With respect to all this, it has to be remembered, as explained earlier, that a MTrP contains a number of dysfunctional motor endplates and the muscle fibres to which these are attached become markedly contracted with the development of several knots. It is possible, therefore, that MTrP-related bands develop because of the increased tension that develops both in these contraction knots and in the elongated sarcomeres on either side of them (Simons et al 1999).

As bands of this type may be found in otherwise healthy people and because it is only possible to palpate them in superficially placed muscles, it necessarily follows that the eliciting of them cannot be made one of the essential criteria required for the diagnosis of the MTrP pain syndrome.

**Local twitch response** If a finger is drawn sharply across a palpable band in a manner similar to that employed when plucking a violin string it is possible to evoke a transient contraction of the muscle fibres. This local twitch response (LTR) may either be visible or detected under the examining finger. In some cases it is both seen and felt.

A LTR may also be elicited when, during the course of carrying out the therapeutic procedure known as deep dry needling (see Ch. 10), a needle is rapidly thrust into a MTrP. The reason for this is thought to be because of needle-induced stimulation of the MTrP's nociceptors giving rise to a sensory afferent barrage which, on reaching the spinal cord, sets up reflex motor efferent activity.

Gerwin & Duranleau (1997) have shown that it is possible to visualize LTRs by means of the use of ultrasound imaging.

**Tender nodules** Tender nodules that are mainly found in muscles in the lower part of the back and, to a lesser extent, in muscles in the neck and shoulder region, have over the years given rise to such considerable controversy concerning both their morphology and their ability to cause pain, that it will be necessary to discuss these structures at some length.

The first to examine them microscopically was Ralph Stockman at the University of Glasgow who, in 1904, as discussed in Chapter 5, reported that on histological examination he had found their connective tissue to show patches of inflammatory hyperplasia. This led him to conclude that the pain from them arises as a result of sensory nerves becoming stretched or compressed both by fibrous tissue proliferation and by inflamed connective tissue infiltrating the walls of nerves.

It has to be said, however, that the inflammatory type of reaction described by him has never subsequently been confirmed.

The next to investigate these nodules was Schade (1919) who carried out his studies in a German field hospital during World War I. He located these structures in the muscles of a number of soldiers and observed that they continued to be palpable in those of them who, for one reason or another, had to be anaesthetized. He also noted that they were palpable in those who died up to the time of the setting in of rigor mortis. Furthermore, when this group were subjected to post-mortem examinations, the muscles containing them were found to be otherwise normal.

As a result of observing that the nodules continued to be palpable both under deep anaesthesia and after death he concluded that they could not have developed as a result of muscle having gone into spasm. Moreover, he considered that the discovery of normal muscle tissue on histological examination ruled out any possibility that nodules of this type might have developed as a result of structural changes in its connective tissue. He, therefore, suggested that they may have done so as a result of a change in the colloidal state of muscle cytoplasm from sol to gel. And in view of this coined the term myogelose (muscle gelling or myogelosis).

The first extensive well-documented study of carefully selected material designed to demonstrate the histological changes associated with myogelosis was carried out by Glogowski & Wallraff (1951) in Germany. They examined 24 biopsies of what they called muscle hardening (muskelharten), but, despite the use of no less than nine tissue stains were unable to demonstrate any significant abnormalities; they, therefore, concluded that myogelosis must occur at the sarcoplasmic level beyond reach of the light microscope.

In the meantime, in Britain, Copeman & Ackerman (1944) added to the confusion by erroneously concluding that nodules felt in the muscles of patients with low-back pain are nothing more than herniated fat lobules.

It was Brendstrup et al (1957) who carried out the first controlled biopsy and biochemical examination of these nodules. In their study the microscopic appearances of biopsies of paraspinal muscles containing palpable tender nodules were compared with those of biopsies taken from normal contralateral paraspinal muscles in patients undergoing operations for prolapsed intervertebral discs. They stressed that, as the subjects were fully anaesthetized and the muscle relaxed with curare, neither painfulness nor muscle spasm could have been factors in choosing the areas for biopsy and that the selection was done entirely by palpating the nodules.

They found a striking difference between the microscopic appearances of the control biopsy material and of the tissue in which these nodules was present. By staining sections of these nodules with toluidine blue they were able to demonstrate the presence in them of much interstitial oedema containing acid mucopolysaccharides and an accumulation of mast cells. In addition, biochemical analysis showed there to be a much higher concentration of hexosamine and hyaluronic acid in them than in the controls. Hyaluronic acid has a strong water-binding capacity and it was believed it was because of this that the extra-cellular content of the nodules was considerably more than that found in the control material.

Wegelius & Absoe-Hansen (1956) suggested that it may be this oedematous change in a nodule that, by distorting the peripheral nerve endings, contributes to the development of the pain produced by it.

The next person to study nodules of this type was Awad (1973), who took biopsies of muscle in which nodules could be felt from 10 patients and examined them with the electron microscope. Firstly, the skin overlying each nodule to be biopsied was carefully marked with an indelible pen, and then muscle fasicles, approximately 1 cm wide and 2 cm long, were dissected out after the tissues involved had been firmly grasped between the opposing jaws of a modified chalazion clamp. The reason for doing that was partly to prevent the development of muscle contraction artefacts but also to ensure that the fluid content of the muscle remained trapped within the biopsy material.

When examined under the light microscope the muscle fibres appeared normal, except that in every case there seemed to be an increase of interstitial nuclei. However, of much greater significance was the discovery in 8 of the 10 cases of a large amount of amorphous material in between the muscle fasicles which, when stained with toluidine blue, was shown to consist of acid mucopolysaccharides. This substance that is known to have enormous water-binding properties is, under normal conditions, only present in small amounts in muscle extracellular tissue.

On electron microscopic examination, it was noted that this amorphous material distended the spaces between muscle fibres that were themselves of normal appearance. In addition, large clusters of platelets were observed and mast cells were seen to be discharging mucopolysaccharide-containing granules into the intercellular space. The next most common finding of any significance was an increased amount of connective tissue in some of the cases.

They concluded that it is this water-retaining mucopolysaccharide amorphous substance in these nodules that causes them to be space-occuping lesions. That it is the accumulation of this substance in their extracellular tissues that impairs the oxygen flow to muscle fibres and increases their acidity. And that it is this increased acidity that sensitizes muscle sensory nociceptors and converts them into pain-producing TrPs.

Awad (1990) some years later came to the conclusion that several questions still remained to be answered, including: does the mucopolysaccharide in these nodules accumulate as a result of an increased production of this normally occurring substance, or a decrease in its degradation, or a change in its quality?

**Nerve root entrapment caused by TrP–induced muscle shortening**    Trp activity in a muscle causes it to become shortened and at certain sites this gives rise to nerve root entrapment.

The following are three common examples of this: (1) TrP-induced shortening of either the scalenus anterior or pectoralis minor is liable to cause compression of the lower trunk of the brachial plexus; (2) TrP-induced shortening of the piriformis muscle is liable to give rise to compression of the sciatic nerve; and (3) Trp-induced shortening of the peroneus longus is liable to be responsible for entrapment of the peroneal nerve with, as a consequence, the development of a foot drop.

**Degree of interexaminer concordance in eliciting the physical signs of the MTrP pain syndrome**    In recent years there have been several studies carried out for the purpose of assessing the degree of concordance among examiners when attempting to elicit physical signs appertaining to the diagnosis of the MTrP pain syndrome.

In the study reported by Wolfe et al (1992), four physicians experienced in locating MTrPs examined eight patients with MTrP pain syndrome, seven patients with fibromyalgia and eight controls for focal tenderness, pressure-induced reproduction of the pain, pain referral, palpable bands and local twitch responses. Agreement with regard to the elicitation of these signs was poor and it was considered by Simons (1996) that the most likely explanation for this was that differing examination techniques were employed by the participants.

In a study reported by Nice et al (1992), 12 physiotherapists examined the thoracolumbar muscles of 50 patients with low-back pain. They did have a uniformly agreed method of examination for it was laid down that a MTrP could only be considered to be present if the application of firm pressure for 10 seconds to a point of maximum tenderness caused the patient to report the onset of pain at a distance or an increase in the intensity of the pain already present at the point. Agreement among the therapists, however, proved to be poor and one possible reason advanced for this by Simons (1996) was that they had not been adequately trained.

In a study reported by Njoo & Van der Does (1994), a general practitioner in Holland experienced in searching for MTrPs, and four final year medical students trained by him in this skill examined muscles in 61 patients with low-back pain and in 63 controls. Their endeavour was to elicit the same physical signs as those sought in Wolfe et al's study. Out of all those various signs, only localized tenderness with its associated 'jump' sign and pain recognition were generally agreed to be reliable ones. Furthermore, it was considered that the high level of concordance among those taking part in this study was a reflection of the satisfactory amount of training each of them had received.

That inter-examiner agreement can be improved by training has been shown by two studies carried out by Gerwin et al (1995). In the first of these, four clinicians examined 25 people for muscle tenderness, palpable bands, local twitch responses, and referred pain. Agreement among them concerning the elicitation of these signs was poor. Twenty-one months later, however, after the same physicians had been given intensive training, a very satisfactory amount of agreement among them was achieved.

## Criteria for the diagnosis of the MTrP pain syndrome

There are currently no generally accepted criteria for the diagnosis of the MTrP pain syndrome, but

what is certain is that there is much to be said for keeping these as simple and as non-controversial as possible.

As previously stated, the palpation of a taut band at a TrP site and the elicitation of a local twitch response by 'plucking' it cannot be included amongst them, as it is only possible to demonstrate these two physical signs when the muscle containing the TrP is a superficially placed one.

The only widely agreed essential one is the presence of one or more points of maximum tenderness detected by the evocation of 'jump' and 'shout' reactions in response to the application of firm pressure. This, however, by itself does not allow a distinction to be made between active and latent TrPs. A further prerequisite, therefore, insisted upon by some authorities is the reproduction of the spontaneously occurring pain by means of the application of sustained pressure to each of the TrPs. However, in my opinion such a procedure subjects the patient to much unnecessary discomfort. My grounds for saying this are because, when in the absence of any other obvious pain-producing disorder, TrPs are found to be present in a region of the body affected by a persistent dull aching type of pain, it is reasonable to assume that this must be emanating from them. And any relief of it obtained by the carrying out of a MTrP-deactivating procedure further helps to confirm the diagnosis.

It must have been considerations such as these that led Yunus (1993) to cogently comment 'why should all patients with regional musculoskeletal pain not be classified as having the myofascial pain syndrome on the basis of pain and tender points alone?' A difficulty arises, however, with respect to this when the pain is generalized for then it is necessary to decide whether the patient is suffering from fibromyalgia or the MTrP pain syndrome affecting several regions of the body simultaneously. Clearly, in order to make this distinction other considerations have to be taken into account including whether or not the various other characteristic clinical manifestations of fibromyalgia are present.

## Regional MTrP pain syndromes

Before concluding this discussion concerning various aspects of the MTrP pain syndrome it is necessary to make clear that this is a term that is employed collectively to include a number of individual regional syndromes that will be considered in turn in Part 3 of this book.

## Investigatory procedures

### Algometry

As, by definition, a MTrP is a point of maximum tenderness, its presence may be determined semi-objectively by measuring the pressure threshold over it and comparing this with that obtained over a corresponding contralateral non-tender point. The pressure threshold is the minimum pressure or force that induces discomfort. The instrument for measuring this, known as an algometer, or pressure threshold meter (Fig. 7.6), is a force gauge fitted with a disc-shaped rubber tip which has a surface area of $1\,cm^2$. The gauge is calibrated in $kg/cm^2$ with a range of measurements up to 11 kg.

Before carrying out pressure threshold measurements on patients with MTrP pain, it is essential for them to be in a relaxed state and to have been given a detailed explanation of the procedure. This involves locating a MTrP by means of manual palpation, and then, whilst the instrument is held

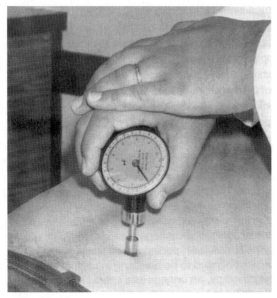

**Figure 7.6** Pressure threshold meter. Reproduced with the permission of Mr R. J. D'Souza.

against it at an angle of 90°, applying steady pressure until the patient reports the onset of discomfort. This should be done before and after the deactivation of a MTrP. For once the latter has been carried out the pressure threshold over a MTrP increases by about 4 kg. (Fischer 1988a).

Although there is little or nothing to be gained by measuring the pressure threshold at a MTrP site in everyday clinical practice, this semi-objective measurement should potentially be of considerable help to those doctors and lawyers involved in making decisions concerning compensation in cases of persistent post-accident MTrP pain. In addition, in clinical trials, its measurement before and after the carrying out of a MTrP deactivation procedure is of much value in assessing the efficacy of this (Fischer 1988b).

Fischer (1998c) and Hong (1998) have provided comprehensive reviews of current knowledge concerning the use of this instrument both for identifying the presence of MTrPs and for assessing the therapeutic effectiveness of various MTrP deactivating procedures.

### Thermography

Thermography may be carried out by one or other of three methods. These are infrared radiometry, a method employing films of liquid crystals and a computer-analysis controlled electronic infrared radiation technique.

This method of investigation is used to study temperature changes in the skin overlying a MTrP and its zone of pain referral.

### Temperature changes in skin at a MTrP site

The typical thermographic finding in the skin immediately overlying a MTrP is a discoid hot spot 5–10 cm in diameter. This is produced as a result of the skin at that site being 0.5–1.0°C warmer than the adjacent skin (Fischer 1986, 1998, Fischer & Chang 1986, Kruse & Christiansen 1992).

A thermographic recorded temperature change of this type, however, is not confined to the skin overlying a MTrP for, as Simons (2001, p. 221) has pointed out, it is equally liable to be found in the presence of a radiculopathy, articular dysfunction, enthesopathy and local subcutaneous inflammation.

It, therefore, follows that this investigation cannot be used specifically for the identification of MTrPs.

### Pressure-induced temperature changes at a MTrP's zone of pain referral

In a controlled study carried out by Kruse & Christiansen (1992), an algometer was used to apply sufficient pressure to MTrPs to produce referred pain. This pressure was maintained for 1 minutes and during this time thermographs were recorded both over the MTrPs and their zones of pain referral every 15 s.

They found a significant lowering of the temperature not only in the zones of pain referral but also well beyond these.

### TrPs in skin, ligaments and periosteum

Although TrPs are most commonly present in muscle they are also liable to be found in the skin, ligaments and periosteum.

**Skin** TrPs may become activated in seemingly normal skin and cause pain of a moderately severe sharp stinging type to be referred either locally or at a distance (Sinclair 1949, Trommer & Gellman 1952). In my experience these are most commonly to be found in skin scars where they give rise to a burning, pricking or electric-shock type of pain. It is particularly important to remember this possibility when investigating the cause of persistent post-operative pain.

With respect to the treatment of this latter type of pain, it should be noted that, although it is impossible to push a needle into a tough fibrous scar, a TrP in such tissue may readily be deactivated by inserting the needle into the healthy subcutaneous tissue immediately lateral to the scar at the appropriate level. The treatment of the following case exemplifies this.

A female (46 year of age) had a very badly infected appendix removed. Five months after this, because of chronic pelvic sepsis, she had to have the right ovary and fallopian tube taken away, and 1 year later she underwent a hysterectomy. Soon after this she started to complain of intermittent but severe jabs of pain in the right lower part of the abdomen. As this continued for several months, she was extensively investigated, but when no visceral cause for it was found, she was referred to me to assess whether or not acupuncture might be of help.

On examination, there were exquisitely tender TrPs in the midline scar. And as a result of deactivating these by the needling technique described above on three occasions the pain disappeared.

**Ligaments** TrPs in the ligaments of joints are also a frequent cause of pain and yet are frequently overlooked despite Leriche in 1930 having drawn attention to the manner in which they develop in these structures following fractures and sprains. Gorrell (1976) has also discussed the diagnosis and treatment of pain emanating from TrPs in ligaments around the ankle. In addition, de Valera & Raftery (1976) have shown that pain emanating from TrPs in strained pelvic ligaments may be relieved by injecting these points with a local anaesthetic.

It has subsequently become evident that TrPs in a structure of this type can equally well be deactivated by means of the far simpler superficial dry needling technique to be described in Chapter 10.

**Periosteum** Kellgren (1939), by experimentally injecting hypertonic saline into periosteum artificially created TrPs in it and observed that pain from these was referred either locally or to a distant site. Inman & Saunders (1944) confirmed this and drew attention to the importance of periosteal TrPs as a source of pain in various musculoskeletal disorders. And Mann (1974) since then has devised a technique he calls periosteal pecking for the alleviation of musculoskeletal pain.

## FIBROMYALGIA SYNDROME

There have been several recently published comprehensive reviews of this commonly occurring syndrome that affects women some 10–20 times more than men. Included amongst these are ones by Bennett (1999), Chaitow (2003), Russell (2001), and Yunus & Inanici (2001).

## Symptoms

### Pain

The pain is most often described as being of a diffuse deep aching in the muscles. In addition, there is sometimes discomfort around the joints in the absence of any objective evidence of these being swollen (Reilly & Littlejohn 1992).

There is also much early morning stiffness with both this and the pain being typically worst between 11 am and 3 pm (Moldofsky 1994).

The intensity of the pain is liable to fluctuate with exacerbations of it being brought on by such factors as excessive exertion, trauma, stress and cold damp weather.

Unlike the MTrP pain syndrome, in which the pain is confined to one region of the body except when several regions are affected concurrently, fibromyalgia syndrome (FS) pain is invariably widespread. The only exception to this is the very occasional case where, at an early stage of the disease, it is localized to one particular site. An example is when it is initially confined to the chest wall (Pellegrino 1990). When this happens, other disorders such as costochondritis, Tietzes's disease and coronary heart disease clearly need to be included in the differential diagnosis.

There is, in addition generalized hyperalgesia (i.e. increased responsiveness to a noxious stimulus such as a pin prick) and widespread allodynia (i.e. pain brought on by some innocuous stimulus such as touch).

## Non-restorative sleep

It is common for there to be a persistent feeling of tiredness due to non-restorative sleep. This sleep disturbance was first investigated electroencephalographically by Moldofsky et al (1975) and again more recently by Hyyppa & Kronholm (1995).

These studies have shown that there is an intrusion of stage 1 rapid eye movement light sleep with fast alpha waves into stage 1V deep restorative sleep with slow delta waves.

Carette et al (1995), however, have only found these electroencephalographic changes to be present in one-third of patients with FS. Moreover, they are not confined to patients with this particular syndrome; Moldofsky et al (1983) have recorded them in a group of patients with rheumatoid arthritis.

## Reactive depression

There are conflicting findings concerning the incidence of reactive depression in patients with

FS but overall there are grounds for believing that about 30–40% of them suffer from it. This is a much higher incidence than that found in the general population, but one that is comparable to that present in patients with rheumatoid arthritis (Ahles et al 1991). However, this is as might be expected considering that these two disorders have similar pain severity, morning stiffness and physical function limitation (Cathey et al 1988), the factors that would seem to be mainly responsible for the development of this particular psychological disturbance.

## Dizziness and light headedness

These symptoms are frequently complained of by people with FS. They tend to be particularly noticeable on getting up from a seated or recumbent position and following long-term immobility. There is often, in addition, a feeling of impending syncope but an overt vasovagal attack is uncommon.

There is now reason to believe that an autonomic nervous system dysfunction present in patients with FS (see p. 95) is most often responsible. Other FS-related causes for it that have to be considered include proprioceptive dysfunction due to MTrP activity in a sternocleidomastoid muscle (see Ch. 16) and drug-induced hypotension. Disorders unrelated to FS, such as brainstem ischaemia and drop attacks of uncertain origin, also have to be included in the differential diagnosis.

## Other complaints

Tension headaches, a subjective feeling of swelling in the small joints and paraesthesiae are also commonly present. In addition, some patients develop a poor memory for recent events and a lack of concentration (Landro et al 1997). It seems likely that both of these are due to the distracting effect of chronic pain and the psychological distress that accompanies this (Kurtze et al 1998, Sletvold et al 1995).

## Associated disorders

### Irritable bowel syndrome

This commonly occurring disorder that affects about one-fifth of the general population has been found to be present in approximately two-thirds of patients with FS (Sivri et al 1996).

### Female urethral syndrome

This disorder, in which there is suprapubic discomfort, frequency, dysuria and urgency is liable to affect about 50% of women with FS (Clauw et al 1997).

### Restless leg syndrome

This syndrome, which was first described by Ekbom (1960) in otherwise fit people, has been found to be present in about one-third of patients with FS (Yunus & Aldag 1996).

In this disorder the patient suffers from numbness and tingling in the legs that is relieved by stretching or walking. It usually comes on when the person is sitting down to relax of an evening and is temporarily relieved by walking around. It then becomes worse again when the patient goes to bed and interferes with any attempt to get off to sleep.

### Raynaud's phenomenon

This is liable to develop in about 40% of patients with FS (Dinerman et al 1986, Vaeroy et al 1988).

## Factors that predispose to the development of FS

When discussing these it has to be said at the outset that despite much extensive research in recent years the aetiology of the disorder remains far from certain.

### Genetic predisposition

There is a strong family prevalence of FS (Buskila et al 1996, Pellegrino et al 1989) suggesting that it may well be genetically determined.

### Trauma

An appreciable number of FS sufferers state that their illness has developed following their subjection to trauma (Aaron et al 1997, Greenfield et al 1992, Waylonis & Perkins 1994).

The strongest evidence to support an association between trauma and FS is that provided by Buskila et al (1997) who observed a high prevalence of FS (22%) in patients who had been subjected to a cervical spine whiplash injury.

It has to be said, however, that in contrast to this he only found that a small number (1% prevalence) of those who had accidents causing them to fracture legs developed it.

Evidence that trauma, in some as yet unexplained way, would seem to be one of the causes for FS developing clearly has important medico-legal implications (Buskila & Neumann 2002).

Bennett (1999) has suggested that one possible reason why patients with whiplash injuries are particularly liable to develop FS is because trauma to the neck muscles may be a particularly potent evoker of central sensitisation which, as discussed later, is known to be a major pathophysiological feature of this disorder.

Clauw (2002) has pointed out that various regional pain syndromes including the MTrP pain syndrome, temporomandibular joint dysfunction, costochondritis and vulvodynia (dyspareunia and vulvar sensitivity) may eventually be followed by the development of FS. He is of the opinion that the most likely reason for this happening is the development of central sensitisation.

### Concomitant inflammatory diseases

FS not infrequently develops in conjunction with rheumatoid arthritis (Urrows et al 1994), systemic lupus erythematosus (Middleton et al 1994) and Sjogren's syndrome (Bonafede et al 1995).

One possible reason for this is that any one of these chronic inflammatory diseases is liable to be responsible for the development of a nociceptor-activity-induced sensory afferent barrage that gives rise to central sensitisation with, as a consequence, the amplification of pain and the development of FS. A genetic predisposition may well be an additional factor.

## Systemic syndromes with similar symptomatology

Disorders with symptoms that are liable to simulate those of FS include chronic fatigue syndrome, somatization disorder (Briquet's syndrome) and conversion disorder. In addition, various exposure disorders have similar symptoms, such as sick building syndrome, Gulf War syndrome and post-silicone breast implant syndrome (Clauw 2002). Also, polymyalgia rheumatica, medication with the cholesterol-lowering statin group of drugs and adult growth hormone deficiency can all cause symptoms seen in FS.

## Diagnostic criteria

The American College of Rheumatology 1990 Criteria for the *classification* of fibromyalgia (Wolfe et al 1990) include a history of widespread spontaneously occurring pain, and pain that is evoked on digital palpation at 11 of 18 specifically defined tender point sites.

### Widespread pain

Pain is considered to be widespread when it affects both sides of the body both above and below the waist. In addition, axial skeletal pain (cervical spine, anterior chest, thoracic spine or low back) must be present. Low-back pain is categorized as lower segment pain.

### Tender points

Pain on digital palpation must be present in at least 11 of the following nine bilateral tender point (TP) sites (Fig. 7. 7):

Occiput: bilateral, at the suboccipital muscle insertions.
Low cervical: bilateral, at the anterior aspects of the intertransverse spaces at C5–C7.
Trapezius: bilateral, at the midpoint of the upper border.
Supraspinatus: bilateral, at origins above the scapula spine near the medial border.
Second rib: bilateral, at the second costochondral junctions.
Lateral epicondyle: bilateral, 2 cm distal to the epicondyles.
Gluteal: bilateral, in upper outer quadrant of buttock in anterior fold of muscle.
Greater trochanter: bilateral, posterior to the trochanteric prominence.
Knee: bilateral, at the medial fat pad proximal to the joint line.

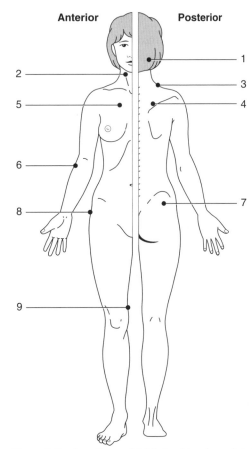

**Figure 7.7** Locations of 9 bilateral tender point sites to be palpated for testing American College of Rheumatology criteria for classification of FMS. 1, occiput; 2, low cervical; 3, trapezius; 4, supraspinatus; 5, second rib; 6, lateral epicondyle; 7, gluteal; 8, greater trochanter; 9, knee. Reproduced from Yunus (1992), with permission.

These classification criteria have proved to be extremely useful when employed for the purpose of standardizing research protocols. However, as pointed out in the consensus document on fibromyalgia – The Copenhagen Declaration (WHO 1993) and again by Wolfe et al (1995) many patients with otherwise typical manifestations of FS have less than 11 tender points (TPs). Furthermore, although the maximum number of these in the above classification is 18, as Bennett (1999) states, this only accounts for about 3% of potential TP locations. Modification of these classification criteria is therefore permissible when diagnosing the disorder in everyday clinical practice.

## The difference between tender points and TrPs

A TrP, as defined in the above criteria, is a point of maximum tenderness with the application to it of firm pressure (i.e. 4 kg or approximately the pressure required to blanch the nail of the palpating finger), giving rise to pain confined to that site. This, therefore, is in contrast to the referral of pain to a distant site as happens when pressure is applied to an active TrP as was discussed earlier when considering the MTrP pain syndrome.

## Conjoint presence of tender points and TrPs

Although those who formulated the currently accepted criteria for the classification of FS drew special attention to the pathognomonic importance of TPs it is evident that TrPs may also be present.

Bengtsson et al (1986) were among the first to report that patients with FS may have both TPs and TrPs having found one or more of the latter to be present in 83.6% of 55 people with this disorder.

Others who have observed this include Granges & Littlejohn (1993) who found that out of a group of 60 patients with FS, 41(68.3%) had TrPs. And Gerwin (1995), who in a study of 25 patients with FS found that 18 (72%) of them had TrPs.

## Pathophysiology of FS

Three important pathophysiological features are central sensitisation, abnormal levels of neurotransmitters and sympathetic hyperactivity.

### Central sensitisation

As discussed in Chapter 6, central sensitisation with hyperexcitability of dorsal-horn-situated nociceptive neurons develops whenever these cells are subjected to a sustained sensory afferent barrage as a result of C-polymodal or Group IV nociceptor activity developing, either because of an inflammatory lesion or a nerve injury (Coderre et al 1993, Devor 1988, Doubell et al 1999, Dubner & Basbaum 1994).

The effects of this central sensitisation include an increased response to a noxious stimulus (hyperalgesia) and the development of pain in response to an innocuous stimulus such as that produced by massaging or touching the skin (allodynia). As both of these phenomena are invariably present in patients with FS, it is clear that this dorsal horn pathophysiological change is an essential feature of this disorder.

In many cases there is an obvious reason for this happening. Trauma is the commonest but other possible causes include either an infection (viral or bacterial) or some inflammatory process such as that brought about by rheumatoid arthritis or systemic lupus erythematosus.

It has to be remembered, with respect to all this, that central sensitisation continues long after its initial peripheral causative stimulus has ceased to be operative (Coderre et al 1993).

Yunus & Inanici (2001) believe that certain susceptible individuals with FS may develop central sensitisation spontaneously in the absence of any peripheral nociceptive stimulation because of 'either a defective inhibitory system or a hyperstimulated facilitatory pathway'.

### Altered serotonin (5–hydroxytryptamine, 5–HT) levels in vascular system

Russell & Vipraio (1994) have shown that there is an abnormally low level of serotonin in the platelets and, consequently, also in the serum of patients with FS.

Wolfe et al (1997) have shown that the serum levels of this neurotransmitter correlate with the number of TPs present in individuals fulfilling the classification criteria for FS.

Klein et al (1992) reported finding high titres of anti 5-HT and immunoglobulin (IgG, IgM) antibodies in the serum of patients with FS. This raised the possibility that an autoimmune process might be responsible for the low levels of 5-HT in the sera and platelets of patients with FS. Subsequent studies, however, have so far failed to show that these serum antibodies are increased in this disorder (Russell et al 1995, Vedder & Bennett 1995).

### Altered serotonin level in central nervous system

When dietary protein is digested in the gut the resultant amino acid tryptophan is absorbed through the intestinal mucosa and conveyed to the nucleus raphe magnus (NRM) in the midbrain.

Neurons in the NRM convert it to serotonin and this then acts as the neurotransmitter in the pain inhibitory system that descends from it.

Although the level of serotonin (5-HT) in the cerebrospinal fluid (CSF) of patients with FS has not been measured, the levels of its precursor, 5-hydroxy-tryptophan, and its metabolic product, 5-hydroxyindole acetic acid, have. And both of them have been found to be significantly lowered (Russell et al 1992, Russell et al 1993). Thus indicating that there must be a deficiency of this neurotransmitter in the central nervous system where its presence is so essential for the regulation of the nociceptive control process.

## Altered substance P level in the central nervous system

This neuropeptide that is released from A-delta, C-polymodal and Group IV sensory afferent terminals in the dorsal horn's Laminae I, II, and V is believed to facilitate the nociceptive processes that take place at these three intra-spinal sites. From these it diffuses out into the CSF and, therefore, measuring the amount of it there provides information concerning the quantity of it present in the dorsal horn.

Vaeroy et al (1988) were the first to report a significant increase in the amount of SP in the CSF of patients with FS in comparison to that found in healthy normal controls. Since then three other studies have confirmed this finding (Bradley et al 1996, Russell et al 1994, Welin et al 1995).

In each of these studies only one test was carried out on each subject and because this provided no indication as to whether SP elevation in the CSF remains constant or fluctuates in accordance with changes in a patient's pain intensity, Russell et al (1998) decided to carry out a study in which CSF samples were collected from FS patients at monthly intervals over the course of 1 year. Their findings led them to conclude that the SP level changes appeared to be integrally related to changes in the severity of the pain experienced by patients with FS.

## Dysfunction of the autonomic nervous system

There is now much evidence to show that dysfunction of the autonomic nervous system has a considerable role in the development of many of the clinical manifestations of FS. Knowledge concerning this has been greatly advanced by the introduction of the technique known as heart rate variability analysis (Martinez-Lavin 2002).

Because the heart rate normally varies frequently and randomly due to the opposing effects of the sympathetic and parasympathetic nervous systems on the sinoatrial node, Martinez-Lavin et al (1998) studied the heart rate variability of 30 patients with FS and 30 age/sex matched controls over 24 hour periods using a Holter monitor. The outstanding advantage of this particular study over previous ones was that the technique allowed the monitoring to be carried out during both normal daytime activities and sleeping.

The results showed that patients with FS had less heart rate variability over 24 hours than did those in the control group. It was considered that this was due to decreased parasympathetic influx and conversely increased sympathetic influx on the sinus node.

These FS patients also had an altered circadian variation of the sympathetic–parasympathetic balance with changes consistent with nocturnal sympathetic hyperactivity.

This circadian variation in the sympathetic–parasympathetic balance with dominant sympathetic hyperactivity, particularly nocturnally, has been confirmed by others (Cohen et al 2000, Cohen et al 2001, Raj et al 2000).

Martinez-Lavin (2002) believes that this sympathetic hyperactivity both day and night, particularly nocturnally, may well offer an explanation for the development of many of FS's clinical manifestations. At night, for example, it would account for the interference with deep sleep. And its unceasing presence both day and night may, he believes, induce pain through the mechanism known as 'sympathetically maintained pain'. An hypothesis that has led him (Martinez-Lavin 2001) to ask 'is FS a generalised reflex sympathetic dystrophy?'.

His reason (Martinez-Lavin 2002) for postulating this is that the pain in FS and in reflex sympathetic dystrophy (complex regional pain syndrome- type 1) has several features in common. He states that these features include: 'post-traumatic onset, relentless pain disproportionate to the underlying tissue damage and unresponsive to analgesic/anti-inflammatory drugs, the presence of allodynia (in FS tender points reflect a generalised state of allodynia), paresthesiae (a typical feature of neuropathic pain) and lastly, in both clinical syndromes, pain improves after sympathetic blockade'.

He concludes that 'Sympathetic nervous system dysfunction is frequent in FS and may explain its multisystem manifestations. It remains to be established if this dysautonomia plays a major role in the pathogenesis of FS. We surmise that it does. If so, new types of non-pharmacological and pharmacological therapeutic interventions intended to restore autonomic nervous system homeostasis may be developed.'

## Origin of the pain in fibromyalgia syndrome

In conclusion, it has to be said that the primary source from which FS's pain arises remains uncertain. Histological studies of the muscles have failed to reveal any evidence that it originates in these. There is, however, much to suggest that the principal pathological changes are in the central nervous system. That most patients with the disorder complain of persistent fatigue and non-restorative sleep is in accord with this. Also in favour of it is the discovery that there are significant abnormalities in the blood and CSF levels of the neuropeptides involved in central pain-modulating mechanisms. All this leads to the belief that progress in the treatment of this disorder will be dependant on the introduction of more effective and less toxic drugs to combat changes in the nervous system, such as those responsible for the development of central sensitisation. In the meantime, much worthwhile symptomatic pain relief may be obtained by suppressing nociceptor activity at TrP and TP sites by one means or another, including the frequent carrying out of superficially directed needle-evoked nerve stimulation at these points on a long-term basis.

## References

Aaron L A, Bradely L A, Alarcon G S et al 1997 Perceived physical and emotional trauma as precipitating events in fibromyalgia. Arthritis and Rheumatism 40: 453–460

Aftimos S 1989 Myofascial pain in children. New Zealand Medical Journal 102: 440–441

Ahles T A, Khan S A, Yunus M B et al 1991 Psychiatric status of patients with primary fibromyalgia, patients with rheumatoid arthritis, and subjects without pain: a blind comparison of DSM-111 diagnoses. American Journal of Psychiatry 148: 1721–1726

Awad E A 1973 Interstitial myofibrositis: hypothesis of the mechanism. Archives of Physical Medicine 54: 440–453

Awad E A 1990 Histological changes in fibrositis. In: Fricton J R, Awad E A (eds) Advances in pain research and therapy. Raven Press, New York, Vol. 17, pp. 249–258

Baldry P E 2001 Myofascial pain and fibromyalgia syndromes. Churchill Livingstone, Edinburgh

Bates T, Grunwaldt E 1958 Myofascial pain in childhood. Journal of Pediatrics 53: 198–209

Becker R O, Reichmanis M, Marino A A, Spadaro J A 1976 Electrophysiological correlates of acupuncture points and meridians. Psychoenergetic System 1: 105–112

Bengtsson A, Henriksson K G, Jorfeldt L et al 1986 Primary fibromyalgia – a clinical and laboratory study of 55 patients. Scandinavian Journal of Rheumatology 15: 340–347

Bennett R M 1999 Fibromyalgia. In: Wall P D, Melzack R (eds) Textbook of pain, 4th edn. Churchill Livingstone, Edinburgh, pp. 579–602

Bonafede R P, Downey D C, Bennett R M 1995 An association of fibromyalgia with primary Sjogren's syndrome: a prospective study of 72 patients. Journal of Rheumatology 22: 133–136

Bonica J J 1957 Management of myofascial pain syndromes in general practice. Journal of the American Medical Association 165: 732–738

Bradley L A, Alberts K R, Alarcon G S et al 1996 Abnormal brain regional cerebral blood flow (rCBF) and cerebrospinal fluid (CSF) levels of Substance P (SP) in patients and non-patients with fibromyalgia (FM). Arthritis and Rheumatism 39 (suppl): S212

Brendstrup P, Jesperson K, Absoe-Hansen G 1957 Morphological and chemical connective tissue changes in fibrositic nodules. Annals of Rheumatic Diseases 16: 438–440

Buskila D, Neumann L 2002 The development of widespread pain after injuries. Journal of Musculoskeletal Pain 10 (1/2): 261–267

Buskila D, Neumann L Hazanov I 1996 Familial aggregation in the fibromyalgia syndrome. Seminars in Arthritis and Rheumatism 26: 605–611

Buskila D, Neumann L, Vaisberg G et al 1997 Increased rates of fibromyalgia following cervical spine injury: a controlled study of 161 cases of traumatic injury. Arthritis and Rheumatism 40: 446–452

Carette S, Oakson G, Guimont et al 1995 Sleep electroencephalography and the clinical response to amitrypyline in patients with fibromyalgia. Arthritis and Rheumatism 38(9): 1211–1217

Cathey M A, Wolfe F, Kleinheksel S M 1988 Functional ability and work status in patients with fibromyalgia. Arthritis Care Research 1: 85–98

Chaitow L 2003 Fibromyalgia syndrome, 2nd edn. Churchill Livingstone, Edinburgh

Cheshire W P, Abashian S W, Mann J D 1994 Botulinum toxin in the treatment of myofascial pain syndrome. Pain 59: 65–69

Chu J 1995 Dry needling (intramuscular stimulation) in myofascial pain related to lumbosacral radiculopathy. European Journal of Physical Medicine and Rehabilitation 5(4): 106–121

Chu J 1997 Twitch-obtaining intramuscular stimulation (TOIMS): effectiveness for long-term treatment of myofascial pain related to cervical radiculopathy. Archives of Physical Medicine and Rehabilitation 78: 1042

Clauw D 2002 Fibromyalgia associated syndromes. In: Bennett R (ed) The clinical neurobiology of fibromyalgia and myofascial pain: therapeutic implications. The Haworth Medical Press, New York, pp. 201–214

Clauw D, Schmidt M, Radulovic D et al 1997 The relationship between fibromyalgia and interstitial cystitis. Journal of Psychiatric Research 31: 125–131

Coderre T J, Katz J, Vaccarino A L, Melzack R 1993 Contributions of central neuroplasticity to pathological pain: review of clinical and experimental evidence. Pain 52: 259–285

Cohen H, Neumann L, Alhosshle A et al 2001 Abnormal sympathovagal balance in men with fibromyalgia. Journal of Rheumatoloigy 28: 581–589

Cohen H, Neumann L, Shore M et al 2000 autonomic dysfunction in patients with fibromyalgia: application of power spectral analysis of heart rate variability. Seminars in Arthritis and Rheumatism 29: 217–227

Cooperative Group of Investigation of PSC 1980 A survey of occurrence of the phenomenon of propagated sensation along channels (PSC). In: Advances in acupuncture and acupuncture anaesthesia: abstracts of papers presented at the National Symposium of Acupuncture, Moxibustion and Acupuncture Anaesthesia, Beijing 1979. The People's Medical Publishing House, Beijing, pp. 258–260

Copeman W S , Ackerman W L 1944 'Fibrositis' of the back. Quarterly Journal of Medicine 13: 37–51

de Valera E, Raftery H 1976 Lower abdominal and pelvic pain in women. In: Bonica J J, Albe-Fessard D (eds) Advances in pain research and therapy. Raven Press, New York, Vol. 1, pp. 935–936

Devor M 1988 Central changes mediating neuropathic pain. Proceedings of the Vth World Congress on Pain. Elsevier Science Publishers BV, Amsterdam, pp. 114–128

Dinerman H, Goldenberg D L, Felson D T 1986 A prospective evaluation of 118 patients with the fibromyalgia syndrome: prevalence of Raynaud's phenomenen, sicca symptoms, ANA, low complement, and Ig deposition at the dermal-epidermal junction. Journal of Rheumatology 13: 368–373

Doubell T P, Mannion R J, Woolf C J 1999 The dorsal horn: state dependent sensory processing, plasticity and the generation of pain. In: Wall P D, Melzack R (eds) Textbook of pain, 4th edn. Churchill Livingstone, Edinburgh, pp. 165–182

Dubner R, Basbaum A 1994 Spinal dorsal horn plasticity following tissue or nerve injury. In: Wall P D, Melzack R (eds) Textbook of pain, 3rd edn. Churchill Livingstone, Edinburgh, pp. 225–241

Ekbom K A 1960 Restless leg syndrome. Neurology 10: 868

Fields H L 1987 Pain. McGraw-Hill, New York, pp. 152–154

Fine P G 1987 Myofascial trigger points in children. Journal of Pediatrics 111: 547–548

Fischer A A 1986 Pressure threshold meter: its use for quantification of tender spots. Archives of Physical Medicine and Rehabilitation 67: 836–838

Fischer A A 1988a Documentation of muscle pain and soft tissue pathology. In: Kraus H (ed) Diagnosis and treatment of muscle pain, Quintessence, Chicago

Fischer A A 1988b Documentation of myofascial trigger points. Archives of Physical Medicine and Rehabilitation 69: 286–291

Fischer A A 1998c Algometry in diagnosis of musculoskeletal pain and evaluation of treatment outcome: an update. Journal of Musculoskeletal Pain 6(1): 5–32

Fischer A A, Chang C H 1986 Temperature and pressure threshold measurements in trigger points. Thermology 1: 212–215

Fricton J, Kroenig R, Haley D, Siegert R 1985 Myofascial pain syndrome of the head and neck. A review of clinical characteristics 264 patients. Oral Surgery, Oral Medicine, Oral Pathology 60(6): 15–23

Gerwin R D 1994 Neurobiology of the myofascial trigger point. In: Masi A T (ed) Fibromyalgia and myofascial pain syndromes. Bailliere's Clinical Rheumatology 8(4): 747–762

Gerwin R D 1995 A study of 96 subjects examined both for fibromyalgia and myofascial pain. Journal of Musculoskeletal Pain 3 (suppl 1): 121

Gerwin R D 1999 Differential diagnosis of myofascial pain syndromes and fibromyalgia. Journal of Musculoskeletal Pain 7(1/2): 209–215

Gerwin R D 2002 Myofascial and visceral pain syndromes: visceral-somatic pain representations. Journal of Musculoskeletal Pain 10(1/2): 165–175

Gerwin R D, Duranleau D 1997 Ultrasound identification of the myofascial trigger point. Muscle and Nerve 20: 767–768 [Letter]

Gerwin R D, Shannon S, Hong C-Z, Hubbard D, Gevirtz R 1995 Identification of myofascial trigger points: inter-rater agreement and effect of training. Journal of Musculoskeletal Pain 3 (suppl 1) 55 (abstract)

Giamberardino M A, Affaitati G, Lerza R, De Laurentis S 2002 Neurophysiological basis of visceral pain. Journal of Musculoskeletal Pain 10(1/2): 151–163

Glogowski G, Wallraff J 1951 Ein beitrag zur Klinik und Histologie der Muskelharten (Myogelosen). Zeitschrift fur Orthopadie 80: 237–268

Gorrell R L 1976 Troublesome ankle disorders and what to do about them. Consultant 16: 64–69

Granges G, Littlejohn G 1993 Prevalence of myofascial pain syndrome in fibromyalgia syndrome and regional pain syndrome: a comparative study. Journal of Musculoskeletal Pain 1(2): 19–35

Greenfield S, Fitzcharles M, Esdaile J M 1992 Reactive fibromyalgia syndrome. Arthritis and Rheumatism 35: 678–681

Heuser J, Miledi R 1971 Effect of lanthanum ions on function and structure of frog neuromuscular junctions. Proceedings of the Royal Society of London B Biological Science 179: 247–260

Hong C-Z 1998 Algometry in evaluation of trigger points and referred pain. Journal of Musculoskeletal Pain 6(1): 47–59

Hong C-Z 1999 Current research on myofascial trigger points – pathophysiological studies. Journal of Musculoskeletal Pain 7(1/2): 121–129

Hong C-Z, Chen Y-N, Twehous D, Hong D H 1996 Pressure threshold for referred pain by compression on the trigger point and adjacent areas. Journal of Musculoskeletal Pain 4(3): 61–79

Hong C-Z, Simons D G 1998 Pathophysiological and electrophysiological mechanisms of myofascial trigger points. Archives of Physical Medicine and Rehabilitation 79: 863–871

Hubbard D R, Berkoff G M 1993 Myofascial trigger points show spontaneous needle EMG activity. Spine 18(13): 1803–1807

Hyyppa M T, Kronholm E 1995 Nocturnal motor activity in fibromyalgia patients with poor sleep quality. Journal of Psychosomatic Research 39(1): 85–91

Inman V T, Saunders R B 1944 Referred pain from skeletal structures. Journal of Nervous and Mental Disease 99: 660–667

Jones R V, Lambert E H, Sayre G P 1955 Source of a type of 'insertion activity' in electromyography with evaluation of a histologic method of localisation. Archives of Physical Medicine and Rehabilitation 35: 301–310

Jose P J, Page D A, Wolstenholme B E, Williams T J, Dumonde D C 1981 Bradykinin- stimulated prostaglandins E2 production of endothelial cells and its modulation by anti-inflammatory compounds. Inflammation 5: 363–378

Kellgren J H 1939 The distribution of pain arising from deep somatic structures with charts of segmental pain areas. Clinical Science 4: 35–46

Kieschke J, Mense S, Prabhaker N R 1988 Influence of adrenaline and hypoxia on rat muscle receptors in vitro. Progress in Brain Research 74: 91–97

Klein R, Bansch M, Berg P A 1992 Clinical relevance of antibodies against serotonin and gangliosides in patients with primary fibromyalgia syndrome. Psychoneuroendocrinology 17: 593–598

Kraft G H, Johnson E W, La Ban M M 1968 The fibrositis syndrome. Archives of Physical Medicine and Rehabilitation 49: 155–162

Kruse R A Jr, Christiansen J A 1992 Thermographic imaging of myofascial trigger points: a follow-up study. Archives of Physical Medicine and Rehabilitation 73: 819–823

Kurtze N, Gundersen K T, Svebak S 1998 The role of anxiety and depression in fatigue and patterns of pain among subgroups of fibromyalgia patients. British Journal of Medical Psychology 71: 185–194

Landro N I, Stiles T C, Sletvold H 1997 Memory functioning in patients with primary fibromyalgia and major depression and healthy controls. Journal of Psychosomatic Research 42: 297–306

Leriche R 1930 Des effetes de l'anaesthésie à la novocaine des ligaments et des insertions tendinuses. Gazette des Hospitaux 103: 1294

Lewis Sir Thomas 1942 Pain. Macmillan, New York

Livingston W K 1943 Pain mechanisms. Macmillan, New York

Lu Gwei-Djen, Needham J 1980 Celestial lancets. Cambridge University Press, Cambridge

Macdonald A J R 1982 Acupuncture from ancient art to modern medicine. George Allen & Unwin, London

Mackenzie J 1909 Symptoms and their interpretation. Shaw & Sons, London

Mann F 1974 The treatment of disease by acupuncture, 3rd edn. Heinmann Medical, London

Martinez-Lavin M 2001 Is fibromyalgia a generalized reflex sympathetic dystrophy? Clinical and Experimental Rheumatology 19: 1–3

Martinez-Lavin M 2002 The autonomic nervous system and fibromyalgia. In: Bennett R (ed) The clinical neurobiology of fibromyalgia and myofascial pain: therapeutic implications. Hayworth Mcaical Press, New York, pp. 221–228

Martinez-Lavin M, Hermosillo A G, Rosas M, Soto M E 1998 Circadian studies of autonomic nervous balance in patients with fibromyalgia. A heart rate variability analysis. Arthritis and Rheumatism 29: 217–227

McCain G A 1994 Fibromyalgia and myofascial pain syndromes. In: Wall P D, Melzack R (eds) Textbook of pain, 3rd edn. Churchill Livingstone, Edinburgh

McMahon S B, Lewin G R, Anand P et al 1989 Quantitative analysis of peptide levels and neurogenic extravasation following regeneration of afferents to appropriate and in appropriate targets. Neuroscience 33: 67–73

McMahon S B, Skyova E, Wall PD et al 1984 Neurogenic extravasation and substance P levels are low in muscle as compared to skin in the rat hindlimb. Neuroscience Letters 52: 235–240

McNulty W H, Gevirez R N, Hubbard D R et al 1994 Needle electromyographic evaluation of trigger point response to a psychological stressor. Psychophysiology 31(3): 313–316

Melzack R, Wall P D 1988 The challenge of pain, 2nd edn. Penguin, Harmondsworth, Middlesex, p. 186

Mense S 1990 Considerations concerning the neurobiological basis of muscle pain. Canadian Journal of Physiology and Pharmacology 69: 610–616

Mense S 1993a Neurophysiology of muscle in relation to pain. In: Voeroy H, Merskey H (eds) Progress in fibromyalgia and myofascial pain. Elsevier Science, Amsterdam, pp. 23–39

Mense S 1993b Nociception from skeletal muscle in relation to clinical muscle pain. Pain 54: 241–289

Mense S 1994 Referral of muscle pain. New aspects. American Pain Society Journal 3: 1–9

Mense S 1997 Pathophysiologic basis of muscle pain syndromes. An update. Physical Medicine and Rehabilitation. Clinics of North America 8(1): 23–52

Mense S 2001 Pain referred from and to muscles. In: Mense S, Simons D, Russell I J (eds) Muscle pain, understanding its nature, diagnosis, and treatment. Lippincott Williams & Wilkins, Philadelphia

Mense S, Simons D G, Russell I J 2001 Muscle pain, understanding its nature, diagnosis and treatment. Lippincott Williams & Wilkins, Philadelphia

Middleton G D, McFarlin J E, Lipsky P E 1994 The prevalence and clinical impact of fibromyalgia in systemic lupus erythematosus. Arthritis and Rheumatism 37: 1181–1188

Moldofsky H 1994 Chronobiological influences on fibromyalgia syndrome: theoretical and therapeutic implications. Bailliere's Clinical Rheumatology 8: 801–810

Moldofsky H, Lue F A, Smythe H A 1983 Alpha EEG sleep and morning symptoms in rheumatoid arthritis. Journal of Rheumatology 10(3): 373–379

Moldofsky H, Scarisbrick P, England R, Smythe H 1975 Musculoskeletal symptoms and non-REM sleep disturbance in patients with 'fibrositis syndrome' and healthy subjects. Psychosomatic Medicine 37(4): 341–351

Nice D A, Riddle D L, Lamb R L, Mayhew T P, Rueker K 1992 Intertester reliability of judgements of the presence of trigger points in patients. Archives of Physical Medicine and Rehabilitation 73: 893–898

Njoo H K, Van der Does E 1994 The occurrence and inter-rater reliability of myofascial trigger points in the quadratus lumborum and gluteus medius: a prospective study in non-specific low back patients and controls in general practice. Pain 58: 317–323

Pellegrino M J 1990 Atypical chest pain as an initial presentation of primary fibromyalgia. Archives of Physical Medicine and Rehabilitation 71(7): 526–528

Pellegrino M J, Waylonis G W, Somner A 1989 Familial occurrence of primary fibromyalgia. Archives of Physical Medicine and Rehabilitation 70: 61–63

Rachlin E S 1994 Myofascial pain and fibromyalgia. Mosby, St Louis

Raj R R, Brouillard D, Simpson C S, Hopman W M, Abdollah H 2000 Dysautonomia among patients with fibromyalgia: A non-invasive assessment. Journal of Rheumatology 27: 2660–2665

Research Group of Acupuncture Anaesthesia, Institute of Medicine and Pharmacology of Fujian Province 1986 Studies of phenomenon of blocking activities of channels and collaterals. In: Zhang X (ed) Research on acupuncture, moxibustion and acupuncture anaesthesia. Science press, Beijing 653–667

Reilly P A, Littlejohn G O 1992 Peripheral arthralgic presentation of fibrositis/fibromyalgia syndrome. Journal of Rheumatology 19(2): 281–283

Ruch T C 1949 Visceral sensation and referred pain. In: Fulton J (ed) Howell's textbook of physiology, 16th edn. Sanders, Philidelphia, pp. 385–401

Russell I J 2001 Fibromyalgia syndrome. In: Mense S, Simons D G (eds) Muscle Pain. Understanding its nature, diagnosis and treatment. Lippincott Williams & Wilkins, Philadelphia Ch 9

Russell I J, Fletcher E M, Vipraio G A et al 1998 Cerebrospinal fluid (CSF) substance P (SP) in fibromyalgia: changes in CSF SP over time parallel changes in clinical activity. Journal of Musculoskeletal Pain 6 (suppl 2): 77

Russell I J, Orr M D, Littman B et al 1994 Elevated cerebrospinal fluid levels of substance P in patients with fibromyalgia syndrome. Arthritis and Rheumatism 37: 1593–1601

Russell I J, Vaeroy H, Javors M et al 1992 Cerebrospinal fluid biogenic amine metabolites in fibromyalgia/fibrositis syndrome and rheumatoid arthritis. Arthritis and Rheumatism 35: 550–556

Russell I J, Vipraio G A 1994 Serotonin (5-HT) in serum and platelets (PLT) from fibromyalgia patients (FS) and normal controls (NC). Arthritis and Rheumatism 37 (suppl): S214

Russell I J, Vipraio G M, Acworth I 1993 Abnormalities in the central nervous system (CNS) metabolism of tryptophan (TRY) to 3-hydroxy kynurenine (OHKY) in fibromyalgia syndrome (FS). Arthritis and Rheumatism 36(9): S222

Russell I J, Vodjani A, Michalek J E et al 1995 Circulating antibodies to serotonin in fibromyalgia syndrome, rheumatoid arthritis, osteoarthrosis, and healthy normal controls. Journal of Musculoskeletal Pain 3 (suppl 1 ): 143

Salpeter M M 1987 Vertebrate neuromuscular junctions: general morphology, molecular organization and functional consequences. In: Salpeter M M (ed) The vertebrate neuromuscular junction. Alan R. Liss, New York, pp. 1–54

Schade H 1919 Beiträge zur Umgrenzung und Klärung einer Lehre von der Erkaltung. Zeitschrift Geselschaft Experimentaler Medizin 7: 275–374

Schiffman E L, Fricton J R, Haley D P, Shapiro B L 1990 The prevalence and treatment needs of subjects with temperomandibular disorders. Journal of the American Dental Association 120(3): 295–303

Sicuteri F 1967 Vasoneuroactive substances and their implications in vascular pain. In: Friedman A P (ed) Research and clinical studies in headache. Karger, Basel, Vol. 1, pp. 6–45

Simons D G 1993 Referred phenomena of myofascial trigger points. In: Vecchiet L, Albe-Fessard D, Lindblom U (eds) New trends in referred pain and hyperalgesia. Elsevier Science, Amsterdam

Simons D G 1996 Clinical and etiological update of myofascial pain from trigger points. Journal of Musculoskeletal pain 4(1/2): 93–121

Simons D G 1999 Diagnostic criteria of myofascial pain caused by trigger points. Journal of Musculoskeletal Pain 7(1/2): 111–120

Simons D G 2001 Clinical correlations. In: Mense S, Simons D G, Russell I J (eds) Muscle pain, understanding its nature diagnosis and treatment. Lippincott, Williams & Wilkins, Philidelphia, p. 221

Simons D G, Hong C-Z, Simons L S 1995a Prevalence of spontaneous electrical activity at trigger spots and control sites in rabbit muscle. Journal of Musculoskeletal Pain 3(1): 35–48

Simons D G, Hong C-Z, Simons L S 1995b Nature of myofascial trigger points active loci. Journal of Musculoskeletal Pain 3 (suppl 1): 62

Simons D G , Hong C-Z, Simons L S 1995c Spontaneous electrical activity of trigger points. Journal of Musculoskeletal Pain 3 (suppl 1) :124

Simons D G, Hong C-Z, Simons L S 1995d Spike activity in trigger points. Journal of Musculoskeletal Pain 3 (suppl 1): 125

Simons D G, Stolov W C 1976 Microscopic features and transient contraction of palpable bands in canine muscle. Archives of Physical Medicine and Rehabilitation 55: 65–88

Simons D G, Travell J G, Simons L S 1999 Myofascial pain and dysfunction. The trigger point manual, 2nd edn. Williams & Wilkins, Baltimore, Vol. 1

Sinclair D C 1949 The remote reference of pain aroused in the skin. Brain 72: 364–372

Sivri A, Cindas A, Dincer F, Sivri B 1996 Bowel dysfunction and irritable bowel syndrome in fibromyalgia patients. Clinical Rheumatology 15: 283–286

Skootsky S, Jaeger B, Oye R K 1989 Prevalence of myofascial pain in general internal medical practice. Western Journal of Medicine 151(2): 157–160

Sletvold H, Stiles T C, Landro N I, 1995 Information processing in primary fibromyalgia, major depression and healthy controls. Journal of Rheumatology 22: 137–142

Sola A E, Kuitert J H 1955 Myofascial trigger point pain in the neck and shoulder girdle. North West Medicine 54: 980–984

Stockman R 1904 The causes, pathology and treatment of chronic rheumatism. Edinburgh Medical Journal 15: 107–116, 223–235

Travell J G 1976 Myofascial trigger points: clinical view. In: Bonica J J, Albe-Fessard D (eds) Advances in pain research and therapy 1. Raven Press, New York, pp. 916–926

Travell J G, Bigelow N H 1946 Referred somatic pain does not follow a simple 'segmental' pattern. Federation Proceedings 5: 106

Travell J G, Simons D G 1992 Myofascial pain and dysfunction. The trigger point manual, (the lower extremities). Williams & Wilkins, Baltimore, Vol 2

Trommer P R, Gellman M B 1952 Trigger point syndrome. Rheumatism 8 : 67–72

Tsigos C, Diemel L T, Tomlinson D R et al 1993 Cerebrospinal fluid levels of substance P and calcitonin-gene-related peptide: correlation with sural nerve levels and neuropathic signs in sensory diabetic polyneuropathy. Clinical Science 84: 305–311

Urrows S, Affleck G, Tennen H, Higgins P 1994 Unique clinical and psychological correlates of fibromyalgia tender points and joint tenderness in rheumatoid arthritis. Arthritis and Rheumatism 37: 1513–1520

Vaeroy H, Helle R, Forre O et al 1988 Elevated CSF levels of substance P and high incidence of Raynaud's phenomenon in patients with fibromyalgia: new features for diagnosis. Pain 32: 21–26

Vedder C I, Bennett R M 1995 An analysis of antibodies to serotonin receptors in fibromyalgia. Journal of Musculoskeletal Pain 3 (suppl 1): 73

Waylonis G W, Perkins R H 1994 Post-traumatic fibromyalgia. A long-term follow-up. American Journal of Physical Medicine and Rehabilitation 73: 403–409

Weeks V D, Travell J G 1957 How to give painless injections. AMA Scientific Exhibits 1957. Grune & Stratton, New York, pp. 318–322

Wegelius O, Absoe-Hansen G 1956 Mast cell and tissue water. Studies on living connective tissue in the hamster cheek pouch. Experimental Cell Research 11: 437–443

Welin M, Bragee B, Nyberg F et al 1995 Elevated substance P levels are contrasted by a decrease in metenkephalin-arg-phe levels in CSF from fibromyalgia patients. Journal of Musculoskeletal Pain 3 (suppl 1): 4

WHO 1993 Consensus document on fibromyalgia: The Copenhagen Declaration 1993. Journal of Musculoskeletal Pain 1 (3/4): 295–312

Wolfe F, Ross K, Anderson J et al 1995 The prevalence and characteristics of fibromyalgia in the general population. Arthritis and Rheumatism 38: 19–28

Wolfe F, Russell I J, Vipraio G A et al 1997 Serotonin levels, pain threshold and FM. Journal of Rheumatology 24: 555–559

Wolfe F, Simons D, Fricton J et al 1992 The fibromyalgia and myofascial pain syndromes-a preliminary study of tender points and trigger points in persons with fibromyalgia, myofascial pain syndrome and no disease. Journal of Rheumatology 19: 944–951

Wolfe F, Smythe H A, Yunus M B et al 1990 The American College of Rheumatology 1990 criteria for the classification of fibromyalgia. Report of the multicenter criteria committee. Arthritis and Rheumatism 33(2): 160–172

Xue 1986 The phenomenon of propagated sensation along channels (PSC) and the cerebral cortex. In: Zhang X (ed) Research in acupuncture, moxibustion and acupuncture anaesthesia. Science Press, Beijing, pp. 668–683

Yunus M B 1989 Fibromyalgia syndrome: new research on an old malady. British Medical Journal 298: 474–475

Yunus M B 1993 Research in fibromyalgia and myofascial pain syndromes – current status, problems and future directions. Journal of Musculoskeletal Pain 1(1): 23–43

Yunus M B, Aldag J C 1996 Restless leg syndrome and leg cramps in fibromyalgia syndrome: a controlled study. British Medical Journal 312: 1339

Yunus M B, Inanici F 2001 Clinical characteristics and biopathophysiological mechanisms of fibromyalgia syndrome. In: Baldry P E (ed ) Myofascial pain and fibromyalgia syndromes. A clinical guide to diagnosis and management. Churchill Livingstone, Edinburgh

Yunus M B, 1992 Fibromyalgia, restless legs syndrome, periodic limb movement disorder, and psychogenic pain. In: McCarty D J, Koopman W J (eds) Arthritis and allied conditions: a textbook of rheumatology, 12th edn. Lea and Febiger, Philadelphia, pp. 1383–1405

# Chapter 8

# Concurrent complex regional and myofascial trigger point pain syndromes

## INTRODUCTION

The main purpose of this chapter is to draw attention to the still not sufficiently well recognized clinical observation that myofascial trigger point (MTrP) pain syndrome and the disorder currently known as complex regional pain syndrome (CRPS) type 1, or what formerly was called reflex sympathetic dystrophy (RSD), not infrequently develop concurrently.

It is particularly regrettable that many otherwise comprehensive current accounts of CRPS type 1 (RSD) make no reference to this association considering that it was as long ago as 1943 that Livingston, in his classical monograph *Pain Mechanisms*, drew attention to the presence of MTrPs in some of his patients suffering from the disorder and stated that deactivation of these points by injecting a local anaesthetic into them provides a significant amount of pain relief.

It is to be hoped that this fundamentally important discovery made by Livingston during World War II will no longer continue to be ignored now that at least five recent studies have confirmed its veracity.

Filner (1989), after looking specifically for MTrPs in 40 patients with this syndrome, then known as RSD, found active pain-producing ones to be present in 36 of them.

Veldman et al (1993 ) discovered MTrPs to be present in 45% of 377 patients with this disorder. Lin et al (1995) searched for MTrPs in 84 patients with CRPS (RSD) and identified pain-producing ones in 82%. Inamura et al (1997) reported the presence of the MTrP pain syndrome in 82% of a series of cases with CRPS (RSD). And Allen et al (1999), in a retrospective study of 134 patients with CRPS (RSD), found that '56% had a myofascial component present at evaluation'.

The following topics will also be discussed: early observations concerning the two closely related disorders originally known as causalgia and reflex sympathetic dystrophy; the reasons why it was considered necessary to revise the terminology and to introduce the terms CRPS type 1 (RSD) and CRPS type 2 (causalgia); the clinical manifestations of CRPS type 1 (RSD); present-day views concerning the pathophysiology of CRPS type 1 (RSD); and, finally, the various methods of treating the syndrome, including deactivating any MTrPs that may be found to be present.

## CAUSALGIA

Pain of a characteristically burning type that affected soldiers with nerve injuries from gun shot wounds sustained during the American Civil War was described by Mitchell et al in 1864. They stated that the pain was 'mustard red hot', that it was made worse by the application of pressure to the skin or the exposure of it to cold air, and that the site affected, usually a hand or a foot, developed vasomotor, sudomotor and trophic changes.

Three years later Mitchell (1867) called this disorder causalgia (from the Greek kausis [burning] and algos [pain]).

During World War I there was a resurgence of interest in nerve injury-evoked causalgia when in 1916 Leriche described the case of a soldier who developed the characteristic burning pain, excessive sweating and skin colour changes of it as a result of a cannon-ball damaging the left clavicle and adjacent nerves and blood vessels. During the course of the operation for this condition Leriche had to resect 12 cm of the adventitia of the brachial artery and as postoperatively all the symptoms were much improved, he concluded that this must have been because this resection had led to the removal of the periarterial sympathetic fibres. He, therefore, carried out a periarterial sympathectomy on other soldiers with similar clinical manifestations of this disorder in the belief that it is a neuritis of the sympathetic nerves (névrite du sympathique).

At the beginning of World War II his further experience of treating nerve injuries (Leriche 1939) led him to modify this view, once he realized that not all patients with these injuries develop causalgia. This led him to conclude that this disorder must be a 'vasomotor and trophic syndrome brought about by the sympathetic reactions personal to the individual in the presence of an external injury'.

Leriche's belief that causalgia must, nevertheless, be essentially sympathetically mediated became widely accepted and was influential in persuading surgeons both in World War II and in wars in various parts of the world since then to perform a sympathectomy on affected patients.

The results of carrying out this procedure proved to be widely variable but it was a long time before the possibility was considered that the reason for this might be because the pathophysiology of the disorder is more complex than was at first thought.

## REFLEX SYMPATHETIC DYSTROPHY

As the years passed it became clear that a disorder with very similar clinical manifestations could be brought about by injury to tissues other than nerves. This led Evans (1946) to introduce the term reflex sympathetic dystrophy, in line with the then prevailing view concerning the pathophysiological changes responsible for both causalgia and this particular disorder, which some referred to as minor causalgia.

## TERMINOLOGICAL REVISION

For the relief of this latter disorder various procedures designed to suppress sympathetic efferent activity have over the years been employed but, as will be discussed when considering current approaches to its treatment, their efficacy in general has proved to be very disappointing and frequently no better than a placebo.

For this and other reasons the aptness of the term reflex sympathetic dystrophy has in recent years been questioned. As Stanton Hicks et al (1995) have pointed out, dystrophic changes in the tissues are not invariably present, and even when they are, it is only at a late stage. In addition, there is no convincing evidence that these or any of the disorder's other manifestations develop as a result of reflex sympathetic activity.

It was in the light of considerations such as these that prompted the International Association for the Study of Pain (IASP) to arrange for a consensus workshop, to be held at Orlando, Florida in 1993, for the purpose of reviewing and, if necessary, revising the terminology. The terms hitherto employed for the two disorders had included a bewilderingly large number of names, not only causalgia and RSD (minor causalgia), but also algodystrophy, traumatic angiospasm, shoulder-hand syndrome, reflex neurovascular dystrophy, post-traumatic osteoporosis and Sudeck's atrophy.

Those participating at this workshop realizing that the pathophysiology of both causalgia and RSD remained far from certain, decided to replace these terms by the strictly non-committal one of complex regional pain syndrome (CRPS) and to divide this into two separate entities, CRPS type 1 (RSD) and CRPS type 2 (causalgia).

This revised terminology has now been officially included in the IASP's classification of chronic pain (Merskey & Bogduk 1994) .

## CLINICAL MANIFESTATIONS OF CRPS TYPE 1 (RSD)

As CRPS type 1 (RSD) and MTrP pain syndrome are liable to develop concomitantly, it follows that those who frequently have to diagnose and treat the latter need to be familiar with the clinical manifestations of the first. For this reason a detailed account of them will be given. They include pain, autonomic disturbances, dystrophic changes, muscle weakness and emotional disorders.

## Pain

Somewhat confusingly, in view of the currently employed name for this syndrome, it has now been shown that pain is not a constant feature.

Blumberg & Janig (1994), from a detailed analysis of 190 patients diagnosed as having this disorder, stated that it was not present in 25% of them. In addition, Veldman et al (1993), who studied 829 patients with this syndrome, found it to be absent in 7% of them.

The spontaneously occurring pain takes the form of a constant or paroxysmal burning, throbbing or aching sensation. In addition, there may be a mechanically evoked hyperalgesia, hyperaesthesia and allodynia. The latter, which develops as a result of central sensitisation (see Ch. 6 ), is liable to cause considerable suffering. However, somewhat surprisingly, considering the intensity of the nociceptive sensory afferent barrage to which dorsal horn transmission neurons must be subjected to in this disorder, Blumberg & Janig (1994) only found it to be present in about 8% of the patients studied by them.

The severity of the spontaneous and evoked types of pain is liable to lead to prolonged immobilization and this, in turn, causes muscles to waste, joints to stiffen and in some cases contractures to develop.

## Autonomic disturbances

Abnormalities of the temperature and colour of the skin are common. These vasomotor changes are variable with the affected part being either unduly warm or unduly cold. Veldman et al (1993) found that the longer the interval between the onset of the disorder and the first examination the more likely it was for the affected limb to be cold.

Sudomotor changes may also be present but these too are variable so that with some patients there is hyperhydrosis but with others hypohydrosis.

In addition, oedema is frequently present from an early stage of the disease. Scadding (1999) is of the opinion that these autonomic changes may, in part, be brought about by prolonged immobilization.

## Dystrophic changes in skin nails and bone

Tissue dystrophy, according to Veldman et al (1993), is mainly a late finding and was only present in a small percentage of the 829 patients studied by them.

The skin may become either thin and shiny or thickened. The nails also may become thickened. In addition, osteoporosis may eventually develop. Initially, the diagnosis of this latter disorder depends on the use of technetium isotope scintigraphy, but at a later stage a plain radiograph is all that is required.

## Muscle weakness

It is common for muscles in the affected limb to become weakened and wasted. Veldman et al (1993), in a prospective study of 829 patients suffering from what at that time they called RSD, found that 95% of them had weakening and wasting of the muscles in the affected limb. Muscles in this state are clearly liable to become overloaded with, as a consequence, the activation of any TrPs they may happen to contain (see Ch. 7). In addition, this loss of muscle strength is not infrequently accompanied by the development of a tremor, especially in cases where it is the upper limb that is affected.

## Emotional disorders

The severity of any pain that may be present, the difficulty in alleviating this, and the suffering caused by other manifestations of the disorder frequently lead to the development of superimposed anxiety and depression.

## AETIOLOGICAL FACTORS COMMON TO CRPS TYPE 1 (RSD) AND MTrP PAIN SYNDROME

## Trauma

It is hardly surprising that these two syndromes may at times be present concurrently considering that the commonest reason for either of them developing is trauma. In addition, as previously stated, the MTrP pain syndrome is liable to develop as a secondary event when muscles in a limb affected by CRPS-type 1 become weakened, wasted and overloaded with, as a consequence, the activation of any TrPs that may be present in them.

Livingston (1943), when discussing the type of trauma responsible for causing what is now called CRPS type 1 (RSD) stated:

> The onset of symptoms may follow the most commonplace of injuries. A bruise, a superficial cut, the prick of a thorn or a broken chicken bone, a strain or even a post-operative scar may act as the causative lesion. The event which precipitates the syndrome may appear both to the physician and the patient as of minor consequence, and both have every reason to anticipate the same

prompt recovery that follows similar injuries. This anticipation is not realised and the symptoms tend to become progressively worse.

## Vascular disorders

Each of these two syndromes may occasionally develop following either a myocardial infarct or a cerebrovascular accident.

## THE PATHOPHYSIOLOGY OF CRPS TYPE 1 (RSD) AND TYPE 2 (CAUSALGIA)

It has to be said that, despite much research having been carried out over the years into the pathophysiology of both types of CRPS, the mechanisms responsible for their clinical manifestations continue to remain highly contentious.

The traditional view that the pathological changes in these two disorders are essentially sympathetically mediated ones has recently been challenged, particularly by Schott (1994, 1995, 1998). He has done this because those symptoms and signs so often encountered in causalgia and related conditions, that have traditionally been assumed to be due to sympathetic dysfunction, can instead be accounted for by the effects of neuropeptides with vasoactive and perhaps trophic properties that are released from C-afferent fibres, as recognized by Ochoa (1986) and Cline et al (1989).

The sensory afferents that are considered by Schott to be the particular ones involved in these disorders, are those that have been found to travel *within* autonomic nerve fibres. These two sets of fibres have the conjoint function of innervating a number of different structures, including those in the peripheral vascular system.

Schott (1995), persuasively argues that the pain and accompanying features in a disorder such as CRPS type 1 (RSD) develop as a result of trauma-evoked activation and sensitisation of these sensory afferents causing the release of neuropeptides such as Substance P (SP) and calcitonin gene-related peptide, which then give rise to an inflammatory type response.

Oyen et al (1993) have provided support for this view by carrying out scintigraphy with indium-111-labelled human non-specific polyclonal immunoglobulin G, as this demonstrated that patients suffering from what they called RSD have increased vascular permeability for macromolecules, an important characteristic of inflammation.

Veldman et al (1993), during the course of discussing this important finding made by Oyen and his co-workers, pertinently comments 'we hope this observation incites physicians to develop new forms of treatment for this disabling disease'.

All this notwithstanding, that there may be a sympathetic efferent component, in addition to this inflammatory one, is suggested by the findings of other studies. It has been found, in animal studies carried out by Gold et al (1994) and by Levine (1986), that noradrenaline released from sympathetic postganglionic neurons brings about the release of neuron-sensitizing prostaglandins. In addition Sanjue & Juu (1989) found that, whereas the effect of noradrenaline on non-sensitized nociceptors is weak, it has considerably enhanced activity when these are in a sensitized state as a result of inflammation evoked by the release of neuropeptides.

## THE PREDISPOSITION OF INDIVIDUALS TO DEVELOPING CRPS

Despite recent advances in knowledge concerning the inflammatory nature of CRPS, it remains difficult to understand why, as Poplawski et al (1983) have pointed out, type 1 (RSD), develops in less than 1% of patients with tissue damage and type 2 in less than 5% of those with peripheral nerve injuries. It has been suggested that this may be because only a small number of people are predisposed to developing a sufficiently exaggerated inflammatory response. At the same time it has to be admitted that it is possible for an individual to have two similar injuries but only to develop a disorder of this type with one of them.

## TREATMENT OF CRPS TYPE 1 (RSD)

Uncertainty concerning the pathophysiology of this disorder has led to difficulties in formulating a rational approach to its treatment.

### Pharmacotherapy

When it became widely accepted that the disorder was essentially due to aberrant sympathetic

efferent activity, the technique of intravenous regional guanethidine block (IVRGB), introduced by Hannington-Kiff (1974), was for a long time commonly employed. However, when over the years those using it found that with many of their patients the response to it was only transient and that a number of them either did not respond at all, or even had a transient exacerbation of pain, its efficacy was questioned and this then led to the carrying out of controlled trials.

Jadad et al (1995) have reviewed four such trials and found that the results in the treatment groups were no better than those in the control groups. They then conducted a study on patients who had reported obtaining an analgesic effect from IVRGB and found no significant difference between the effect of guanethidine and saline.

Ramamurthy & Hoffman (1995), in a randomized controlled trial, also found no significant difference with respect to pain relief between a guanethidine-injected treated group and a control group. Remarkably, however, both those in the treatment group and the control group showed a reduction in trophic and vasomotor changes together with a diminution in the amount of oedema!

Vanos et al (1992) have found an intravenous block using ketorolac, a non-steroidal anti-inflammatory drug that reduces prostaglandin release, to be effective in improving symptoms in a small group of patients with CRPS type 1 (RSD). This is particularly interesting in view of current views concerning the role of inflammatory-evoking chemical substances in the production of this disorder's clinical manifestations and its use, therefore, deserves to be further explored.

There is no doubt, however, that a simple analgesic such as codeine or a non-steroidal anti-inflammatory orally administered drug should be tried first, as one or other of these is often all that is required to relieve the pain.

Mellick & Mellick (1997) have found the administration of gabapentin, a drug more usually employed as an anticonvulsant, to be of value in the treatment of this disorder.

Muizelaar et al (1997) have reported benefit from the use of the calcium channel blocking agent nifedipine; also, from the employment of the alpha-adrenergic blocking agent phenoxybenzamine. They found the latter, however, not infrequently gives rise to various side-effects including dizziness, ortostatic hypotension and diarrhoea with 22% of their patients forced to stop using it because of these.

Unfortunately, both Muizelaar et al (1997) and Paice (1995) have found it necessary to draw attention to the difficulty in assessing the relative value of these different types of drugs due to the regrettable paucity up to now of large scale multicentre comparative trials.

## Physiotherapy

It is generally agreed that early mobilization of the affected limb is essential.

## Psychotherapy

It is also widely accepted (Scadding 1999) that treatment for anxiety and depression is often necessary in view of the considerable disablement brought about by this disorder and the all too frequent failure of various forms of therapy to ameliorate its physical manifestations.

## Deactivation of myofascial MTrPs

The importance of searching for, and when found to be present, deactivating MTrPs by one means or another (see Ch. 11) has been stressed by Filner (1989), Lin et al (1995) and Sola (1999).

## References

Allen G, Guler B S, Schwartz L 1999 Epidemiology of complex regional pain syndrome: a retrospective chart review of 134 patients. Pain 80(3): 539–544

Blumberg H, Janig W 1994 Clinical manifestations of reflex sympathetic dystrophy and sympathetically maintained pain. In: Wall P D, Melzac R (eds) Textbook of pain, 3rd edn. Churchill Livingstone, Edinburgh, pp. 685–698

Cline M A, Ochoa J, Torebjörk H E 1989 Chronic hyperalgesia and skin warming caused by sensitised C nociceptors. Brain 112: 621–647

Evans J A 1946 Reflex sympathetic dystrophy. Surgical Clinics of North America 26: 780–790

Filner B E 1989 Role of myofascial pain syndrome treatment in the management of reflex sympathetic dystrophy syndrome. Communication to the 1st international symposium on myofascial pain and fibromyalgia, Minneapolis

Gold M S, White D M, Ahlgeru S C, Guo M , Levine J D 1994 Catecholamine-induced mechanical sensitisation of cutaneous nociceptors in the rat. Neuroscience Letters 175: 166–170

Hannington-Kiff J G 1974 Intravenous regional sympathetic block with guanethidine. Lancet 1: 1019–1020

Inamura S T , Lin T Y, Teitaria M J, Fischer A A et al 1997 The importance of myofascial pain syndrome in reflex sympathetic dystrophy. Physical Medicine and Rehabilitation Clinics of North America 8: 207–211

Jadad A R, Carroll D, Glynn C J, McQuay H J 1995 Intravenous regional sympathetic blockade for pain relief in reflex sympathetic dystrophy: a systematic review and a randomised double-blind crossover study. Journal of Pain Symptom Management 10: 13–20

Leriche R 1916 De la causalgie envisagée comme une névrite du sympathique et de son traitement par la dénudation et l'excision des plexus nerveux péri-arteriels. Presse Medicin 24: 177–180

Leriche R 1939 The surgery of pain. (Translated by A Young) Baillière, Tindall and Cox, London

Levine J D, Taiwo Y O, Collins S D, Tam J K 1986 Noradrenaline hyperalgesia is mediated through interaction with sympathetic postganglionic neurone terminals rather than activation of primary afferent nociceptors. Nature 323: 158–160

Lin T Y, Teixeira M J, Kaziyama H H S, Pai H J et al 1995 Myofascial pain syndrome (MPS) asasociated with reflex sympathetic dystrophy (RSD). Journal of Musculoskeletal Pain 3 (suppl 1): 150

Livingston W K 1943 Pain mechanisms: a physiological interpretation of causalgia. Macmillan, New York

Mellick G A, Mellick L B 1997 Reflex sympathetic dystrophy treated with gabapentin. Archives of Physical Medicine and Rehabilitation 78: 98–105

Merskey H, Bogduk N (eds) 1994 Classification of chronic pain. Description of chronic pain syndromes and definitions of pain terms, 2nd edn. IASP Press, Seattle

Mitchell S W 1867 On the diseases of nerves resulting from injuries. In: Flint A (ed) Contributions relating to causation and prevention of disease and to camp diseases. US Sanitary Commission Memoirs, New York

Mitchell S W, Morehouse G R, Keen W W, 1864 Injuries of nerves and their consequences. J B Lippincott, Philadelphia

Muizelaar J P, Kleyer M, Hertogs I A M, De Lange D C 1997 Complex regional pain syndrome (reflex sympathetic dystrophy and causalgia): management with the calcium channel blocker nifedipine and/or the alpha-sympathetic blocker phenoxybenzamine in 59 patients. Clinical Neurology and Neurosurgery 99: 26–30

Ochoa J 1986 The newly recognised painful ABC syndrome: thermographic aspects. Thermology 2: 65–66; 101–107

Oyen W J M, Arntz J E, Claessens R A M J, Van der Meer J V M et al 1993 Reflex sympathetic dystrophy of the hand: an excessive inflammatory response? Pain 55: 151–157

Paice E 1995 Reflex sympathetic dystrophy. British Medical Journal 310: 1645–1648

Poplawski Z L, Wiley A M, Murray J F 1983 Post-traumatic dystrophy of the extremities. Journal of Bone and Joint Surgery 65 A; 642–655

Ramamurthy S, Hoffman J 1995 The guanethidine study group. Intravenous regional guanethidine in the treatment of reflex sympathetic dystrophy/causalgia: a randomised double-blind study. Anaesthesia and Analgesia 81: 718–723

Sanjue H , Juu Z 1989 Sympathetic facilitation of sustained discharges of polymodal nociceptors. Pain 38: 85–90

Scadding J W 1999 Complex regional pain syndrome. In: Wall P D, Melzack R (eds) Textbook of pain, 4th edn, Ch. 36. Churchill Livingstone, Edinburgh

Schott G D 1994 Visceral afferents: their contribution to 'sympathetic dependent' pain. Brain 117: 397–413

Schott G D 1995 An unsympathetic view of pain. Lancet 345: 634–636

Schott G D 1998 Interrupting the sympathetic outflow in causalgia and reflex sympathetic dystrophy. British Medical Journal 316: 792–793.

Sola A E 1999 Upper extremity pain. In: Wall P D, Melzack R (eds ) Textbook of pain, 4th edn, Ch. 24. Churchill Livingstone, Edinburgh

Stanton-Hicks M, Janig W, Hassenbuch S, Haddox J D et al 1995 Reflex sympathetic dystrophy: changing concepts and taxonomy. Pain 63: 127–133

Tilman P B J, Stadhouders A M, Jap P H K, Goris R J A 1990 Histopathological findings in skeletal muscle tissue of patients suffering from reflex sympathetic dystrophy. Micron Microscop Acta 21: 271–272

Vanos D N, Ramamurthy S, Hoffman J 1992 Intravenous regional block using ketorolac: preliminary results in the treatment of reflex sympathetic dystrophy. Anaesthesia and Analgesia 74: 139–141

Veldman P H J M, Reynen H M, Arntz I E, Goris R J A 1993 Signs and symptoms of reflex sympathetic dystrophy: prospective study of 82 patients. Lancet 342: 1012–1016

Chapter **9**

# Neurophysiological pain-suppressing effects of acupuncture and transcutaneous electrical nerve stimulation

## INTRODUCTION

Firstly in this chapter brief mention will be made of various pain-suppressing types of treatment employed by primitive man, whose analgesic effects, in retrospect, would seem to have been dependent on bringing into action similar neurophysiological mechanisms to those now believed to be involved in acupuncture.

Following this, current views concerning the mechanisms in the peripheral and central nervous systems considered to be brought into action when electroacupuncture and transcutaneous electrical nerve stimulation are used for pain relief will be discussed.

Then, because in the next chapter the manually applied acupuncture technique known as superficial dry needling (SDN) will be advocated for the routine deactivation of primarily activated myofascial trigger points (MTrPs), and the technique known as deep dry needling (DDN) for the occasional case where the MTrP activity has arisen secondarily to the development of a radiculopathy, it will be necessary to give a detailed account of the pain-relieving mechanisms believed to be brought into action by these two procedures.

Finally, reasons will be given as to why some of the current concepts concerning the manner in which manually applied needle-evoked nerve stimulation techniques bring about their pain-suppressing effects have recently had to be challenged.

## PRIMITIVE PAIN-SUPPRESSING PROCEDURES

There is no doubt that man has always instinctively realized that by applying a painful stimulus to the body it is possible to dispel from it pain of a more persistent nature. As Melzack & Wall (1982) have pointed out, every culture throughout the ages would seem to have come to realize that brief moderate pain tends to abolish severe prolonged pain.

Cupping, a procedure in which a glass cup is heated and then held with its rim against the skin; and scarification, a procedure in which the skin is cut, often in several places, by a sharp instrument such as, originally, a flint, thorn or fish bone, and then eventually a knife, have from time immemorial been employed to induce bleeding in the belief that this would release from the body the devil or evil spirit responsible for some particular malady. In addition, however, because both these procedures happen to be acutely painful, they have also been used to combat pain of a more persistent type such as that which may arise, for example, from joints, viscera and muscles.

Cauterization, a procedure in which intense heat is applied to an affected part of the body, has also been employed since the dawn of civilization for a variety of reasons, including the control of haemorrhage and the alleviation of pain. With respect to the latter it is interesting to find that in Tibet it was at one time used to alleviate lumbago. When employed for this purpose the treatment involved producing several blisters on the back by means of applying a red-hot branding iron to it. Next, cones packed with a mixture of sulphur and saltpetre were placed on the blisters and then lit with a flaming torch. As Graham (1939) has commented, the result must have been a girdle of burns deep enough to banish any thought of afflictions as mild as lumbago!

A less horrific method of blistering the skin for therapeutic purposes is the application of some irritant substance such as cantharides. This was certainly employed by Hippocrates, and used extensively since his time, with, for example, William Wells, a physician at St Thomas's Hospital in the early part of the 19th century, applying it to the skin of the chest wall for the relief of pericardial pain (Baldry 1971).

A form of treatment closely allied to this and one which has been used in the Far East for at least 3000 years, is the application to the body surface of a substance obtained from the leaves of the mugwort plant called moxa. A cone of this is placed on the skin, then set alight and allowed to burn down to its base. This procedure which must, as a result of damaging the tissues, be extremely painful is yet another example of a noxious stimulus being used to combat pain of a more chronic type.

Acupuncture, which has been used in the Eastern world for much the same period of time, is also a form of treatment in which a noxious stimulus is employed to bring about the alleviation of pain.

All these traditional therapeutic methods, which over the centuries have employed acute pain to drive out more protracted and severe pain, are now referred to collectively as counter-irritants. As Wand-Tetley (1956), in an extensive historical review of their clinical application, has pointed out, they have always mainly been used for the alleviation of musculoskeletal pain.

Originally, it was thought that they owed their efficacy to their ability to cast out evil spirits, but then it was considered that the effects might be due to either the power of suggestion or distraction of attention. It is only since the neurophysiology of pain has become better understood that it is now apparent that their analgesic effect lies in their ability to impart a noxious stimulus to the central nervous system and by so doing to evoke activity in complex endogenous pain-modulating mechanisms. An effect which Melzack (1973) has termed hyperstimulation analgesia.

## THE EARLY USE OF ELECTRICITY FOR THE COMBATING OF PAIN

The application of an electrical stimulus in order to alleviate pain also has its origins in antiquity. As Thompson (1998) pointed out, stone carvings that date from the Egyptian Fifth Dynasty (circa 2500 BC) show the electric fish (Malapterurus electricus) being employed for the treatment of painful disorders. And more than 2000 years later the ancient Greeks made use of the electrical discharge that emanates from the skate-like torpedo fish to alleviate headaches and arthralgias.

## THE INTRODUCTION OF ELECTROACUPUNCTURE FOR PAIN RELIEF

When in the middle of the 18th century Pieter van Musschenbroek showed that it is possible to store electricity in what have come to be known as Leyden jars, the possibility of using electricity in the treatment of disease was once again explored. It also happened to be about that time that Jesuit missionaries, on returning from the Far East, brought news concerning the Chinese practice of acupuncture to France, and Salandière (1825), who had been taught how to use this form of treatment by the physician son of the composer Berlioz, decided that rather than applying a noxious stimulus by means of manually manipulating needles he would do so by passing a direct Galvanic current through them. It may be seen from his writings on the subject that he employed this electrical form of acupuncture for the treatment of 'la goutte, les rheumatismes, et les affections nerveuses'.

It was soon found, however, that this galvanic direct type of current is liable to have undesirable electrolytic effects leading, in some cases, to tissue necrosis. It was because of this that Duchenne (1849), 18 years after Faraday had introduced the use of alternating currents, began to use a faradic type of stimulus when employing electricity for therapeutic purposes (Macdonald 1998).

Physicians during the 19th century, however, viewed electroacupuncture with considerable suspicion, due to there being little or no understanding as to how it might work and also because by that time all forms of electrical treatment had been brought into disrepute by charlatans using them inappropriately (Kane & Taub 1975).

Interest in its use was, nevertheless, eventually rekindled in the West once the Chinese, in the middle of the 20th century, began to use what has come to be known as acupuncture analgesia for the purpose of suppressing surgically evoked pain.

## ACUPUNCTURE ANALGESIA

In 1958 doctors at the First Shanghai Peoples' Hospital decided to try to alleviate severe post-tonsillectomy throat pain in one of their patients by vigorously manipulating, by hand, a needle inserted into the first dorsal interosseous muscle.

They chose this point, known in the traditional system of Chinese acupuncture as Hoku (sometimes spelt Hegu) and also known as Large Intestine 4 (see Fig. 15.11), as needle stimulation of it had been used by the Chinese for centuries in the treatment of various painful disorders around the face. This was, however, the first time that any attempt had been made to suppress severe postoperative pain in this manner.

The procedure proved to be so effective that they next decided to use it on a patient immediately prior to the carrying out of a tonsillectomy in an attempt to suppress the pain caused by the operation. This proved to be equally successful and once a report of it was published acupuncture anaesthesia as it was initially called was soon being used throughout China (Macdonald 1982).

However, in order to suppress surgically evoked pain, peripheral nerve endings have to be stimulated very strongly for at least 20 min; it therefore soon became apparent that to do this by means of manually manipulating needles is a very laborious process. Therefore, the Chinese decided to employ electroacupuncture instead.

Although this procedure was initially referred to as acupuncture anaesthesia, it soon became apparent that this was not a particularly appropriate term as it only suppresses pain and has no effect on other sensations such as touch and temperature. For this reason it is now called acupuncture analgesia (AA).

### How news about acupuncture analgesia reached the Western world

People in the West came to learn about the use of AA for the suppression of surgically evoked pain in China when people, principally from America, went there during the early 1970s.

Dimond in 1971 reported how during the course of a visit to Beijing, he witnessed the technique being used on a regular basis for the suppression of pain evoked by a variety of operations, including dental extractions, thoracotomies and Caesarian sections. He also reported how he became particularly impressed by the seeming advantages of this procedure when, on one occasion, he witnessed it being used whilst a thoracic surgeon himself had a lobe of his lung removed. For not only was the patient so unconcerned about the operation that throughout it he talked animatedly, but at one stage he ate some fruit and at the end entered into a detailed discussion with those present concerning the pathological features of the resected lobe!

In 1972, no less a person than President Nixon visited China on a goodwill mission and both he and his entourage were also shown the technique being used to suppress surgically evoked pain. The President's personal physician, Walter Tkach (1972), became so enthusiastic about what he saw that on his return to America he immediately wrote a somewhat emotive six-page article entitled *I Have Seen Acupuncture Work* in a widely read magazine.

It was not long after this that various leading members of the medical profession in the Western world including Bonica (1974) from America and Smithers et al (1974) from Britain visited China to see for themselves the technique being used.

Any initial enthusiasm such people in the West may have had for it must, however, have been severely strained when an article appeared in the Daily Telegraph in 1980 under the title *China Bursts Acupuncture Bubble*. In this Earnshaw (1980) regrettably had to draw attention to a report that had recently appeared in the Shangai newspaper *Wen Hui Bao* revealing that during China's cultural revolution doctors had been forced to use and patients had been cajoled into receiving acupuncture prior to undergoing major surgery as a matter of political expedience, regardless as to whether or not it was likely to be effective. Furthermore, that when the procedure, as so often happened, failed to provide adequate pain relief the patient was ordered not to scream but instead to shout out political slogans! It also stated that any doctor who deliberately defied official policy by employing some alternative form of anaesthesia took the risk of being denounced as a counter-revolutionary and punished. This depressing state of affairs according to Earnshaw was further compounded by those who wielded political power publishing misleading reports concerning the efficacy of the procedure.

It is only right to stress, however, that subsequent to the revolution, doctors in China have done everything in their power to make amends for the shortcomings of their former masters by conducting research into the various aspects of acupuncture with the highest possible standards of integrity and, as will be seen, so far as the relief of pain is concerned, have helped to place acupuncture on a sound scientific basis.

Among the first to do this were Chiang and his co-workers, who in 1973 provided scientific evidence that acupuncture has an analgesic effect by using electrical dolorimetry to measure the pain threshold in normal adults before and after the insertion of acupuncture needles. By this means they were able to show that treatment of this type causes a significant elevation of the pain threshold all over the body, but with this tending to be greatest in the segments into which needles had been inserted. They also proved that the widespread analgesia produced by an acupuncture stimulus is not due to some chemical agent being released locally and then transported around the body through the cardiovascular system, by showing that its production is not interfered with by occluding the blood supply to a limb above the site to which the stimulus has been applied.

Evidence that acupuncture's analgesic effect is dependant on an intact nervous system came from the Peking Medical College's Research Group of Acupuncture Anaesthesia (1973), who showed in experiments on humans that the pain threshold is not elevated should needles be inserted into tissues affected by a loss of sensation. Also, from Chang (1973) who showed that the pain threshold remains unaffected should acupuncture be carried out at a site where a local anaesthetic has been injected. And demonstrated in experimental animals that sectioning of the anterolateral tract of the spinal cord abolishes acupuncture's analgesic effect.

It was also in 1973 that Chang reported having carried out even more sophisticated experiments on rats and rabbits. In these he recorded impulses from single neurons in thalamic nuclei that had been produced as a result of the application of a painful stimulus to an extremity. He showed that inhibition of these impulses could be obtained by squeezing the tendo Achilles and by electrically stimulating cutaneous nerves. Also, by inserting acupuncture needles into the body and that the most effective inhibition was obtained when the latter was carried out in the same segment as the painful stimulus had been applied.

One year later the Research Group of Acupuncture Anaesthesia at Peking Medical College (1974) produced crucially important evidence to show that acupuncture analgesia (AA) may be associated with the release of chemical substances into the central nervous system by showing that the pain threshold in rabbits could be increased by infusing into their brains cerebrospinal fluid obtained from other rabbits who had been subjected to acupuncture stimulation.

## Pioneer research into the neurophysiology of acupuncture analgesia

It was certainly extremely propitious that the evidence just referred to suggesting the possibility that AA may be brought about by the release of chemical substances was published contemporaneously with the discovery firstly of opioid receptors and then of opioid peptides in the body (see Ch. 6). For it quickly occurred to many working in this particular field of research that these peptides might be the ones involved in its production.

Research into this possibility from the 1970s onwards was principally carried out by Professor Han and his colleagues at Beijing Medical University in China, by Professor Pomeranz and his team at the University of Toronto in Canada and by Professors Besser & Rees, together with their co-workers, at St Bartholomews Hospital in London, UK.

It was incidentally the studies carried out at this latter hospital that did so much at that time to persuade various members of the medical profession in Britain to look at acupuncture in a less suspicious manner than formerly and to start investigating the possibility of employing it clinically for the alleviation of pain.

Included among these was myself, who, having just retired from my post as a hospital-based physician in the early 1980s, was so motivated both by this research being carried out at my alma mater and by the work on TrP acupuncture that was being conducted at that time by Dr Alex Macdonald at Charing Cross Hospital in London for the alleviation of myofascial pain, as to lead me to spend the years that have since passed further investigating the use of acupuncture for analgesic purposes.

## Studies involving the use of naloxone, an opioid peptide antagonist

When in 1974 Pomeranz and his team in Toronto began to study the neural mechanisms involved in the development of AA, they induced it in awake mice by means of a 20-minutes application of a low-frequency (4 Hz)/high-intensity electrically applied stimulus delivered through needles inserted into the 1st dorsal interosseous muscle – the traditional Chinese Large Intestine 4 (Ho-Ku) point (Fig. 15.11). The AA was tested by measuring the latency to squeak after applying heat to the noses of these animals. Then, in order to establish whether or not AA induced by this means is endogenous opioid peptide (EOP) mediated, Pomeranz & Chiu (1976) observed the effect of administering naloxone, a specific opioid peptide antagonist. And it was as a result of this experiment that they had the distinction of being the first to confirm that it is.

This was clearly a very significant discovery, but what was even more exciting was when Mayer et al (1977) confirmed 1 year later that what Pomeranz and his team had found in mice also applied to humans. They did this by means of an experiment showing that the analgesic effect of acupuncture on electrically induced tooth pulp pain in man is similarly reversed by naloxone.

Two years after this, the first clue as to whether or not AA is invariably EOP-mediated was provided by Sjölund & Eriksson (1979) when they showed that whilst both high-frequency (>100 Hz) low-intensity and low-frequency (<10 Hz) high-intensity electrical nerve stimulation alleviate pain, it is only the analgesia provided by the latter type of stimulus that is reversed by naloxone.

The situation then became temporarily confused when the following year Chapman et al (1980) reported their inability to reverse with naloxone AA induced in healthy volunteers subjected to experimentally inflicted dental pain. And when, 3 years later, by which time (see Ch. 6) it was known that stress alone is capable of bringing about the release of EOPs, Chapman et al (1983) concluded that any rise in either the cerebrospinal fluid or plasma EOP levels observed when EA is used in either animal or human experiments, does not occur as a direct result of the acupuncture itself but rather as a result of the stress associated with the carrying out of these experiments.

Peets & Pomeranz (1987), however, were able to refute this by showing that AA induced both in anaesthetized and awake animals is similar.

When Han et al (1984), carried out experiments on rats given EA at stimulation frequencies of either 2, 15 or 100 Hz through needles inserted bilaterally into traditional acupuncture points Stomach 36 (Fig. 19.1) and Spleen 6 (Fig. 16.1), they found that naloxone (1 mg/kg) completely abolished the analgesic effect of 2 Hz EA, partially reversed that of 15 Hz EA and had no effect on that of 100 Hz EA. They discovered that the reason for this is that the type of EOP released into the central nervous system (CNS) is dependant on the EA frequency employed, and that metenkephalin is liberated at 2 Hz, dynorphin A at 100 Hz and a mixture of enkephalins and dynorphins at 15 Hz. They also came to the conclusion that the dose of naloxone needed to block EA-induced AA varies according to the type of EOP released and therefore on the frequency of the EA employed.

The basic reason for this variable ability of naloxone to block analgesia produced either by morphine or EOPs is that all three of these substances have different binding affinities for the mu, delta and kappa opioid receptors in the CNS. Both morphine and naloxone attach themselves principally to mu receptors, met- and leu- enkephalins to delta receptors and dynorphins to kappa receptors (Bowsher 1987).

The lesson to be learnt from all this, as Han (1985) has pointed out, is that when attempting to show whether or not the development of EA-induced AA is EOP-mediated, by means of observing whether or not naloxone blocks the analgesia, it is essential to take into consideration both the parameters of the EA stimulus employed and the dose of naloxone administered.

There have been at least 28 reports confirming naloxone blockade of AA and seven reports failing to observe this effect (Stux & Pomeranz 1987).

In view of the results of the experiments carried out by Han et al (1984), it has become easier to understand the reasons for this disparity with it now being generally accepted that the EOP-mediated mechanism responsible for AA, both in humans and animal studies, is best brought into

action with low-frequency/high-intensity stimulation. This accounts for four of the failed experiments, as the one carried out by Chapman et al (1983) involved the use of a low-frequency/low-intensity EA stimulus and the other three involved the employment of a high-frequency/low-intensity stimulus. And the reason why the other three failed may be because naloxone appears to work best when given before the treatment begins and is unable to reverse analgesia once it has already developed (Pomeranz 1989). The implication of this is that EOP-mediated AA is not naloxone reversible as is so often stated but rather naloxone preventable.

It has been shown that a microinjection of naloxone into sites in the spinal cord (Peets & Pomeranz 1985) and brain (Zhou et al 1981), which contain an abundance of opioid peptides and their receptors blocks the development of AA.

With reference to this, Zhou et al (1981, 1982, 1984), in experiments on rabbits, have demonstrated that to block the effect of AA by more than 70%, it only requires an injection of 1 μg of naloxone into one or other of the following structures: the periaqueductal grey area of the midbrain, the nucleus accumbens, the amygdala in the limbic system and the habenular nucleus situated in the dorsomedial aspect of the thalamus. And that also it only requires a microinjection (5–10 μg) of morphine into any one of these four sites to produce marked analgesia.

These particular sites, therefore, are of considerable importance with respect to EOP-mediated AA and will be referred to again when the long-term analgesic effect of manual acupuncture carried out for the alleviation of chronic pain is discussed because Han (1987) has put forward the suggestion it might be sustained activity in the so-called meso-limbic neural loop formed by them and the arcuate nucleus in the hypothalamus that may be one of the reasons for bringing this about.

### Changes in endogenous opioid peptide cerebrospinal fluid levels in response to electroacupuncture

Evidence in support of EOPs having a role in the production of AA has also come from studies of

EOP levels in the cerebrospinal fluid (CSF) of patients before and after EA.

In the first such study, Sjölund et al (1977) collected CSF from patients with chronic pain treated with EA-like transcutaneous nerve stimulation and measured CSF EOP levels before and after treatment. When they applied electrodes to the lumbar region of patients with low-back pain they observed that the CSF levels of these peptides had doubled after 30 minutes of treatment. And that, in contrast to this, when they treated patients with face pain by stimulating in a similar manner the Large Intestine 4 (Ho-Ku) traditional Chinese acupuncture point in the first dorsal interosseous muscle of the hand (Fig. 15.11), no changes in the lumbar CSF EOP levels were observed. This clearly was because the stimulation was being carried out at a cervical segmental level rather than at a lumbar segmental one. It was unfortunate that in this particular study the CSF EOP levels were measured by receptor-binding assays, as this did not reveal which EOPs in particular were involved.

In contrast to this, Clement-Jones et al (1980), in the studies carried out at St Bartholomews Hospital, London, specifically measured CSF concentrations of beta-endorphin and metenkephalin by radioimmuneassay in a group of patients with recurrent pain before and after a 30 minutes application of low-frequency EA. And found that, although the concentrations of metenkephalin remained unchanged, the beta-endorphin levels rose after this particular type of stimulation had been applied.

Morley (1985), however, has issued a warning that care has to be taken in drawing conclusions from measurements of CSF levels of EOPs, because the presence of these substances in the CSF is most likely to arise from overspill of neuronal activity and may, therefore, not necessarily reflect their degree of activity in neurons themselves.

This not withstanding, such measurements before and after 20–30 minutes of low-frequency/high-intensity EA stimulation, and the results of most of the naloxone studies already discussed, make it reasonable to postulate that the analgesic effect of this particular type of acupuncture is associated with the activation of EOP-mediated pain-modulating mechanisms in the central nervous system.

## Development of opioid peptide activity at three sites

It has been shown that low-frequency/high-intensity EA brings about its analgesic effect by the release of EOPs at three sites, the dorsal horn, the midbrain and the hypothalamus/pituitary complex.

**The dorsal horn**  An EA stimulus of this type applied to A-delta skin and Groups II & III muscle sensory afferents causes enkephalin and dynorphin to be released into the dorsal horn with, as a consequence, the blocking of any nociceptive-generated information transmitted to it via C-polymodal skin and Group IV muscle sensory afferents.

**The midbrain**  In the midbrain it leads to the release of enkephalin and this then activates the serotoninergic-mediated pain inhibitory system that descends from its periaqueductal grey area down the dorsolateral funiculus to dorsal horns.

**The hypothalamus/pituitary complex**  Here it causes adrenocorticotrophic hormone (ACTH) to be released from the anterior pituitary into the circulation. It is presumably because of the liberation of cortisol from the adrenal cortex as a consequence of a stimulus of this type that explains why it would seem to have an anti-inflammatory effect on tissues in general and to act as a bronchodilator.

It also causes beta-endorphin to be released into the hypothalamus and because the latter projects to the midbrain the effect of this is to cause activity to develop in the pain inhibitory system that descends from there.

## Augmentation of acupuncture analgesia (AA) by prevention of EOP degradation

It should be noted that the development of AA may be enhanced by preventing EOPs from becoming degraded by the action of various enzymes for Cheng & Pomeranz (1980) have observed that the administration of the enzyme blockers D-leucine and D-phenylalamine augments the development of AA and that a combination of these D-aminoacids and EA produces a greater amount of analgesia than the latter alone.

## Comprehensive reviews

Space does not permit for all of the evidence in support of EOP involvement in AA to be discussed here and therefore those who wish to know more about this subject should consult recently published comprehensive reviews such as those provided by Han (2001), Pomeranz (2001) and White (1998, 1999).

## The role of serotonin (5–hydroxytryptamine) in the development of acupuncture analgesia

When acupuncture needles are inserted into muscles for the purpose of bringing about the development of AA, the consequent needle-induced stimulation of A-delta skin and Groups II & III muscle sensory afferents has several effects, including the creation of activity in the serotonin-mediated descending pain inhibitory system situated in the dorsolateral funiculus (see Ch. 6). And, therefore, in view of this, it is hardly surprising that the development of AA is now known to be influenced by alterations in the central nervous system's serotonin levels.

Han & Terenius (1982) state that those initially engaged in research into the various aspects of AA at the Peking Medical College, reported in 1975 that para-chlorphenylalanine, a serotonin synthesis inhibitor, when injected into the lateral ventricle of the rabbit, inhibits its development. Following this McLennan et al (1977) found that cyproheptadine, a serotonin receptor antagonist also does this. Later, in 1979, Kin et al demonstrated that cianserin, another serotonin receptor blocker, has a similar effect in the cat.

Conversely, Han et al (1979) found that the intraventricular administration of 5-hydroxytryptophan, a serotonin precursor, enhances the production of AA in the rat.

With respect to humans, Han & Terenius (1982) found that the administration of either clomipramine which blocks the re-uptake of serotonin, or pargyline, which blocks its degradation, augmented the effect of AA in patients who were undergoing the removal of impacted molar teeth.

It should be noted in view of what has already been said with regard to the apparent importance of the nucleus accumbens, the amygdala, the habenula and the periaqueductal grey in the development of AA, that during the 1980s Han and his co-workers published several papers showing that analgesia of this type is significantly attenuated when cianserin, the serotonin receptor blocker is microinjected into any one of these four brain nuclei (Han 1989).

Zhang & Han (1985) have also shown that the release of serotonin and its effect on the production of AA is the same no matter whether the EA is carried out employing either a high- or low-frequency current, and regardless as to whether the stimulus is of high or low intensity.

Finally, in view of all that has been discussed, it is hardly surprising to find (Han et al 1980, Zhou et al 1982) that the simultaneous interference with both serotonin and EOP levels results in a dramatic decrease or even complete abolition of any analgesia induced by EA.

## TRANSCUTANEOUS ELECTRICAL NERVE STIMULATION (TENS)

Although transcutaneous electrical nerve stimulation (TENS) has proved to be of considerable help in relieving the pain present in a number of disorders, its place in the alleviation of musculoskeletal pain in general and of myofascial TrP pain in particular would seem to be strictly limited. Nevertheless, in view of this type of treatment's close relationship to electroacupuncture, its mode of action and the main indications for its use will be briefly discussed.

Melzack & Wall (1965), as explained in Chapter 6, based their gate-control theory on the supposition that the stimulation of large diameter A-beta sensory afferents has the effect of blocking the transmission of noxious information generated in skin C-polymodal and muscle Group IV nociceptors when it reaches the dorsal horn via small diameter non-myelinated sensory afferents.

It was this hypothesis that led Wall & Sweet (1967) to conclude that because large diameter A-beta fibres have a lower electrical resistance than small diameter C and Group IV do, it should be possible to suppress the transmission along these latter fibres by electrically stimulating the larger diameter ones – a deduction that led them to discover the pain-suppressing use of TENS.

A form of therapy that over the years has come to be divided into two types: conventional and acupuncture-like.

## Conventional TENS (Fig. 9.1)

With this type A-beta sensory afferents are stimulated by passing a *high*-frequency (40–150 Hz), *low*-intensity current between electrodes attached to the skin overlying a nerve.

It is believed that a stimulus of this type releases gamma-aminobutyric acid and that this inhibitory neurotransmitter blocks the intra-dorsal transmission of noxious information generated in C skin and Group IV muscle nociceptors (Thompson 1989, 1998).

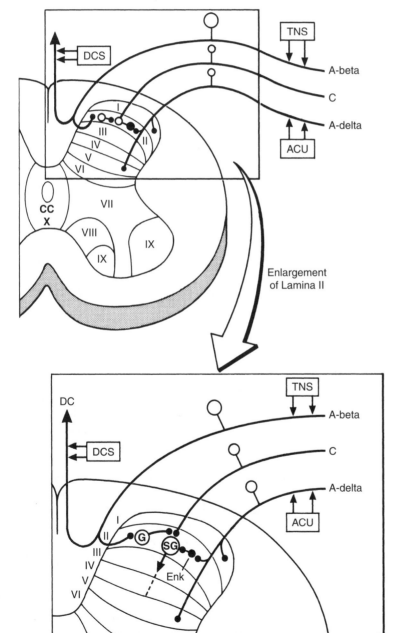

**Figure 9.1** Entry of primary afferents into the dorsal horn of the spinal cord, and circuits involved in TENS and acupuncture. Roman numerals refer to laminae numbers. SG = Substantia gelatinosa cell. G = GABAergic interneuron, presynaptically inhibiting primary afferent C fibre terminal. Enk = Enkephalinergic interneuron, postsynaptically inhibiting substantia gelatinosa neuron. The enkephalinergic interneuron is not only activated, as shown, by A-delta primary afferent terminals, but also by serotoninergic fibres descending from the brainstem (see Fig. 9.2). CC = Central canal. DC = Dorsal column. DCS = Dorsal column stimulation. TNS = Low-threshold, high frequency stimulation. ACU = High-threshold, low frequency stimulation. Dr David Bowsher's diagram in Journal of British Medical Acupuncture Society 1990. Reproduced with permission.

## Acupuncture–like TENS

With this form of TENS a *low*-frequency (1–5 Hz), *high*-intensity current is employed, and because the analgesia produced by it is abolished by the opioid peptide antagonist naloxone, it is believed that a current of this type, like acupuncture, must stimulate A-delta sensory afferents with the result-ant development of opioid peptide-mediated pain suppression. Unfortunately, a strongly applied stimulus of this type is not well tolerated because of it giving rise to strong muscle contractions (Andersson et al 1976, Melzack 1975) and in order to avoid this Eriksson et al (1979) have introduced an apparatus that allows trains of high- and low-frequency stimulation to be applied alternately.

Johnson et al (1991) have shown that it is only possible to decide which of these two forms of TENS best alleviate any particular type of pain by trying each one in turn.

### Indications for the use of conventional and acupuncture-like TENS

Well-conducted clinical trials carried out over the years have provided support for TENS being employed for the suppression of a number of dif-ferent types of pain.

**Orofacial pain**    The use of either high-frequency or acupuncture-like TENS applied to the painful area has been shown to have a pain-relieving effect in patients with a variety of different acute dental disorders such as pulpitis and apical periodontitis (Hansson & Ekblom 1983).

**Angina pectoris**    Borjesson et al (1997), Chauhan et al (1994) and Mannheimer et al (1985) have all demonstrated the usefulness of high-frequency TENS in the alleviation of anginal pain.

**Dysmenorrhoea**    There is good evidence to show that high-frequency TENS is of value in suppress-ing painful menstruation (Dawood & Ramos 1990, Lundeberg et al 1985, Milson et al 1994).

**Peripheral neuropathic pain**    Several studies have demonstrated that TENS has an important place in helping to alleviate the pain in some but not all patients suffering from a peripheral neuropathy (Fishbain et al 1996, Meyler & De Jongste 1994).

The presence of tactile allodynia complicates its employment for this purpose due to the pressure of the pads inducing pain when they are first applied (Hansson & Lundeberg 1999). It should also be noted that with any disorder, such as post-herpetic neuralgia, where there is damage to A-beta fibres, it is essential for the electrodes to be placed above the affected site.

**Postoperative and labour pain**    It was for long thought that TENS had a place in the alleviation of postoperative pain, but a systematic review of controlled trials refutes this (Carroll et al 1996).

Similarly it has been widely used for the sup-pression of labour pain, but again an extensive review of controlled trials has failed to provide sup-port for this (Carroll et al 1997).

**Musculoskeletal pain**    The results of trials to determine the usefulness of TENS in the treatment of chronic low-back pain (Deyo et al 1990) and of acute low-back pain (Herman et al 1994) suggest that it may have a place in the suppression of mus-culoskeletal pain but the non-specificity of the diagnoses in these two studies makes it difficult to come to any firm conclusion about this.

Graff-Radford et al (1989), on the other hand, have shown that treatment of this type is capable of alleviating pain that emanates from MTrPs and, therefore, there is a place for using it for that specific purpose when, as occasionally happens, repeated dry needling carried out at MTrP sites fails to afford any long-term relief.

## TENS – analgesia tolerance

A serious disadvantage of TENS is that any pain relief obtained with it invariably disappears within 30 minutes of the stimulus being discontinued, so that the treatment has to be applied for several hours a day. And, even worse, over the course of time, there is liable to be a declining response to it, a phenomenon Johnson et al (1991) have called TENS analgesia tolerance.

Comprehensive reviews of all aspects of this form of treatment have been provided by Thompson (1986, 1994, 1998).

## THERAPEUTIC ACUPUNCTURE

Felix Mann (1974), during the course of discussing acupuncture analgesia, a procedure in which a very strong needle-evoked nerve stimulus is applied, usually electrically, for up to 20 minutes in order to obtain immediate short-term suppression of surgically induced acute pain, was the first to draw attention to the marked differences between the carrying out of that and of acupuncture employed therapeutically for the relief of symptoms of one type or another. Because, as he said therapeutic acupuncture is one in which a very much lighter needle-evoked nerve stimulus is briefly applied, usually manually, at approximately 7-day intervals, and one that with respect to chronic pain is capable, following successive treatments, of providing gradually increasing long periods of relief.

## The difference in the state of nerve endings at traditional Chinese acupuncture points and at MTrPs

Although Melzack et al (1977) showed that traditional Chinese acupuncture points (TCAPs) and myofascial trigger points (MTrPs) have a very close spatial relationship, the important difference is that a TCAP is only slightly tender due to the nerve endings at such a site being in a quiescent state, but a MTrP is exquisitely tender because of the nerve endings there having become activated and sensitized for one reason or another, with the commonest being the subjection of the muscle containing it to trauma (Ch. 7). This difference concerning the state of the nerve endings at these two types of points is of considerable importance because, when employing manual acupuncture at a TCAP site for the purpose of suppressing chronic pain, the stimulus applied invariably has to be a relatively strong one. In contrast to this, when employing MA at a MTrP site for the specific purpose of alleviating myofascial pain, it is usually only necessary to apply a light one.

## Superficial and deep dry needling for the deactivation of MTrPs

When treating the MTrP pain syndrome there are grounds for believing, as discussed in the next chapter, that manually applied superficial dry needling (SDN) with needles inserted to a depth of 5–10 mm at MTrP sites should mainly be used and that deep dry needling (DDN) should be reserved for the minority of cases where MTrP activity develops as a secondary event such as, for example, because of an underlying radiculopathy. The neurophysiological mechanisms involved during the carrying out of SDN will, therefore, first be considered.

### Superficial dry needling's pain-suppressing mechanisms (Figs 9.1, 9.2)

When SDN is carried out at a MTrP site it is usually only the A-delta sensory afferents that are stimulated for the C-polymodal ones would only be recruited should the stimulus applied happen to be an exceptionally vigorous and prolonged one. Attention will, therefore, be focussed on what is known to happen when A-delta fibres are subjected to needle-evoked stimulation.

Bowsher (1998), in an extremely comprehensive and authoritative review of the mechanisms of acupuncture when employed for the alleviation of chronic pain, has given a detailed account of the effects of stimulating A-delta nerve fibres.

As he states, Kumazawa & Perl (1978) have shown that A-delta nerve fibres in the primate project principally to Waldeyer cells situated in the most superficial zone (Lamina I) of the spinal cord's dorsal horn.

Between Lamina I and II there are very small 'stalked' cells whose presence in the cat was first demonstrated by Bennett et al (1982) and in man by Abdel-Maguid & Bowsher (1984). Stalked cells receive a direct input from A-delta fibres (Gobel et al 1980) and the effect of stimulating sensory afferents of this type with a needle is to cause these cells to release the inhibitory opioid peptide enkephalin (Ruda et al 1984). This in turn then inhibits activity in the substantia gelatinosa cells to which small unmyelinated sensory afferent fibres, such as those connected to MTrP's Group IV nociceptors project. And as a consequence, the input to the dorsal horn of noxious information generated in a MTrP's Group IV nociceptors becomes blocked.

The intra-dorsal-horn flow of this information is also interrupted as a result of manual acupuncture-evoked stimulation of A-delta fibres also having

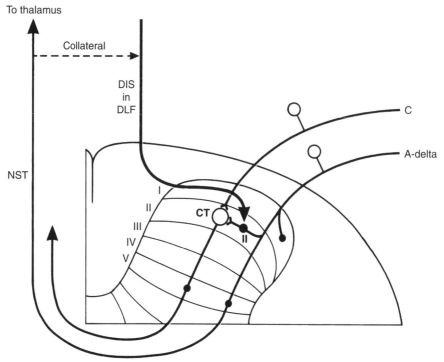

**Figure 9.2** Diagram of dorsal horn to show the local intraspinal connection between A-delta nerve fibres and enkepha-linergic inhibitory interneuron (II), whose function it is to inhibit activity in C afferent terminal cell (CT). Also, to show the indirect A-delta link with inhibitory interneuron via the collateral connecting the A-delta afferent's ascending pathway – the neospinothalamic tract (NST) with the descending inhibitory system in the dorsolateral funiculus (DIS in DLF).

an inhibitory effect on wide dynamic range transmission neurons (Hashimoto & Aikawa 1993).

### Indirect development of pain-suppressing activity in the serotonergic, noradrenergic and diffuse noxious inhibitory systems

Stimulation of A-delta nerve fibres such as when SDN is carried out brings about pain suppression because of it causing local activity to develop in and around Waldeyer cells in the dorsal horn's Lamina I, where these sensory afferents principally terminate. In addition, pain suppression occurs because cells in this lamina, as discussed at some length in Chapter 6, have projections to the periaqueductal grey area in the midbrain at the upper end of the serotonergic-mediated descending pain inhibitory system, to the locus coeruleus in the pons at the upper end of the noradrenergic-mediated descending pain inhibitory system and

to the subnucleus reticularis dorsalis in the medulla at the upper end of the diffuse noxious inhibitory control system.

### Segmental versus non-segmental acupuncture

Should a needle be inserted anywhere in the body the above three descending pain-suppressing systems will be brought into action. It is clearly, however, far better to carry out acupuncture at the same segmental level as any noxiously generated information enters the spinal cord, as this activates not only these three systems, but also the powerful dorsal horn-situated opioid peptide-mediated one.

It is for this reason, as will again be discussed in Chapter 10, that when carrying out SDN for the alleviation of MTrP pain, it is necessary to carefully identify the exact position of each MTrP and then to take care to insert a needle into the tissues at that specific site.

## Deep dry needling's pain-suppressing mechanisms

As will be explained in the next chapter, should a stronger stimulus be required, such as, for example, may happen when MTrP activity arises secondary to the development of a radiculopathy, DDN should be employed.

During the carrying out of this procedure A-delta nerve stimulation must take place as a result of the needle passing through the skin and subcutaneous tissues with, as a consequence, all of the pain-suppressing mechanisms just discussed being brought into action. Then, once the needle enters the substance of the muscle not only are Group II and III afferents stimulated, but also, should the needle be rapidly inserted into a MTrP itself, a local twitch response (LTR) is evoked.

Chu (1995) has postulated that the production of this response and the consequent changes in the lengths of muscle fibres brought about by it leads to the setting up of a large diameter sensory afferent proprioceptive input to the spinal cord which, by virtue of this having a 'gate-controlling' effect, causes blocking of the intra-dorsal horn passage of noxious information generated in the MTrP's nociceptors.

Although this may be one of the mechanisms involved, it would seem that there must also be an EOP-mediated one because Fine et al (1988) have shown that when a needle (together with a small amount of bupivacaine to suppress the discomfort of this procedure – see Ch. 10) is inserted into a MTrP, any alleviation of myofascial pain that may be brought about by this procedure is reversed by the opioid antagonist naloxone.

## CHALLENGE TO CONVENTIONAL VIEWS CONCERNING PAIN-RELIEVING MECHANISMS BROUGHT INTO ACTION BY THERAPEUTIC MANUAL ACUPUNCTURE

Carlsson (2000, 2002 a, b) has compellingly challenged the currently held views concerning therapeutic acupuncture's pain relieving mechanisms.

His grounds for doing so are because the widely accepted modus operandi is only capable of offering an explanation for very short-term pain relief by

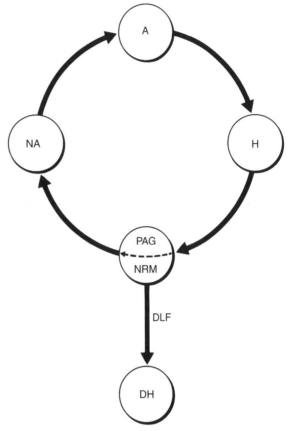

**Figure 9.3**   Han's proposed mesolimbic loop of analgesia – A neuronal circuit involving the nucleus accumbens (NA), the amygdala (A), the habenula (H) and the upper parts of the descending inhibitory system, the periaqueductal grey (PAG) and nucleus raphe magnus (NRM), which are connected to the dorsal horn (DH) by the dorsolateral funiculus (DLF).

virtue of it relying on gate-control mechanisms, which only exert their effect during the time the stimulation is being applied and on descending inhibitory systems, which, he suggests, are unlikely to function for more than about 8 hours.

As he explains, because the gate-control and descending inhibitory mechanisms are so ephemeral, the conventional model cannot account for the following widely recognized clinical observations: (1) that the pain relief often lasts for days after a single treatment, (2) that the pain relief is sometimes delayed for 1–2 days, (3) that the pain is sometimes worse for some days following treatment and then starts to improve, and (4) that there is often a cumulative pain-relieving effect with increasingly long periods of pain relief being obtained in response to successive treatments.

In the light of all this he concludes that the currently accepted neurophysiological model is only capable of providing an explanation for short-term acupuncture analgesia but not for the long-term pain relief afforded by therapeutic acupuncture.

An alternative mechanism put forward by him to explain the latter is the induction of peripheral events that might improve tissue function and induce local pain relief. These include the anti-inflammatory action of neuropeptides like calcitonin gene-related peptide; the local release of endorphins; the induction of segmental mechanisms including

long-term depression of A-delta fibre-evoked excitatory potentials in the dorsal horn (Sandkuhler 2000, Sandkuhler & Randic 1997). Also, the bringing into action of central mechanisms including sympathetic inhibition with a consequent decrease in levels of plasma epinephrine (adrenaline) and cortisone; and possibly the release of oxytocin as this is believed to induce long-term pain threshold elevations and to have effects of an anti-stress nature (Uvnäs-Moberg 2002).

Other mechanisms to account for the sustained analgesic effect of therapeutic acupuncture discussed by White (1999) include Han et al's proposed mesolimbic loop (Fig. 9.3) and the induction of mRNA for opioid peptide expression (Guo et al 1996).

# References

Andersson S A, Hansson G, Holmgren E, Renberg O 1976 Evaluation of the pain – suppressant effect of different frequencies of peripheral electrical stimulation in chronic pain conditions. Acta Orthopaedica Scandinavica 47: 149–157

Abdel-Maguid T E, Bowsher D 1984 Interneurons and proprioneurons in the adult human spinal grey matter and general somatic afferent cranial nerve nuclei. Journal of Anatomy 139: 9–20

Baldry P E 1971 The battle against heart disease. Cambridge University Press, Cambridge, p. 46

Bennett G J, Ruda M A, Gobel S, Dubner R 1982 Enkephalin – immunoreactive stalked cells and lamina 11b islet cells in cat substantia gelatinosa. Brain Research 240: 162–166

Bonica J J 1974 Therapeutic acupuncture in the People's Republic of China. Journal of the American Medical Association 228(12): 1544–1551

Borjesson M, Eriksson P, Dellborg M, Eliasson T, Mannheimer C 1997 Transcutaneous electrical nerve stimulation in unstable angina pectoris. Coronary Artery Disease 8/9: 543–550

Bowsher D 1987 Mechanisms of pain in man. ICI Pharmaceuticals Division

Bowsher D 1998 Mechanisms of acupuncture. In: Filshie J, White A (eds) Medical acupuncture, a Western scientific approach. Churchill Livingstone, Edinburgh

Carlsson C P O 2000 Long-term effects of acupuncture (dissertation), Lund University

Carlsson C P O 2002a Acupuncture mechanisms for clinically relevant long-term effects – reconsideration and a hypothesis. Acupuncture In Medicine 20(2–3): 82–99

Carlsson C P O 2002b Acupuncture mechanisms for clinical long-term effects, a hypothesis. In: Sata A, Li P,

Campbell J (eds) Acupuncture, is there a physiological basis. Excerpta Medica, International Congress Series 1238. Elsevier, Amsterdam, pp. 31–47

Carroll D, Tramer M, McQuay H, Nye B, Moore A 1996 Randomization is important in studies with pain outcomes: systematic review of transcutaneous electrical nerve stimulation in acute postoperative pain. British Journal of Anaesthesia 6: 798–803

Carroll D, Tramer M, McQuay H, Nye B Moore A 1997 Transcutaneous electrical nerve stimulation in labour pain: a systematic review. British Journal of Obstetrics and Gynaecology February: 169–175

Chang H T 1973 Integrative action of thalamus in the process of acupuncture for analgesia. Scientia Sinica 16: 25–60

Chiang C Y, Chang C T, Chu H L, Yang I F 1973 Peripheral afferent pathway for acupuncture analgesia. Scientia Sinica 16: 210–217

Chapman C R, Beneditti C, Colpitts Y H, Gerlach R 1983 Naloxone fails to reverse: pain thresholds elevated by acupuncture. Acupuncture analgesia reconsidered. Pain 16: 13–31

Chapman C R, Colpitts Y M, Benedetti C, Kitaeff R, Gehrig J D 1980 Evoked potential assessment of acupuncture analgesia: attempted reversal with naloxone. Pain 9: 183–197

Chauhan A, Mullins P A, Thurasingham S I, Taylor G, Petch M C, Schofield P M 1994 Effect of trancutaneous electrical nerve stimulation on coronary blood flow. Circulation 2: 694–702

Cheng B, Pomeranz B 1980 A combined treatment with D-amino acids and electroacupuncture produces a greater analgesia than either treatment alone: naloxone reverses these effects. Pain 8: 231–236

Chu J 1995 Dry needling (intramuscular stimulation) in myofascial pain related to lumbosacral radiculopathy. European Journal of Physical medicine and Rehabilitation 5(4): 106–121

Clement-Jones V, Tomlin S, Rees L H, McLoughlin L, Besser G M, Wen H L 1980 Increased beta – endorphin but not met-enkephalin levels in human cerebrospinal fluid after acupuncture for recurrent pain. Lancet 2: 946–948

Dawood M Y, Ramos J 1990 Transcutaneous electrical nerve stimulation (TENS) for the treatment of primary dysmenorrhoea: a randomized crossover comparison with placebo TENS. Obstetrics and Gynaecology 4: 656–660

Deyo R A, Walsh N E, Martin D C, Shoenfield L S, Ramamurthy S 1990 A controlled trial of transcutaneous electrical nerve stimulation (TENS) and exercise for chronic low back pain. New England Journal of Medicine 23: 1627–1634

Dimond E G 1971 Acupuncture anesthesia. Western medicine and Chinese traditional medicine. Journal of the American Medical Association 218(10): 1558–1563

Duchenne G B A 1849 A critical examination of instruments. Comptes Rendus de l' Academie des Sciences

Earnshaw G 1980 China bursts acupuncture bubble. Daily Telegraph, London, 24th October, p. 13

Eriksson M B E, Sjolund B H, Nielzen S 1979 Long term results of peripheral conditioning stimulation as an analgesic measure in chronic pain. Pain 6: 335–347

Fine P G, Milano R, Hare B D 1988 The effects of myofascial trigger point injections are naloxone reversible. Pain 32: 15–20

Fishbain D A, Chabal C, Abbott A, Heine L W, Cutler R 1996 Transcutaneous electrical nerve stimulation (TENS) treatment outcome in long-term users. Clinical Journal of Pain 3: 201–214

Gobel S, Falls W M, Bennett G J, Abdelmoumene M, Hayashi H, Humphrey E 1980 An E. M. analysis of the synaptic connections of horseradish peroxidase filled stalked cells and islet cells in the substantia gelatinosa of the adult cat spinal cord. Journal of Comparative Neurology 194: 781–807

Graff-Radford S B, Reeves J L, Baker R L, Chiu D 1989 Effects of transcutaneous electrical nerve stimulation on myofascial pain and trigger point sensitivity. Pain 37: 1–5

Graham H 1939 Surgeons all. Rich & Cowan, London, p. 24

Guo H-F, Tian J, Wang X, Fang Y et al 1996 Brain substrates activated by electroacupuncture of different frequencies (1): comparative study on the expression of oncogene c- fos and genes coding for three opioid peptides. Molecular Brain Research 43: 157–166

Han J S 1985 Acupuncture analgesia. Pain 21: 307–308

Han J S 1987 Mesolimbic neuronal loop of analgesia. In: Tiengo M, Eccles J, Cuello A C, Ottoson D (eds) Advances in pain research and therapy, Vol. 10. Raven Press, New York

Han J S 1989 Central neurotransmitters and acupuncture analgesia. In: Pomeranz B, Stux K (eds) Scientific bases of acupuncture. Springer-Verlag, Berlin, pp. 7–33

Han J S 2001 Opioid and antiopioid peptides: a model of yin-yang balance in acupuncture mechanisms of pain modulation. In: Stux G, Hammerschlag R (eds) Clinical acupuncture, scientific basis. Springer-Verlag, Berlin

Han J S, Chou P H, Luc C et al 1979 The role of central 5-hydroxytryptamine in acupuncture analgesia. Scientia Sinica 22: 91–104

Han J S, Tang J, Fan S G et al 1980 Central 5-hydroxytryptamine, opiate-like substances and acupuncture analgesia. In: Way E L (ed) Endogenous and exogenous opiate agonists and antagonists. Pergamon, New York, pp. 395–398

Han J S, Terenius L 1982 Neurochemical basis of acupuncture analgesia. Annual Review of Pharmacology and Toxicology 22: 193–220

Han J S, Xie G X, Ding X G, Fan S G 1984 High and low frequency electroacupuncture analgesia are mediated by different opioid peptides. Pain 369(supp): 543

Hansson P, Ekblom A 1983 Transcutaneous electrical nerve stimulation (TENS) as compared to placebo TENS for the relief of acute orofacial pain. Pain 15: 157–165

Hansson P, Lundeberg T 1999 Transcutaneous electrical nerve stimulation, vibration and acupuncture as pain – relieving measures. In: Wall P, Melzack R (eds) Textbook of pain, 4th edn. Churchill Livingstone, Edinburgh

Hashimoto T, Aikawa S 1993 Needling effects on nociceptive neurons in rat spinal cord. Proceedings of the 7th World Congress on Pain. IASP, Seattle, p. 428

Herman E, Williams R, Stratford P, Fargas-Babjak A, Trott M 1994 A randomized controlled trial of transcutaneous electrical nerve stimulation (CODETRON) to determine its benefits in a rehabilitation program for acute occupational low back pain. Spine 5: 561–568

Johnson M I, Ashton C H, Thompson J W 1991 An in-depth study of long term users of transcutaneous electrical nerve stimulation (TENS). Implications for clinical use of TENS. Pain 44: 221–229

Kane K, Taub A 1975 A history of local electrical analgesia. Pain 1: 125–138

Kin K C, Han Y F, Yu L P et al 1979 Role of brain serotonergic and catecholaminergic systems in acupuncture analgesia. Acta Physiologica Sinica 31: 121–132 (In Chinese, English abstract)

Kumazawa T, Perl E R 1978 Excitation of marginal and substantia gelatinosa neurons in the primate spinal cord: indications of their place in dorsal horn functional organization. Journal of Comparative Neurology 177: 417–434

Lundeberg T, Bondesson I, Lundstom V 1985 Relief of primary dysmenorrhea by transcutaneous electrical nerve stimulation. Acta Obstetrica Gynaecologica Scandinavica 64: 491–497

Macdonald A J R 1982 Acupuncture from ancient art to modern medicine. George Allen & Unwin, London

Macdonald A J R 1998 Acupuncture's non-segmental and segmental analgesic effects: the point of meridians. In: Filshie J, White A (eds) Medical acupuncture, a Western scientific approach. Churchill Livingstone, Edinburgh

McLennan H, Gilfillan K, Heap Y 1977 Some pharmacological observations on the analgesia induced by acupuncture in rabbits. Pain 3: 229–238

Mann F 1974 Acupuncture analgesia. Report of 100 experiments. British Journal of Anaesthesia 46: 361–364

Mannheimer C, Carlsson C A, Emanuelsson H, Vedin A, Waagstein F 1985 The effects of transcutaneous electrical nerve stimulation in patients with severe angina pectoris. Circulation 2: 308–316

Mayer D J, Price D D, Raffi A 1977 Antagonism of acupuncture analgesia in man by the narcotic antagonist naloxone. Brain Research 121: 368–372

Melzack R 1973 The puzzle of pain. Basic Books, New York

Melzack R 1975 Prolonged relief of pain by brief intense transcutaneous somatic stimulation. Pain 1: 357–373

Melzack R, Stillwell D M, Fox E J 1977 Trigger points and acupuncture points for pain: correlations and implications. Pain 3: 3–23

Melzack R, Wall P D 1965 Pain mechanisms. A new theory. Science 150: 971–979

Melzack R, Wall P D 1982 The challenge of pain. Penguin, Harmondsworth, Middlesex

Meyler W J, De Jongste M J L 1994 Clinical evaluation of pain treatment with electrostimulation: a study on TENS in patients with different pain syndromes. Clinical Journal of Pain 10: 22–27

Milson I, Hedner N, Mannheimer C 1994 A comparative study of the effect of high-intensity transcutaneous nerve stimulation and oral naproxen on intrauterine pressure and menstrual pain. American Journal of Obstretics and Gynaecology 1: 123–129

Morley J S 1985 Peptides in nociceptive pathways. In: Lipton S, Miles J (eds). Persistent pain. Grune & Stratton, New York, Vol. 5, pp. 65–91

Peets J M, Pomeranz B 1985 Acupuncture-like transcutaneous electrical stimulation analgesia is influenced by spinal cord endorphins but not serotonin: An intrathecal pharmacological study. In: Fields H L, Dutner R, Cervero F (eds) Advances in pain research and therapy, Vol. 9. Raven Press, New York, pp. 519–525

Peets J M, Pomeranz B 1987 Studies of suppression of nocifensive reflexes using tail flick electromyograms and intrathecal drugs in barbiturate anesthetized rats. Brain Research 416: 301–307

Pomeranz B 1989 Acupuncture research related to pain, drug addiction and nerve regeneration. In: Pomeranz B, Stux G (eds) Scientific bases of acupuncture. Springer-Verlag, Berlin, pp. 35–52

Pomeranz B 2001 Acupuncture analgesia – basic research. In: Stux G, Hammerschlag R (eds) Clinical acupuncture, scientific basis. Springer-Verlag, Berlin, pp. 1–28

Pomeranz B, Chiu D 1976 Naloxone blockade of acupuncture analgesia: endorphin implicated. Life Sciences 19: 1757–1762

Research Group of Acupuncture Anaesthesia, Peking Medical College 1973 Effect of acupuncture on the pain threshold of human skin. National Medical Journal of China 3: 151–157 (in Chinese, English abstract)

Research Group of Acupuncture Anaesthesia, Peking Medical College 1974 The role of some neurotransmitters of brain in finger – acupuncture analgesia. Scientia Sinica 17: 112–130 (English translation)

Ruda M A, Coffield J, Dubner R 1984 Demonstration of postsynaptic opioid modulation of thalamic projection neurons by the combined techniques of retrograde horseradish peroxidase and enkephalin immunocytochemistry. Journal of Neuroscience 4: 2117–2132

Salandière 1825 Mèmoires sur l' electropuncture considéreé comme moyen nouveau de traiter efficacement la goutte, les rhumatismes et les affections nerveuses. Paris

Sandkuhler J 2000 Long-lasting analgesia following TENS and acupuncture: spinal mechanisms beyond the gate control. In: Devor M, Rowbotham M C, Weisenfeld-Hallin Z (eds) Proceedings of the 9th World Congress of Pain. Seattle: IASP Press

Sandkuhler J, Randic M 1997 Long-term depression of primary afferent neurotransmission induced by low frequency stimulation of afferent A-delta fibres. In: Jensen T S, Turner J A, Wiesenfield-Hallin Z (eds) Proceedings of the 8th World Congress of Pain. Seattle: IASP Press

Sjölund B H, Erikisson M B E 1979 Endorphins and analgesia produced by peripheral conditioning stimulation. In: Bonica J J, Albe-Fessard D, Liebeskind J C (eds) Advances in pain research and therapy 3. Raven Press, New York, pp. 587–599

Sjölund B H, Terenius L, Eriksson M 1977 Increased cerebrospinal fluid levels of endorphins after electroacupuncture. Acta Physiologica Scandinavica 100: 382–384

Smithers D, Alexander P, Hamilton-Fairley G et al 1974 Report of the British Medical Delegation to China April–May 1974. Unpublished documents. Medical Research Council, London

Stux G, Pomeranz B 1987 Acupuncture textbook and atlas. Springer-Verlag, Heidlberg

Thompson J W 1986 The role of transcutaneous electrical nerve stimulation (TENS) for the control of pain. In: Doyle D (ed) International symposium in pain control. Royal Society of Medicine Services International Congress and Symposium Series 123. Royal Society of Medicine, London

Thompson J 1989 Pharmacology of transcutaneous electrical nerve stimulation (TENS). Journal of the Intractable Pain Society of Great Britain and Ireland 7(1): 33–40

Thompson J 1994 Neuropharmacology of the pain pathways. In: Wells P E, Frampton V, Bowsher D (eds) Pain management and physiotherapy, 2nd edn. Butterworth Heinemann, Oxford

Thompson J 1998 Transcutaneous electrical nerve stimulation (TENS). In: Filshie J, White A (eds) Medical acupuncture, a Western scientific approach. Churchill Livingstone, Edinburgh

Tkach W 1972 I have seen acupuncture work. Today's Health, July, pp. 50–56

Uvnäs-Moberg K 2002 Oxytocin – A possible mediation of anti-stress effects induced by acupuncture. Acupuncture in Medicine 20(2–3): 109–110

Wall P D, Sweet W H 1967 Temporary abolition of pain. Science 155: 108–109

Wand-Tetley J 1956 Historical methods of counter-irritation. Annals of Physical Medicine 3: 90–98

White A 1998 Electroacupuncture and acupuncture analgesia. In: Filshie J, White A (eds) Medical acupuncture, a Western scientific approach. Churchill Livingstone, Edinburgh

White A 1999 Neurophysiology of acupuncture analgesia. In: Ernst E, White A (eds) Acupuncture, a scientific approach. Butterworth-Heinemann, Oxford

Zhang M, Han J S 1985 5-hydroxyytryptamine is an important mediator for both high and low frequency electroacupuncture analgesia. Acupuncture Research 10: 212–215 (In Chinese, English abstract)

Zhou Z F, Du M Y, Wu W Y, Jian Y, Han J S 1981 Effect of intracerebral microinjection of naloxone in acupuncture and morphine analgesia in the rabbit. Scientia Sinica 24: 1168–1178

Zhou Z F, Xuan Y T, Han J S 1982 Blockade of acupuncture analgesia by intraventricular injection of naloxone or cianserin in the rabbit. Acupuncture Research 7: 91–94

Zhou Z F, Xuan Y T, Han J S 1984 Analgesic effect of morphine into habenula, nucleus accumbens and amygdala of rabbits. Acta Pharmacologica Sinica 5: 150–153 (in Chinese, English abstract)

# Chapter 10

# Treatment of myofascial trigger point pain and fibromyalgia syndromes

## INTRODUCTION

In the first part of this chapter the various methods available for the deactivation of myofascial trigger points (MTrPs) will be reviewed.

These include injection either into MTrPs themselves or into the tissues around them of such disparate substances as local anaesthetics, corticosteroids, non-steroidal anti-inflammatory drugs, botulinum toxin, physiological saline and even water alone!

Evidence will be provided to show that all of these forms of treatment, which are now often collectively referred to as 'wet' needling procedures, owe their MTrP pain-relieving effect to one factor, namely the stimulation of nerve endings by the needle employed to inject them.

Reasons will be given for concluding that these 'wet' needling procedures have no advantages over, and many disadvantages compared to the employment of 'dry' needling ones. In view of this, attention will be focussed in particular on the two acupuncture (acus (L)-needle) procedures, called superficial dry needling (SDN) and deep dry needling (DDN) that are now widely used for the deactivation of MTrPs. The measures that sometimes have to be taken to prevent the reactivation of these points will also be outlined.

In the second part of this chapter, the various forms of therapy that are currently being employed in the management of fibromyalgia will be discussed, including the carrying out of needling at tender and TrP sites.

## 'WET' NEEDLING MTrP DEACTIVATING TECHNIQUES

### Injection of a local anaesthetic into MTrPs

As already discussed in Chapter 4, when during the 1930s John Kellgren found that pain in the disorder he called myalgia emanates from points that have since come to be called MTrPs, he alleviated it by injecting a 1% solution of procaine (novocain) into each of them in turn.

He presumably employed a local anaesthetic because of its nerve blocking effect. Yet, although the latter only lasts for some hours he found it was possible to obtain pain suppression for at least 24 hours and often for even longer. Such prolonged periods of relief, therefore, could not have been due to the action of the local anaesthetic but, with hindsight, must have been due to the bringing into action of the various needle-evoked pain suppressing mechanisms discussed at some length in the last chapter. Thus, although Kellgren did not realize it at the time, his observations in retrospect served to re-affirm what physicians like Churchill and Sir William Osler in the latter part of the 19th century and Sun Ssu-mo in the 6th century had discovered concerning the pain-alleviating effect of inserting needles into points of maximal tenderness.

With respect to all this it has to be said that Janet Travell, the American physician, who from the 1940s onwards, took over the study of MTrP pain from where Kellgren left off, was quick to realize that the prolonged analgesia produced by injecting a local anaesthetic into a MTrP could equally well be attained by simply inserting a needle into it (Travell & Rinzler 1952). On finding, however, that a needle on entering a MTrP gives rise to an unacceptable amount of acute pain, she decided to continue to inject a small amount of procaine (0.25%) through it in order to suppress this treatment evoked discomfort.

Her method of carrying out the procedure was succinctly described in a classic paper entitled 'The Myofascial Genesis of Pain' (Travell & Rinzler 1952) as follows:

> By pressing on trigger area, demonstrate pain reference to patient.
>
> Ask patient to announce when pain radiation is felt during infiltration. When needle hits trigger

area, pepper region by moving it in and out of muscle, injecting 1–2 cc continuously.

> Use 0.25 to 0.5% procaine hydrochloride in physiological saline (unless history of procaine allergy).
>
> Use a sharp 22–24 gauge needle, 1–3 in long, depending on site of trigger area.
>
> Apply haemostasis promptly.
>
> Check success of injection. If trigger area is still tender, reinfiltrate at different depths and angles.

### Hong's modification of Travell's technique

Travell's procedure just described has in recent years been modified by Hong (1994a) as a result of him finding that when a needle is rapidly inserted into different parts of a MTrP it is possible to evoke a succession of local twitch responses. He concluded from this that a MTrP must be made up of a number of separate loci and that, in order for it to be satisfactorily deactivated, each locus has to be penetrated in turn.

In order to avoid damaging the muscle whilst doing this, Hong advises pushing the needle in and out of the MTrP at the very fast speed of 100–200 mm/s. A manoeuvre of this type clearly demands much manual dexterity. Furthermore, it inevitably causes much bleeding into the tissues with, because of this, an appreciable amount of post-treatment soreness.

Hong (1994b) has carried out a trial to compare the MTrP pain-relieving effectiveness of either using a needle alone or of injecting a local anaesthetic through it and from the results of this concluded that the latter is preferable.

Hong's method of deactivating MTrPs is now much used (Simons et al 1999), but despite the use of a local anaesthetic the repeated insertion of a needle into each TrP causes a considerable amount of pain; also, much bleeding with, as a consequence, the development of post-treatment soreness. Furthermore, there is at present no evidence to show that the results obtained with it in alleviating pain arising as a result of the primary activation of MTrPs are any better than those obtained with the far simpler and very much less painful superficial dry needling technique advocated later in this chapter.

## Injection of normal saline into MTrPs

Because a local anaesthetic may at times give rise to undesirable side-effects the American physician Anders Sola decided during the 1950s to see whether it is possible to deactivate a MTrP by injecting normal saline into it.

From a trial on 100 consecutive patients with neck and shoulder MTrP pain Sola & Kuitert (1955) came to the conclusion that 'the use of normal saline has none of the disadvantages often associated with the use of a local anaesthetic but appears to have the same therapeutic value'.

One year later Sola & Williams (1956) reported similarly good results from treatment in the same way of 1000 patients with MTrP pain in various parts of the body.

Interestingly enough, it does not seem to have occurred to them that the effectiveness of this type of treatment might have been due to the effect of the needle itself rather than to that of injecting isotonic saline.

Unlike them Frost et al (1980) clearly thought that physiological saline was unlikely to have any specific pain relieving effect because, when carrying out a trial to assess the efficacy of injecting the long-acting local anaesthetic mepivacaine into MTrPs present in 28 patients in an active treatment group, they injected normal saline into the MTrPs of 25 patients in a control group. They were therefore at first somewhat surprised to find that 76% in the 'control' group and only 57% in the 'treatment' group had pain relief. A result, however, which on refection led them to conclude:

> … the more favourable effect of physiological saline may be due to the longer duration of irritation since nerve impulses are not blocked by saline … the study therefore raises questions about the mechanism by which local injections into muscles relieve pain, since there is a possibility that a similar effect might also be achieved by merely inserting a needle into a trigger point. …

Support for this belief has come from three further trials comparing the pain-relieving effect of saline with that of a local anaesthetic.

Tfelt-Hansen et al (1981), injected either lidocaine (lignocaine) or normal saline into tender points of two groups of patients with migraine and showed, according to the patients' assessments using visual analogue scales, that both were equally effective.

Tschopp & Gysin (1996), in patients with MTrPs pain in the head and neck regions, compared the pain-relieving effectiveness of injecting lidocaine (lignocaine) into MTrPs in one group of patients, the longer-acting local anaesthetic bupivicaine into them in a second group and saline into them in a third group. Subjective assessments by the patients led to the conclusion that all three substances are of equal efficacy.

McMillan et al (1997) divided patients with craniofacial MTrP pain into three groups. One group was treated by having both procaine injected into their MTrPs, plus the carrying out of superficial dry needling at these sites. A second group had dry needling of their MTrPs plus injection of saline into the superficial tissues at these sites. And a third group had a superficial injection of saline and superficial dry needling at their MTrP sites. All three groups had similarly significant pain relief as judged by a variety of tests including the use of visual analogue scales and algometers.

## Injections of steroidal and non-steroidal anti-inflammatory drugs into MTrPs

Although histological examination of tissues at MTrP sites have never shown any evidence of an inflammatory lesion, trials have, nevertheless, been carried out to assess the value of injecting either a non-steroidal anti-inflammatory drug (NSAID) or a steroid into MTrPs. This having been said, it has to be admitted that NSAIDs have an inhibitory effect on cyclooxygenase and as a result depress the production of prostaglandins that assist in sensitizing MTrPs' nociceptors.

Frost (1986), in patients with myofascial pain in the neck, shoulder or lower back, compared the effect of injecting the NSAID diclofenac into MTrPs in one group of patients with that of injecting lidocaine (lignocaine) into points of this type in another group. From an assessment employing visual analogue scales the pain relief in both groups was equally good.

Drewes et al (1993) have carried out a study to compare the effectiveness of relieving myofascial pain from injecting either diclofenac or prednisolone into MTrPs. Both forms of treatment proved to be equally effective with 84% of patients in the two groups being significantly improved as judged by verbal pain questionnaires and a physician's evaluation.

The possibility, however, cannot be excluded that the pain relief in both groups was due to the one factor common to both namely the effect of inserting a needle into the MTrPs. Moreover, as was pointed out by those carrying out the trial, the use of these drugs is not without risks. Diclofenac, particularly if injected into the superficial tissues, is liable to cause necrosis of the skin. And the repeated injection of a steroid drug into a muscle is liable to result in its fibres becoming damaged. Also, when given more superficially it is liable to cause the skin to become pitted and depigmented. For these reasons alone the injection into MTrPs of either a non-steroidal anti-inflammatory drug or a corticosteroid as advocated by Bourne (1979, 1984) cannot be recommended.

Despite this there have been two other corticosteroid trials.

Frost et al (1984), divided patients with chronic myofascial pain into three groups and over a period of 6–12 days treated them on three occasions as follows. One group was given injections of isotonic saline (8 ml) into MTrPs, a second group, injections of isotonic saline (2 ml) into MTrPs, and a third group injections of isotonic saline (1 ml) plus prednisolone (1 ml) into points of this type. As judged by visual analogue scales all three groups did equally well with overall 84% of the patients still obtaining some relief 2 months after the treatments had finished.

Garvey et al (1989) divided patients with myofascial low back pain into three groups. They injected 1.5 ml of 1% lidocaine (lignocaine) into MTrPs in one group; 0.75 ml of 1% lidocaine (lignocaine) plus a corticosteroid (Aristospan) into MTrPs in a second group; and inserted needles into MTrPs in a third group. From information obtained with pain scales they concluded that there was no significant difference in the pain-alleviating effect of these three forms of treatment.

The results of these two trials, therefore, confirmed what had already been established, that there is no advantage to be obtained from the use of a corticosteroid when deactivating MTrPs. As Travell & Simons (1983) have pointed out, the only justification for the employment of a steroid injection so far as the management of musculoskeletal pain disorders is concerned is in the treatment of an inflammatory lesion such as a rotator cuff tendinitis or lateral epicondylitis.

## Injection of botulinum A toxin into MTrPs

Tsui et al (1986), because of botulinum A toxin's ability to relax muscle when injected into it, successfully used this toxin for the treatment of spasmodic torticollis.

Cheshire et al (1994) then decided in view of this to see whether it had any place in the treatment of MTrP pain. And on comparing the effect of normal saline with that of this toxin in six patients with myofascial pain found that four of them obtained benefit from the toxin.

Following this, Yue (1995) carried out a retrospective study of 112 patients who had had this substance injected into MTrPs and found that 86% of them reported having been helped, with an average pain reduction of 36.5%. Seventeen per cent of the patients, however, complained of moderate to severe side-effects, with the commonest of these being muscle weakness sufficient to impair motor functions and the eventual onset of muscle atrophy.

Since then Wheeler et al (1988) have divided patients with refractory cervicothoracic paraspinal myofascial pain into three groups and injected into their MTrPs either botulinum toxin (50 units in 2 ml of normal saline); botulinum toxin (100 units in 2 ml of normal saline): or 2 ml of normal saline alone. The effectiveness of the three treatments as judged by subjective assessments made by the patients was equally good and thus showed that the pain alleviation in all three groups was primarily due to the one factor they had in common, namely the application of a needle-evoked nerve stimulus.

In view of this and because of the side-effects of this toxin, contrary to what Lang (2002) has had to say on the matter, there would seem to be no place for its use in the routine treatment of MTrP pain.

It is, nevertheless, extremely interesting to find that this substance, which is know to block the release of acetycholine from motor nerve terminals at neuromuscular junctions, has the ability to deactivates MTrP for, as Simons (1996) has said, this is a 'strong indicator that the MTrP mechanism is intimately associated with the neuromuscular junction'.

## SYSTEMATIC REVIEW OF 'WET' AND 'DRY' NEEDLING CLINICAL TRIALS

Cummings & White (2001) have carried out an extremely valuable systematic review of all the randomized controlled trials in which the treatment of myofascial pain has involved the use of either 'wet' needling or 'dry' needling. Some of these trials are referred to in this chapter and others will be discussed in Chapter 11 when the evaluation of acupuncture's ability to relieve nociceptive pain in general will be considered.

Their search led them to state: 'The principal findings of this review are that, when treating myofascial pain with TrP injections, the nature of the injected substance makes no difference to the outcome, and that wet needling is not therapeutically superior to dry needling.

Thus they, as a result of meticulously analysing the results of clinical trials carried out during the latter part of the 20th century, have now confirmed what Sir William Osler (1909) at the beginning of it intuitively concluded from his own clinical observations, that in order to alleviate what is currently called myofascial pain it is necessary to do no more than simply stimulate nerve endings at points of maximum tenderness with a needle!

## Deep dry needling MTrP deactivating techniques

The person who during the latter part of the 20th century pioneered the use of deep dry needling (DDN) at MTrP sites was the Czech physician Karel Lewit. He, unlike Travell & Rinzler (1952), was not deterred by it being a painful procedure, on the contrary, in his paper on the subject (Lewit 1979) entitled 'The Needle Effect in the Relief of Pain' he stated that 'the effectiveness of the treatment is related to the intensity of pain produced at the trigger zone and to the precision with which the site of maximum tenderness is located by the needle'.

In this paper he reported the results of treating 241 patients with pain emanating from what he variously called trigger zones, pain spots and sites of maximal tenderness by means of inserting dry needles into these points. He called the immediate analgesia produced by this procedure 'the needle effect'. He also reported having obtained it in 86.8% of the patients. A finding that led him to state that

'the pain relieving effect previously ascribed to local anaesthetics may in fact be due to needling'. He thus had come to the same conclusion as had been reached by Travell & Rinzler 30 years earlier.

Chen Gunn (1989, 1996, 1998), a physician working in Vancouver, has since then written extensively in support of the use of DDN. He calls his particular technique 'intramuscular stimulation' (IMS). When employing it he inserts a needle deep into the belly of a muscle, but unlike Lewit, does not believe it is necessary to penetrate the MTrPs themselves.

His method is widely used, but one of its main disadvantages is that it is a very painful procedure, with he himself (Gunn 1989) stating that when a needle is inserted into a tightly contracted band of muscle the 'patient experiences a peculiar cramp-like sensation as the needle is grasped … the intensity of the cramp parallels that of the spasm: it can be excruciatingly painful, but gradually resolves as the spasm eases'. He also points out that the spasm is frequently so prolonged and the needle, because of this, so firmly grasped that it is often 10–30 minutes before it can be released.

This notwithstanding he employs this particular type of DDN routinely in all patients suffering from MTrP pain.

Jennifer Chu, on the other hand, uses a form of DDN specifically for the alleviation of MTrP pain that arises as a secondary event following the development of either a cervical (Chu 1997) or lumbar (Chu 1999) radiculopathy.

Chu, like Hong (see p. 128), is of the opinion, that for the best results, the needle should be repeatedly inserted into various parts of an MTrP for the purpose of evoking a succession of local twitch responses. A procedure she calls twitch-obtaining intramuscular stimulation (TOIMS).

## Disadvantages

DDN is not only extremely painful but is also liable to cause damage to nerves, blood vessels and other structures.

For these reasons and because experience has led me to believe that for the purpose of deactivating a primarily activated MTrP superficial dry needling (SDN) is not only just as effective, but far simpler to carry out and much less likely to cause tissue damage, my personal preference (Baldry 2002b) is to employ SDN for the vast majority of my patients with MTrP pain and to reserve DDN for the small number of them in which MTrP actively arises secondary to the development of a radiculopathy.

## SUPERFICIALLY APPLIED MTrP DEACTIVATING TECHNIQUES

### The application of a vapocoolant spray to the skin

Travell & Rinzler (1952) found that they could deactivate MTrPs by spraying the local anaesthetic ethyl chloride across the skin overlying them whilst at the same time stretching the affected muscle. This substance, however, is potentially explosive and, therefore, Travell (1968) eventually employed instead the safer alternative fluori-methane, a mixture of two fluorocarbons.

Those who have since given detailed accounts of the indications for and the manner of carrying out this muscle stretch and spray technique include Rachlin (1994) and Travell & Simons (1983).

The present position however is that, whilst stretching the muscles after deactivating TrPs in them is still considered to be of considerable importance, the application of a vapocoolant is not any longer widely employed.

## THE INJECTION OF WATER INTRADERMALLY AT MTrP SITES

Byrn et al (1991), in a preliminary uncontrolled trial carried out in Gothenburg, Sweden, found that injecting sterile water into the skin overlying active MTrPs in the necks of patients suffering from whiplash injuries relieved the pain emanating from them for appreciable periods of time.

### Subcutaneous injections of either water or normal saline at MTrP sites

Unfortunately water injected into the skin gives rise to an intense and extremely distressing burning sensation. Therefore, Byrn et al (1993), in a much larger trial, decided to compare the effectiveness of injecting either sterile water or isotonic saline (0.3–0.5 ml) into the subcutaneous tissues overlying active TrPs present in the neck muscles of patients with whiplash injuries.

Their conclusion was that of the two, water injected into the subcutaneous tissues at MTrPs sites gives most pain relief and for this reason have since continued to use it extensively.

The one considerable disadvantage, however, is that water, when injected into the subcutaneous tissues, like when injected into the skin, gives rise to an intense burning sensation similar to that caused by a wasp sting.

Wreje & Brorsson (1995) found this when carrying out a multicentre randomized controlled trial to compare the effectiveness of combined subcutaneous and intracutaneous injections of either sterile water or physiological saline at MTrP sites for chronic myofascial pain. For this reason its use for this particular purpose is unlikely to be widely adopted.

## SUPERFICIAL DRY NEEDLING AT MTrP SITES

Initially it was my practice to use DDN for the deactivation of MTrPs until the early 1980s when a patient was referred to me with pain down the arm from a TrP in the scalenus anterior muscle. In view of the proximity of the lung it was considered wiser not to push the needle into the MTrP itself but rather to insert it more superficially into the tissues immediately overlying it. This proved to be all that was required for after leaving the needle in situ for a short time and then withdrawing it the exquisite tenderness at the MTrP site was found to have been abolished and the spontaneous occurring pain alleviated.

This superficial dry needling (SDN) technique was then used to deactivate TrPs elsewhere in the body where it proved to be equally effective even when the muscles containing them were deep lying. Another interesting observation was that any palpable bands found to be present at the MTrP sites before such treatment disappeared after it.

At about the same time Macdonald et al (1983) confirmed the efficacy of SDN in alleviating pain arising from MTrPs in the lumbar region by means of a trial carried out at Charing Cross Hospital, London, UK. In this study 17 consecutive patients with chronic lumbar MTrP were divided into two groups. One group was treated by means of SDN, with the needles inserted to a depth of 4 mm at

MTrP sites. And a control group was treated by having electrodes applied to the skin overlying MTrPs connected by non-current carrying wires to a purposely impressive TENS machine replete with dials, flashing lights and cooling system that made a 'whirring' sound. The results of this trial were such as to allow unbiased 'blinded' observers to conclude that the effectiveness of SDN is significantly superior to that of a placebo.

## DETERMINATION OF THE OPTIMUM STRENGTH OF NEEDLE–EVOKED NERVE STIMULATION

The responsiveness of people to the needle-evoked nerve stimulation procedure known as acupuncture is widely variable (Mann 1992). Whilst most are average responders there are some who are strong reactors and others who are weak ones. Thus when carrying out SDN at MTrP sites it is essential to establish the optimum strength of stimulation for each individual patient, as a stimulus that is not sufficiently powerful to alleviate a weak reactor's MTrP pain may be enough to cause a strong responder to experience a distressing albeit temporary exacerbation of it.

The reason for this variability amongst people is not certain but there are grounds for believing that weak reactivity may be genetically determined.

In support of this is that Peets & Pomeranz (1978) have identified a strain of mice (CXBX) who, because they are genetically deficient in endogenous opioid peptide receptors, respond poorly to needle-evoked nerve stimulation. And that Murai & Takeshige (1986) had difficulty in producing analgesia by this means in a strain of rats deficient in endorphins.

Another possibility that has to be considered when attempting to explain why some people are weak responders to needle-evoked nerve stimulation is that they may have excessive amounts of endogenous opioid peptide antagonists in their nervous systems. Subsequent to the ancient Chinese putting forward their belief in a yin-yang balance in the body it has been confirmed that every type of physiological activity is regulated by an opposing one. Examples of these include the counterbalancing effects of insulin and glucagon; of calcitonin and parathyroid hormone; and generally speaking

of the sympathetic and parasympathetic nervous systems (Han 2001). It was in view of this that the discovery of endogenous opioid peptides in the 1970s (see Ch. 6) prompted a search for substances in the body possessing antiopioid activity. Several have since been found including orphanin FQ (Yuan et al 1999), nocistatin (Okuda-Ashitaka et al 1998), and angiotensin 11 (Kaneko et al 1985), but as already discussed in Chapter 6, the most powerful one is cholecystokinin-8 (CCK-8).

With respect to this, Han (1995) has shown that an electroacupuncture stimulus accelerates the release of endogenous opioid peptides and that these then stimulate neurons to release CCK-8 as a negative feedback mechanism.

There are therefore grounds for believing that the reason why some people are weak responders to needle-evoked nerve stimulation is because of various genetically determined factors including an inherent tendency to secrete excessive amounts of opioid antagonists.

## TECHNIQUE RECOMMENDED FOR THE CARRYING OUT OF SDN IN THE TREATMENT OF A PRIMARILY ACTIVATED MTrP POINT

A MTrP is of such exquisite tenderness (see Ch. 7) that the application of **firm** pressure to it gives rise to a flexion withdrawal (the 'jump' sign) and often, in addition to this, the utterance of an expletive (the 'shout' sign).

Clinical experience has led me to believe that the optimum strength of needle stimulation required to alleviate an individual patient's MTrP pain is the minimum amount necessary to abolish these two reactions.

In view of this it is my practice (Baldry 1995, 1998, 2001, 2002 a, b) on **first treating** someone, to insert an acupuncture needle (0.3 mm × 30 mm) into the tissues overlying each MTrP to a depth of about 5–10 mm (i.e. sufficient to allow it to be self-standing). The needle is then left in situ for 30 seconds. And on withdrawing it pressure equal to that exerted before treatment is reapplied to the MTrP site to see whether the 'jump' and 'shout' reactions have been abolished. This usually proves to be so but if not the needle is reinserted and left in situ for 2–3 minutes. In a small minority of cases re-testing for the above two reactions shows it is necessary to increase the stimulation still more by means of yet once again re-inserting the needle and not only leaving it in situ for some time but also intermittently twirling it.

The purpose of adopting this step-by-step approach when determining each individual patient's responsiveness to SDN at a MTrP site is to reduce the risk of causing a temporary but, nevertheless, distressing exacerbation of pain as a result of exceeding that person's optimum needle stimulation requirement. Nevertheless, it has to be admitted that there is a small group of patients who are such very strong reactors that even a needle left in situ for 30 seconds proves to be more than necessary. For these people all that is required is for the needle to be inserted into the superficial tissues and then immediately withdrawn.

During subsequent treatments the optimum amount of stimulation found initially to be needed for each patient should be strictly adhered to.

## THE NUMBER OF TREATMENT SESSIONS

There would seem to be general agreement amongst those health professionals in the Western world who use needle-evoked nerve stimulation for the relief of chronic pain that treatment should not be carried out more often than once a week. This is because the full effect of such treatment often does not become apparent for several days and it may, therefore, be misleading to try to assess how much response there has been to it before the end of that time.

## INFORMATION TO BE GIVEN TO A PATIENT AT THE END OF THE FIRST TREATMENT WITH SDN

The patient should be told that any pain relief obtained from the first treatment may only last for 1–2 days; and that occasionally there is a delay of 12–14 hours before this is obtained or conversely but rarely, in view of the particular technique employed, there may be a temporary exacerbation of it. And that should the latter happen the amount of stimulation given on subsequent occasions may have to be reduced.

The patient should also be informed that treatment will initially be given at weekly intervals and the length of time for which relief is obtained after each session should hopefully increase to the extent that after the third one it may well last for 7 days or more and that following this a decision will be made as to whether further treatment is required and if so for how long.

It should be explained that in general the number of sessions required and the interval between them varies according to a person's individual responsiveness and, in particular, to how long the pain has been present prior to starting treatment. That because of this people with chronic pain may have to have SDN repeated every 4 weeks for an indefinite period and conversely, those who have only had pain for a relatively short duration may only require two to three treatments at weekly intervals.

It should also be made clear that should progress not appear to be satisfactory after the third session both the diagnosis and the method of treatment may need to be reviewed.

## SYSTEMATIC SEARCH FOR MTrPs

It is important for needling to be carried out at every active MTrP site. The failure of primary MTrP pain to respond to SDN is often because one or more points have been overlooked. Prior to starting treatment therefore it is essential for the search for them to have been carried out in a systematic manner. Then once all the obviously active MTrPs have been deactivated it is important to check that none have been overlooked. This should be done by ascertaining the range of movements now possible and by systematically palpating the muscles in the affected region again.

## THE SEPARATE OR SIMULTANEOUS DEACTIVATION OF MTrPS

It is my practice when first treating a patient, and on all occasions with strong reactors, to deactivate each MTrP in turn so that the time for which the needle is left in situ can be accurately determined. Then on subsequent occasions, in those cases where the response to the initial treatment has shown that needles can be left in situ for an appreciable period of time without fear of exacerbating the pain, all of the MTrPs are deactivated simultaneously.

## JAPANESE SHALLOW NEEDLING

The SDN method just described needs to be distinguished from the shallow needling one currently used in the traditional Japanese channel type of therapy known as *keiraku chiryo*. During the carrying out of this very thin needles (0.12–0.14 mm) are inserted into the skin to a depth of not more than 1–2 mm at traditional Chinese acupuncture point sites (TCAPs). And in some cases this lightly applied stimulus is augmented by pairs of needles being linked together by an ion pumping cord. This device, according to Birch & Felt (1999), 'connects one shallowly inserted needle into another, allowing for a tiny electrical current to flow between the two needles'.

Trials employing this shallow needling procedure for the alleviation of myofascial pain include one by Birch & Jamison (1998) and another by Ceccherelli et al (2002).

Birch & Jamison divided 46 patients with chronic myofascial neck pain into two groups. Group I had needles (connected by IP Cords) inserted to a depth of 2–3 mm (shallow needling) at what were deemed to be relevant TCAPs. Group II had needles inserted to the same depth at what were deemed to be irrelevant TCAPs. And Groups III was a medication-only control one.

Their conclusion was that 'the results of this study suggest that combined treatment with relevant acupuncture, heat and IP cords is more helpful in relieving myofascial neck pain than irrelevant acupuncture or medication alone'.

Ceccherelli and his co-workers divided 42 patients with lumbar myofascial pain into two groups. Group I had needles inserted to a depth of 2 mm (shallow needling) and Group II had needles inserted into muscle. In both groups the needling was carried out at five predetermined TCAPs and four arbitrarily chosen MTrP sites. They concluded that their clinical results showed that their deep stimulation technique had a better analgesic effect than their shallow needling one.

It may therefore be seen that the shallow needling techniques employed in these two trials were very different from the one called SDN by me, in that needles are not only inserted to a significantly greater depth (5–10 mm) but also, this is done at *all* active MTrP sites found to be present in any particular patient.

## COMPLICATIONS OF ACUPUNCTURE

A prospective survey carried out by White et al (2001) showed that when acupuncture is carried out by doctors and physiotherapists the incidence of side-effects is minimal and that the ones that do occur are far less harmful than those produced by many of the drugs currently being prescribed for combating pain.

The various adverse effects of acupuncture have also been extensively and comprehensively reviewed by Rampes (1998) and by Rampes & Peuker (1999).

### Vaso–vagal attacks

Some people faint at the sight of a needle let alone when it is inserted into them. People who are apprehensive about being needled or have a past history of passing out when being inoculated should not be persuaded against their will to have any form of acupuncture. Moreover, as a liability to fainting is often unpredictable, it is important that everyone on the first occasion should be treated lying down. Having said this, it has to be admitted that the incidence of this complication would seem to be low, as Chen et al (1990) have reported it only occurring 55 times during the course of carrying out 28,285 acupuncture treatments (0.19%).

### Convulsions

Very occasionally a person who has fainted in response to needle stimulation may proceed to have an epileptic fit. Over the past 20 years this complication has only arisen in one of my patients, a known epileptic. Hayhoe & Pitt (1987), however have reported two cases.

### Post-treatment drowsiness

It is not uncommon for a patient to feel sleepy following dry needling. The greater the amount of stimulation given the more likely is this to occur, but with a strong reactor it may happen with only a lightly applied stimulus.

As such a reaction is impossible to predict it is wise for a patient when first treated to be accompanied by a friend who can, if necessary, drive the car on the journey home. A study carried out by Brattberg (1986) on 122 patients treated with acupuncture in a hospital in Sweden revealed that 56% of them were deemed to be so drowsy as to be unsafe to drive themselves home after it.

## Damage to viscera

Visceral damage has been reported to occur during the carrying out of DDN, but is most unlikely to happen when SDN is employed. Nevertheless, care must be taken in both the chest wall and lower neck regions to always insert the needle at an oblique angle in order to avoid inducing a pneumothorax for, as Rampes & Peuker (1999) have pointed out, post-mortem examinations have shown that a puncture depth of as little as 10 mm either parasternally or in the region of the midclavicular line can reach the lung.

In the popliteal region care must be taken not to rupture a Baker's cyst. When this happened to one of my patients during the course of inserting needles into periarticular tender points in the popliteal space for the treatment of osteoarthritis of the knee the considerable pain, tenderness and swelling of the calf that took place simulated that which arises with a deep vein thrombosis. Gray (1996) has also reported a similar case where this happened.

## Haemorrhage

With SDN bleeding into the tissues is uncommon and when it does occur may readily be controlled by the application of firm pressure. Occasionally, however, a haematoma may develop. This is particularly liable to happen with elderly people and with patients on steroids as a result of capillary fragility.

People on anticoagulants should not be treated with dry needling. Smith et al (1989) reported how a man taking warfarin, on being needled, bled so much that pain and swelling in the leg developed to such an extent as to require the carrying out of an anterior compartment decompression fasciotomy.

## Needles lost or forgotten

It is easy to overlook a needle, especially when it has been inserted into a part of the body covered by hair such as the upper part of the neck or scalp of a woman. Therefore, in all cases needles should be counted when being inserted and again when being taken out.

## Transmission of infection

Due to the now universal usage of disposable needles by doctors and physiotherapists when carrying out acupuncture there is no longer any risk of this procedure causing hepatitis B to be transmitted. In the past, however, there were some serious outbreaks of this mainly due to poor hygienic techniques employed by non-medically qualified practitioners. The first to be documented in the UK was reported by the Communicable Disease Surveillance Centre of the Public Health Laboratory Service in 1977. And up until the end of the 1980s there were several other outbreaks in various parts of the world including ones reported by Kent et al (1988) and by Slater et al (1988).

The transfer of AIDS by acupuncture needles has not proved to be a problem. One possible case reported by Vittecoq et al (1989) was not subsequently substantiated.

## Skin disinfection

Routine disinfection of the skin before the carrying out of needling is not considered to be necessary as bacteria resident in it are not liable to cause infection provided host immunity is not seriously impaired. However, as Hoffman (2001) has stated, in any case where the skin is manifestly dirty it should be washed and if there is overt evidence of infection it should be disinfected with alcohol. Laurence & Bennett (1987) recommended using 70% ethyl or isopropyl alcohol for this purpose.

## PHYSIOLOGICAL REACTIONS TO NEEDLING

### Wheal and flare

Sir Thomas Lewis (1942) observed that following a superficial injury to the skin there is often an intense vasodilation at the site of injury followed by the development of oedema (wheal) and a spreading redness (flare). As Fields (1987) has said, this is probably due to Substance P (SP) causing histamine to be released from mast cells. This reaction, which is commonly observed when a needle is inserted into or through the skin, often provides the patient with a pleasant warm feeling but occasionally it is so excessive as to cause a protracted burning sensation.

## Needle-evoked sensations

The Chinese from the earliest days have described various sensations that arise in response to needle stimulation. In the Western literature they are often referred to as de qi, although the sinology scholars Lu & Needham (1980) have stated that the Chinese traditionally called them tê chhi (obtaining the chhi) or chen kan (responding to the needle).

These sensations include first of all ma (a feeling of numbness), then chang (a feeling of distension), followed by chung (a feeling of heaviness) and after this suan (a feeling of soreness).

Wang et al (1985), from studies in which direct microelectrode recordings were made from single fibres in the median nerve during the time that needling was being carried out distally, confirmed that stimulation of Group II muscle afferents produces numbness, stimulation of Group III ones gives rise to sensations of distension and heaviness, and stimulation of unmyelinated Group IV ones causes soreness to develop. De qi may also be produced in response to needle-evoked stimulation of A-delta nerves in the skin (see Ch. 11).

These subjective responses are not only felt at the needle site but may on occasions travel slowly up or down a limb. Lu & Needham (1980) during the course of discussing this drew attention to a statement concerning the cure of headache which appeared in a book entitled *Chi Sheng Pa Sui*, published in 1315. It said, … Ask the subject to cough, then insert the needle at Ho-Ku (Large intestine 4 – see Fig. 15.11) on both sides to a depth of 5 fen (1.53 cm) and turn it counter-clockwise while the patient inhales three times. Then clockwise again for three deep breaths. Repeat the counter-clockwise turning only this time for five inhalations and the contrary ones again in the same way. The patient will then feel the sensation (suan) rising slowly from the hands right up to the shoulders like a thread. Finally ask the patient to take one more breath and withdraw the needle. …

As Lu & Needham (1980) commented:

This strongly suggests that the conception of the acu-tracts may have arisen, at least in part, from the subjective sensations of those who were undergoing acupuncture. It would have been natural enough to envisage thread-like lines of communication after such experiences and what more reasonable than to suppose that the almost indefinable *chhi* flowed along them.

## PREVENTION OF MTrP REACTIVATION

### Identification of causative factors

In every case it is essential to take a detailed history aimed at identifying the factors responsible for causing the MTrPs to become active in order to ascertain whether any of them can be avoided in the future.

### Muscle stretching exercises

Exercises to stretch muscles that have become shortened as a result of MTrP activity should invariably be taught and carried out by the patient on a regular basis. For the effect of these is to activate A-beta nerve fibres with, as a consequence, the evocation of pain-suppressing activity in large diameter nerve fibres, similar to that brought about by conventional TENS (see Ch. 9).

Exercises designed to strengthen muscles should, however, be avoided as these are liable to cause them to become overloaded with, as a consequence, the risk of reactivating any TrPs that may be present.

### Correction of postural and structural disorders

It is particularly important to correct any postural or structural disorder that may be present especially in cases where there is TrP activity in either the neck or lower back muscles.

Following the deactivation of TrPs in the cervical muscles the patient should be advised to avoid situations where the neck is liable to become

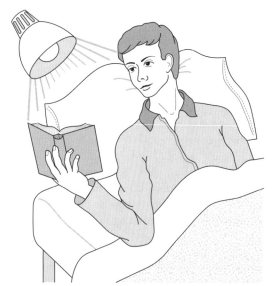

**Figure 10.1** Overloading of the right sternocleidomastoid muscle as a result of prolonged kinking of the neck.

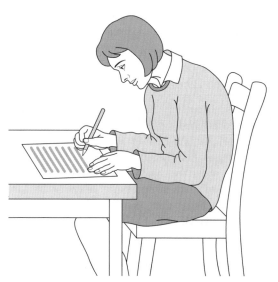

**Figure 10.2** Overloading of the posterior cervical group of muscles as a result of sitting crouched over a desk.

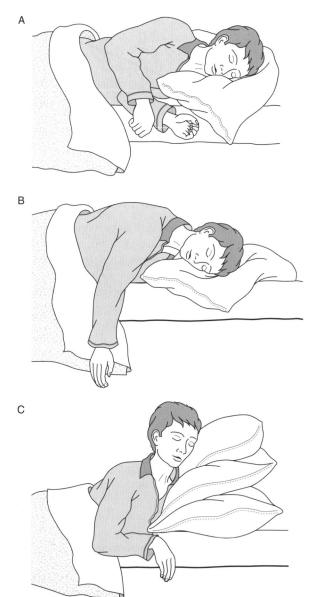

**Figure 10.3** Pillow arrangement. A patient with TrPs in muscles of the neck must ensure that the pillow arrangement is such as to avoid it becoming kinked during sleep. A, Correct pillow arrangement. B and C, Incorrect pillow arrangement.

persistently hyper-extended, kinked (Fig. 10.1) or flexed (Fig. 10.2). And the patient should be told that when using a computer for any length of time to check that the position of the screen is such as not to cause the shoulders to be kept in a persistently elevated position.

Attention should also be drawn to the importance of avoiding kinking of the neck during sleep as a result of resting the head on either too many or too few pillows (Fig. 10.3).

Should the initial physical examination of the patient have revealed that one of the shoulders is lower than the other, then the length of the two

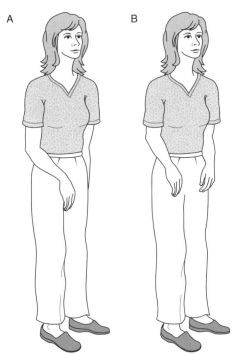

Figure 10.4    A: Person whose arms are of sufficient length in relation to the height of the torso for the elbows to reach the iliac crest. B: Person with abnormally short arms so that in the relaxed standing position the elbows do not reach the level of the iliac crest.

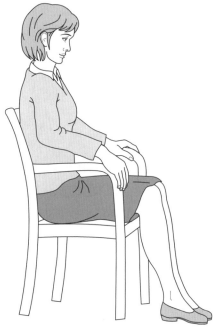

Figure 10.5    A person with abnormally short upper arms may be unable to place elbows on the arm rest of a chair.

legs should be compared as this deformity may be due to a scoliosis brought about as a result of a lower-limb length inequality (Fig. 10.4) which, if left uncorrected (see below) will cause the overloading of the neck muscles to persist.

The length of the upper arms should also be checked because if these in a relaxed standing position do not reach the level of the iliac crest (Fig. 10.4), then on sitting, it may not be possible to place the elbows on the arm rest of a chair (Fig. 10.5) with, as a consequence, strain being imposed on the muscles of the neck and the reactivation of any TrPs that may be present in them. Therefore, should they be found to be abnormally short the height of the arm rest should be suitably adjusted.

Following the deactivation of TrPs in muscles of the lower back an examination should be carried out to exclude a lower limb length inequality, a small hemipelvis, short upper arms and a Morton's foot deformity.

## Lower–limb length inequality

Lower-limb length inequality (LLLI) may be a congenital deformity. In such a case one side of the body tends to be smaller than the other. Also, there is liable to be upper arm length inequality, asymmetry of the two halves of the pelvis and a slight but discernible asymmetry of the face. Alternatively, it may be acquired as a result of an injury or a badly fitting hip prosthesis.

A LLLI tends to cause the patient to stand with the weight of the body shifted to the side of the shorter limb and the knee on the contralateral side slightly flexed. On walking there is also tilting of the torso.

It also leads to the development of a scoliosis. This tends to be C-shaped when the leg length difference is 6 mm (1/4 inch) or less and causes sagging of the shoulder on the side opposite to that of the short leg (Fig. 10.6). Conversely, should the leg length difference be 1.3 cm (1/2 inch) or more the scoliosis which develops is S-shaped and this causes sagging of the shoulder on the same side as the short leg (Fig. 10.7).

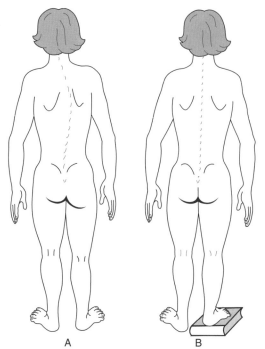

**Figure 10.6**   A: Diagram to show C-shaped scoliosis and sagging of the left shoulder produced by right leg being 6 mm (1/4 inch) or less shorter than the left one.
B: Correction of scoliosis by raising the right heel.

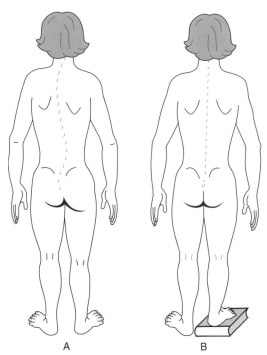

**Figure 10.7**   A: Diagram to show S-shaped scoliosis and sagging of the right shoulder produced by right leg being 1.3 cm (1/2 inch) or more longer than the left one.
B: Correction of scoliosis by raising the right heel.

When assessing whether or not there is a LLLI the patient should stand with the legs straight and the feet together in order that the relative heights of both the iliac crests and the greater trochanters may be compared.

Travell & Simons (1992) have described how to assess LLLI by means of the carrying out of a radiological examination, but, although this is a more accurate procedure, it is not one which need be employed routinely.

Should a LLLI be found to be present it has to be decided whether this is a true inequality that requires the heel on the short side to be raised, or an apparent one due to the leg-raising effect of TrP-induced shortening of the quadratus lumborum muscle, as in the latter case it is correctable by deactivating TrPs in this muscle. Whenever it proves to be a true inequality, then it should be corrected by placing filing cards or pages of a journal under the foot on the shorter side so that a cobbler can increase the thickness of the heel of the shoe accordingly.

## Inequality of the two halves of the pelvis

In some patients with a LLLI one side of the pelvis is smaller than the other. This leads to the development of a compensatory scoliosis and a corresponding sagging of the shoulder on that side. The scoliosis may be corrected by the person concerned sitting on a cushion placed under the ischial tuberosity on the affected side (Fig. 10.8).

## Short upper arms

This abnormality not only puts a strain on the muscles in the neck and shoulder girdle, but is also liable to cause the development and perpetuation of TrP activity in the quadratus lumborum muscle. Therefore, whenever such activity is found to be present in this muscle an examination to establish whether or not this particular structural disorder may be contributing to it should be carried out.

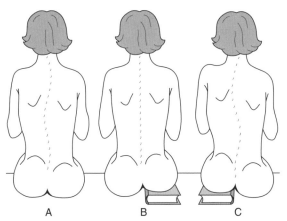

**Figure 10.8**    A: Hemipelvis on the right side smaller than on the left side causing S-shaped scoliosis. B: Scoliosis corrected by raising right buttock. C: Scoliosis made worse by raising left buttock.

## Morton's foot deformity

This disorder, which was described by Morton in 1935, is one in which there is a short first metatarsal bone and a relatively long second one. Harris & Beath (1949) found it to be present in about 40% of people. The deformity causes medio-lateral rocking of the foot with a consequent strain being imposed on a number of muscles including the gluteus medius maximus in the buttock and the peroneal muscles vastus medialis in the lower limb. Its correction requires the placing of a pad under the first metatarsal head.

## ALLEVIATION OF STRESS

There is now good evidence to show that stress may not only cause MTrP activity to develop but may also cause it to persist (McNulty 1994).

As Gerwin & Dommerholt (2002) have pointed out 'trigger point EMG activity has been shown to increase dramatically in response to mental and emotional stress, whereas adjacent non-trigger point muscle activity remains normal'.

Treatment directed towards reducing stress following the deactivation of MTRPs is therefore in certain cases essential.

Banks et al (1998) showed that autogenic relaxation training significantly and dramatically reduced the needle-evoked EMG activity in TrPs

in the upper trapezius muscles of 21 chronic pain patients.

My preferred method is to employ hypnotherapy and to teach the patient to practice autohypnosis once or twice a day on a regular basis (Hilgard & Hilgard 1994).

## CORRECTION OF BIOCHEMICAL DISORDERS

Gerwin (1992) has stressed the importance of recognizing the presence of certain biochemical disorders as, in his experience, a failure to correct any one of these may cause MTrP activity to persist. These include sub-clinical hypothyroidism, iron deficiency, vitamin B12 insufficiency and a low serum folic acid level.

Gerwin (1995), during the course of examining 96 subjects for both fibromyalgia and myofascial pain found that 16% of those with MTrP pain syndrome had a vitamin B12 deficiency and 10% had biochemical evidence of hypothyroidism.

Gerwin & Dommerholt (2002), with reference to iron deficiency, have stated that 'of women with a chronic sense of coldness and chronic myofascial pain, 65% have a low normal or below normal serum ferritin, largely from an iron intake insufficient to replace menstrual iron loss. Other causes of low serum ferritin include blood loss associated with chronic intake of mixed cyclooxygenase 1 & 2 non-steroidal anti-inflammatory drugs'.

## TREATMENT OF FIBROMYALGIA SYNDROME

The management of the fibromyalgia syndrome (FS) involves the use of a large number of different types of treatment. Each of these will be briefly discussed.

More comprehensive reviews of this subject include amongst others those published by Bennett (1999), Inanici & Yunus (2001), Russell (2001) and Simms (1994). Because FS at the present time remains a very disabling one with no known cure it requires long-term skilled management that includes patient education, the prescribing of symptom-relieving drugs, psychotherapy and the employment of various physical modalities.

## Education of the patient

When FS is first diagnosed it is essential to reassure the patient that, although it is a chronic disorder, it is not one that reduces life expectancy and that the various forms of treatment currently available enable its symptoms to be kept under sufficient control as to allow a reasonably active life to be led both in the home and at the work place.

It is also essential to explain to the patient that successful management of it cannot only depend on physician-based therapeutic regimes but must also include patient-orientated self-help programmes (Burckhardt & Bjelle 1994).

## Symptom-relieving drugs

Drugs are mainly required for the relief of sleep disturbances, pain and affective disorders.

### Sleep disturbances

**Non-restorative sleep** Non-restorative sleep which not only contributes so much to FS patients' feelings of persistent tiredness but also exacerbates their pain should be treated with a tricyclic antidepressant. The one most widely used is amitryptyline given 1–3 hours before going to bed. This initial recommended dose is 10 mg and it can gradually be increased to 50–75 mg if necessary, but often, especially in older people, 20 mg proves to be sufficient.

The commonest side-effect, as with all drugs in this group, is a dry mouth.

Contraindications to it being prescribed include a history of urinary retention, prostatic hypertrophy, narrow angle glaucoma, impaired liver function and epilepsy.

Its main disadvantage is that tolerance builds up after 3–4 months use but discontinuing it for a 2–4 week period usually allows sufficient CNS re-adaptation to take place for its use to be resumed. During the break from it Russell (2001) recommends the use of aprazolam.

The possibility of using the pineal hormone melatonin in FS because of its sleep-promoting property has been explored by Citera et al (2000) in a 4 week open study of 25 patients with this disorder. They found that this hormone given in a dose of 3 mg at night lowered the tender point count and significantly improved the quality of sleep.

Further studies are therefore clearly indicated to confirm the value of this drug.

**Sleep apnoea** It has been estimated that about 25% of males and 15% of females with FS have sleep apnoea (Bennett 1999), which requires treatment with positive airway pressure or surgery.

**Restless leg syndrome** In this disorder first described by Ekbom in 1960 there is an intolerable discomfort in the legs which first comes on when sitting down at the end of a day and the involuntary movements of them then prevent the person concerned from getting off to sleep. Yunus & Aldag (1996) have reported an appreciable incidence of this syndrome in patients with FS.

Its treatment includes the use of either L-dopa (Montplaisir et al 1986) or clonazepam (Boghen et al 1986).

### Pain

Amitryptyline at night not only helps to provide restorative sleep but also by so doing helps to ameliorate the pain in patients with FS.

The analgesic most widely prescribed is paracetamol (acetaminophen), but there is no convincing evidence of its efficacy in this disorder (Wolfe et al 2000).

It is also generally agreed that most patients do not derive much benefit from a non-steroidal anti-inflammatory drug such as ibuprofen and there is no case for prescribing a corticosteroid one like prednisolone (Clark et al 1985).

Tramadol, a weak opioid agonist and a noradrenaline uptake inhibitor, is, however, proving to be moderately effective (Biasi et al 1998), although unfortunately it is poorly tolerated by about 20% of patients with this disorder (Russell 2001).

In view of the marked hyperalgesia and allodynia present in patients with FS as a result of central sensitisation there are grounds for believing that a N-methyl-D-aspartate (NMDA) antagonist should be helpful. Support for this comes from a double-blind train carried out by Sorensen et al (1995) in which the pain suppressing effects of intravenous infusions of isotonic saline and ketamine were compared, and the latter was shown to provide a significantly greater reduction of pain intensity.

Unfortunately ketamine not only has to be given intravenously but is also liable to give rise to a number of particularly undesirable adverse effects. The routine use of a NMDA antagonist for treatment in FS and other pain disorders will, therefore, have to await the discovery of a far less toxic one.

## Affective disorders

As with patients suffering from chronic pain disorders those with FS are liable to become anxious and depressed.

**Anxiety**    As with any other chronic disorder the use of a benzodiazepine drug is not recommended because of the risks of dependence and withdrawal seizures (Leventhal 1999).

In view of this, it has been my practice for some years, as previously stated, to employ hypnotherapy in patients with this and similar chronic pain disorders and to teach them how to practice autohypnosis for 10 minutes once or twice a day on a regular basis. It is, therefore, gratifying to find that Haanen et al (1991), in a randomized controlled trial carried out for the purpose of comparing physical therapy with hypnotherapy in patients with FS, have provided objective evidence of the ability of the latter form of treatment to lower the intensity of pain, improve sleep and lessen morning fatigue.

**Depression**    When depression is a prominent feature in patients with this disorder, fluoxetine, a selective serotonin reuptake inhibitor has been shown in controlled studies to both relieve it and to improve sleep (Wolfe et al 1994).

With respect to this it should be noted that Goldenberg et al (1996) have provided evidence to suggest that a combination of amitryptyline and fluoxetine may be better than either drug alone.

## Physical modalities

### Muscle stretching and aerobic exercises

It is important for patients with FS to be taught how to carry out on a regular daily basis both muscle stretching and aerobic exercises. The latter should initially be for 10 minutes periods three times a day and should include regular walking and the use of a stationary exercise bicycle.

Some hospitals provide group exercise programmes for patients with this disorder. An interesting alternative recently reported by Richards & Scott (2002) is the carrying out of such a programme in the 'healthy living centres' recently set up with the help of grants from the UK's National Lottery Fund. A randomized controlled trial conducted by them led to the conclusion that 'the carrying out of graded aerobic exercise is a simple, cheap, effective, and potentially widely available treatment for fibromyalgia'.

### Electroacupuncture

Deluze et al (1992) carried out a randomized controlled trial of this particular type of acupuncture in 54 women and 16 men with FS.

In the 'treatment' group (36 patients), electroacupuncture with a variable high-/low-frequency and an intensity sufficient to induce visible muscular contractions was applied to needles inserted to a depth of 10–25 mm into the first dorsal interosseous muscle (i.e. Hegu or Large Intestine 4) bilaterally, into a point in the anterior tibial muscle know as Stomach 36 (Zusanli) bilaterally and into various other points which they said 'depended on the patient's symptoms and pain pattern and according to the empirical efficacy of the sites in the treatment of pain'. This is a somewhat imprecise description which in my opinion makes it difficult to be certain which points in particular were used!

The 'control' groups had the same number of needles inserted but only to a depth of 3–4 mm and 20 mm away from the points chosen for the 'treatment' group. They stated that 'the current used was similar to but weaker than that used in the real procedure … (so that) … there was no muscular contraction'.

They found that the 'pain threshold which was considered to be the main parameter improved by 70% in the treatment group and 4% in the control group'.

As Lewis (1993) has pointed out, this is a very surprising result not because the treatment group did so well, but because the 'control' group did so badly. The reason for him saying this is because the points into which needles were inserted in this latter group of patients were only 20 mm away from those used in the treatment group and despite the stimulus being weaker, from what is know concerning the pain-alleviating neurophysiological mechanisms of acupuncture, it is very unlikely that it did not have some therapeutic effect. Furthermore, that four patients in this 'control' group had to withdraw from the trial because of an exacerbation of their pain is an added reason for believing that the electrical stimulus employed in their 'treatment' had more than a placebo effect.

Although the result of this trial clearly shows that electroacupuncture with needles inserted into traditional Chinese points is capable of alleviating the pain of FS, there are in my opinion three reasons for not using it. One is that the stimulus provided by this particular type of acupuncture is liable to be more powerful than the optimum required by FS patients who, as a group are widely recognized to be strong reactors to needle-evoked nerve stimulation procedures. The second is that it requires the use of a machine not normally available to, and special training not usually undertaken by those who treat this disorder. And the third reason is because manually applied dry needling carried out either at traditional Chinese acupuncture point sites or at tender point sites are far simpler procedures and seemingly equally effective ones.

## Manual acupuncture at traditional Chinese acupuncture point sites

Sandberg et al (1999) chose manual acupuncture when carrying out a cross-over designed pilot study in 10 patients with FS because as they stated 'this is a milder form of sensory stimulation than electroacupuncture and our clinical experience has led us to believe that FS pain is liable to be aggravated by too strong a stimulus'.

The first five referred patients, group I, received acupuncture treatment over a period of 2–3 months. The subsequent five patients, group II, acted as controls for 2–3 months, after which treatment was given as in group I. Six months after the end of the treatment, group I crossed over to form a control group.

The traditional Chinese acupuncture points employed were Large Intestine 4 (Hegu) in the first dorsal interosseous muscle of the hand, Stomach 36 in the tibialis anterior muscle and what they described as 'points in the upper part of the body … within the most painful area'. Also they said, 'for additional stimulation from the lower part of the body one or two more points in the lower extremities were used'. Yet another imprecise statement, similar to that employed in the trial just previously discussed, which makes it extremely difficult to determine which points in particular were used. They furthermore stated that 'the strength of the needle stimulation was enough to elicit the sensation of 'de Qi' but … noxious painful stimulation … was avoided'. A very important feature of the study was that the treatment parameters were varied according to the optimum amount of stimulation required by each individual patient; this is a consideration not sufficiently often included in the protocols of acupuncture trials. A very interesting and encouraging finding in this pilot study was that not only did 78% of the patients report considerable pain relief immediately after completion of the treatment, but 56% continued to experience this 1 month later and 33% after 2–3 months.

Their particular method of treatment, therefore, even when the shortcomings of a crossover study are taken into account, shows considerable promise. Its only disadvantage is that it relies on inserting needles into traditional Chinese acupuncture points and, therefore, cannot be used by the majority of health professionals who treat FS as they have no knowledge as to where these points are situated!

Sprott et al (1998) also confirmed the value of manually applied traditional Chinese type acupuncture in the alleviation of FS pain when they used it to treat 29 patients (25 women, 4 men) suffering from this disorder over a 6-week period (six single treatments once a week), according they said 'to an individually adapted therapy strategy following acupuncture rules'.

They found that the treatment '… was associated with decreased pain levels and fewer positive tender points as measured by VAS and dolorimetry…' And in addition confirmed that, '… this was accompanied by decreased serotonin and substance P levels in serum, suggesting that acupuncture therapy is associated with changes in the concentrations of pain-modulating substances in serum …'

## Tender point injections

Another approach to the treatment of FS pain and one which is proving to be helpful is to inject a local anaesthetic into tender points (Yunus et al 1998).

In an open study carried out by Reddy et al (2000) 41 patients with FS had a mixture of 1% lidocaine (lignocaine) (1/2 cc) and triamcinolone diacetate (1/4 cc) injected into tender points. They admitted that the inclusion of a corticosteroid was more because of the continuation of a 'tradition' than because it had any scientific basis for, as has been shown by Yunus et al (1989), there is no evidence of an inflammatory lesion in the muscles of FS patients in electron microscopic studies.

A tender point injection of this type gratifyingly led on average to a 12-week-long period of pain relief at each injected site.

A serious disadvantage though was that the stimulus was so strong that in order to combat any resultant post-injection soreness the treated areas had to be rested for 48 hours and ice had to be applied to them for 20–30 minutes/hour for 4–8 hours. Because of this the treatment had to be restricted to no more than five sites or, in patients with particularly bad pain, to no more than eight sites.

Figuerola et al (1998) have studied plasma met-enkephalin (ME) levels in 15 women with FS before and after the following different forms of treatment to tender points – 5 patients had lidocaine (ligno-caine) hydrochloride injected into them, 5 had injections of saline into them and 5 had dry needles inserted into them.

Significant increases in plasma ME concentrations were observed in all groups 10 minutes after finishing each treatment session irrespective of the procedure employed. A finding strongly suggesting that this biochemical change was brought about by the effect of the needle was that this was the one stimulus common to all of the three groups.

## Superficial dry needling at tender and TrP sites

In view of it having been found that an injection of a local anaesthetic/corticosteroid mixture into tender points is liable to give rise to such a considerable amount of soreness at that site that the number of them treated has to be strictly limited, there is clearly a case for either injecting a local anaesthetic alone, as Inanici & Yunus (2001) now do, or for simply inserting a needle into the superficial tissues overlying it.

The main advantage of carrying out SDN is that the strength of the stimulus applied, rather than being the same for everyone, can readily be adjusted to suit each individual patient's optimum requirement. This is particularly important when treating patients with FS because in general they tend to be strong reactors to needle-evoked nerve stimulation. And because, due to the lack of treatment-induced tenderness, providing the stimulus applied is a light one the needling can be carried out at all the tender and TrPs present in turn.

It is, therefore, my practice to insert a needle to a depth of about 5 mm at a tender/TrP site and to leave it in situ for from 10–30 seconds according to what is found by trial and error to be the time necessary to abolish the exquisite tenderness at the point being treated.

With SDN carried out in this way it is usually necessary to repeat it once a week for 3–4 weeks, then at 2-week intervals, and finally at 4–6 week intervals on a long-term basis. Although due to the nature of the underlying disorder, the treatment has perforce to be protracted, most patients find it to be worthwhile as the pain relief afforded by it appreciably improves the quality of their lives (Baldry 2000).

## Training required in order to carry out superficial and deep dry needling

In concluding this chapter it is felt necessary to say that whilst SDN carried out at either tender points or TrP sites, and DDN carried out at these latter sites are forms of acupuncture, the employment of these two needle-evoked nerve stimulation techniques does not require knowing where traditional Chinese acupuncture points are situated, or for that matter any particular training in the carrying out of traditional Chinese acupuncture in general. All that a physician or physiotherapist who wishes to make use of them has to have is the skill required to locate TrPs and tender points, and the ability to insert needles into the tissues at these particular sites.

Having said this, it behoves all health professionals who employ these two techniques to familiarize themselves with the principles and practice of traditional Chinese acupuncture (TCA). This is because, as has already been shown in this book, much of what is known concerning the neurophysiological mechanisms involved in the pain-alleviating effects of needle-evoked nerve stimulation techniques in general has come from experiments involving the insertion of needles into TCA points. And because without having knowledge of TCA in general it is impossible to be able to fully comprehend and evaluate clinical trials carried out to ascertain what place if any it may have in the treatment of a muscle pain disorder such as fibromyalgia.

# References

Baldry P E 1995 Superficial dry needling at myofascial trigger point sites. Journal of Musculoskeletal Pain 3(3): 117–126

Baldry P E 1998 Trigger point acupuncture. In: Filshie J, White A (eds) Medical acupuncture. A Western scientific approach. Churchill Livingstone, Edinburgh

Baldry P E 2000 Acupuncture treatment of fibromyalgia and myofascial pain. In: Chaitow L (ed) Fibromyalgia syndrome A practitioner's guide to treatment. Churchill Livingstone, Edinburgh

Baldry P E 2001 Myofascial pain and fibromyalgia syndromes. Churchill Livingstone, Edinburgh

Baldry P E 2002a Management of myofascial trigger point pain. Acupuncture in Medicine 20(1): 2–10

Baldry P E 2002b Superficial versus deep dry needling. Acupuncture in Medicine 20(203): 78–81

Banks S L, Jacobs D W, Gervitz R, Hubbard D R 1998 Effects of autogenous relaxation training on electromyographic activity in active myofascial trigger points. Journal of Musculoskeletal Pain 6(4): 23–32

Bennett R 1999 Fibromyalgia. In: Wall P D, Melzack R (eds) Textbook of pain. Churchill Livingstone, Edinburgh

Biasi G, Manca S, Manganelli S, Marcolongo R 1998 Tramadol in the fibromyalgia syndrome: a controlled clinical trial versus placebo. International Journal of Clinical Pharmacology Research 18(1): 13–19

Birch S J, Felt R L 1999 Understanding acupuncture. Churchill Livingstone, Edinburgh

Birch S, Jamison R N 1998 Controlled trial of Japanese acupuncture for chronic myofascial neck pain: assessment of specific and non-specific effects of treatment. Clinical Journal of Pain 14: 248–255

Boghen D, Lamothe L, Elie R, Godbout R, Montplaisir J 1986 The treatment of the restless legs syndrome with clonazepam: a prospective controlled study. Canadian Journal of Neurological Sciences 13(3): 245–247

Bourne I H J 1979 Treatment of backache with local injections. The Practitioner 222: 708–711

Bourne I H J 1984 Treatment of chronic back pain, comparing corticosteroid-lignocaine injections with lignocaine alone. The Practitioner 228: 333–338

Burckhardt C S, Bjelle A 1994 Education programmes for fibromyalgia patients: description and evaluation. In: Masi A T (ed) Fibromyalgia and myofascial pain syndromes. Baillière's Clinical Rheumatology 8(4): 935–956

Brattberg G 1986 Acupuncture treatments: a traffic hazard? American Journal of Acupuncture 14: 265–267

Byrn C, Borenstein P, Linder L-E 1991 Treatment of neck and shoulder pain in whiplash syndrome with intracutaneous sterile water injections. Acta Anaesthetica Scandinavica 35: 52–53

Byrn C, Olsson I, Falkheden L et al 1993 Subcutaneous sterile water injections for chronic neck and shoulder pain following whiplash injuries. Lancet 341: 449–452

Ceccherelli F, Rigoni M T, Gagliardi G, Ruzzante L 2002 Comparison of superficial and deep acupuncture in the treatment of lumbar myofascial pain; A double-blind randomised controlled study. The Clinical Journal of Pain 18: 149–153

Citera G, Arias M A, Maldronado-Cocco J A et al 2000 The effect of melatonin in patients with fibromyalgia: a pilot study. Clinical Rheumatology 19(1): 9–13

Chen F, Hwang S, Lee H et al 1990 Clinical study of syncope during acupuncture treatment. Acupuncture and Electrotherapy Research 15: 107–119

Cheshire W P, Abashian S W, Mann J D 1994 Botulinum toxin in the treatment of myofascial pain syndrome. Pain 59: 65–69

Chu J 1997 Twitch – obtaining intramuscular stimulation (TOIMS): effectiveness for long-term treatment of myofascial pain related to cervical radiculopathy. Archives of Physical Medicine and Rehabilitation 78: 1042

Chu J 1999 Twitch – obtaining intramuscular stimulation. Observations in the management of radiculopathic chronic low back pain. Journal of Musculoskeletal Pain 7(4): 131–146

Clark S, Tindall E, Bennett R M 1985 A double-blind crossover trial of prednisone versus placebo in the treatment of fibrositis. Journal of Rheumatology 12: 980–983

Communicable Diseases Surveillance Centre of the PHLS 1977 Acupuncture associated hepatitis in the West Midlands in 1977. British Medical Journal 2: 1610

Cummings T M, White A R 2001 Needling therapies in the management of myofascial trigger point pain: a systematic review. Archives of Physical Medicine and Rehabilitation 82(7): 986–992

Deluze C, Bosia L, Zirbs A, Chantraine A, Vischer T L 1992 Electroacupuncture in fibromyalgia; results of a controlled trial. British Medical Journal 305(6864): 1249–1252

Drewes A M, Andreasen A, Poulson L H 1993 Injection therapy for treatment of chronic myofascial pain. A double-blind study comparing corticosteroid versus diclofenac injections. Journal of musculoskeletal Pain 1(3/4): 289–294

Ekbom K A 1960 Restless leg syndrome. Neurology 10: 969

Fields H 1987 Pain. McGraw-Hill, New York

Figuerola M L, Loe W, Sormani M, Barontini M 1998 Met-enkephalin increase in patients with fibromyalgia under local treatment. Functional Neurology 13(4): 291–295

Frost A 1986 Diclofenac versus Lidocaine as injection therapy in myofascial pain. Scandinavian Journal of Rheumatology 15: 153–156

Frost F A, Jessen B, Siggaard-Anderson J 1980 A controlled double-blind comparison of mepivacaine injection versus saline injection for myofascial pain. Lancet 1: 499–450

Frost F A, Toft B, Aaboe T 1984 Isotonic saline and methylprednisolone acetate in blockade treatment of myofascial pain. A clinical controlled study. Ugeskrift For Laeger 146: 652–654

Garvey T A, Marks M R, Wiesel S W 1989 A prospective, randomised, double-blind evaluation of trigger point injection therapy for low-back pain. Spine 14: 962–964

Gerwin R D 1992 The clinical assessment of myofascial pain. In: Turk D C, Melzack R (eds) Handbook of pain assessment. Guildford Press, New York

Gerwin R D 1995 A study of 96 subjects examined both for fibromyalgia and myofascial pain. Journal of Musculoskeletal Pain 3 (suppl 1): 121

Gerwin R D, Dommerholt J 2002 Treatment of myofascial pain syndromes. In: Weiner R (ed) Pain management, a practical guide for clinicians. CRC Press, Boca Raton, pp. 235–249

Goldenberg D, Mayskiy M, Mossey C, Ruthazer R, Schmid C 1996 A randomised double-blind crossover trial of fibromyalgia. Arthritis and Rheumatism 39(11): 1852–1859

Gray P 1996 Baker's cyst bursts after acupuncture. Acupuncture in Medicine 14(1): 41–42

Gunn C C 1989 Treating myofascial pain – intramuscular stimulation (IMS) for myofascial pain syndromes of neuropathic origin. Health Science Center for Educational Resources, University of Washington, Seattle

Gunn C C 1996 The Gunn approach to the treatment of chronic pain. Churchill Livingstone, Edinburgh

Gunn C C 1998 Acupuncture and the peripheral nervous system. In: Filshie J, White A (eds) Medical acupuncture, a Western scientific approach. Churchill Livingstone, Edinburgh, pp. 137–150

Haanen H C, Hoenderdos H T, van Romunde L K et al 1991 Controlled trial of hypnotherapy in the treatment of refractory fibromyalgia. Journal of Rheumatology 18(1): 72–75

Han J S 1995 Cholecystokinin octapeptide (CCK-8): a negative feedback control mechanism for opioid analgesia. Progress in Brain Research 105: 263–271

Han J S 2001 Opioid and antiopioid peptides: A model of yin-yang balance in acupuncture mechanism of pain modulation. In: Stux G, Hammerschlag R (eds) Clinical acupuncture, scientific basis. Springer-Verlag, Berlin

Harris R I, Beth T 1949 The short first metatarsal: its incidence and clinical significance. Journal of Bone and Joint Surgery (Am) 31: 553–565

Hayhoe S, Pitt E 1987 Case reports. Complications of acupuncture in Medicine 4: 15

Hilgard E R, Hilgard J R 1994 Hypnosis in the relief of pain. Brunner-Mazel, New York

Hoffman P 2001 Skin disinfection and acupuncture. Acupuncture in Medicine X1X (2): 112–116

Hong C-Z 1994a Considerations and recommendations regarding myofascial trigger point injections. Journal of Musculoskeletal Pain 2(1): 29–59

Hong C-Z 1994b Lidocaine injection versus dry needling to myofascial trigger point. American Journal of Physical Medicine and Rehabilitations 73: 256–263

Inanici F, Yunus M 2001 Management of fibromyalgia syndromes. In: Baldry P E (ed) Myofascial pain and fibromyalgia syndromes. Churchill Livingstone, Edinburgh

Kaneko S, Tamura S, Takagi H 1985 Purification and identification of endogenous antiopioid substance from bovine brain. Biochemical and Biophysical Research Communications: 587–593

Kent G P, Brondrum J, Keenlyside R A et al 1988 A large outbreak of acupuncture associated hepatitis B. American Journal of Epidemiology 127: 591–598

Lang A M 2002 Botulinum toxin therapy for myofascial disorders. Current Pain Headache Reports 6(5): 355–360

Laurence D R, Bennett P N 1987 Clinical pharmacology, 6th edn. Churchill Livingstone, Edinburgh, p. 735

Leventhal L J 1999 Management of fibromyalgia. Annals of Internal Medicine 7131(11): 850–858

Lewis P 1993 Electroacupuncture in fibromyalgia. British Medical Journal 306: 393 (letter)

Lewis Sir Tomas 1942 Pain. Macmillan, New York

Lewit K 1979 the needle effect in the relief of myofascial pain 6: 83–90

Lu G-D, Needham J 1980 Celestial lancets. Cambridge University Press, Cambridge

Macdonald A J R, Macrae K D, Master B R, Rubin A P 1983 Superficial acupuncture in the relief of chronic low-back pain. Annals of the Royal College of Surgeons of England 65: 44–46

Mann F 1992 Reinventing acupuncture. Butterworth-Heinemann, Oxford

McNulty W H, Gervirtz R N, Hubbard D R et al 1994 Needle electromyographic evaluation of trigger point response to a psychological stress. Psychophysiology 31(3): 313–316

McMillan A S, Nolan A, Kelly P J 1997 The efficacy of dry needling and procaine in the treatment of myofascial pain in the jaw muscles. Journal of Orofacial Pain 11: 307–314

Montplaisir J, Godbout R, Poirier G, Bedard M A 1986 Restless leg syndrome and periodic limb movements in sleep; physiology pathology and treatment with L-dopa. Clinical Neuropharmacology 9: 956–463

Morton D J 1935 The human foot: its evolution, physiology and functional disorders. Columbia University Press, New York

Murai M, Takeshige C 1986 Correlation between individual variations in effectiveness of acupuncture analgesia and those in contents of brain endogenous morphine-like factors (Japanese with English summary). In: Takeshige C (ed) Studies on the mechanism of acupuncture analgesia based on animal experiments. Showa University Press, Tokyo, p. 542

Okuda-Ashitaka E, Minami T, Tachibana S et al 1988 Nocistatin, a peptide that blocks nociceptive action in pain transmission. Nature 392: 286–289

Osler W 1909 The principles and practice of medicine, 7th edn. Appleton, New York

Peets J, Pomeranz B 1978 CXBX mice deficient in opiate receptors show poor electroacupuncture analgesia. Nature 273: 675–676

Rachlin E S 1994 Myofascial pain and fibromyalgia. Mosby, St Lewis

Rampes H 1998 Adverse reactions to acupuncture. In: Filshie J, White A (eds) Medical acupuncture, a western scientific approach. Churchill Livingstone, Edinburgh

Rampes H, Peuker E 1999 Adverse effects of acupuncture. In: Ernst E, White A (eds) Acupuncture: A scientific appraisal. Butterworth Heinemann, Oxford

Reddy S S, Yunus M B, Inanici F, Aldag J C 2000 Tender point injections are beneficial in fibromyalgia syndrome: A descriptive open study. Journal of Musculoskeletal Pain 8(4): 7–17

Richards S C M, Scott D L 2002 Prescribed exercise in people with fibromyalgia: parallel group randomised controlled trial. British Medical Journal 325: 185–187

Russell I J 2001 Fibromyalgia syndrome. In: Mense S, Simons D G (eds) Muscle pain. Lippincott Williams & Wilkins, Philadelphia

Sandberg M, Lundeberg T, Gerdle B 1999 Manual acupuncture in fibromyalgia: a long-term pilot study. Journal of Musculoskeletal Pain 7(3): 39–58

Simms R W 1994 Controlled trials of therapy in fibromyalgia syndrome. In: Masi A T (ed) Baillière's Clinical Rheumatology 8/4: 917–934

Simons S D 1996 Clinical and etiological update of myofascial pain from trigger points. Journal of Musculoskeletal Pain 4 (1/2): 93–121

Simons D G, Travell J G, Simons L S 1999 Travell & Simons Myofascial pain and dysfunction, the trigger point manual, 2nd edn. Williams & Wilkins, Baltimore

Slater P E, Ben-Ishai P, Leventhal A et al 1988 An acupuncture-associated outbreak of hepatitis B in Jerusalem. European Journal of Epidemiology 4: 322–325

Smith D L, Walczyk M H, Campbell S 1989 Acupuncture needle induced compartment syndrome. Western Journal of Medicine 144: 478–479

Sola A E, Kuitert J H 1955 Myofascial trigger point pain in the neck and shoulder girdle. Northwest Medicine 54: 980–984

Sola A E, Williams R L 1956 Myofascial pain syndromes. Neurology (Minneapolis) 6: 91–95

Sorensen J, Bengtsson A, Backman E, Henriksson K G, Bengtsson M 1995 Pain analysis in patients with fibromyalgia. Effects of intravenous morphine, lidocaine and ketamine. Scandinavian Journal of Rheumatology 24(6): 360–365

Sprott H, Franke S, Kluge H, Hein G 1998 Pain treatment of fibromyalgia by acupuncture. Rheumatology International 18: 35–36

Tfelt-Hansen P, Lous I, Olesen J 1981 Prevalence and significance of muscle tenderness during common migraine attacks. Headache 21: 49–54

Travell J G 1968 Office Hours – day and night. The Word Publishing Company, New York

Travell J G, Rinzler S H 1952 The myofascial genesis of pain. Postgraduate Medicine 11: 425–434

Travell J G, Simons D G 1983 Myofascial pain and dysfunction. The trigger point manual. Williams & Wilkins, Baltimore

Travell J G, Simons D G 1992 Myofascial pain and dysfunction. The trigger point manual. Williams & Wilkins, Baltimore

Tschopp K P, Gysin C 1996 Local infection therapy in 107 patients with myofascial pain syndrome of the head and neck. Journal of Otorhinolaryngology 58: 306–310

Tsui J K E, Stoessal A J, Eisen A, Calne S, Calne D B 1986 Double-blind study of botulinum toxin in spasmodic torticollis. Lancet ii: 245–246

Vittecoq D, Meltetal J F, Rouzioux C et al 1989 Acute HIV infection after acupuncture treatments. New England Journal of Medicine 320: 250–251

Wang K, Yao S, Xian Y, Hou Z 1985 A study of the receptive fields of acupoints and the relationship between characteristics of needle sensation and groups of afferent fibres. Scientia Sinica 28: 963–971

Wheeler A H, Goolkasian P, Gretz S S 1998 A randomised, double-blind, prospective pilot study of botulism toxin injection for refractory, unilateral, cervicothoracic, paraspinal, myofascial pain syndrome. Spine 23: 1662–1666

White A, Hayhoe S, Hart A, Ernst E 2001 Survey of adverse events following acupuncture (SAFA): a prospective study of 32,000 consultations. Acupuncture in Medicine 19(2): 84–92

Wolfe F, Cathey M A, Hawley D J 1994 A double-blind placebo controlled trial of fluoxetine in fibromyalgia. Scandinavian Journal of Rheumatology 23(5): 255–259

Wolfe F, Zhao S, Lane N 2000 Preference for nonsteroidal anti-inflammatory drugs over acetaminophen by rheumatic disease patients. Arthritis and Rheumatism 43(2): 378–385

Wreje U, Brorsson B 1995 a multicenter randomized controlled trial of injections of sterile water and saline for chronic myofascial pain syndromes. Pain 61: 441–444

Yuan L, Hah Z, Chang J K, Han J S 1999 Accelerated release and production of orphanin F Q in the brain of chronic morphine tolerant rats. Brain Research 826: 330–334

Yue S K 1995 Initial experience in the use of botulinum toxin A for the treatment of myofascial related muscle dysfunctions. Journal of Musculoskeletal Pain 3(suppl 1): 22

Yunus M B, Aldag J C 1996 Restless leg syndrome and leg cramps in fibromyalgia syndrome: a controlled study. British Medical Journal 312: 1339

Yunus M B, Kalyan-Raman U, Masi A T, Aldag J C 1989 Electron microscopic studies of muscle biopsy in primary fibromyalgia syndrome; a controlled and blinded study. Journal of Rheumatology 16: 97–101

Yunus M B, Reddy S S, Inanici F, Aldag J C 1998 Tender point injections are beneficial in fibromyalgia (abstract). Journal of Rheumatology 25(suppl 52): M58

Chapter **11**

# Scientific evaluation of acupuncture's ability to relieve nociceptive pain

## INTRODUCTION

The future of acupuncture for the relief of nociceptive pain and the decision as to whether or not this particular type of treatment will eventually become readily incorporated within the framework of orthodox Western medical practice for this purpose will largely depend on clinical trials showing its ability to do this is significantly greater than that of a powerful placebo.

This, however, presents a considerable challenge because, as Belgrade (1994) has cogently commented:

> … The complexity of testing a therapeutic modality like acupuncture is an order of a magnitude greater than for testing drugs. Look at the variables involved: definition of acupuncture, choice of points, type of stimulation, technique of the acupuncturist, frequency and duration of treatment and the problems of choosing an appropriate placebo that is similar enough to acupuncture but would not be expected to have a significant acupuncture effect. These variables create overwhelming problems for research design and implementation …

Such difficulties have been extensively reviewed by many reflective clinicians well skilled in the principles and practice of this needle-evoked nerve stimulation type of therapy. These include, amongst others Ernst (1999a, 1999b), Ernst & White (1997, 1999), Filshie & Cummings (1999), Han (1994), Lewith & Machin (1983), Lewith & Vincent (1995, 1998), Richardson & Vincent (1986),

Vincent (1989), Vincent & Lewith (1995), Vincent & Richardson (1986).

The purpose of this chapter is to provide an overview of this complex subject.

## POINT SPECIFICITY

The first question that has to be asked when attempting to assess the pain-relieving efficacy of traditional Chinese acupuncture is – does its effectiveness with respect to this depend on needling being carried out at specifically designated sites?

My main reason for advocating this when deactivating trigger points (TrPs) is that experience has taught me that it only requires one such point to be left in an active state for a certain amount of pain to persist.

What, however, has to be considered is whether this precision is also required when needling traditional Chinese acupuncture points, now that both Mann (1992) and Campbell (1999, 2001) have astutely observed that needling carried out anywhere within a sizeable area provides as good analgesia as does needling at specifically nominated sites.

This it has to be said is not some new discovery for Melzack as long ago as 1984 wrote with considerable perspicacity on the subject as follows:

> … An impressive number of studies show that acupuncture stimulation need not be applied at the precise points indicated on acupuncture charts. It is possible, for example, to achieve as much control over dental pain by stimulating an area between the fourth and fifth fingers, which is not designated on acupuncture charts as related to facial pain, as by stimulating the Hoku point between the thumb and index finger which is so designated (Taub et al 1977). The decreases in pain obtained by stimulation at either site are so large and occur in so many patients that it is unlikely that the pain relief is due to placebo effects. Rather, the results suggest that the site that can be stimulated is not a discrete point but a large area, possibly the whole hand.
>
> The same conclusion can be drawn from another study – a double-blind experiment on the efficacy of acupuncture on osteoarthritic pain – in which the control patients received 'placebo' acupuncture stimulation at sites just adjacent to the 'real' acupuncture sites (Gaw et al 1975). Patients in both

groups showed significant improvement in tenderness and subjective report of pain as evaluated by two independent observers, as well as in activity of the joint. Because there was no difference between the two groups the improvement was attributed to a placebo effect. It is more likely, however, that it is stimulation within a large area and not merely at a point that has an effect. Similar conclusions can be drawn from an excellent study of acupuncture control over pain in patients with sickle-cell anaemia (Co et al 1979). In fact, intense stimulation at many sites of the body may be effective. It is the intense stimulation rather than the precise site that appears to be the crucial factor… . That the pain relief produced by acupuncture cannot be attributed simply to a placebo effect is also indicated by the fact that analgesia can be produced in animals such as monkeys and mice (Vierck et al 1974, Pomeranz et al 1977, Sandrew et al 1978) …

All this leads to the posing of two further questions. What is a placebo? And what placebo in particular is best for use in trials to assess the pain-relieving efficacy of acupuncture?

## PLACEBOS

Before discussing placebo-controlled trials for the evaluation of the pain-relieving properties of acupuncture, it is first necessary to say something about them in general. The term placebo, which is derived from the Latin word *placere* (to please), has an established ecclesiastical usage in the phrase Placebo Domino (I shall please the Lord) that appears in the opening antiphon of the vespers for the dead. According to the Shorter Oxford Dictionary it has, in addition, been used by the medical profession since 1811 to describe some medical substance given more to please than benefit a patient. However, it has always seemed to me that it would have been more apposite for the word in the medical sense to have been derived from the Latin *placare* (to placate) because therapeutically it is given more to pacify or appease than it is to give pleasure to a patient!

Wall (1994, p. 1301) has commented, 'the myth is widely quoted in papers and textbooks that a fixed fraction of patients respond to placebos, with the figure of 33% being commonly quoted'. He also pointed out that:

> … Where these sources quote the origin of the myth, they refer to Beecher (1955) who indeed gives the figure of 35.2%. However, had they bothered to read the paper, they would have found that this figure is an average of Beecher's own 11 studies, each of which varied widely from the average. Scanning a large number of double-blind studies shows the fraction of placebo responders varying from close to 0% (Tyler 1946) to near 100% (Liberman 1964) depending on the circumstances of the trial. Clinical pains are associated with a larger number of placebo responders than experimental pains are (Beecher 1959)… There is no fixed fraction of the population who respond to placebos …

Wall (1994, p. 1034) also stated:

> … By far the commonest proposal is that the placebo effect depends on the expectation of the subject. There is nothing subtle about this. Placebo reactors can be identified before the trial by simply asking the subject what they expect to be the outcome of the therapy. Those who doubt do not respond to the placebo while those with high expectations do. The very extensive literature on this is reviewed by Bootzin (1985). Lasagna et al (1954) investigated many aspects of postoperative patients who responded to placebos and to analgesic drugs and concluded that 'a positive placebo response indicated a psychological set predisposing to anticipation of pain relief' …
>
> … Expectation is a learned state and therefore young children do not respond to placebos as adults do since they have had neither the time nor the experience to learn. Similarly in adults, the learning of expected effects will depend on culture, background, experience and personality. A desire to believe, please and obey the doctor will increase the effect while hostility decreases it. Obviously, part of the expectation of the patient will depend on the expectation, enthusiasm and charisma of the therapist, and therefore there are many reports on this doctor–patient interaction. Expectation in a laboratory experiment may be more limited than in a clinical setting; this may explain why rates and intensities of placebo effects

tend to be less in the laboratory than in the clinic (Beecher 1959) …

## Credible placebos

Controlled trials may entail comparing a group treated with acupuncture with either a waiting-list group, a group given an alternative treatment, or a group given a placebo. As Vincent (1989) has pointed out when discussing the methodology of controlled trials of acupuncture, the main problem is to select a credible placebo. It is, therefore, necessary to discuss this subject at some length.

In the past it was common for patients in the placebo control group to be treated by means of needling carried out at sites some distance away from traditional Chinese acupuncture points. The use of these so-called sham points should, however, be discontinued (Richardson & Vincent 1986) because, as previously discussed, it is now known that needling anywhere in the body has an analgesic effect mainly because of the bringing into action of the diffuse noxious inhibitory control system identified by Le Bars et al (1979, 1991).

It was because of this that Ezzo et al (2000), after having carried out an extensive review of 51 randomized controlled trials carried out between 1980 and 1999, concluded that 'there is limited evidence that acupuncture is more effective than no treatment for chronic pain; and inconclusive evidence that it is more effective than placebo, sham acupuncture or standard care'.

In recent years, therefore, much effort has been put into trying to find a credible placebo. Borkovec & Nau (1972) were the first to study the credibility of analogue therapy rationales in the treatment of psychological disorders. As Lewith & Vincent (1998) have pointed out, the main questions identified by Borkovec & Nau in their 'Credibility treatment rating scale' were:

1. How confident do you feel that this treatment can alleviate your complaint?
2. How confident would you be in recommending this treatment to a friend who suffered from similar complaints?
3. How logical does this treatment seem to you?
4. How successful do you think this treatment would be in alleviating other complaints?

## Placebos currently employed

### Inactivated transcutaneous electrical nerve stimulation machine

Macdonald et al (1983) were the first to use an inactivated transcutaneous electrical nerve stimulation (TENS) machine especially fitted with a number of flashing lights in an attempt to increase any expectation of its efficacy. Petrie & Langley (1983) also used this device in a pilot study carried out to assess the value of acupuncture in the treatment of chronic cervical pain.

Petrie & Hazleman (1985), however, were the first to employ Borkovec & Nau's credibility scale when comparing the relative plausibility of acupuncture and sham TENS in patients suffering from chronic neck pain. As they stated:

> ... the potent analgesic effect of placebo is well recognised (Evans 1974). Such an effect, however, is variable (Doongaji et al (1978), and is influenced by a number of factors, not least of which are the physical appearance of the placebo and the manner in which it is presented (Buckalew & Ross 1981) ...

They concluded that 'the present study shows by means of a questionnaire designed to measure patient expectation of effectiveness that a placebo TENS treatment offers equal suggestibility to that of acupuncture'.

### Inactivated laser

Irnich et al (2001, 2002), in trials carried out on patients with chronic neck pain, used a laser pen that had been purposely deactivated by the manufacturer. And in order to ensure double 'blinding' (see p. 154) neither the patients nor therapist were informed about this.

### Non-invasive needling techniques

Placebos of this type have been used in the past but which in no way could be considered by a patient to be credible. They include rubbing needles against the skin (Borglum-Jensen et al (1979) and gluing needles to the skin (Gallacchi et al 1981).

More credible ones have included the employment of a pencil-like probe (Molsberger & Hille

1994), the tapping of a needle's guide tube against the skin (Lao et al 1995), and the insertion of a blunted cocktail skin through such a tube (White et al 1996).

Recently, two even more credible but unfortunately slightly more invasive needling techniques have been invented.

Stretberger & Kleinhenz (1998), working at the Clinic of Anesthesiology in Heidlberg, have designed a needle with a blunt tip which, by moving inside its handle, gives rise to a pricking sensation on touching the skin similar to that felt when a needle penetrates the skin. In a study which involved 60 volunteers divided into a 'needle' group and a 'placebo needle' group none of them in either group suspected that the instrument employed had not penetrated the skin. The only difficulty, as will be discussed again later, was that the needle-evoked sensation known as de qi was felt by some of these volunteers both with placebo needling and real acupuncture. A finding that led them to comment, 'De qi in placebo needling could be caused by the pressure of the ring and plastic cover, by psychological influences, or by pain produced by direct pressure on a pain receptor in the skin.'

Park et al (1999) at the University of Exeter, UK, have invented a sham needle (Park Sham Device (PSD) that, by telescoping on making impact with the skin, avoids penetration of it (Fig. 11.1).

This PSD has now been subjected to two randomized controlled trials (Park et al 2002). In the first study carried out in a district general hospital, 58 patients were enrolled in a clinical trial of acupuncture for acute stroke. Not one of these patients realized they had not been subjected to penetrative needling but as Park and his co-workers stated, 'this finding may be limited by the facts that these patients may have had abnormal sensations because of their recent stroke and were possibly disorientated from hospital admission ... Experience in other clinical settings will be required for further validation of the device.'

In the second study carried out in a university laboratory, 40 healthy acupuncture-naive adult volunteers were tested. In this trial the surrogate measure of activity adopted was experience of the specific needle sensation known as de qi. And as judged by that none of the participants realized

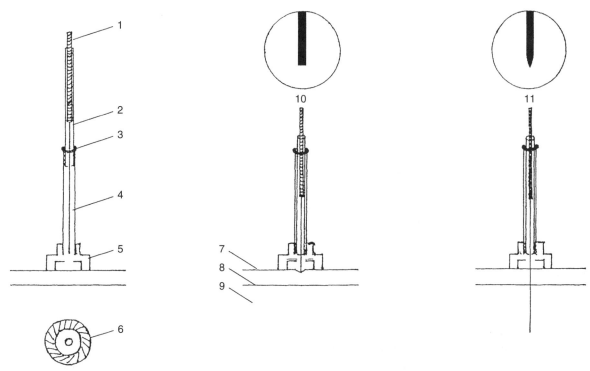

**Figure 11.1**    Park's sham needle unit: 1. Needle handle, 2. Guide tube, 3. Guide o-ring, 4. Park tube, 5. Flange, 6. Double-sided tape, 7. Skin, 8. Dermis, 9. Muscle, 10. Dull tip of sham needle, 11. Sharp tip of needle. (Reproduced with permission of Park J. et al (1999) Development of a new sham needle. Acupuncture in Medicine 17(2): 111)

they had not been subjected to acupuncture. These findings led them to conclude 'that the newly developed PSD is valid as a control procedure for trials of the efficacy of acupuncture, or more specifically, the needle penetration aspect of treatment'. They also, however commented, 'further investigation of this device will be required to establish its performance in the hands of different clinicians, in different acupuncture points particularly with a different anatomical configuration (e.g. in more curved skin or in hairy regions), and with sham needles made to match different manufacturers' styles'.

All this notwithstanding, that these two types of non-penetrative needling employed in both the trial carried out in Germany and the one in England caused a significant number of participants to experience the needle-evoked sensation of de qi shows that they cannot be considered to be entirely inactive forms of treatment because presumably this sensory effect must have been brought about as a result of pressure applied to the skin causing A-delta nerves to be stimulated which, as discussed in Chapter 10, is a sine qua non for the evoking of needle-induced analgesia.

## Placebo analgesia

The greatest hindrance to proving or disproving whether or not the analgesic effect produced by acupuncture is no more than a placebo effect is that a placebo itself is now known to afford pain relief in response to cues that suggest it is an effective treatment. Furthermore, it has recently been confirmed that this placebo-evoked analgesia, like acupuncture-evoked analgesia, is opioid peptide-mediated (ter Reit 1998) and because of this, as was shown some years ago, is naloxone reversible (Levine et al 1978, Levine & Gordon 1984).

As Fields & Basbaum ( 1999) have pointed out, it is possible in experiments using tourniquet-induced ischaemic pain as a model, to demonstrate a significant placebo analgesic effect. And that, whilst naloxone does not affect pain in subjects who have not been given a placebo, it has been shown to significantly reduce placebo analgesia (Amanzio & Benedetti 1999).

The weight of current evidence, therefore, supports a role for endogenous opioids in the production of placebo analgesia particularly now that Lipman et al (1990) have reported finding endogenous opioid-like material in the cerebral spinal fluid (CSF) of chronic pain patients after their pain levels had dropped following placebo administration. And now that Benedetti (1996) has demonstrated not only a reduction of placebo analgesia by naloxone but an enhancement of it by the cholecystokinin antagonist proglumide.

In the light of all this, it is perhaps possible that the prevailing preoccupation with trying to find a suitable placebo for the purpose of comparing its analgesic effect with that produced by acupuncture might be misconceived and it may be better instead to test acupuncture against other analgesics as Loh et al (1984) did in a trial to determine the place of this needle-evoked nerve stimulation therapy in the prevention of migraine.

In that study patients were randomly assigned either to Group A, who received acupuncture for 3 months followed by drug therapy for the next 3 months, or to Group B, who were given drug therapy first followed by acupuncture treatment for the same periods of time. The two groups were switched at the end of each 3-month period after a 2-week interval to allow for the effects of acupuncture to have worn off and for the excretion of any residual drugs.

The outcome of all this was that the frequency and duration of migraine was found to be significantly less during the period of acupuncture treatment and that most patients much preferred having that particular form of therapy.

## OTHER ACUPUNCTURE TRIAL–RELATED FACTORS REQUIRED TO BE TAKEN INTO CONSIDERATION

### Blinding

In drug trials it has for long been accepted that both the patient and therapist should not be able to distinguish between the active substance being tested and the inert one, as the expectations of either of them are liable to strongly influence the results, as Noseworthy et al (1994) showed in a randomised placebo-controlled multiple sclerosis drug trial.

In acupuncture trials such double-blinding is not possible for whilst the patient can readily be 'blinded' it is clearly not possible to 'blind' the therapist who by word or action may unwittingly communicate bias. Hansen & Hansen (1983) sought to overcome this difficulty by the employment of so-called 'standardised minimal interaction', but in general, the best that can be achieved is to have a 'blinded' independent evaluator.

### Randomization

The random placing of patients into a treatment group and a control group is a well-established practice in all clinical trials since its first successful use by the UK's Medical Research Council in a trial carried out in 1948 to ascertain the efficacy of streptomycin in the treatment of pulmonary tuberculosis.

In that trial, because only one disease was involved the employment of this procedure was relatively straightforward. With many acupuncture trials, however, as Hansson & Lundeberg (1999) have pointed out, difficulties in ensuring that patients with exactly the same type of pain are evenly distributed between an active and a control group have arisen when attempts have been made to assess the efficacy of this type of treatment in patients with conditions such as dental, neck or low-back pain that lack diagnostic precision. This is because they are liable to be suffering from either myofascial TrP nociceptive pain, nociceptive pain from some other cause, radiculopathic pain, neuropathic pain or a combination of these making the assessment of results, even when randomization is employed, virtually impossible due to the responsiveness of these different types of pain to acupuncture almost certainly being very different.

There is therefore a pressing need when attempting to assess the value of acupuncture in patients with any regional pain disorder to ensure that the pain suffered by those randomized to either an active treatment group or a control group is of the same type.

## Needle stimulation strength

For the purpose of conducting acupuncture trials it might seem essential for the strength of the dry needle-evoked stimulus applied to each patient in the treatment group to be kept constant. In trials where manual acupuncture is employed, this would mean keeping the needles in situ for the same length of time in everyone; also, either not twirling them or twirling them, and in the case of the latter, this being carried out in exactly the same manner and to the same extent. It is, however, apparent from everyday clinical practice that, so far as manual acupuncture is concerned, the optimum amounts of stimulation required for individual patients are widely different and can only be found for each person by a process of trial and error.

Therefore, the insistence on a fixed amount of stimulation for every patient is liable to result in some patients being overstimulated, with as a consequence, exacerbation of their pain and others being understimulated with, as a result, the treatment not given a chance to exert its maximum effect.

Macdonald et al (1983) are therefore in my opinion to be commended, for in their study on patients with low-back pain, they made provisions in their trial protocol for the strength of stimulus to be varied according to individual patients' requirements.

## Number of treatment sessions

With acupuncture treatment it is rare for there to be any appreciable benefit after only one treatment and, therefore, in my opinion, it is not appropriate to attempt to evaluate the effectiveness of this type of therapy in a trial in which it is only given on one occasion as has been the case in a number of trials, such as the ones carried out by Irnich et al (2002), Jensen et al (1979) and Moore & Berk (1976).

It usually requires 3–4 sessions before a decision can be made as to whether a patient's pain is likely to respond to acupuncture (Lewith 1985) and often more than these before any long-term relief is obtained. This, however, it has to be admitted varies according to both the type of pain disorder being treated and the person's individual responsiveness to acupuncture.

In acupuncture trials, therefore, it would not seem prudent to allow only a fixed number of sessions to be given to every patient for fear that with some individuals this may not be sufficient to allow them to achieve their maximum response. A more realistic approach might be to allow each patient to receive up to a maximum of 10 treatments depending on their individual requirements, as was done in the traditional Chinese acupuncture trial carried out by Coan et al (1980) and the TrP one carried out by Macdonald et al (1983).

## Design of acupuncture trials

Of the various trials so far completed in which the effect of acupuncture has been compared either with that of some other type of treatment in current use such as physiotherapy or with that of a placebo treatment, the design of most of them has been one in which the comparison has been made between two groups, one receiving acupuncture and the other serving as a control.

A few trials, however, have been of the crossover type in which the treatments being compared have been given sequentially in random order to each patient in turn. A trial of this type though has certain disadvantages when the effect of acupuncture is being assessed because the speed of response to such treatment and the immediate duration of relief from it varies widely from person to person, with in some cases there being a considerable delay before its full effect manifests itself. For this reason acupuncture and then some other form of treatment should be given with only a short interval in between, any delayed response from the acupuncture may cause confusion when attempting to assess the effectiveness of the second treatment. Such a problem is not confined to acupuncture trials alone but applies to any trial in which some type of physical treatment is being evaluated. It is, therefore, apparent that if a cross-over design is used in trials of this kind it is essential for there to be a long interval of up to several months in between each type of treatment (Lewith & Machin 1983).

A further problem with a cross-over trial is that a person who seems to be doing well with the initial treatment may be reluctant or even unwilling to change from this to some other form of treatment.

On balance, therefore, with acupuncture trials, group comparison is preferable.

## Numbers required in trials for the evaluation of acupuncture

The number of patients required in order to make an acupuncture trial statistically valid depends on several factors including the anticipatory clinical differences between the treatments being compared, the level of statistical significance considered appropriate and what are considered to be the chances of detecting such differences. Advice therefore should always be taken from a statistician with special training in this particular type of work ( Lewith & Machin 1983).

## The assessment of results

Assessments of the results of an acupuncture trial should be made immediately at the end of a laid down course of treatment and then at varying intervals after this, depending on the disorder being treated and in particular on its natural history.

Whilst agreeing with Richardson & Vincent (1986) in their reference to trials already completed that 'the relative paucity of long-term follow-up data is especially disappointing with chronic pain patients where the need to demonstrate lasting benefits from a new treatment is of paramount importance', exception has to be taken to their view that 'temporary relief of pain in such a group may be of theoretical interest but will have little significance' for it has to be remembered that even when the relief from chronic pain with acupuncture or for that matter any form of treatment is found to be only short lasting, this is not necessarily a failure so far as the patient is concerned as the quality of life is often improved by repeating the treatment at frequent intervals. And within this context, it has to be borne in mind that, whilst it may be possible to demonstrate that acupuncture, so far as the alleviation of chronic pain is concerned, is a valuable symptomatic form of treatment, the very nature of the condition makes it unlikely that it will often be shown to be a 'cure'.

## Methods of measuring pain relief

Unfortunately there are no objective means of measuring changes in the character and intensity of pain because, as Scott & Huskisson (1976) pointed out over 20 years ago, 'measurement of pain must always be subjective since pain is a subjective phenomenon – only the patient can therefore measure its severity.'

The pain-measuring devices that have proved to be of value include the visual analogue scale, the graphic rating scale (Huskisson 1974a, b) and the McGill Pain Questionnaire (Melzack 1975).

As patients find it extremely difficult to remember any changes that may occur in their perception of pain over a period of time, it is very helpful for them to be issued with diaries so that they can record details concerning pain levels, medication intake and sleep on a daily basis (Lewith et al 1983). In addition to information provided by the patient, the assessor should take into account such factors as changes in mobility and time off work. Finally, with certain disorders such as, for example, shoulder-cuff lesions, use should be made of a goniometer for measuring joint movements (Fernandes et al 1980).

These subjective and objective methods of assessment clearly apply to pain trials in general and as there is nothing particular about them in relation to acupuncture trials they will not be discussed further, but anyone who requires more detailed information should consult an extensive review of measuring and assessing pain in general provided by Melzack & Katz (1999) and an account of how methods of measuring pain should be employed in the assessment of acupuncture treatment in particular provided by Vincent & Chapman (1989).

## FUTURE ACUPUNCTURE CLINICAL TRIALS

## Trial protocols

From what has already been said in this chapter it is obvious that the carrying out of acupuncture clinical trials in the future will demand the employing of methodology of a higher standard than heretofore with, as an essential component of this, the drawing up of well-designed protocols (White & Park 1999).

### Recommended standards for the reporting of acupuncture trials

In an attempt to improve the quality of acupuncture trials an international group of experienced acupuncturists have devised a set of recommendations called Standards for Reporting Interventions in Controlled Trials of Acupuncture (STRICTA), which all those engaged in investigating the efficacy of this type of therapy are urged to adopt (Macpherson et al 2002).

These recommendations are meant to be employed in conjunction with the Consolidated Standards for Reporting Trials (CONSORT) statement. This statement, which was originally drawn up by Begg et al (1996) and then subsequently shown by Moher et al (2001a) to have a positive influence on the quality of trial reporting, was not only revised by Moher et al (2001b), but also ultimately further explained and elaborated by Altman et al (2001).

These STRICTA recommendations are considered to be of such fundamental importance that it has been decided to publish them concurrently in all the principal journals devoted to the study of acupuncture. The hope is that the implementation

of these will so improve the reporting of acupuncture trials as to make both their critical appraisal and the interpretation of their results far easier than when, for example, ter Reit et al in 1990 carried out a criteria-based meta-analysis of them.

They are therefore reproduced here (Table 11.1) to serve as a benchmark for all those wishing to participate in the carrying out of future trials.

It should be emphasized that these STRICTA guidelines are not immutable for the intention is to re-draft them as and when subsequent experience and debate dictates.

My only comment concerning this matter is that the giving of multiple types of acupuncture to those in the 'treatment' group, as Irnich et al (2002) recently did when they needled not only trigger and traditional Chinese acupuncture points but also auricular ones in a study of patients with chronic neck pain, is best avoided as it makes the relative contribution of each of them to the overall results of such a trial difficult to assess.

### Table 11.1

| Intervention | | Description |
|---|---|---|
| Acupuncture rationale | 1 | Style of acupuncture<br>Rationale for treatment (e.g. syndrome patterns, segmental levels, trigger points) and individualization if used. And literature sources to justify rationale |
| Needling details | 2 | Points used (uni/bilateral)<br>Numbers of needles inserted<br>Depths of insertion (tissue level, mm or cun)<br>Responses elicited (e.g. de qi or twitch response)<br>Needle stimulation (manual or electrical)<br>Needle retention time<br>Needle type (gauge, length, and manufacturer ) |
| Treatment regime | 3 | Number of treatment sessions<br>Frequency of treatment |
| Co-interventions | 4 | Other interventions (e.g. moxibustion, cupping, herbs, exercises, lifestyle advice) |
| Practitioner background | 5 | Duration of relevant training<br>Length of clinical experience<br>Expertise in specific condition |
| Control interventions | 6 | Intended effect of control intervention and its appropriateness to research question and, if appropriate, blinding of participants (e.g. active comparison, minimally active penetrating or non-penetrating sham, inert)<br>Explanations given to patient of treatment and control interventions<br>Details of control intervention (precise description, as for Item 2 above, and other items if different)<br>Sources that justify choice of control |

## Prospective participants in acupuncture clinical trials

The time has passed when acupuncture clinical trials can continue to be carried out by practitioners in private practice with inadequate numbers, difficulty in finding suitable controls and little or no statistical advice. For as Filshie & Cummings (1999) have so rightly said 'too much time has been spent by lone enthusiasts and inexperienced research teams who may have repeated previous errors made by academics unfamiliar with the subject'.

The carrying out of clinical trials requires considerable expertise and can only in the future be adequately conducted by university-based research teams with money for it provided either by the government or charitable research trusts. However, as Ernst & White (1997) have commented, 'research including that appertaining to acupuncture is expensive, there are no sponsors from industry and official funding bodies do not view acupuncture as a priority'.

Regrettably, we are currently in the unfortunate position that hospital-based physicians will not use acupuncture without clinical-trial-based evidence to support this but at the same time such trials cannot be carried out by them without them first becoming experienced in the practice of it!

There is however light on the horizon for as Hayhoe (1998) has pointed out, several British universities now provide lectures on acupuncture for their medical students and one, Exeter, has a chair in Complementary Medicine. In addition, there has recently been a strong move to integrate complementary medicine within the UK's National Health Service (Foundation for Integrated Medicine 1997). And in the USA a conference organized by the National Institute of Health (1997) has published a consensus statement concluding that there is now sufficient evidence of acupuncture's value to justify its incorporation within the framework of conventional medicine.

Moreover, in the UK the numbers of doctors practising acupuncture is steadily rising, with the membership of the British Medical Acupuncture Society now being over 1400 medical practitioners. Also, acupuncture is now available in 86% of hospital-based chronic pain services (Clinical Standards Advisory Group Report 1999) and is used in 37% of hospices (Wilkes 1992).

There are therefore sound grounds for believing that clinicians with access to research facilities may well be increasingly persuaded to enter into the difficult domain of assessing acupuncture's pain-relieving capability including, so far as the myofascial trigger point pain and fibromyalgia syndromes are concerned, the conducting of large scale trials to provide evidence-based data concerning the relative efficacy of and indications for superficial and deep dry needling at trigger and tender point sites.

## Possible future therapeutic advances relevant to the practice of acupuncture

Before closing this chapter it should be pointed out that over the course of time the practice of acupuncture for the relief of pain may become greatly changed by future pharmaceutical innovations that then, in turn, will themselves have to be subjected to the rigours of carefully conducted clinical trials.

There are at least two possibilities. One is the introduction into clinical practice of a cholecystokinin octapeptide receptor antagonist as this would have the effect of tilting the opioid and antiopioid balance in the central nervous system (CNS) and, by so doing, would considerably assist with the treatment of chronic pain with acupuncture (Han 1994). The other is the introduction of a ketamine-like non-toxic N-methyl-D-aspartate receptor antagonist, which would significantly decrease dorsal horn central sensitisation and thus reduce the chronicity of such disorders as the myofascial trigger point pain and fibromyalgia syndromes.

## References

Altman D G, Schulz K F, Moher D, Egger M et al 2001 The revised CONSORT statement for reporting randomized trials: explanation and elaboration. Annals of Internal Medicine 134(8): 663–694

Amanzio M, Benedetti F 1999 Neuropharmacological dissection of placebo analgesia: expectation-activated opioid systems versus conditioning-activated specific sub-systems. Journal of Neuroscience 19: 484–494

Beecher H K 1955 The powerful placebo. Journal of the American Medical Association 159: 1602–1606

Beecher H K 1959 The measurement of subjective responses. Oxford University press, Oxford

Begg C, Cho M, Eastwood S, Horton R, Moher D, Olkin I 1996 Improving the quality of reporting of randomized controlled trials. The CONSORT statement. Journal of the American Medical Association 276(8): 637–639

Belgrade M 1994 Two decades after ping-pong diplomacy. Is there a role for acupuncture in American pain management? American Pain Society Journal 3(2): 73–83

Benedetti F 1996 The opposite effects of the opiate antagonist naloxone and the cholecystokinin antagonist proglumide on placebo analgesia. Pain 64: 535–543

Bootzin R R 1985 The role of expectancy in behaviour change. In: White L P, Tursky B, Schwarz G E (eds) Placebo: theory, research and mechanism. Guildford Press, New York

Borglum-Jensen L, Melson B, Borglum-Jensen S 1979 Effect of acupuncture on headache measured by reduction in number of attacks and use of drugs. Scandinavian Journal of Dental Research 87: 373–380

Borkovec T D, Nau S D 1972 Credibility of analogue therapy rationales. Journal of Behavior Therapy and Experimental Psychiatry 3: 257–260

Buckalew L W, Ross S 1981 Relationship of perceptual characteristics to efficacy of placebos. Psychological Reports 49: 955–958

Campbell A 1999 Acupuncture: where to place the needles and for how long. Acupuncture in Medicine 17(2): 113–117

Campbell A 2001 Acupuncture in practice: beyond points and meridians. Butterworth-Heinmann, Oxford

Clinical Standards Advisory Group Report 1999 National Review of Pain Services and Standards. London: The Stationary Office

Co L L, Schmitz T H, Havdala H, Reyes A, Westerman M P 1979 Acupuncture : An evaluation in the painful crises of sickle cell anaemia. Pain 7: 181–185

Coan R M, Wong G, Su L K, Yick C C, Wang L, Ozer F T, Coan P L 1980 The acupuncture treatment of low-back pain: a randomized controlled study. American Journal of Chinese Medicine 8: 181–189

Doongaji D R, Vahia V N, Bharucha M P E 1978 On placebos, placebo responses and placebo responders (a review of psychological, psychopharmacological and psychophysiological factors). Psychological factors. Journal of Postgraduate Medicine 24: 91–96

Ernst E 1999a An evidence-based approach to acupuncture. Acupuncture in Medicine XV11(1): 59–61

Ernst E 1999b Clinical effectiveness of acupuncture; an overview of systematic reviews. In: Ernst E, White A (eds) Acupuncture, a scientific appraisal. Butterworth-Heinemann, Oxford Ch5

Ernst E, White A 1997 A review of problems in clinical acupuncture research. American Journal of Chinese Medicine XXV(1): 3–11

Ernst E, White A 1999 Acupuncture, a scientific appraisal. Butterworth-Heinemann, Oxford

Evans F J 1974 The placebo response in pain reduction. In: Bonica J J (ed) Advances in neurology, Vol. 4. Raven Press, New York, pp. 289–296

Ezzo J, Berman B, Hadhazy V A, Jadad A R et al 2000 Is acupuncture effective for the treatment of chronic pain? A systematic review. Pain 86: 217–225

Fernandes I, Berry H, Clark R J, Bloom B, Hamilton E B D 1980 Clinical study comparing acupuncture, physio-therapy, injection, and anti-inflammatory therapy in shoulder cuff lesions. Lancet 1: 208–209

Fields H L, Basbaum A I 1999 Central nervous system mechanisms of pain modulation. In: Wall P D, Melzack R (eds) Textbook of pain, 4th edn. Churchill Livingstone, Edinburgh

Filshie J, Cummings M 1999 Western medical acupuncture. In: Ernst E, White A (eds) Acupuncture, a scientific appraisal. Butterworth-Heinemann, Oxford

Foundation for Integrated Medicine 1997 Integrated healthcare: a way forward for the next five years/a discussion document

Gallacchi G, Mueller W, Plattner G R, Schnorrenberger C C 1981 Akupunktur und laserstrahlbehandlung beim zervikal und lumbalsyndrom. Schweizerische Medizinische Wochenschrift 111: 1360–1366

Gaw A C, Chang L W, Shaw L C 1975 Efficacy of acupuncture in osteoarthritic pain. New England Journal of Medicine 21: 375–378

Han J -S 1994 Scientific study may pave the way for the use of acupuncture in pain medicine. American Pain Society Journal 3(2): 92–95

Hansen P E, Hansen J H 1983 Acupuncture treatment of chronic facial pain – a controlled cross-over trial. Headache 23: 66–69

Hansson P, Lundeberg T 1999 Transcutaeous electrical nerve stimulation, vibration and acupuncture as pain-relieving measures. In: Wall P D, Melzack R ( eds) Text book of pain, 4th edn. Churchill Livingstone, Edinburgh

Hayhoe S 1998 The future. In: Filshie J, White A ( eds) Medical acupuncture. A Western scientific approach. Churchill Livingstone, Edinburgh

Huskisson E C 1974a Measurement of pain. Lancet 2: 1127–1131

Huskisson E C 1974b Pain mechanisms and measurements. In: The treatment of chronic pain. Medical and Technical Publishing, Lancaster

Irnich D, Behrens N, Molzen H et al 2001 Randomised trial of acupuncture compared with conventional massage and 'sham' laser acupuncture for treatment of chronic neck pain. British Medical Journal 322: 1574–1577

Irnich D, Behrens N, Gleditsch J M et al 2002 Immediate effects of dry needling and acupuncture at distant points in chronic neck pain: results of a randomized, double-blind, sham- controlled cross-over trial. Pain 99: 83–89

Jensen B L, Melsen B, Jensen S B 1979 The effects of acupuncture on headache measured by reduction in number of attacks and use of drugs. Scandinavian Journal of Dental Research 87: 373–380

Lao L, Bergman S, Langenberg P et al 1995 Efficacy of Chinese acupuncture on postoperative oral surgery pain. Oral Surgery, Oral Medicine, Oral Pathology, Oral Radiology 79: 423–428

Lasagna L, Mosteller F, Von Felsinger J M, Beecher H K 1954 A study of the placebo response. American Journal of Medicine 16: 770–779

Le Bars D, Dickenson A H, Besson J 1979 Diffuse noxious inhibitory controls (DNIC). 1 – Effects on dorsal horn convergent neurones, supraspinal involvement and theoretical implications. Pain 6: 283–327

Le Bars D, Villaneuva L, Willer J C, Bouhassira D 1991 Diffuse noxious inhibitory controls (DNIC) in animals and man. Acupuncture in Medicine 9: 47–56

Levine J D, Gordon N C 1984 Influence of the method of drug administration on analgesic response. Nature 312: 755–756

Levine J D, Gordon N C, Fields H L 1978 The mechanism of placebo analgesia. Lancet 2: 654–657

Lewith G T 1985 Acupuncture and transcutaneous nerve stimulation. In: Lewith G T (ed) Alternative therapies. Heinemann Medical, London, p. 33

Lewith G T, Field J, Machin D 1983 Acupuncture compared with placebo in post-herpetic pain. Pain 17: 361–368

Lewith G T, Machin D 1983 On the evaluation of the clinical effects of acupuncture. Pain 16: 111–127

Lewith G T, Vincent C A 1995 On the evaluation of the clinical effects of acupuncture: a problem reassessed and a framework for future research. Pain Forum 4(1): 29–39

Lewith G T, Vincent C A 1998 The clinical evaluation of acupuncture. In: Filshie J, White A (eds) Medical acupuncture. A Western scientific approach. Churchill Livingstone, Edinburgh

Liberman R 1964 An experimental study of the placebo under three different situations of pain. Journal of Psychiatric Research 2: 233–246

Lipman J J, Miller B E, Mays K S, Miller M N, North W C, Byrne W L 1990 Peak B endorphin concentration in cerebrospinal fluid: reduced in chronic pain patients and increased during the placebo response. Psychopharmacology 102: 112–116

Loh L, Nathan P W, Schott G D, Zilkha K J 1984 Acupuncture versus medical treatment for migraine and muscle tension headaches. Journal of Neurology and Psychiatry 47: 333–337

Macdonald A J R, Macrae K D, Master B R, Rubin A P 1983 Superficial acupuncture in the relief of chronic low-back pain. Annals of the Royal College of Surgeons of England 65: 44–46

Macpherson H, White A, Cummings M, Jobst K, Rose K, Niemtzow R 2002 Standards for reporting interventions in controlled trials of acupuncture. The STRICTA recommendations. Acupuncture in Medicine 20(1): 22–25

Mann F 1992 Reinventing acupuncture. A new concept of ancient medicine. Butterworth-Heinemann, Oxford

Melzack R 1975 Prolonged pain relief by brief intense transcutaneous somatic stimulation. Pain 1: 357–373

Melzack R 1984 Acupuncture and related forms of folk medicine. In: Wall P D, Melzack R (eds) Textbook of

pain, 1st edn. Churchill Livingstone, Edinburgh, pp. 691–700

Melzack R, Katz J 1999 Pain measurements in persons in pain. In: Wall P D, Melzack R (eds) Textbook of pain, 4th edn. Churchill Livingstone, Edinburgh

Moher D, Jones A, Lepage L 2001a Use of the CONSORT statement and quality of reports of randomized trials: a comparative before-and-after evaluation. Journal of the American Medical Association 285(15): 1992–1995

Moher D, Schulz K F, Altman D G 2001b For the CONSORT Group. The CONSORT statement: revised recommendations for improving the quality of reports of parallel-group randomised trials. Lancet 357(9263): 1191–1194

Molsberger A, Hille E 1994 The analgesic effect of acupuncture in chronic tennis elbow. British Journal of Rheumatology 33: 1162–1165

Moore M E, Berk S N 1976 Acupuncture for chronic shoulder pain: an experimental study with attention to the role of placebo and hypnotic susceptibility. Annals of Internal Medicine 84: 381–384

National Institutes of Health (NIH) Consensus Statement Online 1997 http://odp.od.nih.gov/consensus/ statements/cdc/107/107stmt.html Question 1

Noseworthy J H, Ebers G C, Vanderoort M K, Farquhar R E, Roberts R 1994 The impact of blinding on the results of a randomized placebo-controlled multiple sclerosis trial. Neurology 44: 16–20

Park J, White A, Lee H, Ernst E 1999 Development of a new sham needle. Acupuncture in Medicine 17(2): 1210–112

Park J, White A, Stevenson C, Ernst E, James M 2002 Validating a new non-penetrating sham acupuncture device. Two randomised controlled trials. Acupuncture in Medicine 20(4): 168–174

Petrie J, Hazleman B 1985 Credibility of placebo transcutaneous nerve stimulation and acupuncture. Clinical and Experimental Rheumatology 3: 151–153

Petrie J, Langley G B 1983 Acupuncture in the treatment of chronic cervical pain. A pilot study. Clinical and Experimental Rheumatology 1: 333–335

Pomeranz B, Cheng R, Law P 1977 Acupuncture reduces electrophysiological and behavioral responses to noxious stimuli: pituitary is implicated. Experimental Neurology 54: 172–178

Richardson P H, Vincent C A 1986 acupuncture for the treatment of pain: a review of evaluative research. Pain 24: 15–40

Sandrew B B, Yang R C C, Wang S C 1978 Electroacupuncture analgesia in monkeys: a behavioral and neurophysiological assessment. Archives Internationales de Pharmacodynamie et de Therapie 231: 274–284

Scott J, Huskisson E C 1976 Graphic representation of pain. Pain 2: 175–184

Stretberger K, Kleinhenz J 1998 Introducing a placebo needle into acupuncture research. Lancet 352: 364–365

Taub H A, Beard M C, Eisenberg L, McCormack R K 1977 Studies of acupuncture for operative dentistry. Journal of American Dental Association 95: 555–561 ter Reit G, de Craen A J M, de Boer, Kessels A G H 1998 Is placebo analgesia mediated by endogenous opioids? A systematic review. Pain 76: 273–275

ter Reit G, Kleijnen J, Knipschild P 1990 Acupuncture and chronic pain: a criteria-based meta-analysis. Journal of Clinical Epidemiology 43(11): 1191–1199

Tyler D B 1946 The influence of a placebo and medication on motion sickness. American Journal of Physiology 146: 458–466

Vierck C J, Lineberry C G, Lee P K, Calderwood H W 1974 Prolonged hypalgesia following 'acupuncture' in monkeys. Life Sciences 15: 1277–1289

Vincent C A 1989 The methodology of controlled trials of acupuncture. Acupuncture in Medicine 6: 9–13

Vincent C A, Chapman C R 1989 Pain measurement and the assessment of acupuncture treatment. Acupuncture in Medicine 6: 14–19

Vincent C A, Lewith G T 1995 Placebo controls for acupuncture studies. Journal of the Royal Society of Medicine 88: 199–202

Vincent C A, Richardson P H 1986 The evaluation of therapeutic acupuncture. Concepts and models. Pain 24: 1–13

Wall P D 1994 The placebo and placebo response. In: Wall P D, Melzack R (eds) Textbook of pain, 3rd edn. Churchill Livingstone, Edinburgh, pp. 1301, 1304

Wilkes E 1992 Complementary therapy in hospice and palliative care. Report for Trent Palliative Care Centre

White A, Eddleston C, Hardie R et al 1996 A pilot study of acupuncture for tension headaches using a novel placebo. Acupuncture in Medicine 14: 6–10

White A, Park J 1999 Protocols for clinical trials of acupuncture. Acupuncture in Medicine 17(1): 54–58

# PART 3

# The practical application of trigger point acupuncture

# Chapter 12

# Chest pain

## CHAPTER CONTENTS

## INTRODUCTION

In discussing the practical applications of trigger point (TrP) acupuncture in Part Three of this book, the indications for its use in the alleviation of certain types of chest pain will firstly be considered because, historically, some of the earliest clinical observations concerning the referral of pain from TrPs were made just before World War II on patients with these in the muscles of the chest wall.

Attention will mainly be directed to cardiac pain and to musculoskeletal pain in this chapter because, so far as chest pain is concerned, it is in the alleviation of these two types of pain that acupuncture has its main application.

At the outset it has to be made clear that clinically there is often difficulty in distinguishing between cardiac and TrP pain because their patterns of distribution are often identical. Furthermore, the added difficulty is that both may be present together.

Attention was fist drawn to the phenomenon of secondary TrP activation in the muscles of the chest wall in patients with coronary heart disease by two University of Pennsylvania physicians, Joseph Edeiken and Charles Wolferth, when in 1936 they reviewed some cases of coronary thrombosis in which pain in the shoulder had developed during the course of strict bed rest.

Edeiken & Wolferth reported that on examination of the muscles around the scapula in two of their patients, they found focal areas of exquisite tenderness, or what they called trigger zones in view of the fact that by applying pressure to these zones they were able to reproduce the spontaneously occurring pain in the shoulder. They further stated that one of their patients had noticed for himself that pressure over one of these so-called trigger zones caused pain to be referred to the left shoulder, up the left side of the neck and down the left arm.

The significance of such observations might readily have been overlooked had it not been that this report came to the attention of Janet Travell, the American physician who has since contributed so much to the subject of referred pain from TrPs, at a time when she herself was suffering from a painful shoulder, not following a coronary thrombosis, but after having strained some muscles during the course of her work. As she said in her autobiography, *Office Hours: Day and Night* (1968):

> Poking around at night on the muscles over my shoulder blade, trying to give some 'do-it-yourself' massage, I was astonished to touch some spots that intensified, or reproduced my pain, as though I had turned on an electric switch. It was my first introduction to the enigmatic trigger area. No nerve existed, I knew, to connect those firing spots directly with my arm. I was baffled, but I did not discard the observation on the grounds that I could not explain it.

It was because Travell found that she could reproduce pain in herself in exactly the same manner as Edeiken & Wolferth had done in patients with myocardial infarction that prompted her to study the subject further. The opportunity to do this arose almost immediately when, in 1936, she was appointed to work under Dr Harry Gold in the Cardiac Consultation Clinic at Sea View Hospital on Staten Island, New York. At this hospital, which specialized in the treatment of tuberculosis, a large number of patients, having been kept in bed for long periods, suffered severe pain in their shoulders and arms. As she says in her autobiography:

> When I examined them by systematic palpation of the scapula and chest muscles, I easily uncovered the presence of trigger areas. I knew what to look for . . .

Her interest in the referral of pain from what are now called myofascial TrPs having been aroused

in this manner, she was prompted to read the various other important contributions to the subject published over the next few years including those of Kellgren (1938), Steindler & Luck (1938) and Steindler (1940). From these she learnt that such pain may be alleviated by injecting procaine into 'tender spots' (trigger zones) in the muscles.

As a result of reading these reports Travell decided in 1940 to persuade Dr Myron Herman, the medical resident at Sea View Hospital, to inject procaine into trigger areas in the chest walls of patients with painful shoulders at that hospital (Travell et al 1942). It was because the results of this treatment were so impressive that Travell and her cardiologist colleague, Seymour Rinzler, decided to investigate a number of other patients under their care in the general medical wards at the Beth Israel Hospital. The outcome of this was that in 1948 they published two outstanding papers. In one they drew attention to the fact that TrPs may develop in the muscles of the chest wall as a secondary event in patients with cardiac pain and reported that it is possible to relieve the latter by injecting procaine into these points, or by spraying the skin overlying them with ethyl chloride (Rinzler & Travell 1948). In the other they showed how closely the pattern of pain, occurring as a result of the primary activation of chest wall TrPs, may simulate that of ischaemic heart disease (Travell & Rinzler 1948). They were not, however, the first to recognize this, as Gutstein (1938), Kelly (1944) and Mendlowitz (1945) had previously described how pain from 'tender spots' in the muscles of the chest wall may have a similar pattern of distribution to that of cardiac pain.

## ANTERIOR CHEST WALL MTrP PAIN SYNDROME

This syndrome (Baldry 1997, 2001) mainly arises as a result of either trauma-induced or stress-induced activation of TrPs in muscles of the anterior chest wall. It may also develop as a secondary event in patients with coronary artery disease as a result of TrPs in muscles present in the zone of cardiac pain referral becoming activated as a result of cardiac pain-evoked muscle spasm. In addition, it is liable to arise, for some as yet unexplained reason, in patients with mitral valve prolapse (see p. 179).

## SIMILARITIES BETWEEN THE REFERRAL PATTERNS OF ANTERIOR CHEST WALL TrP PAIN AND CARDIAC PAIN

Pain from TrPs in muscles on the left side of the neck and chest wall and cardiac pain may have similar referral patterns.

Primary TrP pain referral may simulate that of cardiac pain referral when there is TrP activity in only one muscle. More often, however, such activity develops in several muscles simultaneously, or spreads from one muscle to another until ultimately several are involved.

As pointed out by Travell (1976), a good example of such a chain reaction is when TrP activity arises in the sternal division of the sternocleidomastoid muscle causing pain to be referred down the length of the sternum. Pain in this distribution may then lead to the development of TrP activity in the sternalis muscle, with, as a result of this, pain being referred to the pectoral region and the development of secondary TrP activity in the pectoralis major muscle. These TrPs may then be responsible for pain being referred to the left shoulder and down the left arm. This, therefore, is a good example as to how doing nothing more serious than straining a muscle in the neck may lead to the development of pain with a referral pattern exactly similar to that of coronary heart disease pain.

As it cannot be stressed too strongly it will be reiterated that what makes the differential diagnosis difficult is that not only may primary TrP pain have a similar pattern of referral to that of ischaemic heart disease pain, but secondary TrP activity may also develop in muscles that happen to lie within an area affected by the pain of this cardiac disorder.

The various muscles liable to be involved include those in the neck, the sternal division of the sternocleidomastoid and the scaleni; in the chest, the sternalis, the subclavius, the pectoralis major, the pectoralis minor and the serratus anterior; and in the abdomen, the rectus abdominis and the external oblique muscles. The clinical manifestations and treatment of TrP activity in each of these muscles will therefore be considered in turn.

## Sternocleidomastoid muscle

TrP activity in the lower end of the sternal division of the muscle may cause pain to be referred over the upper part of the sternum (Fig. 16.6). TrPs elsewhere in this muscle refer pain to the face and scalp. Therefore, any discussion concerning the activation and deactivation of them will be deferred until Chapter 16.

## Scalene muscles

### Activation of TrPs

TrP activity in any of the three scalene muscles may develop as a primary event by straining the neck such as when pulling with the hands against a strongly resistant force, or when lifting or carrying awkwardly some heavy object. Also, TrP activity may develop as a result of the muscle strain brought about by severe bouts of coughing, or by holding the neck in some awkward position either when lying or standing; and as a secondary event when there is TrP activity in the sternocleidomastoid muscle.

### Specific pattern of pain referral

Pain from TrPs in either the scalenus anterior, medius, or posterior (Fig. 12.1) is liable to be referred anteriorly over the pectoral region; posteriorly along the medial border of the scapula; and laterally across the front of the shoulder and down the arm. When the latter occurs, it is felt both in the front and back of the arm, and extends to the thumb and index finger (Fig. 12.2).

Pain from TrP activity in one or other of these muscles on the left side because of its distribution and because it sometimes only comes on with exertion may closely simulate coronary heart disease pain.

In differentiating between the two it is helpful to remember that referred pain from the scalenus anterior muscle is relieved when both the arm and clavicle are elevated by placing the forearm on the affected side across the forehead (Ochsner et al 1935); and it is aggravated by contracting the muscle by rotating the head as far as possible to the side of the pain whilst pulling the chin down into the supraclavicular fossa.

With regard to the effect the position of the arm has on this type of pain, it is of interest to note that a man under my care, with pain in the chest and

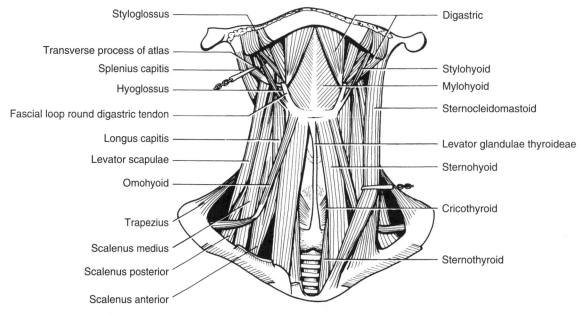

**Figure 12.1** Muscles of the front of the neck. On the right the sternocleidomastoid has been removed.

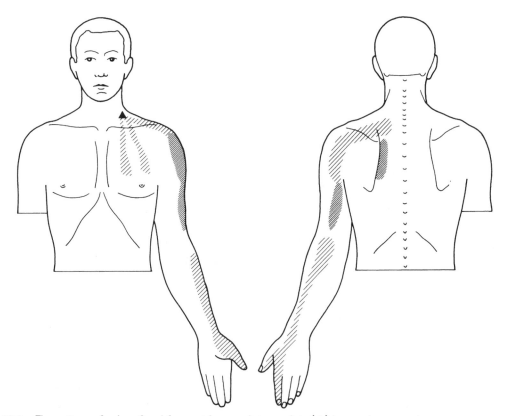

**Figure 12.2** The pattern of pain referral from a trigger point or points (▲) in a scalene muscle.

down the right arm from TrP activity in the right scalenus anterior muscle, found that, although the pain was always aggravated by carrying heavy loads with the arm hanging down at the side of the body, it was never present when, with the arm held high, he carried the British Legion banner at ex-Servicemen's parades.

## TrP examination

TrPs in the scalenus anterior are found by palpating the muscle where it lies behind the posterior border of the sternocleidomastoid muscle. It is useful to distend the external jugular vein by putting pressure on it at the base of the neck, as the vein crosses the scalenus anterior muscle usually just about the level where TrP activity in this muscle occurs.

The scalenus medius lies lateral to the scalenus anterior and at a much deeper level against the transverse processes of the vertebrae. TrPs in it may readily be identified by pressing against these structures. The scalenus posterior is far more difficult to palpate, but, fortunately, TrP activity in it seems to be much less common than in the other two.

TrP activity often develops in the scalenus anterior and medius concomitantly.

## Associated TrPs

Satellite TrPs may develop in the various muscles situated in the regions to which pain from TrP activity in the scalene muscles is referred. Anteriorly referred pain may cause TrPs in the pectoralis major to become activated. Pain referred to the back of the arm may cause TrPs to become activated in the triceps, and pain referred down the front of the arm may cause similar activity to develop in the brachioradialis and the extensor carpi radialis. TrP activity in the scalene muscles may also occur in association with it developing in the levator scapulae muscle (see Ch. 14).

## Deactivation of TrPs

Deactivation of TrPs in the scalenus anterior and medius should be carried out with the patient in the supine position, with the head supported by a pillow and turned towards the opposite side. In deactivating TrPs in the scalenus anterior, care has

to be taken not to puncture the external jugular vein, or to damage the cervical spinal nerve roots and part of the brachial plexus where they emerge in the groove between the scalenus anterior and medius. It must, however, be remembered that needling a scalene TrP itself may cause momentary intense pain to shoot down the arm and that therefore this alone does not necessarily imply that a nerve root has been irritated.

## Thoracic outlet entrapment syndrome

Compression of the brachial plexus and subclavian vessels as a result of TrP-evoked shortening of the scalene muscles will be discussed in Chapter 15.

## Sternalis muscle

### Activation of TrPs

TrP activity arises in this muscle as a primary event usually as a result of trauma to the front of the chest. And as a secondary event when pain is referred to the region of the sternum as a result of coronary heart disease or the development of TrP activity in either the lower end of the sternocleidomastoid muscle or a scalene muscle.

### Specific pattern of pain referral

This muscle is only present in about one in 20 people, but when it does exist, the development of TrP activity in it is liable to give rise to deep substernal pain with, at times, radiation of this across the left or right pectoral region and down the inner side of the arm to the elbow (Fig. 12.3).

### TrP examination

TrPs occur anywhere along the length of this muscle and are found by systematically palpating it against both borders of the underlying sternum. Firm pressure on a TrP causes considerable local tenderness and at times the referral of pain in a lateral direction.

### Associated TrPs

TrP activity in this muscle is rarely an isolated event. It usually occurs in conjunction with similar

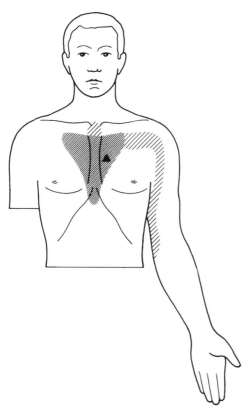

**Figure 12.3**   The pattern of pain referral from a trigger point or points (▲) in the sternalis muscle.

activity in the pectoralis major muscle. And, as stated earlier, pain from TrP activity in the sternal division of the sternocleidomastoid muscle may be referred downwards over the sternum and cause TrPs in it to become activated.

### TrP deactivation

A TrP in this muscle is readily located by flat palpation. A needle is then inserted into the tissues overlying it after it has first been trapped between two fingers.

## Subclavius muscle

### Activation of TrPs

TrPs in this muscle are liable to become activated for the same reasons as, and often in conjunction with, points in the pectoralis major muscle.

### Specific pattern of pain referral

TrP activity in this muscle causes pain to be referred across the front of the shoulder, down the front of the arm in the midline, the front of the forearm on the radial side, and the radial side of the palmar surface of the hand and fingers. As Travell & Simons (1983) have pointed out, pain for some curious reason is not felt at either the elbow or the wrist (Fig. 12.4).

### TrP examination

TrPs in this muscle are usually to be found at its medial end around the site of its insertion into the 1st rib (Fig. 12.4).

### Associated TrPs

TrP activity in this muscle invariably occurs in association with similar activity in the pectoralis major muscle.

### Deactivation of TrPs

A needle should be inserted superficially at any points of maximum tenderness found to be present just below the clavicle.

## Pectoralis major

### Activation of TrPs

The factors which may cause primary TrP activity to develop in this muscle include lifting a heavy weight or holding it for a sustained period; any task that involves either repeated adduction of the arm, such as when cutting a hedge with manually operated shears, or sustained adduction of it, such as when the arm is placed in a sling for any length of time. Also, exposure of the muscle to draughts or damp; persistent contraction of the muscle as a result of chronic anxiety; and, in particular, the adoption of a faulty slouching posture when reading, writing or the carrying out of some task at a work bench.

Secondary TrP activity may develop in this muscle when pain from coronary heart disease is referred to the left side of the chest anteriorly.

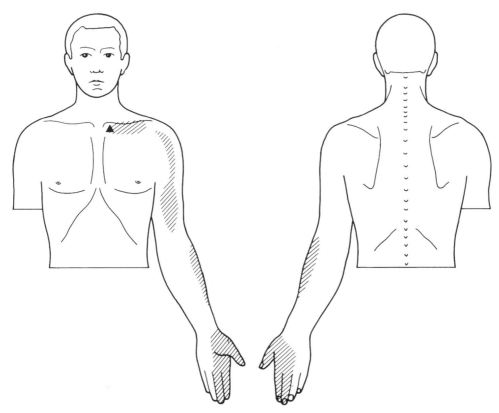

**Figure 12.4** The pattern of pain referral from a trigger point or points (▲) in the subclavius muscle.

## Specific patterns of pain referral

This muscle is divided according to its various attachments into a clavicular section, a sternal section, and a costo-abdominal section. These merge together to be inserted by means of a tendon into the lateral lip of the bicipital groove of the humerus (Fig. 12.5). The specific patterns of TrP pain referral vary according to the particular section affected.

TrP activity in the clavicular section of the muscle causes pain to be referred both locally and, even more markedly, over the shoulder as far as the anterior part of the deltoid muscle (Fig. 12.6).

TrP activity in the sternal section is found mainly along the parasternal and mid-clavicular lines, with TrPs along the parasternal line referring pain locally and over the sternum. TrPs in the mid-clavicular line give rise to severe pain over the anterior part of the chest and thus, on the left side, over the praecordium. From there it often spreads down the inner aspect of the arm and is felt particularly strongly over the medial epicondyle. It then terminates in the ring and little fingers (Fig. 12.7).

TrP activity along the lateral free margin of the muscle, where it forms the anterior axillary fold, gives rise to pain and tenderness in the breast, as well as tenderness of the nipple. In women this not infrequently leads to an erroneous diagnosis of mastitis, even when the texture of the breast is normal (Fig. 12.8).

## TrP examination

TrPs in all sections of this muscle should be located by flat palpation with the patient lying down.

## Associated TrP activity

TrP activity in the pectoralis major may occur in conjunction with similar activity in the sternalis, sternocleidomastoid, and scalene muscles. Satellite

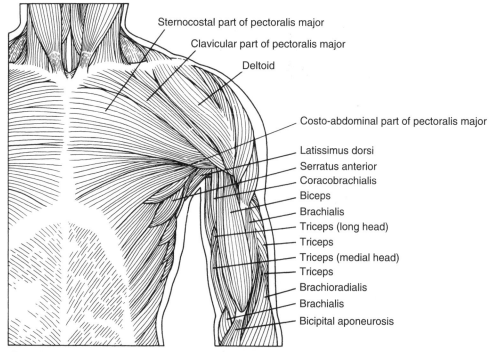

**Figure 12.5**   Superficial muscles of the front of the chest and upper arm. Left side.

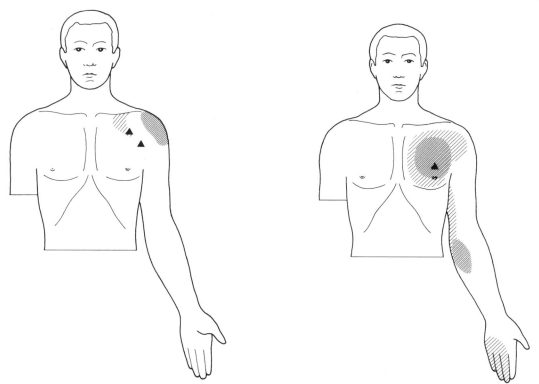

**Figure 12.6**   The pattern of pain referral from a trigger point or points (▲) in the clavicular section of the pectoralis major muscle.

**Figure 12.7**   The pattern of pain referral from a trigger point or points (▲) in the sternal section of the pectoralis major muscle.

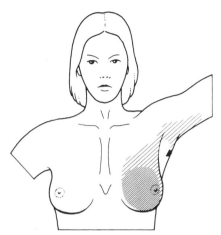

**Figure 12.8** The pattern of pain referral from a trigger point or points (▲) in the lateral free margin of the pectoralis major muscle.

TrPs may also be found in the anterior deltoid muscle due to it lying within the pectoralis major's pain referral zone.

## Deactivation of TrPs

When deactivating TrPs in the pectoralis major or any other muscle covering the chest wall, needles should never be inserted vertically for fear of penetrating the pleura and producing a pneumothorax, but should always be inserted in an oblique direction.

## Bilateral TrP activity

When TrP activity occurs in both the right and left pectoralis major muscles simultaneously the pain may be said by the patient to be 'across the chest', a description that immediately raises the possibility of it being due to coronary heart disease. However, the circumstances prevailing prior to the development of the pain may be of diagnostic help as shown by the following case history.

A maintenance fitter (47 years of age) sent for his general practitioner in the middle of the night because of pain across the chest and shortness of breath. A pain-relieving injection was given. Blood specimens were taken that night and the next 2 days for cardiac enzyme studies. These proved to be normal as did a subsequent ECG both at rest and after exercise.

However, as he continued to get episodes of pain across his chest most days he was at first given nifedipine (Adalat), but when it became obvious he was not suffering from angina, he was put on to naproxen (Naprosyn). And when this did not prove particularly helpful, he was given clomipramine (Anafranil) as it was thought the persistence of the pain might be associated with nervous tension and depression. After 7 months he was referred to me for further assessment. On going back over the history it became apparent that the initial attack of nocturnal pain had started after lifting a particularly heavy piece of machinery. Also, that the subsequent episodes of pain that he described as stabbing in character were not brought on by walking, but usually came on after having exerted himself carrying out some heavy task at work. They were also particularly troublesome on adopting certain positions in bed.

From the history, therefore, it was most likely that the pain was of muscular origin. And on examination, TrPs were found to be present in the sternal section of the pectoralis major, along the parasternal line on the right side and mid-clavicular line on the left side, also along the free edge of the costo-abdominal section of the muscle on the left side.

Once these TrPs had been deactivated by means of the carrying out of superficial dry needling on three occasions at weekly intervals and one further time 2 weeks later lasting relief from the pain was obtained.

## Pectoralis minor

### Activation of TrPs

The factors responsible for the development of TrP activity in this muscle (Fig. 12.9) are similar to those responsible for this happening in the pectoralis major and therefore it often develops simultaneously in both of these muscles.

### Specific pattern of pain referral

Pain from TrP activity in this muscle is referred widely over the front of the chest so that on the left side it is felt over the praecordium, over the front of the shoulder, and at times down the ulnar side

**Figure 12.9** The deep muscles of the front of the chest and arm. Left side.

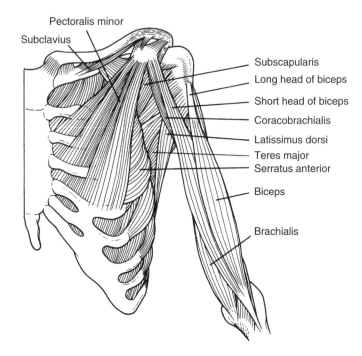

Pectoralis minor
Subclavius
Subscapularis
Long head of biceps
Short head of biceps
Coracobrachialis
Latissimus dorsi
Teres major
Serratus anterior
Biceps
Brachialis

of the arm to the hand, where it is felt in the middle, ring and little fingers (Fig. 12.10).

## TrP examination

When locating TrPs in this muscle the patient may either be seated or lying in the supine position. In either case the pectoralis major should be slackened by having the patient's arm lying comfortably to the side with the forearm across the abdomen. The pectoralis minor is then put on the stretch by getting the patient to brace the shoulder backwards. TrPs are usually to be found in the lower part of the muscle where it is attached to the ribs, or in the upper part close to its attachment to the coracoid process.

## Deactivation of TrPs

This is the same as for the pectoralis major muscle.

## Serratus anterior muscle

### Activation of TrPs

TrP activity may develop in this muscle (Fig. 12.9) when it is strained either as a result of the carrying

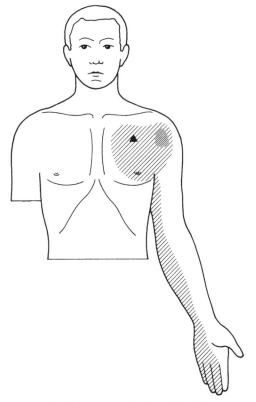

**Figure 12.10** The pattern of pain referral from a trigger point or points (▲) in the pectoralis minor muscle.

out of some athletic pursuit or during the course of severe coughing. Anxiety, with the muscles of the chest wall held in a persistently contracted state, is another cause.

## Specific pattern of pain referral

Pain from TrP activity in this muscle which wraps itself closely around the rib cage is referred to the side and back of the chest, and, at times, down the ulnar aspect of the arm (Fig. 12.11). The patient may also complain that it is painful to take a deep breath – the so-called stitch in the side.

## TrP examination

With the patient lying down and turned so that the affected side is uppermost, the muscle is put on the stretch by pulling the arm backwards. TrPs in it are usually located in the mid-axillary line at about the level of the 5th and 6th ribs in line with the nipple (Fig. 12.11).

## Associated TrPs

TrP activity in this muscle is often an isolated event. After a time, however, TrPs in its main antagonist the latissimus dorsi may also become activated.

## Deactivation of TrPs

The TrPs are deactivated by superficial dry needling carried out with the patient lying with the affected side uppermost. The needle should be directed at a shallow angle almost parallel to the chest wall towards an underlying rib so as to avoid entering the pleural space.

## Rectus abdominis and external oblique muscles

The effects of TrP activity developing in these two muscles will be discussed in detail when considering abdominal pain in Chapter 20. It is necessary to state here, however, that TrP activity in the upper part of the rectus abdominis muscle and in the upper part of the external oblique muscle may cause pain to be referred upwards over the lower part of the chest anteriorly. When this occurs, either on the left or right side, it is liable to be misdiagnosed as being pleural in origin in spite of the absence of either a pleural rub or any signs of intrapulmonary disease. And on the left side it may closely mimic the pain of coronary heart disease (Kelly 1944).

## Activation of TrPs

This commonly occurs either as a result of acute trauma or chronic overloading with the latter often having an occupational basis.

## TrP examination

The patient should be placed in the supine position and instructed to stretch the muscles by holding the breath in deep inspiration. TrPs in the upper part of the rectus abdominis are usually to be found in the angle between the costal margin and the xiphisternum. In the upper part of the external oblique muscles they are either along or under the lower border of the rib cage (Figs 20.3 and 20.4).

## Deactivation of TrPs

Each TrP should be trapped between two fingers prior to inserting a needle into the tissues overlying it.

## ANTERIOR CHEST WALL MTrP PAIN AND CARDIAC PAIN – THE DIFFERENTIAL DIAGNOSIS

As has already been stated, muscles in the chest wall when subjected to trauma of one kind or another may develop TrP activity with the pattern of pain referral resulting from this being identical with that seen in coronary heart disease. Also, the same chest wall muscles may develop satellite TrP activity as a result of being within the area affected by pain from coronary heart disease.

It is, therefore, easy to see that diagnostic confusion may readily occur and, whilst it is obviously important not to overlook angina when present, it

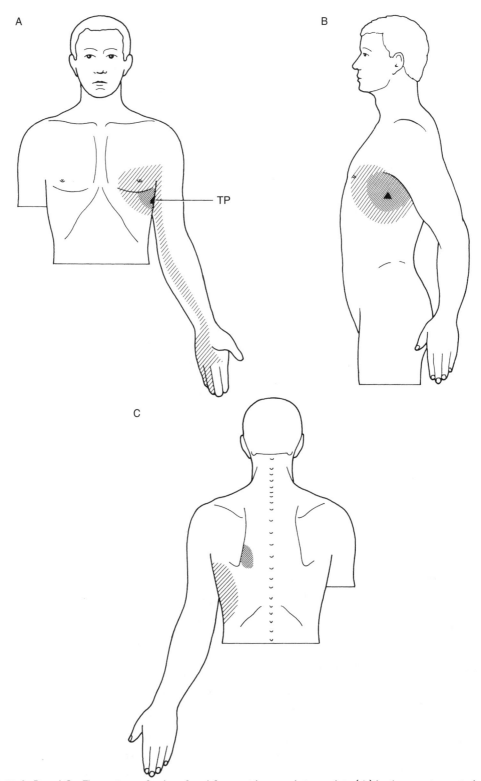

**Figure 12.11 A, B and C** The pattern of pain referral from a trigger point or points (▲) in the serratus anterior muscle.

is equally essential not to diagnose chest pain as being anginal when it is only muscular in origin. This is a mistake as frequently made today as it was when Allison (1950) wrote in reference to non-cardiac chest pain:

> ... the frequency with which such patients are seen in routine out-patient work emphasizes the need for a reorientation towards pain in the chest, and suggests that in clinical teaching pride of place is too often given to angina pectoris in explanation of the pain, and too little regard is paid to local structural causes.

One particular circumstance when primary anterior chest wall TrP pain may be overlooked is when it occurs in someone known to have a history of coronary heart disease. Chest pain arising soon after recovery from a myocardial infarction, if accompanied by fever and a pericardial rub, is readily recognized to be part of the post-infarction syndrome (Dressler 1959). If, however, it occurs by itself, there is a tendency to assume it must be anginal, and to overlook the possibility that it may have arisen as a result of the activation of TrPs. Similarly, anterior chest wall TrP pain may erroneously be assumed to be anginal when it occurs at some time following coronary by-pass surgery.

The relevance of all this to the practice of TrP acupuncture is that, whilst pain arising as a result of the primary activation of TrPs is readily alleviated by means of superficial dry needling carried out at these points, and whilst, as will be explained later, treatment of this type may have a limited place in the overall management of coronary heart disease, clearly before using it for the alleviation of any type of chest pain, it is essential to have made an exact diagnosis as to its cause. For this reason the various problems that arise in differentiating between cardiac pain and TrP pain will now be discussed.

When attempting to distinguish between these two types of pain careful history-taking is clearly of prime importance, but this by itself may be inconclusive. This is because, whilst with ischaemic heart disease there is substernal tightness and frequently radiation of pain up into the neck, across the chest to the shoulder and down the left arm, what is less well known is that pain emanating from TrPs in anterior chest wall muscles may have a referral pattern exactly the same as this. And, moreover, although angina is characteristically brought on by exertion, chest wall TrP pain may also be aggravated by this. The difference is that whereas with angina the amount of effort required to produce the pain is fairly constant, with TrP pain it is liable to vary widely from day to day. Also, pain of this type is often aggravated by stretching and twisting movements of the chest wall muscles.

Furthermore, angina may on occasion come on at rest. When this is due to the heart rate increasing in response to some emotional upset, it usually only lasts for a relatively brief period, whereas, in contrast to this, when TrP pain develops at rest it is liable to persist for a long time. Also, both types of pain may disturb sleep. With ischaemic heart disease this is sometimes because of a tachycardia brought on by dreaming, and with non-cardiac TrP pain, it is due to the adoption of some posture that puts the muscles on the stretch.

The finding of TrPs on clinical examination is clearly only of limited value as it does not help to distinguish between cardiac pain with superimposed TrP pain and primary myofascial TrP pain.

The response to a therapeutic trial of sublingual glyceryl trinitrate may also be misleading since the placebo effect of this ensures that up to 30% of patients with chest pain from any cause may be improved.

Electrocardiography, too, has its limitations, as it is not uncommon for a patient with widespread coronary heart disease to have a normal tracing. Conversely, any abnormal changes seen may only be a reflection of what has happened in the past and have no relevance to the pain under investigation. An ECG taken after exercise testing may also occasionally be misleading.

It therefore follows that there are times when in order to distinguish between coronary artery disease pain and a non-cardiac chest wall pain such as that which emanates from primarily activated TrPs either a coronary arteriogram, or assessment of left-ventricular function by the more recently introduced technique of radionuclide technetium angiography performed at rest and during exercise (Borer et al 1977, Petch 1986) may be necessary.

## THE USE OF TRADITIONAL CHINESE AND TrP ACUPUNCTURE IN THE TREATMENT OF CORONARY HEART DISEASE

### Angina

The use of traditional Chinese acupuncture for the treatment of angina has, over the years, been extensively investigated by Ballegaard and his co-workers (Ballegaard 1998). Nevertheless, in view of the various highly effective anti-anginal agents now available, the place for this in its routine management must be strictly limited.

If, however, superimposed upon episodes of anginal pain, a more persistent type of pain develops with tenderness of the chest wall, then TrPs should be sought and, if found, should be deactivated by means of the carrying out of superficial dry needling at these TrP sites.

### Myocardial infarction

The pain of myocardial infarction, although severe, is generally of relatively limited duration and usually satisfactorily controlled by analgesics. However, at times, in spite of a patient's general condition improving, the pain persists for an unusually long time. One reason for this is the secondary development of TrP activity in the muscles of the chest wall (Rinzler & Travell 1948, Kennard & Haugen 1955). And when this is so, it may readily be alleviated by means of dry needle stimulation of nerve endings in the tissues immediately overlying these points.

### Coronary by-pass surgery

When chest pain recurs soon after a coronary by-pass operation, there is an instinctive tendency, particularly on the part of the patient, to assume it must be anginal and that the operation has been a failure. It has to be remembered, however, that trauma to the chest wall muscles whenever a thoracotomy is performed for any purpose is very liable to activate TrPs in these muscles and for this to be the cause of the pain. In such circumstances, therefore, a search for TrPs should always be made and, if found, deactivated by the carrying out of superficial dry needling.

## ANTERIOR CHEST WALL MTrP PAIN SYNDROME AND OTHER MUSCULOSKELETAL PAIN DISORDERS – THE DIFFERENTIAL DIAGNOSIS

There are several anterior chest wall musculoskeletal disorders which, because of the distribution of their pain and the presence of focal areas of exquisite tenderness, have to be distinguished from the MTrP pain syndrome (Baldry 1997, 2001).

These include, amongst others, pathological fractures of the ribs, costochondritis, Tietze's disease and fibromyalgia.

### Pathological rib fractures

Multiple pathological fractures of the ribs with focal areas of pain and tenderness may be due to metastases from carcinoma of the breast, kidney, lung, prostate or thyroid; also to osteomalachia, osteoporosis or Pagets disease of bone.

### Costochondritis (syns: costosternal chondrodynia, costosternal syndrome, chest wall syndrome)

The pathogenesis of this disorder is uncertain but possibly trauma is a contributory factor. With it a number of costal cartilages, usually the second to the fifth become painful and extremely tender. The pain may remain localized, but frequently it radiates across the chest towards the shoulder, down the arm and, in some cases, up into the neck (Bonica & Sola 1990). On either side of the chest, therefore, its pain referral pattern may simulate pain from anterior chest wall TrPs, and on the left side that of coronary heart disease. Furthermore, at times it may develop in conjunction with this latter disorder (Wolf & Stern 1976, Epstein et al 1979).

### Tietze's syndrome

This much rarer syndrome, first described by the German physician Tietze in 1921, is one where, unlike with costochondritis, the pain is confined to one or more of the upper four costal cartilages. It also differs from that disorder in so much that the affected cartilages are not only tender but swollen (Kayser 1956).

With both costochondritis and Tietze's syndrome, pecking the costal cartilage with a dry needle often provides temporary pain relief and the advantage of it over the alternative of injecting a corticosteroid is that it can be repeated as often as is found to be necessary.

## Fibromyalgia

Patients with fibromyalgia are liable to have tender points at their second costochondal junctions. This rarely causes any diagnostic difficulty as there are usually, in addition to pain in many regions of the body, various other characteristic manifestations of this disorder. However, as discussed in Chapter 10, very occasionally the pain at an early stage of this disease may be confined to the chest wall (Pellegrino 1990).

## THE DEVELOPMENT OF MTrP PAIN IN ASSOCIATION WITH MITRAL VALVE PROLAPSE

When Maresca et al (1989) examined 30 patients with mitral valve prolapse, they found that 30 of them had TrPs in muscles of the chest wall and that 12 of them had pain emanating from these points. The reason for TrP activity developing in this disorder is not known.

## POSTERIOR CHEST WALL MYOFASCIAL TrP ACTIVITY

TrP activity in certain muscles of the posterior chest wall such as the supraspinatus and infraspinatus cause pain to be referred mainly to the shoulder region and down the arm. These muscles will, therefore, be discussed in Chapter 13. And TrP activity in others, such as the levator scapulae, trapezius, and rhomboids causes pain to be felt predominantly in the neck, shoulder girdle and down the arm; a detailed account of these muscles will, therefore, be given in Chapter 14.

The two muscles in the posterior part of the chest in which TrP activity causes pain to be felt in the upper part of the back itself as well as down the arm are the serratus posterior superior and the latissimus dorsi. It is to these two muscles, therefore, that attention will now be directed.

## Serratus posterior superior

### Activation of TrPs

Primary activation of TrPs in this muscle may occur as a result of protracted bouts of coughing. This may also happen when the scapula is pressed hard against it by the shoulders being persistently elevated and rotated forwards such as may occur when sitting for long periods at a desk or working surface that is too high. Also, satellite TrPs may develop in this muscle when TrP activity in the scalene muscles causes pain to be referred to the posterior chest wall around the inner part of the scapula (Fig. 12.2).

### Specific pattern of pain referral

This thin quadrilateral muscle, situated beneath the trapezius and the rhomboids, and attached medially to the spines of the 7th cervical vertebra and the first three dorsal vertebrae, and inferolaterally by four fleshy digitations to the 2nd, 3rd, 4th and 5th ribs near to their angles behind the upper part of the scapula, is liable to develop TrP activity at various sites near to this inferolateral insertion (Fig. 12.12). When this occurs, pain is felt as a dull

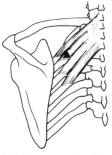

**Figure 12.12** With the arm to the side, a trigger point in the inferolateral part of the serratus posterior superior cannot be palpated as it lies behind the upper inner part of the scapula. To palpate a trigger point at this site, therefore, the scapula has to be pulled forwards as shown.

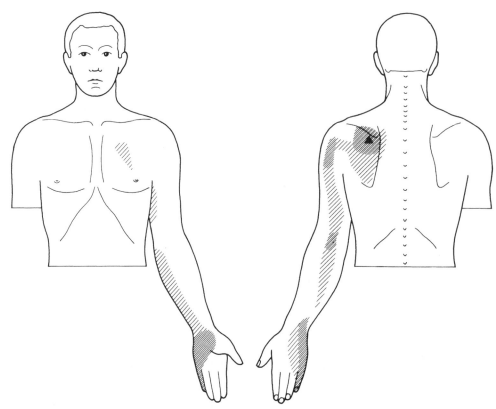

**Figure 12.13** The pattern of pain referral from a trigger point or points (▲) in the serratus posterior superior muscle.

ache around the insertion of the muscle into the ribs behind the scapula. From there it radiates to the back of the shoulder and down the back of the arm to be felt particularly around the medial epicondyle. Occasionally, it is felt down the inner side of the forearm and hand as far as the little finger (Fig. 12.13). This pain pattern is similar to that produced by compression of the 8th cervical nerve root (Reynolds 1981). It is distinguished from this by there being no objective neurological signs and by pressure on these TrPs reproducing the characteristic pain pattern.

### TrP examination

The patient sits forwards with the arm stretched across the front of the chest in order to bring the scapula out of the way so that the muscle can be palpated where it lies behind the upper part of this bone deep to the trapezius and rhomboid muscles. The muscle is then examined by rolling a finger over it against an underlying rib. Associated TrPs may also be found in the rhomboids and in some of the nearby paraspinal muscles.

### Associated TrPs

TrPs in this muscle are often associated with TrP activity in the synergistic inspiratory scalene muscles in the neck, the nearby erector spinae muscles, and overlying rhomboids.

### Deactivation of TrPs

With the patient lying on the opposite side and with the scapula brought well forwards, a needle is inserted at an angle of 45° into the tissues overlying the TrP whilst fixing this between two fingers over a rib. Care must be taken not to insert the needle perpendicularly into an intercostal space as this may result in the pleura being penetrated.

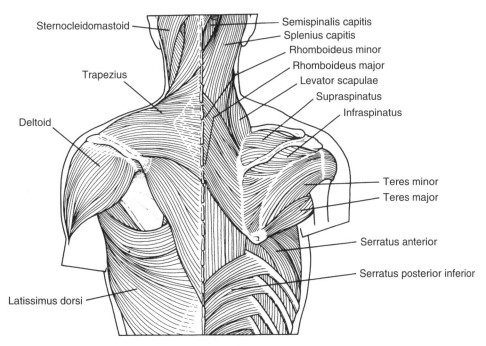

Sternocleidomastoid

Trapezius

Deltoid

Latissimus dorsi

Semispinalis capitis
Splenius capitis
Rhomboideus minor
Rhomboideus major
Levator scapulae
Supraspinatus
Infraspinatus

Teres minor
Teres major

Serratus anterior

Serratus posterior inferior

**Figure 12.14**  Superficial muscles of the back of the neck and upper part of the trunk. On the left, the skin, superficial and deep fasciae have been removed. On the right, the sternocleidomastoid, trapezius, latissimus dorsi and deltoid have been dissected away.

## Latissimus dorsi muscle

Latissimus dorsi, which translated from the Latin means 'widest of the back', is an appropriate name for this muscle with its extensive fan-shaped attachment to the trunk that stretches from the spinous processes of the lower six thoracic, and all the lumbar vertebrae and sacrum in the midline to the crest of the ilium and to the last four ribs. And which then sweeps upwards into the axilla to form with the teres major muscle the posterior axillary fold prior to the tendons of these two muscles then joining together to be inserted into the bicipital groove of the humerus (Fig. 12.14). For some reason, despite this muscle covering such a large area of the back, TrPs usually only become activated in the part of it that is situated in the posterior axillary fold.

### Activation of TrPs

These TrPs in the posterior axillary fold become activated when the upper part of the muscle at its insertion into the humerus is subjected to strain.

Examples of when this may occur include reaching forwards and upwards with the arm whilst carrying some heavy object; stretching the arm such as when hanging on to a rope; or straining the arm whilst engaging in some unusually heavy task such as digging or weeding.

### Specific pattern of pain referral

From TrPs in the posterior axillary fold, pain of a dull aching type is referred to the inferior angle of the scapula and the part of the back immediately around this; it may also extend to the posterior aspect of the shoulder, and down the inner side of the arm, forearm and hand, to terminate in the ring and little fingers (Fig. 12.15).

The pain is persistent and is neither aggravated nor relieved by any type of movements. It is because of this lack of relationship to movements and because the TrPs responsible for it are tucked away in the posterior axillary fold that probably accounts for its myofascial origin being both easily and commonly overlooked.

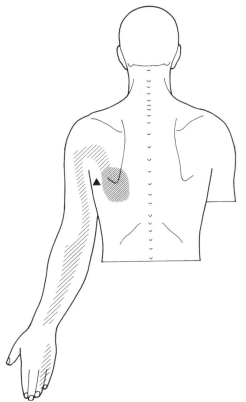

**Figure 12.15** The pattern of pain referral from a trigger point or points (▲) in the latissimus dorsi muscle where this muscle together with the teres major muscle forms the posterior axillary fold.

## TrP examination

TrPs in this muscle are most readily found by placing the patient in the supine position and putting it on the stretch by means of abducting the arm and placing the hand behind the head.

Both the superficial and deep parts of the muscle in the posterior axillary fold should be examined, because when Simons & Travell (1976) inserted 7.5% saline into the muscle at this site, an injection into the deep fibres referred pain to the back around the lower part of the scapula, whilst an injection into the superficial ones referred pain down the arm.

## Associated TrPs

TrP activity is likely to develop at the same time in the anatomically closely related teres major and the long head of the triceps.

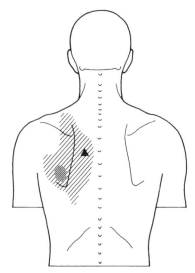

**Figure 12.16** The pattern of pain referral from a trigger point (▲) in the iliocostalis thoracis muscle.

## Deactivation of TrPs

Once a TrP is located it is held between the thumb and fingers whilst a needle is inserted into the tissues overlying it. As TrPs in this muscle tend to be grouped together, both in its superficial and deep parts, this procedure may have to be repeated several times.

## Paraspinal muscles

Myofascial pain in the posterior chest wall may also arise from TrP activity in superficial paraspinal muscles (erector spinae) such as the iliocostalis thoracis and in deep paraspinal muscles such as the multifidius.

The pain from TrP activity in the iliocostalis thoracis muscle at the mid-thoracic level is concentrated around the inferior angle of the scapula, but it also spreads upwards and downwards (Fig. 12.16).

The pain that emanates from a TrP in the multifidus at the mid-thoracic level remains localized around it deep in the paravertebral region (Fig. 12.17).

## Rectus abdominis muscle

Myofascial pain in the lower part of the posterior chest wall may, at times, be referred there from

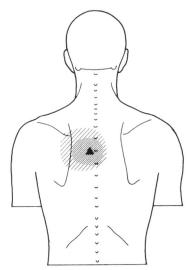

**Figure 12.17** The pattern of pain referral from a trigger point (▲) situated deep in the paravertebral gutter in the multifidus muscle at the mid-thoracic level.

TrPs in the upper part of the rectus abdominis at the site where the muscle becomes inserted into the rib cage at the junction of the costal margin and xiphisternum (Fig. 20.3).

## INTERCOSTAL PAIN

Pain that radiaties from the back to the front of the chest in a direction parallel with the ribs and from the lower part of the chest to the anterior abdominal wall may be due to a vertebral disorder causing irritation of an intercostal nerve root. In all such cases, therefore, radiographs of the dorsal spine are mandatory. It should be remembered, however, that in the early stages of metastatic involvement of vertebrae, the radiographic appearances may remain normal.

The possibility that the pain is the precursor of a herpes zoster rash also has to be considered.

Alternatively, and what for long has been known, but somehow lost sight of, is that pain in this distribution may be due to the development of TrP activity in an intercostal muscle. Kellgren in 1938 produced it experimentally by injecting hypertonic saline into intercostal muscles. And Kelly in 1944 reported that pain around the chest in several

patients under his care emanated from foci of exquisite tenderness in these particular muscles.

The following case illustrates how TrP activity in an intercostal muscle may be overlooked unless specifically looked for.

A farmer (36 years of age) developed severe pain radiating from the back to the front of the right side of the chest in the 5th intercostal space. When after 2 years he continued to complain of this in spite of having been given analgesics for most of this time, his general practitioner referred him to a pain clinic in order to exclude the possibility of nerve root entrapment. There were no objective neurological signs; also, chest and spine X-rays were normal. In spite of this an intercostal nerve block was carried out but with no significant improvement. When subsequently he was seen by me there were two foci of exquisite tenderness to be found, one in the multifidus muscle at the level of the 5th thoracic vertebra, and one in an intercostal muscle in the posterior axillary line. Deactivation of these two TrPs by dry needle stimulation resulted in temporary relief for a few days and after repeating this on two subsequent occasions at weekly intervals permanent relief was obtained.

## POST-THORACOTOMY PAIN

Pain around the chest that develops following a thoracotomy may be due to the development of trauma-evoked TrP activity either in the surgical scar itself or in the muscles of the chest wall. Alternatively, it may develop as a result of the division of an intercostal nerve.

## THORACOTOMY SCAR PAIN

It is not uncommon for persistent pain to develop in and around a thoracotomy scar. One and an often overlooked reason for this happening is the development of TrP activity in the scar tissue.

It often requires deactivation of these TrPs by means of needles inserted into the tissues immediately lateral to the scar (see Ch. 10) to be repeated several times before such pain is brought under control as shown by the following case.

A man (56 years of age), discovered to have an opacity in the right lung on a routine chest radiograph, was submitted to a thoracotomy. Histological examination of the lesion proved it to be benign. One month later he began to complain of pain along the scar. He was reassured that there was no evidence of a stitch abscess but was offered no specific treatment. The pain persisted and eventually he was given Distalgesic to take as and when required. In spite of this, the pain gradually became worse and by the time he was referred to me 12 months later, in addition to the chest pain, he was getting severe attacks of cramp-like pain in the upper part of the anterior abdominal wall.

On examination, four TrPs were found in the scar. It required deactivation of these to be carried out on six occasions at weekly intervals before any lasting pain relief was obtained.

## SECTION OF AN INTERCOSTAL NERVE

Persistent post-thoracotomy pain may also occur as a result of the division of an intercostal nerve. This is often associated with a severe burning and marked hyperaesthesia of the chest wall. This does not, in my experience, respond to acupuncture. Transcutaneous electrical nerve stimulation (TENS), however, is sometimes helpful.

# References

Allison D R 1950 Pain in the chest wall simulating heart disease. British Medical Journal 1: 332–336

Baldry P E 1997 Cardiac and non-cardiac chest wall pain. Acupuncture in Medicine 15(2): 83–90

Baldry P E 2001 The chest wall. In: Myofascial pain and fibromyalgia syndromes, Ch. 14. Churchill Livingstone, Edinburgh

Ballegaard S 1998 Acupuncture and the cardiovascular system: a scientific challenge. Acupuncture in Medicine 16(1): 2–9

Bonica J J, Sola A 1990 Anterior chest wall syndrome. In: Bonica J J (ed) The management of pain, Vol. 2, 2nd edn. Lea & Febiger, Philadelphia, pp. 1126–1128

Borer J S, Bacharach S L, Greer M V, Kent K M, Epstein S E, Johnston G S 1977 Real-time radionuclide cineangiography in non-invasive evaluation of global and regional left ventricular function at rest and during exercise in patients with coronary artery disease. New England Journal of Medicine 286: 839–844

Dressler W 1959 Flare-up of pericarditis complicating myocardial infarction after two years of steroid therapy. American Heart Journal 57: 501

Edeiken J, Wolferth C 1936 Persistent pain in the shoulder region following myocardial infarction. American Journal of Medical Science 191: 201–210

Epstein S E, Gerber L H, Borer J S 1979 Chest wall syndrome: a common cause of unexplained cardiac pain. Journal of the American Medical Association 241: 2793–2797

Gutstein M 1938 Diagnosis and treatment of muscular rheumatism. British Journal of Physical Medicine 1: 302–321

Kayser H L 1956 Tietze's syndrome. A review of the literature. American Journal of Medicine 21: 982–989

Kellgren J H 1938 A preliminary account of referred pain arising from muscle. British Medical Journal 1: 325–327

Kelly M 1944 Pain in the chest: Observations on the use of local anaesthesia in its investigation and treatment. Medical Journal of Australia 1: 4–7

Kennard M A, Haugen F 1955 The relation of subcutaneous focal sensitivity to referred pain of cardiac origin. Anaesthesiology 16: 297–311

Maresca M, Galanti G, Castellani S, Procacci P 1989 Pain in mitral valve prolapse. Pain 36: 89–92

Mendlowitz M 1945 Strain of the pectoralis minor, an important cause of praecordial pain in soldiers. American Heart Journal 30: 123–125

Ochsner A, Gage M, Debakey M 1935 Scalenus anticus (Naffziger) syndrome. American Journal of Surgery 28: 669–695

Pellegrino M J 1990 Atypical chest pain as an initial presentation of primary fibromyalgia. Archives of Physical Medicine and Rehabilitation 71(7): 526–528

Petch M C 1986 Investigation of coronary artery disease. Journal of the Royal College of Physicians of London 20(1): 21–24

Reynolds M 1981 Myofascial trigger point syndromes in the practice of rheumatology. Archives of Physical Medicine and Rehabilitation 62: 111–114

Rinzler S, Travell J 1948 Therapy directed at the somatic component of cardiac pain. American Heart Journal 35: 248–268

Simons D G, Travell J 1976 The latissimus dorsi syndrome. A source of mid-back pain. Archives of Physical Medicine and Rehabilitation 57: 561

Steindler A 1940 The interpretation of sciatic radiation and the syndrome of low-back pain. Journal of the American Medical Association 110: 106–113

Steindler A, Luck J V 1938 Differential diagnosis of pain low in the back. Journal of the American Medical Association 110: 106–113

Travell J 1968 Office hours: day and night. World Publishing Company, New York

Travell J 1976 Myofascial trigger points: clinical view. In: Bonica J J, Albe-Fessard D (eds) Advances in pain research and therapy, Vol. 1. Raven Press, New York

Travell J, Rinzler S 1948 Pain syndromes of the chest muscles. Resemblance to effort angina and myocardial infarction, and relief by local block. Canadian Medical Association Journal 59: 333–338

Travell J, Rinzler S, Herman M 1942 Pain and disability of the shoulder and arm: treatment by intramuscular infiltration with procaine hydrochloride. Journal of the American Medical Association 120: 417–422

Travell J, Simons D 1983 Pectoralis major muscle (subclavius muscle) in myofascial pain and dysfunction. The trigger point manual. Williams & Wilkins, Baltimore, p. 577

Wolf E, Stern S 1976 Costosternal syndrome. Its frequency and importance in differential diagnosis of coronary heart disease. Archives of Internal Medicine 136: 189–191

# Chapter 13

# The painful shoulder

## CHAPTER CONTENTS

## INTRODUCTION

When presented with a case of persistent pain in the shoulder region, rheumatoid arthritis, other inflammatory arthritides, crystal arthropathy and haemarthrosis of the glenohumeral joint, osteo-arthritis of the acromioclavicular joint and, occasionally, of the glenohumeral joint, and diseases of the bone all have to be included in the differential diagnosis. Far more often, however, such pain occurs either as a result of a soft-tissue disorder in the vicinity of the glenohumeral joint, or because it is referred to the shoulder region from trigger points (TrPs) in nearby muscles.

The purpose of this chapter is to discuss the clinical manifestations and treatment of these latter more commonly occuring causes of shoulder pain.

## SOFT-TISSUE DISORDERS

The soft-tissue disorders in and around the glenohumeral joint that will be considered are rotator cuff tendinitis, subacromial bursitis, bicipital tendinitis and capsulitis.

### Rotator cuff tendinitis

#### The rotator cuff

The musculotendinous cuff muscles, the supraspinatus, the infraspinatus, the teres minor, and the subscapularis have a conjoined tendinous insertion into the humerus. The supraspinatus tendon is attached to the laterally placed greater tuberosity; the infraspinatus and teres minor tendons are attached immediately below this, and the sub-scapularis tendon is attached to the medially placed lesser tuberosity. As a result of their attachments to the humerus these tendons act as rotators of the joint and in addition, by combining with the del-toid muscle, abduct the arm.

Inflammation is liable to develop in any of these rotator cuff muscles' tendons but the supraspinatus tendon is the one that is most commonly affected.

### Pathogenesis

In young adults this disorder is liable to develop suddenly when oedematous and haemorrhagic changes take place in these tendons as a result of the sudden overloading of the cuff muscles with the arm in the elevated position such as, for example, when throwing a cricket ball.

In older people the disorder develops more insidiously with slowly progressive degenerative and ischaemic changes eventually causing the cuff to become so weakened that the acromion, cos-toacromial ligament and acromioclavicular joint impinge on it (Matsen et al 1990). This impinge-ment is liable to be made worse should degenera-tive changes take place in the acromion and humeral head. Eventually, attrition of the cuff may cause it to rupture.

### Symptoms and signs

With tendinitis affecting any part of the cuff, there is a nagging ache at rest and an increase in the pain on the carrying out of certain movements. The ones affected depend on which tendon or tendons in particular are involved. In addition, sudden severe pain may develop should the cuff become torn.

With supraspinatus tendinitis, active abduction of the arm is painful through the intermediate range (60–120°). The painful arc is probably due to the inflamed tendon rubbing against the acromion because it is abolished by externally rotating the arm, thus placing the greater tuberosity behind the acromion, before carrying out abduction. The pain is also aggravated by resisted abduction. Tenderness is maximal over the tendon where it blends with the anterior part of the capsule of the shoulder joint.

The clinical presentation with infraspinatus and teres minor tendinitis is similar. In both conditions

the pain is also localized around the greater tuberosity, but it is resisted external rotation that makes it worse. Pain from subscapularis tendinitis is experienced over the lesser tuberosity and is aggravated by resisted medial rotation.

### Natural history of the disorder

When attempting to assess the effectiveness of any form of treatment, including acupuncture, in relieving the pain of this disorder, it is important to realize that its natural history is usually that of a mild ache at rest and pain brought on by certain movements which persists for weeks or months and then eventually undergoes spontaneous reso-lution. On occasions, however, the pain may sud-denly become more intense due to the development of an acute inflammatory reaction in the tendon and the tissues adjacent to it, including those in the wall of the subacromial bursa. Calcium is liable to become deposited in a degenerative ten-don and when, in the case of the supraspinatus tendon, this suddenly bursts into the subacromial bursa, there is very severe pain and marked restric-tion of movements, with abduction and external rotation in particular aggravating the pain.

## Subacromial bursitis

Subacromial (subdeltoid) bursitis used to be included amongst the primary causes of shoulder pain, but it is now generally recognized that inflam-matory changes in the bursa do not occur as a primary event but are always secondary to an inflammatory lesion in an adjacent tendon. As Cailliet (1981) says, 'any adjacent inflammation of the tendon causes inflammation of the bursa. It is inconceivable that bursitis could exist without ten-dinitis and vice versa'.

### Cuff tears

It is generally agreed that cuff tears are far com-moner than previously supposed. It is now recog-nized that it only requires some minor injury to cause partial or complete tear of a tendon that has already been weakened by degenerative changes. The patient who is often in the 40–70 age range experiences a tearing sensation in the shoulder followed immediately by severe pain that often increases in intensity until it reaches a peak about 2 days later. It then remains very acutely painful for a further 4–7 days. On examination there is usually exquisite tenderness on palpation over the greater tuberosity. There is marked aggravation of pain on resisted abduction, and most significant of all, once the patient has raised the arm, there is an inability to control the lowering of it to the side. This, however, does not occur exclusively with a rotator cuff tear but may also be observed with a 5th cervical nerve root lesion.

It is essential to confirm the diagnosis and assess the extent of a tear by contrast radiography. Minor tears usually heal spontaneously within 2 months and require only symptomatic treatment. Extensive tears may need to be repaired surgically.

## Bicipital tendinitis

The tendon of the long head of the biceps, attached above to the superior rim of the glenoid fossa, passes downwards enclosed in a sheath of synovium through the glenohumeral joint to emerge from it through an opening in the capsule close to the latter's humeral attachment. The tendon then descends in the bicipital groove situated between the greater and lesser tuberosities (Fig. 12.9). This structure is liable to develop a degenerative tendinitis that clinically presents with pain and tenderness to pressure over the bicipital groove. Moreover, the pain is characteristically aggravated by attempting to supinate the arm against resistance.

### Acromioclavicular joint strain

When the acromioclavicular joint becomes mechanically strained, the pain that develops is limited to the tip of the shoulder and aggravated by full passive adduction of the arm across the chest.

## Treatment of a tendinitis in the glenohumeral joint region

The principal object of treatment both for acute and chronic tendinitis in the vicinity of the glenohumeral joint is to symptomatically relieve pain and to ensure that full movements of the joint are restored as quickly as possible, for the longer they remain

restricted, the more likely it is that a disabling capsulitis or so-called frozen shoulder may develop.

### Anti-inflammatory drug therapy

A widely adopted regime (Barry & Jenner 1996, Dalton 1995) is firstly to employ an orally administered non-steroidal anti-inflammatory drug. And then, if necessary, to inject a corticosteroid/local anaesthetic mixture into the subacromial bursa. Such treatment may have to be repeated at intervals. Therefore, rather than using a long-acting steroid such as methylprednisolone, which is liable to cause tissue atrophy, it is better to employ shorter acting hydrocortisone acetate (Hazleman 1990).

Unfortunately, a steroid injection not infrequently gives rise to appreciable post-treatment pain. In addition, repeated injections are liable to damage the soft tissues and when injected into a joint may destroy it (Bentley & Goodfellow 1969). Repeated injections may also have systemic effects; Koehler et al (1974) have shown that the hypothalamic/pituitary/adrenal axis is affected 48 hours after an injection of 80 mg of methyl prednisolone acetate into a knee with plasma cortisol levels being suppressed for 3–6 days. In addition, there is always the small but definite risk of infection developing at the site of a steroid injection.

### TrP acupuncture

The examination of a patient with rotator cuff tendinitis should include a search for TrPs in both the vicinity of the cuff itself and in the muscles of the neck, shoulder girdle, upper arm and anterior chest wall, as deactivation of these by means of the carrying out of superficial dry needling at regular intervals is often sufficient by itself to alleviate the pain.

## Capsulitis (frozen shoulder)

Frozen shoulder is one of the great enigmas of medicine with there being no general agreement as to its nature, diagnosis or treatment, and with the situation still further confounded by a confusing terminology.

Duplay (1896) first termed the condition periarthrite scapulohumerale. It has also been known as periarthritis and pericapsulitis. Then in 1945 Neviaser coined the term adhesive capsulitis because of appearances he found at operation on 10 cases. These included thickening and contraction of the capsule; also adhesions between opposed synovial surfaces were observed, particularly in the inferior part of the joint. It was not, however, because adhesions were a striking feature that he described the capsulitis as being adhesive, but rather because he noted that during manipulation of the shoulder after an incision through the anterior capsule, the capsule separated from the head of the humerus in the same manner as adhesive strapping peels from the skin.

There is undoubtedly a widespread acute inflammatory reaction involving the capsule and the rotator cuff, with the latter being reported at operation to be extremely friable (Bunker 1985). It is not surprising, therefore, that radioisotope scans show gleaming hot spots in the shoulder region (Binder et al 1984).

## Pathogenesis

The disorder is liable to develop whenever movements at the shoulder joint are restricted. It may, therefore, occur either following some injury to the shoulder including repeated episodes of minor trauma (Wright & Haq 1976), or as a complication of a tendinitis, or when the arm remains immobile for some appreciable period of time such as with a hemiplegia.

It is particularly liable to develop in patients with diabetes mellitus and when it does so is often present bilaterally (Satter & Luqman 1985). Why it is prone to develop as a complication of this disorder is not known. Possible reasons suggested include the predilection of diabetics to infection or because of the development of a vasculitis (Nash & Hazleman 1989). Patients with hyper and hypothyroidism are also susceptible to developing it (Bowman 1988, Wolgethan 1987).

## Clinical diagnosis

Capsulitis is a condition in which there is considerable pain and stiffness around the shoulder with marked restriction of all glenohumeral joint movements, both passive and active. External rotation is more severely affected than abduction or internal rotation. An important characteristic of the pain is that it is particularly liable to disturb sleep.

It was because of this marked restriction of all movements that Codman (1934) introduced the term 'frozen shoulder', and, although that has since had much popular appeal, as Bunker (1985) pointed out, the acute inflammatory nature of the condition makes it somewhat of a misnomer.

The clinical diagnosis may be confirmed by arthrography, which shows a marked reduction in the volume of the glenohumeral joint so that it only accommodates a few millilitres of contrast medium instead of the normal 10–15 ml (Bruckner 1982).

## Natural history of the disorder

It is important when considering the influence of various forms of treatment on this disorder, including the possible place of acupuncture in its management, to have a clear knowledge of its natural history for, as Lloyd-Roberts & French (1959) when writing about this said:

> A knowledge of the average time between onset and recovery is of outstanding importance if the effects of treatment are to be assessed in a disease which usually resolves spontaneously.

The pain usually remains severe for about 3 months, after which it begins to abate, but the restriction of movements continues for much longer. The condition is usually eventually self-limiting, burning itself out within 2 years in the absence of any treatment (Grey 1977). A minority of cases, however, have some permanent disability.

## Treatment

A variety of different treatments have been advocated, including local steroids, oral steroids, ultrasound, radiotherapy and sympathetic ganglion block, but the reports concerning these have been confusingly inconclusive and conflicting, and as the condition is a naturally resolving one, only those studies that have included controls will be considered.

Lloyd-Roberts & French (1959), in studying a series of patients suffering from what they termed periarthritis or capsulitis of the shoulder, treated one group with an intra-articular injection of hydrocortisone combined with forcible manipulation under anaesthesia followed by active supervised movements; and another group with oral cortisone for 1 month plus active supervised movements. They concluded that the group treated with manipulation and local hydrocortisone did better than the group treated with oral cortisone.

Kessel et al (1981) from a carefully controlled trial concluded that manipulation in combination with systemic steroids is of value. As Bruckner (1982) has pointed out, however, manipulation together with steroids is generally reserved for those patients who have made no improvement 9–12 months from the onset, and, therefore, after the acute phase of the disease is over. As he says 'it would be very helpful if a simple treatment could be shown to cut short this common and often extremely painful condition'.

The administration of corticosteroids, either locally or systemically, has been popular in the treatment of frozen shoulder ever since they first became available for therapeutic use. Cyriax & Troisier (1953), in treating what they termed 'freezing arthritis', recommended giving an intra-articular injection of hydrocortisone, but the results of this were poor. Subsequently, Cyriax (1980) advocated the use of multiple intra-articular injections of hydrocortisone at weekly or biweekly intervals. The dangers inherent in this, however, have already been alluded to when discussing the management of tendinitis.

Lee et al (1974) compared the effects of three forms of treatment (heat plus exercises; intra-articular hydrocortisone plus exercises; hydrocortisone around the biceps tendon plus exercises) with the effect of treatment with analgesics alone. All three groups in which exercise was used obtained a significantly improved range of movements to a similar degree. The analgesic group's response was not as good.

Richardson (1975) showed no difference in relief of pain in one group treated with steroid injections and in another treated with a placebo. And finally, Bulgen et al (1984) have shown that there is no long-term advantage of steroid injection over mobilization, ice, or no treatment in the management of the frozen shoulder.

It is in the light of these conflicting reports that Bruckner (1982) concludes that in the majority of cases, reassuring the patient that it is a self-limiting condition, advising the use of simple 'pendulum' mobilizing exercises, and, in the early stages of the condition, controlling the pain by some simple means, is as much as can be hoped for.

Acupuncture also has a place in alleviating the pain present at the early stage of this disorder. Camp (1986), one of the few British rheumatologists with experience in the use of it, has found this form of therapy to be certainly as helpful as corticosteroid injections in the treatment of the frozen shoulder. She advocates 'acupuncture as the treatment of choice in preference to the very painful cortico-steroid injections and the largely useless physiotherapy', but makes it clear that, in her opinion, acupuncture, like local steroids, is only of symptomatic benefit and does not alter the natural history of the condition.

There is no doubt, as Bruckner (1982) has said in discussing the shortcomings of numerous reports on the treatment of the 'frozen shoulder', that 'it is essential to design prospective trials that will give definite answers, by carefully defining the condition under study (excluding shoulder pain without passive limitation of movement), treating patients only in the acute stage (first 6 months) and including a proper control group'. It would also seem reasonable, in view of Camp's observations, to include in any such trial one group treated with acupuncture. Firstly, however, it is necessary to establish which particular acupuncture technique is most suitable for the alleviation of this type of pain. My reason for saying this is because, in my experience, the pain of frozen shoulder can be aggravated by carrying out superficial dry needling at TrP sites too vigorously. Gentle brief stimulation of nerve endings in the tissues overlying these points is often all that is necessary. This is similar to what Camp (1986) has found, as she states: 'sometimes attempts at needling trigger points simply produces more pain and a violent reaction to acupuncture. Moving the needle away from the trigger points and treating more peripheral points, results almost in complete loss of symptoms in these cases'.

The matter, however, is far from straightforwards for undoubtedly there are some patients who only respond to strong stimulation and it is for this reason that Mann (1974) has found that on occasions patients with a persistently painful shoulder require the powerful stimulus provided by 'pecking' the periosteum over the coracoid process.

There is no doubt, as stressed throughout this book, that patients' individual responsiveness to needle-evoked nerve stimulation varies widely and it is essential to take account of this, not only in everyday clinical practice, but also when drawing up clinical trial protocols.

## Secondary activation of myofascial TrPs in tendinitis and capsulitis

It is common for the persistent pain and restricted movements associated with tendinitis and, in particular, with capsulitis to lead to the secondary activation of TrPs in muscles in the anterior and posterior axillary folds, the upper arm, the shoulder girdle and neck.

## REFERRAL OF PAIN TO THE SHOULDER REGION

Pain in the shoulder region may occur in the absence of any lesion in or around the glenohumeral joint and be due to it being referred there, either because of nerve root entrapment, or because of the primary activation of TrPs in muscles in the neck and shoulder girdle, or because of a lesion around the diaphragm irritating the phrenic nerve.

### Nerve root entrapment pain referral

Pain in the shoulder and upper extremity can occur as a result of pressure on a cervical nerve root such as may occur with cervical disc herniation or cervical spondylosis. For reasons to be given in Chapter 14, there are grounds for believing that these disorders are not responsible for this as often as is commonly supposed. Certainly cervical spondylosis cannot be assumed to be the cause just because the characteristic appearances of this degenerative condition are demonstrable radiographically. The only circumstances in which the diagnosis of a nerve root lesion can be made with any confidence is when there are objective neurological signs and when in particular the electromyogram (EMG) is abnormal.

On clinical examination, movements of the shoulder are free and do not aggravate the pain,

whereas neck movements with, in particular, forced extension and sideways rotation commonly do.

With a C6 nerve root lesion there is usually pain and stiffness in the neck as well as pain in the outer part of the shoulder. Pain may also radiate down the arm to the thumb and first finger. In addition, there is weakness and wasting of the biceps muscle and depression of the biceps jerk.

A C7 nerve root lesion is associated with pain in the upper scapular region and the outer side of the shoulder. It may also radiate down the arm to the middle and index fingers. In addition, there is weakness and wasting of the triceps muscle and depression of the triceps jerk. A C8 nerve root lesion causes pain to be felt in the outer part of the shoulder and mid-scapular regions.

Muscles in the areas affected by radiculopathic pain are often found to contain secondarily activated TrPs and these need to be deactivated by means of the carrying out of superficial dry needling.

### Primary myofascial TrP pain referral

It is well known that pain may be referred to the shoulder region from some disorder around the diaphragm irritating the phrenic nerve. In addition, it may be referred to this site from TrPs that have become primarily activated when muscles in the upper part of the chest wall and neck have become acutely strained or chronically overloaded. For some reason, this is still not generally recognized, in spite of attention having first been drawn to it by Edeiken & Wolferth as long ago as 1936. Also, Kellgren described cases of it 2 years later, and since then it has been the subject of several detailed reports.

These include one by Kelly (1942), which he wrote whilst serving in the Australian Army Medical Corps and another by Travell et al (1942). In addition, Sola et al (1955) and Sola & Kuitert (1955) gave descriptons of it based on observations made by them whilst serving as medical officers in the United States Air Force.

Unfortunately when these reports were first published they were for some reason largely ignored, but in recent years the importance of this particular cause of shoulder pain has once again been stressed, so that, hopefully, it may now begin to receive the recognition it deserves (Baldry

1998, 2001, Bonica & Sola 1990, Simons et al 1999, Sola 1999).

The muscles most frequently involved include the supraspinatus, infraspinatus, levator scapulae, trapezius, deltoid, long head of triceps, latissimus dorsi, teres major, biceps and subscapularis. TrPs in these muscles can only be found by systematically examining each muscle in turn. The search for these, however, is greatly assisted by every muscle having its own specific pattern of TrP pain referral.

## Supraspinatus muscle (see Fig. 12.14)

*Activation of TrPs* TrP activity may develop in the supraspinatus muscle when it is subjected to strain, as for example, by the carrying of a heavy load such as a suitcase with the arm hanging by the side. Alternatively, by pulling a heavy object or lifting it to, or above, the shoulder level with the arm outstretched. In addition, the repeated overloading of the muscle by such means is liable to convert an acute condition into a chronic one.

*Specific pattern of pain referral* TrP activity in this muscle causes pain to be referred to the region of the deltoid muscle. Because of its distribution this pain is often erroneously diagnosed as being due to subdeltoid (subacromial) bursitis, which, as explained earlier, is a condition that rarely, if ever, occurs as a primary event. The pain frequently extends down the arm and forearm and, as Travell & Simons (1983, p. 368) stated, it is often felt particularly strongly over the lateral epicondyle (Fig. 13.1).

*Movements aggravating the pain* This referred pain is usually a dull ache at rest that is made worse by abducting the arm, and by passively stretching the muscle by adducting the arm behind the back.

Some of the commoner types of movements likely to aggravate the pain include reaching upwards either to brush the hair, shave, or clean the teeth.

*TrP examination* The patient should sit comfortably, or lie with the affected side uppermost. As the TrPs have to be palpated through the trapezius

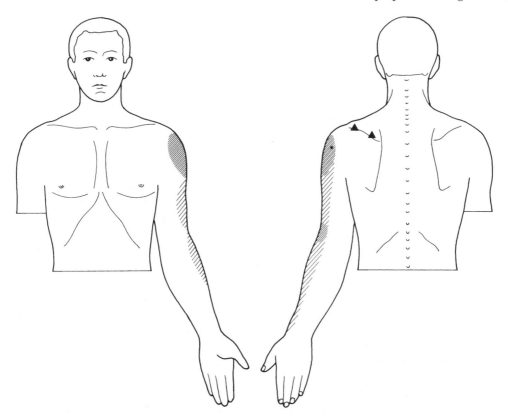

**Figure 13.1** The pattern of pain referral from a trigger point or points (▲) in the supraspinatus muscle.

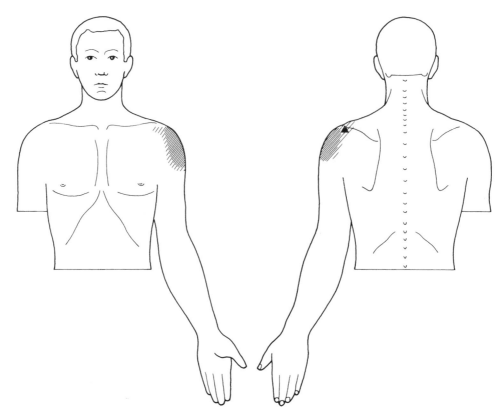

**Figure 13.2**   The pattern of pain referral from a trigger point or points (▲) in the supraspinatus tendon.

muscle they are often found more readily if the muscle is put on the stretch by placing the forearm of the patient behind the back at waist level. Their location is either at the medial or lateral parts of the muscle, or in both places (Fig. 13.1). In addition, there may be one in the tendon of the muscle near to its insertion (Fig. 13.2).

*Associated TrPs*   TrP activity may develop in the supraspinatus muscle alone, but more often it develops in the infraspinatus at the same time, and also quite often in the trapezius, levator scapulae and deltoid muscles.

*Similarity to radiculopathic pain distribution*   Referred pain from supraspinatus TrPs is similar in distribution to that from a C5 nerve root lesion (Reynolds 1981). There is, however, an absence of objective neurological signs, and electromyography shows no abnormality.

*Deactivation of TrPs*   The deactivation of TrPs in this muscle presents no problem despite it lying behind the trapezius muscle.

### Infraspinatus muscle (see Fig. 12.14)

*Activation of TrPs*   This is usually brought about by the muscle being subjected to some sudden strain such as, for instance, when reaching backwards for support when falling; or when it is repeatedly put on the stretch, such as when reaching backwards to pick up objects from the back of a car when sitting in the front of it.

*Specific pattern of pain referral*   Referred pain from TrPs in this muscle is felt deep inside the front of the shoulder joint and for this reason is sometimes erroneously thought to be due to an arthritis of the glenohumeral joint which, as stated earlier, is rare. It may also radiate down the antero-lateral aspect of the arm and forearm to the radial aspect of the hand, sometimes reaching the thumb and first two fingers (Fig. 13.3) (Travell et al 1942, Travell 1952, Sola & Williams 1956, Pace 1975, Rubin 1981).

This particular type of shoulder pain is particularly disturbing at night because it not only prevents

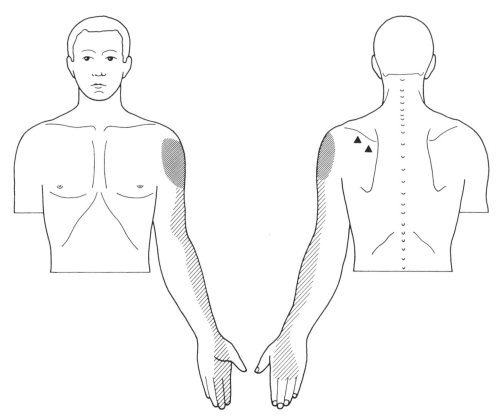

**Figure 13.3**    The pattern of pain referral from a trigger point or points (▲) in the infraspinatus muscle.

the patient from lying on the affected side, but is also troublesome when lying on the unaffected side.

*Characteristic disorder of movements*    There is an inability to internally rotate and adduct the arm at the shoulder. The hand-to-shoulder blade test in which a normal individual's finger tips can reach the spine of the scapula reveals this typical restriction of movement (Fig. 13.4). A sufferer from this has difficulty in doing up buttons, manipulating a zip fastener, or putting a hand into a back trouser pocket.

*TrP examination*    With the patient sitting in a chair, the muscle should be stretched by bringing the hand and arm across the front of the chest to grasp the contralateral arm rest of the chair.

Flat palpation of the infraspinatus fossa should then be carried out systematically. One or more TrPs are usually to be found somewhere along a line immediately beneath the spine of the scapula.

*Differential diagnosis*    Referred pain to the shoulder from TrP activity in the infraspinatus muscle may closely simulate that arising from gleno-humeral joint disease. Also, as it causes pain to radiate down the arm in a similar distribution to that occurring with irritation of the 5th, 6th and 7th cervical nerve roots, a full neurological examination is essential and, at times, an EMG may be necessary to distinguish between them. Confusion is particularly likely to occur in patients who also have neck pain (see Ch. 14).

*Deactivation of TrPs*    This should be done with the patient lying on the opposite side, with the arm resting on a pillow placed against the chest. The needle is inserted into the tissues overlying a TrP whilst fixing the latter between two fingers pressed against the scapula. Care must be taken not to push the needle too hard against the scapula as penetration of the infraspinatus fossa with the production of a pneumothorax has been reported (Travell & Simons 1983, p. 385).

**Teres minor (Fig. 13.4)**    This muscle with its attachments immediately adjacent to and just below

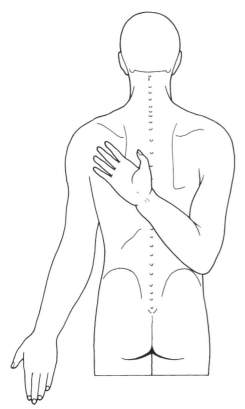

**Figure 13.4**   To illustrate how a normal person, on placing an arm behind the back, is able to reach the spine of the contralateral scapula with the finger tips. With trigger point activity in either the supraspinatus or infraspinatus or both, this is not possible.

those of the infraspinatus, and having actions that are almost identical to the latter, has TrP activity brought about by exactly similar stresses, i.e. stretching and reaching behind the shoulder.

However, unlike the infraspinatus, it is one of the less commonly involved muscles. Sola & Kuitert (1955) found only about 7% of their patients with shoulder pain had TrPs in this muscle.

Teres minor is rarely involved without simultaneous involvement of the infraspinatus, and usually notice is drawn to it by the patient continuing to complain of pain in the posterior part of the shoulder, once pain deep in the front of the shoulder has been satisfactorily alleviated by deactivating TrPs in the infraspinatus.

**Levator scapulae and trapezius muscles**   These muscles are discussed in detail in Chapter 14 as TrP activity in them is mainly responsible for pain

and limitation of movement of the neck. It is, however, also liable to cause pain to be referred to the posterior part of the shoulder (see Figs 14.1 & 16.6).

**Deltoid muscle (see Fig. 12.14)**   The deltoid muscle, so-called because being triangular in shape it resembles the Greek letter Δ (delta), is made up of three parts: the anterior, middle and posterior.

*Activation of TrPs*   This occurs mainly in the anterior and posterior parts of the muscle, either as a secondary or a primary event. It often occurs as a secondary phenomenon, both in the anterior and posterior parts simultaneously, when pain is referred to that area from TrPs in the supraspinatus and infraspinatus muscles. The pain that arises as a result of TrP activity in this muscle remains localized to that area, and is not projected to some distant site.

In the case of primary activity, the clinical picture differs according to whether the anterior or posterior part is involved and so each will be considered separately.

ANTERIOR PART   Primary TrP activity may be brought about by direct trauma to the upper part of the arm such as may occur with a fall, or when it is damaged by the impact of a ball, or the recoil of a gun. Also, when the muscle is subjected to sudden overload such as when grasping a rail to break a fall, or when the muscle is recurrently overloaded such as may occur when some heavy object such as a tool or instrument is repeatedly held at shoulder level.

**Symptoms**   The patient complains of pain at rest over the anterior part of the deltoid muscle (Fig. 13.5). This is made worse by movement, and, in particular, there is difficulty in raising the arm to the horizontal so that drinking becomes troublesome.

**Signs**   Pain is aggravated by asking the patient to abduct the arm with the elbow straight and the palm to the front. The patient also has difficulty in passing the hand across the small of the back. Normally, it is possible to rest the hand on the back of the opposite arm. With anterior deltoid TrP activity, it may only be possible to reach the midline (Fig. 13.6).

**Differential diagnosis**   Pain arising as a result of TrP activity in the deltoid muscle has be distinguished from that arising because of a sprain of

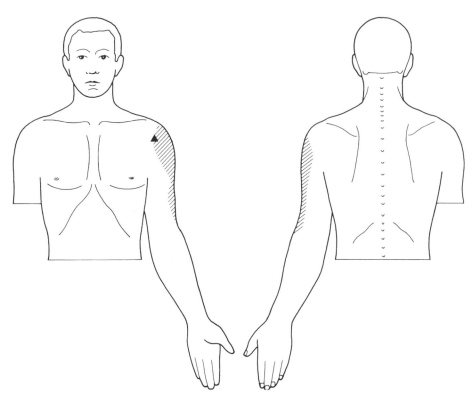

**Figure 13.5** The pattern of pain referral from a trigger point (▲) in the anterior part of the deltoid muscle.

the acromioclavicular joint that lies underneath the proximal attachment of the anterior part of this muscle. This injury, common in rugby players, is characterized by pain and tenderness localized to the shoulder tip and there are of course no TrPs to be found in the deltoid muscle itself.

**POSTERIOR PART** Primary TrP activity may occur as a result of injecting some irritant substances such as an antibiotic, vitamin or vaccine into this part of the muscle, or when it is subjected to excessive strain during sporting activities.

**Symptoms** The patient complains of pain at the back of the shoulder at rest, and this is made worse by movement (Fig. 13.7). External rotation is also limited so that whilst the hand can be brought up to the head it cannot be wrapped around the back of the head.

**Signs** Pain is aggravated by asking the patient to abduct the arm with the elbow straight and the palm facing backwards.

*TrP examination* This is carried out by flat palpation preferably with the muscle under moderate tension by slightly abducting the arm. Because the muscle is superficially situated taut bands at TrP sites are often felt and local twitch responses readily elicited.

TrPs present in the front of this muscle are usually to be found in its upper part. This is in contrast to those present at the back of it which are usually situated in its lower part (Fig. 13.8).

*TrP deactivation* This should be done with the patient lying on the opposite side.

*Associated TrPs* TrP activity is rarely confined to the deltoid alone. In addition to the muscles already mentioned, anterior deltoid TrP activity may be associated with similar activity in the biceps brachii, the clavicular section of the pectoralis major, and the coracobrachialis. Posterior deltoid TrP activity is often associated with the development of similar activity in TrPs in the long head of the triceps, and in the two muscles that form the posterior axillary fold – the latissimus dorsi and the teres major. Each of these muscles will, therefore, be discussed in turn.

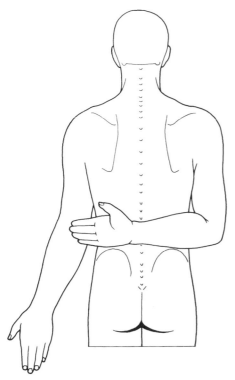

**Figure 13.6**   To illustrate how a normal person on putting the arm behind the back can reach across to rest the back of the hand on the opposite arm. With trigger points in either the anterior deltoid or coracobrachialis muscle it is usually not possible to reach past the midline.

**BICEPS BRACHII MUSCLE (see Fig. 12.9)**   TrPs are to be found in the lower part of this muscle just above the elbow (Fig. 13.9).

**Activation of TrPs**   These TrPs are liable to become activated when the muscle is strained by lifting a heavy object with the arm outstretched. By carrying out some task with the elbow flexed for a long time such as occurs when cutting a hedge. When supinating against resistance such as when using a screwdriver. And, as with the infraspinatus muscle, when suddenly reaching backwards for support to prevent a fall.

**Specific pattern of pain referral**   TrP activity in the distal part of the muscle near to the elbow causes pain to be referred upwards to the anterior surface of the shoulder joint, and sometimes to a lesser extent to the suprascapular region (Fig. 13.10). There is no restriction of movement at the shoulder joint

but pain is aggravated by raising the hand above the head.

**TrP examination**   The examination is carried out with the patient seated and with the elbow resting on a table. With the hand supinated, the elbow is slightly flexed to slacken the biceps muscle. TrPs in elongated tense bands are usually found in the distal part of the muscle (Winter 1944) and may, therefore, be located by sliding the examining finger across the lower part of both heads.

**Deactivation of TrPs**   Once a TrP has been located in this part of the muscle it should be trapped between two fingers whilst a needle is inserted into the tissues overlying it. Care should be taken to avoid penetrating either the median or radial nerves; the one lying along the medial and the other along the lateral border of the lower part of this muscle.

**CLAVICULAR SECTION OF THE PECTORALIS MAJOR MUSCLE**   A detailed discussion concerning the activation of TrPs in this muscle is given in Chapter 12, but attention must be drawn here to the fact that any in the clavicular section of this muscle may be responsible for pain in the front of the shoulder, and may also cause abduction of the arm at the shoulder joint to be restricted (see Fig. 12.6).

**CORACOBRACHIALIS (see Fig. 12.9)**   This muscle, together with the pectoralis minor and the short head of the biceps, is attached at its upper end to the coracoid process, and at its lower end to the middle of the humerus.

TrP activity in it usually does not become evident until TrPs in other shoulder muscles, particularly the anterior deltoid, have first been successfully deactivated. As Travell & Simons (1983, p. 440) have pointed out, TrP activity in this muscle should be suspected when despite deactivating TrPs in neighbouring muscles the patient continues to complain of pain over the anterior deltoid region, and down the back of the arm to the dorsum of the hand, but sparing for some reason the elbow and wrist (Fig. 13.11). TrPs in this muscle are usually to be found in in the upper part of it deep to the anterior deltoid (Fig. 13.11).

In order to deactivate TrPs in this muscle the patient should be placed in the supine position with the arm externally rotated.

**TRICEPS (LONG HEAD)**   A detailed account of the various parts of the triceps muscle and their patterns

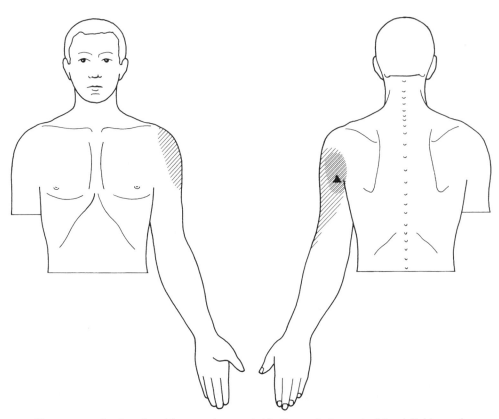

**Figure 13.7**    The pattern of pain referral from a trigger point in the posterior part of the deltoid muscle.

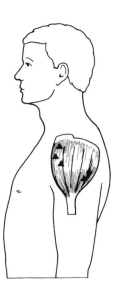

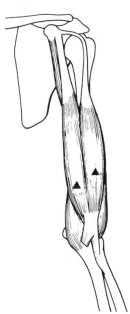

**Figure 13.8**    To illustrate the usual location of trigger points in the upper anterior part and lower posterior part of the deltoid muscle.

**Figure 13.9**    To show the usual location of trigger points in the lower part of the biceps muscle just above the elbow.

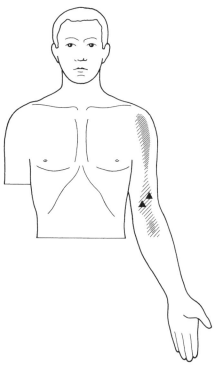

Figure 13.10 The pattern of pain referral from trigger points (▲) in the lower part of the biceps muscle.

of TrP pain referral will be given when discussing pain around the elbow joint in Chapter 15. Reference, however, must be made here to the long head of this muscle (Fig. 13.12) because when TrP activity develops in the posterior part of the deltoid it may also arise in this and in the latissimus dorsi and the teres major. TrPs in the long head cause pain to be referred upwards over the back of the arm to the posterior part of the shoulder and sometimes downwards along the back of the forearm (Fig. 13.13).

A person with TrP activity in this muscle, when instructed to raise both arms above the head with the elbows straight and palms to the front, finds it impossible to hold the arm on the affected side tight against the side of the head (Fig. 13.14).

**TrP examination**   TrPs when present are usually to be found in the mid third of the long head (Fig 13.13).

**TrP deactivation**   A detailed discussion of this will be given in Chapter 15.

**LATISSIMUS DORSI AND TERES MAJOR (see Fig. 12.14)** These muscles, which together form the posterior axillary fold, often have TrP activity in them at the same time.

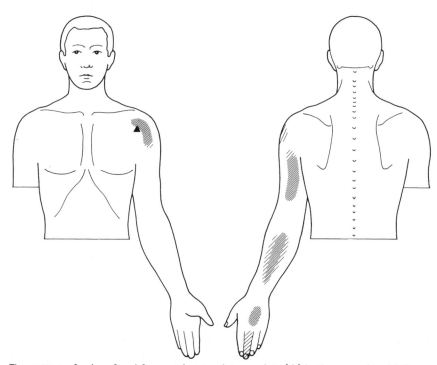

Figure 13.11   The pattern of pain referral from a trigger point or points (▲) in the coracobrachialis muscle.

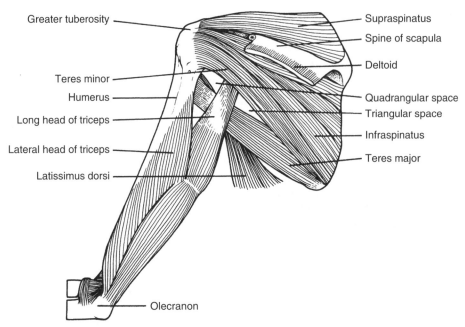

Greater tuberosity
Supraspinatus
Spine of scapula
Deltoid
Teres minor
Humerus
Quadrangular space
Long head of triceps
Triangular space
Lateral head of triceps
Infraspinatus
Teres major
Latissimus dorsi
Olecranon

**Figure 13.12**   The dorsal scapular muscles and triceps. Left side. The spine of the scapula has been divided near its lateral end and the acromion has been removed together with a large part of the deltoid.

TrP activity in the latissimus dorsi muscle has already been discussed in Chapter 12 as it mainly causes pain to be felt in the chest wall around the inferior angle of the scapula. The pain, however, may also be referred to the back of the shoulder and down the inner side of the arm (see Fig. 12.15).

Teres major is attached medially to the lower part of the scapula; and laterally converges with the latissimus dorsi muscle to form the posterior axillary fold before being inserted into the tuberosity close to the latissimus dorsi in the bicipital groove (see Fig. 12.14). TrP activity in it causes pain to be felt in the posterior part of the shoulder when reaching forwards and upwards and occasionally along the back of the forearm (Fig. 13.15).

A person with TrP activity in this muscle has difficulty in pressing the raised outstretched arm tightly against the side of the head in the same way as someone with TrP activity in the long head of the triceps does. (Fig. 13.14).

**TrP examination**   TrPs are liable to be found both at the inner and outer ends of the muscle (Fig. 13.16). Those present medially at the insertion of the muscle into the lower lateral border of the

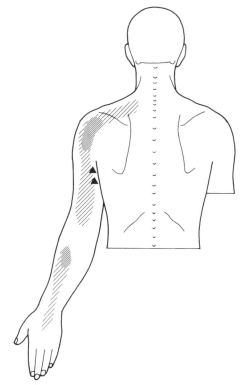

**Figure 13.13**   The pattern of pain referral from a trigger point or points (▲) in the long head of the triceps muscle.

scapula may be located by applying pressure against the underlying scapula. Those occurring laterally in the posterior axillary fold may be located by gripping the fold between the thumb and fingers but my preference is to use flat palpation (see Ch. 7). This may be done with the patient sitting but is easier to do with the patient lying supine and the arm abducted to 90°.

**Deactivation of TrPs**  TrPs in the vicinity of where this muscle inserts into the scapula are most readily deactivated with the patient lying on the contralateral side. TrPs in the posterior axillary fold should be deactivated with the patient lying in the supine position and the arm abducted at a right angle.

**SUBSCAPULARIS MUSCLE**  It is important not to overlook TrPs hidden away in the subscapularis muscle in anyone with persistent pain in the shoulder (Fig. 13.17).

**Activation of TrPs**  TrPs are liable to become active in this muscle when repeated movements involving a considerable amount of internal rotation are carried out. Also, as a result of direct

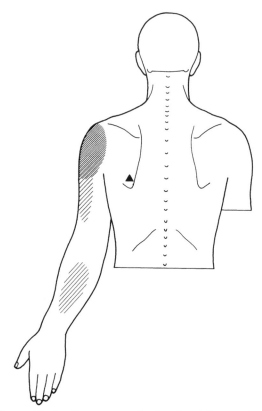

**Figure 13.15**  The pattern of pain referral from a trigger point at the inner end of the teres major muscle.

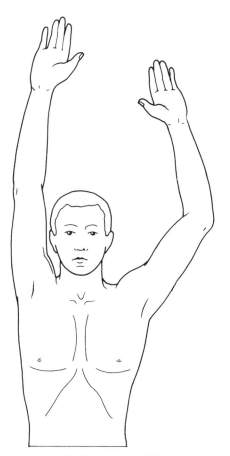

**Figure 13.14**  To illustrate the difficulty experienced in bringing the ipsilateral arm up against the ear when there is trigger point activity in either the long head of the triceps or the teres major muscle.

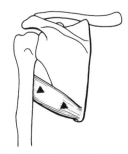

**Figure 13.16**  To show sites at which trigger points are liable to become activated in the teres major muscle.

trauma to the shoulder. And when the shoulder joint is immobilized for any length of time in the adducted and internally rotated position.

**Specific pattern of TrP pain referral**    Pain emanating from TrPs in this muscle is very severe even at rest and is made worse by movement. It is predominantly felt over the back of the shoulder but also extends up towards the scapula and down the back of the arm to the elbow. There may also be some pain around the back of the wrist (Fig. 13.18).

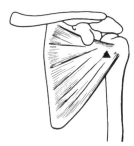

Figure 13.17    The subscapularis muscle with a trigger point (▲) near to the insertion of this muscle into the humerus.

**Characteristic disturbance of movements**    TrP activity in this muscle gives rise to progressively painful restriction of abduction and external rotation of the shoulder joint.

**Associated TrPs**    When TrPs become active in this muscle similar activity is liable to develop in the pectoralis major, latissimus dorsi, teres major, long head of the triceps, and the anterior and posterior part of the deltoid muscles.

**TrP examination**    TrPs in this muscle are usually to be found along the axillary border of the subscapular fossa. These are difficult to palpate unless the arm is well abducted and traction is put on it for the purpose of abducting the scapula. Unfortunately, however, severe pain and limitation of movement often makes this difficult.

**Deactivation of TrPs**    The patient should be placed in the supine position with the arm abducted if possible to 90°, with the hand placed behind the head and anchored beneath the pillow. When a TrP is located it should be fixed between two fingers and a needle inserted parallel to the rib cage into the tissues overlying it.

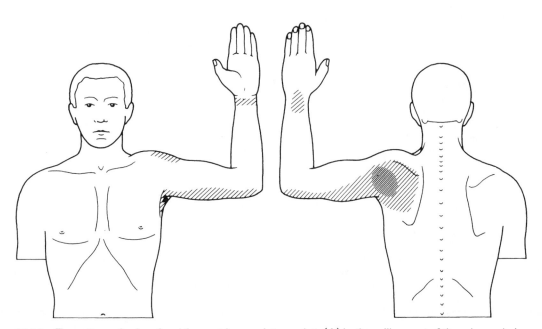

Figure 13.18    The pattern of pain referral from a trigger point or points (▲) in the axillary part of the subscapularis muscle.

# References

Baldry P E 1998 Pain in and around the shoulder's glenohumeral joint. In: Filshie J, White A (eds) Medical acupuncture, a Western scientific approach. Churchill Livingstone, Edinburgh, pp. 44–48

Baldry P E 2001 The shoulder. In: Myofascial pain and fibromyalgia syndromes. Churchill Livingstone, Edinburgh

Barry M, Jenner J R 1996 Pain in the neck, shoulder and arm. In: Snaith M I (ed) ABC of rheumatology. BMA Publishing Group, London

Bentley G, Goodfellow J W 1969 Disorganization of the knees following intra-articular hydrocortisone injections. Journal of Bone and Joint Surgery 51B: 498–502

Binder A I, Bulgen D Y, Hazleman B L, Tudor J, Wraight P 1984 Frozen shoulder: an arthrographic and radionuclear scan assessment. Annals of Rheumatic Diseases 43: 359–369

Bonica J J, Sola A E 1990 Other painful disorders of the upper limb. In: Bonica J J (ed) The management of pain, 2nd edn. Lea & Febiger, Philadelphia, Vol 1, p. 955

Bowman C, Jeffcoate W, Patrick M, Doherty M 1988 Bilateral adhesive capsulitis, oligoarthritis and proximal myopathy as presentation of hypothyroidism. British Journal of Rheumatology 27: 62–64

Bruckner F E 1982 Frozen shoulder (adhesive capsulitis). Journal of the Royal Society of Medicine 75: 688–689

Bulgen D Y, Binder A E, Hazelman B, Dutton J, Roberts S 1984 Frozen shoulder: prospective clinical study with an evaluation of three treatment regimens. Annals of Rheumatic Diseases 43: 353–360

Bunker T D 1985 Time for a new name for 'frozen shoulder'. British Medical Journal 290: 1233–1234

Cailliet R 1981 Shoulder pain, 2nd edn. Davis, Philadelphia, p. 48

Camp V 1986 Acupuncture for shoulder pain. British Medical Acupuncture Society Journal iii: 28

Codman E A 1934 The shoulder. Todd, Boston

Cyriax J 1980 Textbook of orthopaedic medicine, Vol 2. Baillière Tindall, London

Cyriax J, Troisier O 1953 Hydrocortisone and soft tissue lesions. British Medical Journal 11: 966–968

Dalton S E 1995 The shoulder. In: Klippel J, Dieppe P (eds) Practical rheumatology. Mosby, London

Duplay S 1896 De la periarthrite scapulo-humerale. L'Abeille Medicale 53: 226

Edeiken J, Wolferth C C 1936 Persistent pain in the shoulder region following myocardial infarction. American Journal of Medical Science 191: 201–210

Grey R G 1977 The natural history of 'idiopathic' frozen shoulder. Journal of Bone and Joint Surgery 60A: 564

Hazleman B 1990 Musculoskeletal and connective tissue disease. In: Souham R L, Moxham J (eds) Textbook of medicine. Churchill Livingstone, Edinburgh, p. 1037

Kellgren J H 1938 A preliminary account of referred pains arising from muscle. British Medical Journal 1: 325–327

Kelly M 1942 New light on the painful shoulder. Medical Journal of Australia 1: 488–493

Kessel L, Bayley I, Young A 1981 The frozen shoulder. British Journal of Hospital Medicine 25: 334–338

Koehler B E, Urowitz M B, Killinger D W 1974 The systemic effects of intra-articular corticosteroid. Journal of Rheumatology 1: 117–125

Lee P N, Lee M, Haq A M, Longton E B, Wright V 1974 Periarthritis of the shoulder. Annals of Rheumatic Diseases 33: 116–119

Lloyd-Roberts G C, French P R 1959 Periarthritis of a shoulder. British Medical Journal 1: 1569–1571

Mann 1974 The treatment of disease by acupuncture. Heinemann Medical, London, p. 196–197

Matsen F A, Bonica J J, Franklin J 1990 Pain in the shoulder and elbow. In: Bonica J J (ed) The management of pain, 2nd edn, Vol 1. Lea & Febiger, Pennsylvania

Neviaser J S 1945 Adhesive capsulitis of the shoulder. Journal of Bone and Joint Surgery 27: 211–222

Nash P, Hazleman B L 1989 Frozen shoulder. In: Hazleman B L, Dieppe P A (eds) The shoulder joint. Baillière's Clinical Rheumatology, London, pp. 551–556

Pace J B 1975 Commonly overlooked pain syndromes responsive to simple therapy. Postgraduate Medicine 58: 107–113

Reynolds M D 1981 Myofascial trigger point syndromes in the practice of rheumatology. Archives of Physical Medicine and Rehabilitation 62: 111–114

Richardson A T 1975 The painful shoulder. Proceedings of the Royal Society of Medicine 68: 731–736

Rubin D 1981 An approach to management of myofascial trigger point syndromes. Archives of Physical Medicine and Rehabilitation 62: 107–110

Satter M A, Luqman W A 1985 Periarthritis: another duration-related complication of diabetes mellitus. Diabetes Care 8: 507–510

Simons D G, Travell J G, Simons L S 1999 Myofascial pain and dysfunction. The trigger point manual, Vol 1, 2nd edn. Williams & Wilkins, Baltimore, pp. 267–274

Sola A 1999 Upper extremity pain. In: Wall P D, Melzack R (eds) Textbook of pain. Churchill Livingstone, Edinburgh

Sola A E, Kuitert J H 1955 Myofascial trigger point pain in the neck and shoulder girdle. Northwest Medicine 54: 980–984

Sola A E, Rodenberger M L, Gettys B B 1955 Incidence of hypersensitive areas in posterior shoulder muscles. American Journal of Physical Medicine 34: 585–590

Sola A E, Williams R L 1956 Myofascial pain syndromes. Neurology 6: 91–95

Travell J 1952 Pain mechanisms in connective tissue. In: Ragan C (ed) Connective tissues, transactions of the second conference 1951. Josiah Macy Jnr Foundation, New York

Travell J, Rinzler S, Herman M 1942 Pain and disability of the shoulder and arm: treatment by intramuscular infiltration with procaine hydrochloride. Journal of the American Medical Association 120: 417–422

Travell J G, Simons D G 1983 Myofascial pain and dysfunction. The trigger point manual. Williams & Wilkins, Baltimore

Winter S P 1944 Referred pain in fibrositis. Medical Record 157: 34–37

Wolgethan J R 1987 Frozen shoulder in hyperthyroidism. Arthritis and Rheumatism 30: 936–939

Wright V, Haq A M M 1976 Periarthritis of the shoulder. I. Aetiological considerations with particular reference to personality factors. Annals of the Rheumatic Diseases 35: 213–219

## INTRODUCTION

Persistent pain in the neck with restriction of its movements, with or without referral of the pain down the arm, is a commonly occurring disorder, and before deciding on whether or not to use acupuncture in an attempt to relieve it, it is obviously essential to first of all establish its cause.

Some of the less common causes and ones that require other forms of treatment include primary or secondary malignant disease infiltrating nerve roots or vertebral bodies; a variety of other disorders affecting the vertebrae such as fractures, infective lesions and rheumatoid arthritis; and some disorders of the muscle such as polymyalgia rheumatica. The exclusion of these clearly requires the taking of a detailed history, a carefully conducted clinical examination, and some basic investigations including an erythrocyte sedimentation rate (ESR) and cervical radiographs.

It is hardly necessary to cite cases illustrating the importance of making an accurate diagnosis before embarking upon treatment of any type but the following one, although it occurred a long time ago, is worth quoting as it is firmly imprinted on my mind for reasons that will become obvious.

A man (56 years of age) developed persistent pain in the neck with restricted movements. He was treated for several months symptomatically but when, in spite of this, the pain became progressively worse, he was referred to my outpatient clinic for assessment. On examination there were no abnormal neurological signs, but whilst he was having X-rays of his neck and chest, he suddenly collapsed due to the development of a quadriplegia! The appearances on the radiographs of the neck at first sight seemed to be normal until it was realized that only six cervical vertebrae were visible, one having collapsed so completely as a result of metastatic infiltration as to have virtually disappeared. The chest radiograph revealed the site of the primary growth.

This having been said it is now necessary to discuss some of the common causes of persistent neck pain as it is in the treatment of these that acupuncture has much to offer.

It is now evident that persistent neck pain with or without referral of this down the arm is often due to the primary activation of trigger points (TrPs) in muscles in the neck and shoulder region (Michele et al 1950, Sola & Kuitert 1955, Long 1956, Sola & Williams 1956, Michele & Eisenberg 1968, Travell & Simons 1983). Neurologists, however, continue to put most emphasis on nerve root entrapment as being the principal cause of this type of pain. With patients under the age of 40 years, pain is ascribed to acute rupture of an intervertebral disc, and with those older than this, it is considered to be due to cervical spondylosis (Posner 1982, Matthews 1983). These two conditions will, therefore, be considered first.

## ACUTE RUPTURE OF THE ANNULUS FIBROSUS OF AN INTERVERTEBRAL DISC WITH HERNIATION OF THE NUCLEUS PULPOSUS

From early adult life to middle age the intervertebral disc undergoes a degenerative process. Among the various biochemical changes which take place in the nucleus pulposus is a gradual decrease of its water content with a consequent progressive loss of its fluidity (Urban & Maroudas 1980).

Eventually as a result of this degenerative process the annulus fibrosus may rupture. When this happens the nucleus pulposus, provided it is still in a sufficiently fluid state, herniates through it and impinges on a nerve root. This, however, is relatively rare (Waddell 1982) as by the time an annulus fibrosus is liable to tear the nucleus pulposus tends to be too inspissated to flow through it.

It therefore follows that, although in adults under the age of 40 years, the sudden onset of severe pain in the neck and arm is often considered to be due to the entrapment of a nerve from a ruptured intervertebral disc, except in the minority of cases where there are definite physical signs of this, such as weakness of muscles, sensory changes and the loss of a tendon jerk, together with evidence of disc protrusion on magnetic resonance imaging (MRI) at a level corresponding with that shown by the physical signs, such an assumption is unjustified.

The commonest cause for acute neck pain would seem to be the primary development of TrP activity in the muscles in that region. In support of this belief are the observations that pain of this type usually develops when these muscles have been subjected to some acute strain, and that in such circumstances careful examination of various neck muscles, including the levator scapulae, splenius cervicis and trapezius reveals the presence of TrPs with pressure on them aggravating the spontaneously occurring pain. In addition, should acute neck pain be associated with considerable muscle spasm causing the neck to be pulled to one side (acute wry neck) TrPs are likely to be found in the sternocleidomastoid muscle.

TrP activity may also develop as a secondary event in muscles to which pain has been referred as a result of nerve root entrapment caused by either a cervical disc prolapse or cervical spondylosis.

## Cervical spondylosis

Cervical spondylosis is liable to develop from the age of 40 years upwards. It is a very commonly occurring degenerative condition affecting the discs and facet joints of the 5th, 6th and 7th cervical vertebrae. A striking feature of the condition is the development of osteophytes, both anteriorly and posteriorly. It is the posterior osteophytes that are of particular importance because, if sufficiently big, they may cause narrowing of the spinal canal with the gradual onset of a spastic paraplegia, or the narrowing of one or other of the intervertebral foramina with the development of nerve root entrapment, giving rise to pain in the neck and arm and the eventual appearance of neurological signs in the arm. In contrast to this, anterior osteophytes and also narrowing of the intervertebral spaces, although often seen on lateral radiographs in this condition, are not a cause of either symptoms or signs.

It needs to be stressed that radiographic appearances of cervical spondylosis are frequently seen in asymptomatic elderly people (Pallis et al 1954, Friedenberg & Miller 1963, Heller et al 1983).

Pallis et al (1954) carried out a detailed clinical and radiographic study of asymptomatic cervical spondylosis in a random group of 50 inpatients over the age of 50 years suffering from a variety of other medical and surgical disorders. A number of these patients, despite having no neurological symptoms were found to have pyramidal tract and posterior column signs, together with radiographic evidence of moderate or severe narrowing of their spinal canals from posterior osteophytic, kyphotic, and subluxation changes of cervical spondylosis. What, however, was of particular relevance, when considering neck pain and the part that cervical spondylosis may play in producing this, was that they found that a number of patients with no pain in the neck or arm had severe osteophytic narrowing of one or another intervertebral foramen. And that approximately one-third of these had neurological evidence of nerve root involvement in an arm.

Heller et al (1983) compared the cervical radiographs of two groups of patients. One group included all patients over the age of 60 years referred to their department of radiology during the course of one particular year specifically for X-ray examinations of the neck. The other group consisted of all of the patients, also over the age of 60 years, referred to the department that year for barium studies. They not only found that 85% of those specifically referred for neck X-rays had radiographic evidence of cervical spondylosis, but also that there was no significant difference in the prevalence and extent of the radiographic changes in the two groups. Furthermore, there was no consistent relationship between symptoms and X-ray appearances.

There are therefore certain enigmas associated with this commonly occurring condition. Foremost amongst these is that whilst the condition causes pain in the neck and arm to develop in some people, others with equally severe radiographic changes remain symptomless. Furthermore, as a corollary to this, the presence of radiographic changes of cervical spondylosis in a person suffering from pain in the neck does not necessarily imply that the latter is due to this disorder as these X-ray appearances of it are often no more than a fortuitous finding in someone whose pain is due to some other cause including in particular the primary development of TrP activity in muscles of the neck.

Nerve root entrapment from cervical spondylosis is of course the most likely cause of persistent pain in the neck and arm *when the latter occurs in association with objective neurological signs* of it such as muscle wasting, sensory loss, and depression of one or other of the tendon jerks in an arm (biceps jerk – C5 root; supinator jerk – C6 root; triceps jerk – C7 root) together with, in particular, an electromyographic abnormality. In such circumstances the presence of posterior osteophytes on the lateral view of a cervical radiograph helps to confirm the diagnosis. It, nevertheless, has to be remembered that osteophytes are not the only cause of nerve entrapment in cervical spondylosis as this may also develop as a result of fibrosis in a dorsal root sleeve, a tissue reaction that requires a myelogram for its detection (Frykholm 1951).

Unlike what one might expect with nerve root entrapment, either from well-developed posterior osteophytes or peri-radicular fibrosis in cevical spondylosis, the pain arising as a result of it is not persistent but episodic, with each bout lasting from a few weeks to a few months, with the average being about 6 weeks. As pointed out by Hopkins (1993) it is not known why pain suddenly arises from a root or roots that must have been compressed for some considerable time or why, as is usually the case, it spontaneously disappears. One possible explanation he suggests is that trauma to the nerve leads to the development of inflammatory oedema of the tissues around the root or roots that over the course of time spontaneously subsides.

## CERVICAL MYOFASCIAL TrP PAIN SYNDROME

A far commoner and frequently overlooked cause of persistent neck and shoulder girdle pain, with or without pain down the arm, is the primary development of TrP activity in muscles in the neck and shoulder girdle.

Muscles in which this TrP activity is liable to cause neck and shoulder girdle pain to develop are the levator scapulae, the splenius cervicis, other posterior cervical muscles, the trapezius and rhomboids. The ones in which TrPs are liable to cause pain to be referred down the arm include the levator scapulae, the scalene muscles (Ch. 12), the supraspinatus and the infraspinatus (Ch. 13). The sternocleidomastoid muscle, although situated in the neck, will be discussed in Chapter 16 as its TrP pain referral is to the head and face.

Each of these muscles, other than those dealt with elsewhere, will be considered in turn with regard to the sites at which TrPs arise in them and their specific patterns of pain referral. This will be followed by a discussion concerning the factors responsible for causing this TrP activity to develop and its treatment.

## Levator scapulae muscle

When persistent pain in the neck with restriction of its movements is due to TrP activity, this usually develops in several muscles at the same time, either on one side or, as is often the case, on both sides of the neck. It is, however, this muscle that is the one most frequently involved (Fig. 12.14).

### Specific pattern of pain referral

The pain from TrP activity in this muscle is mainly felt at the base of the neck, but it may also extend upwards towards the occiput, outwards to the back of the shoulder and downwards along the inner border of the scapula (Fig. 14.1).

The pain may also radiate anteriorly around the chest wall along the course of the 4th and 5th intercostal nerves when it may erroneously be diagnosed as being either anginal or pleural, or even more frequently, as being due to intercostal nerve-root entrapment. In addition, it quite commonly extends down the arm along the posteromedial aspect of the upper arm and the ulnar border of the forearm and hand to terminate in the ring and little fingers. A pattern of referral that coincides with the

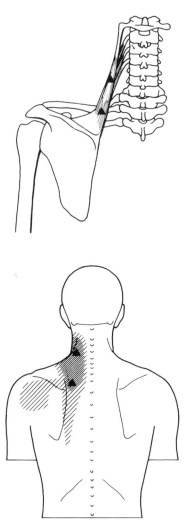

**Figure 14.1** The pattern of pain referral to the neck, shoulder and inner border of the scapula from a trigger point or points (▲) in the levator scapulae muscle. Pain in this distribution occurs as a result of activity in either a trigger point at the angle of the neck or one near to the insertion of this muscle into the superior angle of the scapula, or in both.

cutaneous areas of distribution of spinal segments C8, T1 and T2 (Fig. 14.2).

Of those patients in whom levator scapulae TrP pain is referred to these distant parts of the body some only experience it down the arm, some only feel it around the chest wall, whilst others are aware of it at both sites simultaneously.

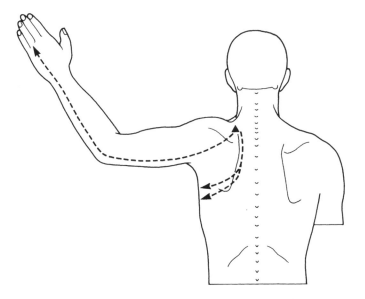

**Figure 14.2**  Some other patterns of pain referral from a trigger point (▲) in the levator scapulae near to its insertion into the superior angle of the scapula. These include referral down the inner side of the arm to the ring and little fingers. And referral around the chest wall along the course of the 4th and 5th intercostal nerves.

**Scapulocostal and scapulohumeral syndromes**
Michele et al (1950), Russek (1952) and Michele & Eisenberg (1968), in describing the condition in which pain is referred down the arm and around the chest wall as a result of TrP activity in the levator scapulae muscle, call it the scapulocostal syndrome. Long (1956) more appropriately divides it into the scapulocostal and scapulohumeral syndromes, because, as he states, 'trigger point pain around the chest wall and down the arm, although commonly occurring in consort, does not always do so'.

*TrP examination*

TrPs may be found at two separate sites in this muscle. One is at the angle of the neck where the muscle emerges from beneath the anterior border of the trapezius muscle. The other is situated lower down the back at the attachment of the muscle to the superior angle of the scapula (Fig. 14.1).

The point at the angle of the neck where the upper TrP is situated is best palpated with the patient sitting comfortably with the elbows supported on arm rests. This helps to relax both the levator scapulae and trapezius, and allows the clinician to pull the trapezius out of the way. Once the levator scapulae muscle has been identified, the TrP is most readily located by gently turning the

head to the opposite side as this puts the muscle on the stretch. The lower placed TrP may also be located with the patient in the sitting position and is best identified by rolling the fingers across the muscle fibres just above the superior angle of the scapula.

## Splenius cervicis

*Specific pattern of pain referral*

TrP activity may be found in the upper part of the muscle and in the lower part. The TrP in the upper part refers pain to the head and will, therefore, be considered in greater detail in Chapter 16.

It is the TrP in the lower part of the muscle that causes pain to be felt locally around the base of the neck.

*TrP examination*

This TrP may be located at the angle of the neck where the muscle lies between the trapezius medially and the levator scapulae laterally. It is advisable to rotate the head and neck to the opposite side in order to put the muscle on the stretch when attempting to identify it (Fig. 14.3).

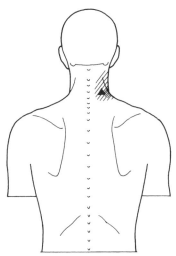

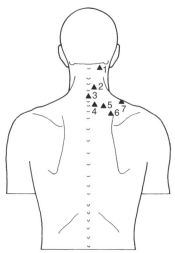

**Figure 14.3**   The pattern of pain referral from a trigger point (▲) at the base of the neck in the lower part of the splenius cervicis muscle.

**Figure 14.4**   To show the positions of some commonly occurring trigger points at the back of the neck and shoulder girdle.
1. Trigger point in a depression between the upper ends of the trapezius and sternocleidomastoid muscles close to the mastoid process and coinciding in position with the traditional Chinese acupuncture point Gall Bladder 20 (see Ch. 16).
2. Trigger point in a posterior cervical muscle at the level of the 4th cervical vertebra. The particular muscle involved depending on the depth at which the trigger point lies – see text.
3. Trigger point in the ligamentum nuchae.
4. Trigger point in the splenius cervicis muscle at the angle of the neck.
5. and 6. Trigger points in the levator scapulae muscle.
7. Trigger point in the upper free border of the trapezius muscle halfway between the spine and acromion and corresponding in position with the traditional Chinese acupuncture point Gall Bladder 21.

## Posterior cervical muscles halfway down the back of the neck

The paravertebrally situated posterior cervical muscles are arranged in four layers. In descending order of depth, these layers consist of the upper part of the trapezius; the splenius capitis and cervicis; the semispinalis capitis and cervicis; and the multifidi and rotatores. With a painful stiff neck there is frequently an exquisitely tender TrP close to the spine in one or other of these posterior cervical muscles at about the level of the 4th or 5th cervical vertebra (Fig. 14.4). The depth at which the TrP lies and therefore the muscle involved varies from person to person.

### Specific pattern of pain referral

Pain from a TrP in one of these posterior cervical muscles at this level is referred upwards towards the base of the skull and downwards over the shoulder girdle towards the upper part of the scapula (Fig. 14.5).

## Trapezius muscle

TrP activity in this muscle is very common. There are several sites where this may develop and therefore

reference will first be made to some anatomical features of the muscle. It will be remembered that the two trapezius muscles together take the shape of a diamond. They extend in the midline from the occiput above, to the 12th thoracic vertebra below, and fan out on both sides to be attached to the clavicle in front and the spine of the scapula behind.

For descriptive purposes the muscle may therefore be conveniently divided into an upper part extending from the occiput down to the 5th cervical spine, a middle part extending from the 6th cervical spine to the 3rd dorsal vertebra, and a

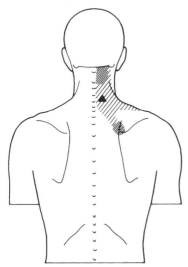

**Figure 14.5**   The pattern of pain referral from a trigger point (▲) in a posterior cervical muscle at the level of the 4th cervical vertebra.

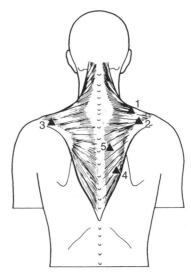

**Figure 14.6**   Trigger points (▲) in the trapezius muscle.

lower part extending from the 4th to the 12th dorsal vertebra (Fig. 12.14).

### Upper part of the muscle

The most frequently occurring TrP in the trapezius muscle is to be found along the upper border of the shoulder girdle about half way between the spine and the tip of the shoulder. This point, therefore, coincides in position with the well-known traditional Chinese one known as Gall Bladder 21.

TrP activity at this site is the cause of pain being referred up the side of the neck to the base of the skull, and on occasions around the side of the head to reach the temple and back of the eye (TP1 Figs 14.6 & 16.6D).

Sometimes there is a further TrP in this upper part of the muscle situated just below the one already described (TP2 Fig. 14.6). This also causes pain to be referred up the side of the neck.

### Middle part of the muscle

A TrP near to the acromion may be responsible for pain being referred to the posterior part of the shoulder (TP3 Fig. 14.6).

### Lower part of the muscle

A TrP (TP4 Fig. 14.6) may be found in the outer border of the lower part just above the level of the inferior angle of the scapula. Also another one may occur just below the inner end of the scapular spine (TP5 Fig. 14.6). These two TrPs are not often involved but when they are, they may cause pain to be referred to the upper scapular and neck region. They are, therefore, always worth looking for if neck pain persists after activity in the other TrPs already described has been adequately suppressed.

## Rhomboids (major and minor) (see Fig. 12.14)

### Activation of TrPs

This occurs less frequently than in the other shoulder girdle muscles, but factors that cause it include prolonged working in a round-shouldered position; also strain on the muscles from an upper thoracic scoliosis, such as may occur idiopathically, or following chest surgery.

It may also occur when these muscles, together with the trapezius, become overloaded by having to counteract tension in the pectoralis major and minor brought about by TrP activity developing in these latter two muscles.

### Specific pattern of pain referral

Pain from TrPs in these muscles (Fig. 14.7) is confined mainly to an area immediately medial to the inner border of the scapula (Fig. 14.8).

### TrP examination

With the patient seated and the arms wrapped tightly around the front of the chest in order to bring the scapulae forwards the TrPs are located by means of deep palpation through the trapezius muscle.

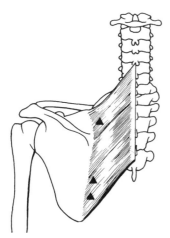

**Figure 14.7** Trigger points (▲) along the medial border of the scapula in the rhomboid muscles.

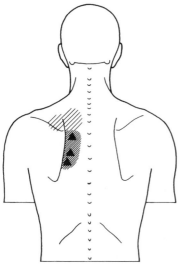

**Figure 14.8** The pattern of pain referral from a trigger point or points in the rhomboid muscles.

## ACTIVATION OF MID-LINE TrPS IN THE LIGAMENTUM NUCHAE

Pain on extending or flexing the neck is often associated with the presence of one or more TrPs in the ligamentum nuchae connecting the apices of the cervical vertebral spines (Fig. 14.4). In all such cases therefore it is important to palpate along the length of this ligament from the occiput above to the spine of the 7th cervical vertebra below.

## FACTORS RESPONSIBLE FOR THE PRIMARY ACTIVATION OF TrPS IN THE NECK

These include trauma to the neck such as that sustained as a result of a whiplash injury; postural disorders; sagging of, tilting of and persistent pressure applied to the shoulder girdle; strain transmitted to the neck as a result of a lower limb disorder; and anxiety-evoked contraction of muscles. Each of these will be considered in turn.

### Whiplash injury

TrPs in the muscles of the neck may become activated as a result of various forms of trauma such as that incurred when falling from a horse or tripping whilst going downstairs, but one of the commonest nowadays is the whiplash injury liable to affect the occupants of a stationary car when this is hit from behind by another car.

As previously discussed by me (Baldry 1996, 2001), all the various aspects of this particular type of injury have over the years given rise to considerable controversy.

Extensive reviews of the literature concerning it have been provided by Barnsley et al (1994); by the Quebec Task Force on Whiplash Associated Disorders (Spitzer et al 1995); by The World Congress on Whiplash Associated Disorders held in Vancouver during February 1999 (Anton 2000); by Ryan (2000) and by Galasko et al (2000).

### Factors responsible for the development of pain

*Activation of myofascial TrPs*    It is still not sufficiently well recognized that the commonest reason for pain in this disorder developing is trauma-induced activation of TrPs in the muscles of the neck (Baldry 1996, 2001, Byrn et al 1991, 1993, Evans 1992, Fricton 1993, Mailis et al 1995, Simons et al 1999) and in muscles of the upper anterior chest wall including, in particular, the pectoralis minor (Hong & Simons 1993).

It therefore follows that in all cases of whiplash injury a systematic search for TrPs in these muscles is mandatory.

*Facet joint damage*   The reason why pain may arise from facet joints following a whiplash injury is still not certain (Gibson et al 2000). Some of the possible causes include occult fractures, capsular ruptures and intra-articular haemorrhages (Taylor & Twomey 1993).

Bogduk & Simons (1993) have shown that because an individual facet joint and the muscle around it share the same nerve supply, the pattern of pain referral from TrPs in that muscle and from the joint is the same. In view of this any TrP found to be present should first be deactivated. If despite doing this the pain persists, then the possibility that it may also be arising from the facet joint has to be considered and a diagnostic block of the nerves supplying it carried out (Bogduk & Marsland 1988).

*Intervertebral disc damage*   There are grounds for believing that persistent localized pain in the neck following a whiplash injury may develop as a result of tears in the richly innervated outer third of a disc's annulus fibrosus, as these have been shown to be present in patients with this disorder by means of the carrying out of cineradiograms (Buonocore et al 1996) and MRI scans (Davis et al 1991). The latter have shown that avulsion of the disc from the vertebral endplate may be yet another cause.

RADIOGRAPHIC AND MRI FINDINGS   The carrying out of radiography and MRI are widely employed for identifying the above skeletal causes of pain in this disorder but interpreting the significance of abnormalities found by this means demands considerable caution. This is because, as Ryan (2000) has pointed out, the Quebec Task Force (Spitzer et al 1995) reported that MRI and radiographic examinations are confounded by age-related changes in bony and soft tissues. And because Boden et al (1990), from the carrying out of MRI on 63 asymptomatic volunteers, observed an abnormality such as a herniated disc, bulging disc or foraminal stenosis in 19% of these people and found that the frequency of abnormalities in those aged 40 years or more was 28%.

Conversely, it has to be said that an all too frequent cardinal error is to conclude that because a radiographic or MRI examination fails to show any significant abnormality that any persistent pain that may be present in someone with this disorder must be due to either neuroticism or compensation-seeking avarice without considering the possibility that the pain may be emanating from TrPs in the muscles.

*Pain in the head*   The commonest reason for this developing in someone with a whiplash injury is TrP activity in one or more of the following muscles. The posterior cervical muscles, the upper part of the trapezius and the sternocleidomastoid.

*Paraesthesiae in the fingers*   There are three reasons why paraesthesiae in the fingers may arise in this disorder. One is because of the development of a thoracic outlet syndrome as a result of TrP-evoked shortening of the pectoralis minor muscle and the scalenus anterior muscle causing compression of underlying vessels and the brachial plexus; a second is the development of a cervical radiculopathy; and a third is the development of a carpal tunnel syndrome. This latter disorder may be brought about as a result of perineural oedema of the median nerve occuring either because of vascular compression at the thoracic outlet, because of a hyper-extension injury to the wrist caused by excessive gripping of the steering wheel, or because of bracing the hands on the dashboard during the collision (Evans 1992).

*Spatial disorientation*   The type of spatial disorientation that most often affects patients with a whiplash injury is dizziness and light-headedness with a sudden loss of balance and a tendency to veer to one side when walking. This may on occasions be due to vertebrobasilar insufficiency (Schneider & Schemm 1961) but far more often (see Ch. 16) it is due to a change in the tension and shortening of the clavicular part of the sternocleidomastoid muscle brought about as a result of trauma-induced TrP activity (Travell 1967, Weeks & Travell 1955).

*Cognitive impairment*   Psychometric assessment of patients with whiplash injuries have shown that some of them have impaired attention, concentration and memory (Kischka et al 1991, Radanov et al 1991). Possible reasons for these cognitive disorders include the distracting influence of persistent neck and head pain, together with the anxiety and depression produced by this and the effects of drugs given to combat these symptoms (Shapiro et al 1993).

*Emotional disturbances* Persistent whiplash injury-evoked pain, like any other chronic pain, may lead to the development of anxiety and depression. These two disorders of the affect, furthermore, are liable to be made worse by any job insecurity, marital disharmony or social disruption that may be brought about by the physical disability.

*Late whiplash syndrome* It has been estimated that approximately 75% of patients with whiplash injuries recover within 3–6 months and that the remaining may develop what is known as the late whiplash syndrome – a condition in which symptoms, including in particular pain, persist for longer than 6 months.

Factors that Radanov et al (1991) have identified as being predictive of this developing include the severity of the initial neck pain, the presence of cognitive disorders, and the effects of ageing.

Pettersson et al (1995), from MRI studies, have shown that the syndrome is particularly likely to develop in those who have an antecedent narrowing of the cervical canal.

This syndrome is also more liable to develop when the trauma to the neck is so severe that pain comes on immediately after it rather than being delayed for 24–48 hours, as is more usually the case. This notwithstanding, it has to be said that patients who have been subjected to no more than mild or moderate injury may also develop it. Possible reasons for this include undiagnosed and therefore untreated causes of the pain such as TrP activity, facet joint injury or disc damage. Another is the central sensitisation of dorsal horn-situated nociceptive neurons that develops as a result of the sensory afferent barrage set up when there is persistent activation and sensitisation of nociceptors in either TrPs or other structures.

A clear understanding of these various causative factors is of considerable importance because the prolongation of symptoms in a patient with a whiplash injury has for all too long been attributed to either neuroticism or a subconscious or even conscious exaggeration of them for the purpose of obtaining financial compensation (Pearce 1989). The following case typefies this.

A builder (46 years of age), as a result of a car accident, was admitted to hospital unconscious and with severe bruising of the right side of the neck, right shoulder and right elbow.

He recovered consciousness within a matter of hours, the bruising disappeared over the next few weeks, but he was left with much pain in and restricted movements of the right side of the neck and in spite of physiotherapy, neck traction and the wearing of a collar he still had this pain when seen by an orthopaedic specialist 3 months after the accident. The patient was told at this stage that no further treatment was likely to be helpful but that the pain would disappear spontaneously with time.

When, at follow-up 6 months later, he still had considerable pain and limitation of movements of the neck, and had also by then developed headaches and unsteadiness on sudden movements, the same specialist told him that with patience it would all settle down and that certainly he was unlikely to have trouble once a compensation claim had been settled! The patient felt the implications of such a remark to be totally unjustified particularly as being a self-employed person he was desperately anxious to get back to work. His general practitioner wondered if he might be helped by acupuncture and when seen by me 12 months after the accident he was obviously having much genuine pain in the neck causing him to take large amounts of analgesics.

On examination, there were many exquisitely tender TrPs to be found in several muscles of the neck, and after these had been deactivated by means of the carrying out of superficial dry needling at weekly intervals on six occasions, his pain was sufficiently well controlled to allow him to return to work, and after two further treatments over the next month it disappeared.

This response to acupuncture was gratifying but of course it would have been possible to have relieved his pain much more quickly if only the development of TrP activity had been recognized at a much earlier stage.

## Postural disorders

TrP activity may arise in the neck muscles when some faulty posture is persistently adopted. This not infrequently occurs occupationally as a result of a desk or workbench not being adjusted to an individual's body build. Machine operators and typists are some of those particularly at risk.

A draughtsman (29 years of age) had two attacks of severe rightsided neck pain with restricted movements. Each time he was told he must have 'slipped a disc' and was treated by having his neck intermittently stretched and immobilized in a collar.

On each occasion he obtained little or no benefit from these measures, had to take much time off work, and the pain persisted for about 6–8 weeks. In view of this experience, when 1 year later it recurred a third time, he asked his general practitioner about the possibility of acupuncture and was referred to me. I saw him within a week of the pain developing, and found TrPs to be present in the right levator scapulae muscle at the angle of the neck; in the free border of the trapezius half-way between the angle of the neck and the tip of the shoulder; and a third half-way down the side of the neck in a posterior cervical muscle.

When these were deactivated by means of the carrying out of superficial dry needling the pain immediately abated and full movement of the neck was restored. It was only necessary to repeat the procedure once again a week later before lasting improvement was obtained. However, what was of particular importance to him was that he did not have to take any time off work. It is not sufficient to content oneself with effectively alleviating pain, without at the same time seeing whether there is anything that has to be done in order to prevent a recurrence. In this case it was found that each attack had occurred at a time when pressure of work demanded that he sat at his drawing board for a particularly long period on a chair that was too low with, because of this, his shoulder girdle abnormally elevated.

TrP activity in neck muscles may develop too when the neck has to be turned to one side for long periods such as when a secretary has to read shorthand notes whilst typing, or when the neck is kept fixed in one position for a long time, such as when watching a play or driving a car, also when it is repeatedly rotated such as watching a tennis match.

It also may occur during sleep when the neck becomes kinked at an acute angle either due to the pillow being too high or too low.

A girl (14 years of age) suffered from severe neck pain that much affected her schooling for 3 years because the significance of too high a pillow was not recognized. During that 3 years she was given several courses of physiotherapy, had had her neck stretched and from time to time had worn a collar. When eventually she was seen by me it only required the deactivation of TrPs on three occasions to bring the pain under control. On investigating the cause of the pain it became apparent that the child for many years had insisted on sleeping with the head resting on three pillows. Since this habit has been changed, she has had no recurrence of pain.

## Sagging of the shoulder girdle

The activation of TrPs commonly occurs in those, who because of occupational strains, obesity, or even laziness, have become round shouldered with drooping of the shoulder girdle – the so-called syndrome of the sagging shoulders.

## Tilting of the shoulder girdle

This is not an uncommon reason for TrP activity to develop. It occurs either secondary to a pelvic tilt in someone who because of a congenital or acquired defect has one leg longer than the other, or because of the habitual use of a walking stick which is too long.

## Transmitted strain to the neck

Any painful disorder affecting the lower limb may, by putting a strain on all parts of the spine, cause not only the development of TrP activity in the muscles of the lower back but also in the muscles of the neck.

## Persistent pressure on the shoulder girdle

TrP activity may develop in the neck muscles when they are subjected to persistent strain from the wearing of unsuitable clothing, such as an overcoat that is too heavy, or shoulder straps that are too tight.

## Environmental factors

These include exposure either to draughts or to damp.

## Anxiety

A common cause of TrPs developing in neck muscles is when these are persistently held in a contracted state because of nervous tension. When this is the predominant cause the patient often also complains of headaches.

## PREVENTATIVE MEASURES

It must be stressed that, although pain from any of the above causes may readily be alleviated by means of the carrying out of superficial dry needling at TrP sites, such pain will recur unless the reasons for it developing are identified and measures are taken to avoid the re-activation of the TrPs.

## TREATMENT OF PERSISTENT NECK PAIN

Because of the traditional belief that persistent pain and stiffness of the neck are mainly due to nerve-root entrapment, either from an acute prolapse of an intervertebral disc, or from cervical spondy-losis, treatment usually includes continuous or more often intermittent traction; the wearing of a specially designed collar; and the use of various forms of physiotherapy.

Pain of this type may persist for many months or years but often it subsides spontaneously after about 6–8 weeks, and it is now generally agreed that none of the standard forms of treatment, such as neck traction (Steinberg & Mason 1959, British Association of Physical Medicine Trial 1966), the wearing of a collar (Matthews 1983), or different types of physiotherapy including diathermy and ultrasound (Rogers & Williams 1981), significantly influence its course.

There is, therefore, much need for a different approach to the treatment of persistent neck pain and now that it is realized that often it is associated with the development of TrP activity in the muscles, we have in superficial dry needling at TrP sites one of considerable promise. This first became apparent to me some years ago now, when, as it so happened, one of the first patients to be treated by me with this particular form of therapy had pain of this type.

A housewife (61 years of age) was referred to my outpatient clinic with angina, but what troubled her

even more was that for the past 6 months, since she and her husband had been in a car accident, she had had persistent pain in the neck with marked restriction of its movements. She further informed me that she had not mentioned this to her general practitioner as she could not face having to wear a collar! An X-ray of the cervical spine showed, as might be expected at that age, the characteristic appearances of cervical spondylosis. In addition, however, examination of her neck muscles revealed the presence of TrPs and she was, therefore, asked to attend my outpatient clinic again for me to attempt to relieve her pain by means of deactivating these.

It must have been with a certain amount of trepidation that she kept her appointment for this as she brought her husband with her for moral support! TrPs were found at three similar sites on both sides of her neck and deactivated by means of needles being inserted into the tissues immediately overlying them for a short period. Much to her surprise (and to a certain extent mine also!) on withdrawing the needles she found that her neck was very much more comfortable and that she could move it through a full range of movements. She said that her husband would never believe this and so asked if he could come into the treatment room to witness it!

After expressing pleasure at his wife's response to treatment, he revealed that he too, since the car accident, had had persistent pain in his neck and had experienced severe limitation of its movements. Further, he said that he had had two courses of intensive treatment for what he had been told was severe arthritis of the neck, and wondered whether as an act of desperation he also might be allowed to try the effects of acupuncture.

Examination showed him to have several TrPs in both sides of his neck and once these had been deactivated in a similar manner the immediate results were as gratifying as in the case of his wife.

Ultimately the wife had to have treatment on four occasions and the husband on six in order to obtain lasting relief from their pain. My memory, however, of those two walking down the hospital corridor after their first treatment both joyfully moving their heads from side to side in evident amazement at their new-found freedom of neck movements will forever be indelibly imprinted on my mind, and at the time the sight of it did much to strengthen my resolve to study acupuncture further!

There can be no doubt that in both these cases the neck pain was due to TrP activity developing in muscles that had become strained as a result of the car accident and that the radiographic appearances of degenerative skeletal changes observed in both of them were chance findings. It is interesting to note that the husband had been told that the reason for his failure to respond to physiotherapy was because the arthritis in his neck was so bad!

## Identification and deactivation of TrPs

The two cases just quoted once again serve to illustrate how important it is in all cases of persistent neck pain to examine the muscles of the neck for TrPs. Moreover, such an examination has to be carried out in a systematic manner as it is essential to avoid overlooking any of them that may be contributing to the pain.

The patient should therefore be seated comfortably in a chair but with the head and arms suitably positioned to put the muscles on the stretch. Each muscle should then be examined in turn in order to ensure that no TrPs are overlooked and that each in turn has a needle inserted into the tissues overlying it. Particular care, however, must be taken when putting needles into muscles around the base of the neck and chest wall, never to insert them in a vertical direction but always at an angle so as to avoid penetrating the pleura.

As previously stated (see Ch. 8), when treating myofascial pain by the carrying out of superficial dry needling at TrP sites this needle-evoked nerve stimulation procedure should never be carried out so energetically as to cause a temporary exacerbation of the pain. For some reason it would seem that this is especially likely to happen when deactivating TrPs in muscles around the head and neck. Therefore, in carrying out such treatment in this particular part of the body, it is advisable to be especially careful not to keep needles in situ for longer than is necessary and to keep any manipulation of them down to a minimum (see Ch. 10).

## Results of employing acupuncture for the treatment of neck pain

Everyday clinical experience would appear to suggest that the treatment of persistent neck pain with acupuncture is very rewarding. It would seem that approximately 70% of patients obtain long-term relief from repeating this type of treatment on several occasions but the number of times this has to be carried out is largely dependent on the length of time the pain has been present before it is started. A minority of cases only obtain relief for short periods and the treatment, therefore, has to be repeated on a regular basis at fairly frequent intervals. Such patients however find this a small price to pay for having their pain kept under control. A small group of patients obtain no benefit from it. These are usually people who have not only had pain of muscular origin for many years but also have some other underlying chronic skeletal pain disorder.

When considering results, however, it is difficult to generalize, for in the treatment of persistent neck pain with acupuncture the effectiveness of this not only depends on the underlying pathology, but also on a person's individual degree of responsiveness to needle-evoked nerve stimulation (see Chs 9 & 10).

### Clinical trials

White & Ernst (1999) have carried out a systematic search of randomized controlled trials of acupuncture for neck pain. During the course of discussing this, Ernst (1999) stated that 'twenty-four studies met our predefined inclusion and exclusion criteria. The trials were highly heterogenous and few were of acceptable quality as estimated by the Jadad score (Jadad et al 1996) ... Of the five sham-controlled studies, one was positive and four were negative. On the basis of these findings, we concluded that data are insufficient to state with certainty that acupuncture is more effective than sham acupuncture or other controlled interventions in the treatment of neck pain'.

A major criticism of all the trials reviewed by them is that they had been carried out on patients with non-specific chronic neck pain so that the treatment and control groups studied could well have contained people suffering from pain that may have been either of muscular origin, skeletal origin or a combination of these and which also may have been either nociceptive, neuropathic or a mixture of both. The response to acupuncture of pain of such disparate types is likely to be very different so as to make the interpretation of results when trials are carried out on patients with ill-defined heterogeneous chronic neck pain virtually impossible.

It is clearly essential when carrying out an acupuncture clinical trial to do so on patients with a single well-defined disorder. At first sight it might be thought, for example, that Loy (1983) fulfilled this criterion in a trial in which the relative pain-relieving efficacy of electroacupuncture and physiotherapy was compared in patients diagnosed as having pain due to cervical spondylosis, mainly on the grounds of there being evidence of this radiographically. However, as stated earlier in this chapter, pain in the neck cannot be assumed to be due to this degenerative disorder without evidence of nerve root entrapment because, in most cases, without this the changes of it seen on an X-ray are usually no more than a chance finding and the pain due to some other cause, the commonest being TrP activity in the neck muscles. Thus, chronic neck pain diagnosed as being due to cervical spondylosis on radiographic evidence alone, as in Loy's trial, may well be due to any one of a variety of disorders making randomization into homogenous 'treatment' and 'control' groups impossible.

There have been up to now few trials to assess the efficacy of TrP acupuncture alone in the treatment of the cervical myofascial TrP pain syndrome.

As previously discussed in Chapter 10, Hong (1994) carried out a well-planned trial to compare the effectiveness of lidocaine (lignocaine) injections with that of deep dry needling at myofascial TrP sites in the upper trapezius muscle. And Chu (1997) compared the effects of deep dry needling at TrP sites and at non-specific sites in patients who had cervical nerve root irritation pain and the secondary development of myofascial TrP pain.

Most other acupuncture trials carried out on patients with this TrP syndrome have had needles inserted either at traditional Chinese acupuncture sites alone or at a combination of both these and TrP sites. The following are examples of this.

Birch & Jamison in 1998 reported the results of a controlled trial carried out to assess the value of Japanese acupuncture in the treatment of chronic myofascial neck pain. The treatment, however, was not carried out at myofascial TrP sites but instead needles connected together by ion pumping cords

(see Ch. 10) were inserted very shal-lowly at what were deemed to be either 'relevant' or 'irrelevant' traditional Chinese acupuncture points. Their conclusion was that 'relevant traditional Chinese acupuncture ... contributes to modest pain reduction in persons with myofascial neck pain.'

Irnich et al in 2001 reported the results of a randomized trial of acupuncture in patients with chronic neck pain that was considered to have either emanated from TrPs or to have arisen as a result of a whiplash injury. No mention is made in the report as to how many with this latter disorder had active TrPs.

Three procedures were employed in the 'treatment' group. These were dry needling carried out at some of the TrP sites, acupuncture carried out 'according to the rules of traditional Chinese medicine' and ear acupuncture. There were two 'control' groups. One of them had an inactivated laser pen applied to similar points and the other was treated with massage.

The conclusion was that 'acupuncture is an effective short term treatment for patients with chronic neck pain.'

It may be seen therefore that despite there having been a large number of patients in this trial with pain emanating from myofascial TrPs, the design of it precluded any information being obtained concerning the value of dry needling carried out on these points alone.

Irnich et al in 2002 reported the results of a randomized double-blind sham-controlled trial in patients with chronic neck pain that had arisen either as a result of TrP activity or what they called 'the cervical irritation syndrome'.

The aim of the trial was to compare the immediate effects on motion-related pain and cervical spine mobility of three types of treatment given to each patient on single occasions. These treatments were: (1) needles inserted into traditional acupuncture points and one or two ear points; (2) dry needling carried out at myofascial TrP sites; and (3) sham laser carried out at traditional Chinese acupuncture points. There was a 1 week wash-out period between the carrying out of each of these procedures.

The results showed that 'acupuncture is superior to sham in improving motion-related pain and range of movements following a single session of treatment in chronic neck pain patients'. Unfortunately, once again the design of the trial was such that they had to admit that 'it is not possible to conclude from our data whether needling classical acupuncture points is more effective than needling other sites'.

It may therefore be seen that there remains a pressing need for suitably designed trials to be carried out to assess the relative efficacy, advantages and disadvantages of, Japanese shallow needling, superficial dry needling and deep dry needling carried out at TrP sites for the alleviation of cervical myofascial pain.

## References

Anton H A 2000 Whiplash associated disorders: yesterday-today-tomorrow. Journal of Musculoskeletal Pain 8(1/2): 1–2

Baldry P E 1996 Whiplash injuries. Acupuncture in Medicine XIV (1): 22–28

Baldry P E 2001 cervical whiplash injuries. In: Myofascial pain and fibromyalgia syndromes. Churchill Livingstone, Edinburgh, pp. 134–145

Barnsley L, Lord S M, Bogduk K 1994 Whiplash injury. Pain 58: 283–307

Birch S, Jamison R N 1998 Controlled trial of Japanese acupuncture for chronic myofascial neck pain: assessment of specific and nonspecific effects of treatment. The Clinical Journal of Pain 14: 248–255

Boden S D, McCowin P R, Davis D O, Dina T S, Mark A S, Wiesel S 1990 Abnormal magnetic resonance scans of the cervical spine in asymptomatic subjects. Journal of Bone and Joint Surgery 72A: 1178–1184

Bogduk N, Marsland A 1998 The cervical zygapophysial joint as a source of neck pain. Spine 13: 610–617

Bogduk N, Simons D G 1993 Neck pain: joint pain or trigger points? In: Voeroy H, Merskey H (eds) Progress in fibromyalgia and myofascial pain. Elsevier, Amsterdam, pp. 267–273

British Association of Physical Medicine Trial 1966 Pain in the neck and arm. A multicentre trial of the effects of physiotherapy. British Medical Journal 1: 253–258

Buonocore E, Hartman J T, Nelson C L 1966 Cineradiograms of cervical spine in diagnosis of soft-tissue injuries. Journal of American Medical Association 198: 143–147

Byrn C, Borenstein P, Linder L E 1991 treatment of neck and shoulder pain in whiplash syndrome patients with intracutaneous sterile water injections. Acta Anaesthesiologica Scandinavica 35: 52–53

Byrn C, Olsson I, Falkheden L et al 1993 Subcutaneous sterile water injections for chronic neck and shoulder pain following whiplash injuries. Lancet 341: 449–452

Chu J 1997 Does EMG (dry needling) reduce myofascial pain symptoms due to cervical nerve roor irritation? Electromyography and Clinical Neurophysiology 37: 259–272

Davis S J, Teresi L M, Bradley W G J, Ziemba M A, Bloze A C 1991 Cervical spine hyperextension injuries. MR findings. Radiology 180: 245–251

Ernst E 1999 Clinical effectiveness of acupuncture: an overview of systematic reviews. In: Ernst E, White A (eds) Acupuncture, a scientific appraisal. Butterworth-Heinmann, Oxford

Evans R W 1992 Some observations on whiplash injuries. Neurologic Clinics 10(4): 975–997

Friedenberg Z B, Miller W T 1963 Degenerative disc disease of the cervical spine. A comparative study of asymptomatic and symptomatic patients. Journal of Bone and Joint Surgery 45A: 1171–1178

Fricton J 1993 Myofascial pain and whiplash. Spine: State of the Art Reviews 7: 403–422

Frykholm R 1951 Cervical nerve root compression resulting from disc degeneration and root-sleeve fibrosis. Acta Chirurgica Scandinavica Supplement 160

Galasko C S B, Murray P A, Pitcher M 2000 Prevalence and long-term disability following whiplash – associated disorder. Journal of Musculoskeletal Pain 8(1/2): 15–27

Gibson T, Bogduk N, MacPherson J, McIntosh A 2000 Crash characteristics of whiplash associated chronic neck pain. Journal of Musculoskeletal Pain 8(1/2): 87–95

Heller C A, Stanley P, Lewis-Jones B, Heller R F 1983 Value of X-ray examinations of the cervical spine. British Medical Journal 287: 1276–1278

Hong C-Z 1994 Lidocaine injection versus dry needling to myofascial trigger point. American Journal of Physical Medicine and Rehabilitation 73: 256–263

Hong C-Z, Simons D G 1993 Response to treatment for pectoralis minor myofascial pain syndrome after whiplash. Journal of Musculoskeletal Pain 1(1):89–131

Hopkins A 1993 Clinical neurology. University Press, Oxford, p. 336

Irnich D, Behrens N, Gleditsch J M et al 2002 Immediate effects of dry needling and acupuncture at distant points in chronic neck pain: results of a randomized, double-blind, sham- controlled crossover trial. Pain 99: 83–89

Irnich D, Behrens N, Molzen H et al 2001 Randomised trial of acupuncture compared with conventional massage and 'sham' laser acupuncture for treatment of chronic neck pain. British Medical Journal 322: 1574–1577

Jadad A R, Moore R A, Carrol D et al 1996 Assessing the quality of reports of randomized clinical trials: is blinding necessary? Controlled Clinical Trials 17: 1–12

Kischka V, Ettlin T, Heim S, Schmid G 1991 Cerebral symptoms following whiplash injury. European Neurology 31: 136–140

Long C 1956 Myofascial pain syndromes. Part 2 – syndromes of the head, neck and shoulder girdle. Henry Ford Hospital Medical Bulletin 4: 22–28

Loy T T 1983 Treatment of cervical spondylosis. Electroacupuncture versus physiotherapy. Medical Journal of Australia 2: 32–34

Mailis A, Papagapiou M, Vanderlinden R G et al 1995 Thoracic outlet syndrome after motor vehicle accidents in a Canadian pain clinic population. Clinical Journal of Pain 11: 316–324

Matthews W B 1983 Lesions of the spinal roots. In: Weatherall D J, Ledingham J G G, Warrell D A (eds) Oxford textbook of medicine. Oxford University Press, Oxford, p. 43–44

Michele A A, Davies J J, Krueger F J, Lichtor J M 1950 Scapulocostal syndrome (fatigue-postural paradox). New York State Journal of Medicine 50: 1353–1356

Michele A A, Eisenberg J 1968 Scapulocostal syndrome. Archives of Physical Medicine and Rehabilitation 49: 383–387

Pallis C, Jones A M, Spillane J D 1954 Cervical spondylosis. Incidence and implications. Brain 77: 274–289

Pearce J M 1989 Whiplash injury: a reappraisal. Journal of Neurology, Neurosurgery and Psychiatry 52: 1329–1331

Pettersson K, Karrholm J, Toolanen G, Hildingsson C 1995 Decreased width of the spinal canal in patients with chronic symptoms after whiplash injury. Spine 20: 1664–1667

Posner J 1982 Diseases compressing nerve roots or spinal cord. In: Wyngaarden James B, Smith Lloyd H (eds) Cecil's textbook of medicine, 16th edn. Saunders, Philadelphia, pp. 2148–2150

Radanov B P, Stefano G, Schnidrig A, Ballinari P 1991 Role of psychosocial stress in recovery from common whiplash. Lancet 338: 712–715

Rogers M, Williams N 1981 Rheumatology in general practice. Churchill Livingstone, Edinburgh, p. 109

Russek A S 1952 Diagnosis and treatment of scapulocostal syndrome. Journal of the American Medical Association 150: 25–27

Ryan G A 2000 Etiology and outcomes of whiplash: review and update. Journal of Musculoskeletal Pain 8(1/2): 3–14

Schneider R C, Schemm G W 1961 Vertebral artery insufficiency in acute and chronic spinal trauma. Journal of Neurosurgery 18: 348–360

Shapiro A P, Roth R S 1993 The effect of litigation on recovery from whiplash. Spine: State of the Art Reviews 7(3): 531–556

Simons D G, Travell J G, Simons L S 1999 Myofascial pain and dysfunction. The trigger point manual, Vol. 1, 2nd edn. Williams & Wilkins, Baltimore, pp. 439–440

Sola A E, Kuitert J H 1955 Myofascial trigger point pain in the neck and shoulder girdle. Northwest Medicine 54: 980–984

Sola A E, Williams R L 1956 Myofascial pain syndromes. Neurology (Minneapolis) 6: 91–95

Spitzer W O, Skovron M L, Salmi LR et al 1995 Scientific monograph of the Quebec Task Force on whiplash – associated disorders: Redefining 'whiplash' and its management. Spine 20(8S): 2–73

Steinberg V L, Mason R M 1959 Cervical spondylosis. Pilot therapeutic trial. Annals of Physical Medicine 5: 37

Taylor J R, Twomey L T 1993 Acute injuries to cervical joints. An autopsystudy of neck sprain. Spine 18: 1115–1122

Travell J 1967 Mechanical headache. Headache 7: 23–29

Travell J G, Simons D G 1983 Myofascial pain and dysfunction. The trigger point manual. Williams & Wilkins, Baltimore

Urban J, Maroudas A 1980 In: Graham R (ed) Clinics in rheumatic diseases, Vol. 6, No. 1. Saunders, Philadelphia

Waddell G 1982 An approach to backache. British Journal of Hospital Medicine 28(3): 187–219

Weeks V D, Travell J 1955 Postural vertigo due to trigger areas in the sternocleidomastoid muscle. Journal of Pediatrics 47: 315–327

White A R, Ernst E 1999 a systematic review of randomized controlled trials of acupuncture for neck pain. Rheumatology 38: 143–147

# Chapter 15

# Pain in the arm

## CHAPTER CONTENTS

## INTRODUCTION

In this chapter brachial pain occurring as a result of the primary activation of trigger points (TrPs) in neck, shoulder girdle, chest wall, upper arm, forearm and hand muscles will be discussed. Also, the necessity for carefully distinguishing between TrP pain and radiculopathic pain in those cases where their referral patterns happen to be similar and when TrP pain arises as a secondary event following the development of radiculopathic pain.

In addition, attention will be drawn to a number of disorders including lateral and medial epicondylalgia, neuralgic amyotrophy, shoulder–hand syndrome, and repetitive strain injury where the pathogenesis of the brachial pain is complex and TrP activity is only one of the factors responsible for its development.

## NECK AND ARM PAIN FROM CERVICAL SPONDYLOSIS, CERVICAL DISC PROLAPSE OR MYOFASCIAL TrP ACTIVATION

As already stated in Chapter 14, and repeated now, as it cannot be too strongly emphasized, there is no justification for assuming that pain in the neck and down the arm, in the absence of objective evidence of nerve root involvement, is necessarily due to either cervical disc prolapse or spondylosis. The commonest cause for its development is primary myofascial TrP (MTrP) activity.

Furthermore, even if there should be evidence of nerve root entrapment both clinically, electromyographically and from the carrying out of magnetic resonance imaging (MRI), it has to be remembered that TrP activity not uncommonly develops as a secondary event in a region affected by radiculopathic pain.

## PARAESTHESIAE AS A RESULT OF NERVE ROOT COMPRESSION OR TrP ACTIVITY

A diagnostic pitfall is to assume that because pain down a limb is accompanied by various paraesthesiae such as numbness, burning, and pins and needles, such symptoms must inevitably be due to nerve root entrapment. That this is not necessarily so and they at times are complained of by patients with primary MTrP pain was first pointed out by Sola & Kuitert (1955) and again more recently by Simons et al (1999, p. 20). The following case exemplifies this.

A publican's wife (56 years of age) with a 12-year history of intermittent neck pain for which she had frequently worn a collar, once again developed pain in the neck and down the left arm. However, what disturbed her most this time was a feeling of 'pins and needles' spreading down both sides of that arm on moving it. She was informed by her doctor that this was because she had a trapped nerve and was given some physiotherapy and told to wear a collar once again, but when after 5 months her symptoms had not improved, she herself asked for some acupuncture.

The most striking feature in this case was that whenever pressure was applied to a TrP in the supraspinatus muscle, it invariably brought on the sensation of pins and needles in the outer arm, and when pressure was applied to a TrP in the levator scapulae muscle a similar sensation travelled down the inner side of the arm to the ring and little fingers. There were no abnormal neurological signs. After deactivation of these TrPs by means of superficial dry needling carried out on four occasions at weekly intervals both the pain and paraesthesiae disappeared.

## REFERRAL OF PAIN DOWN THE ARM FROM TrPs IN THE NECK AND SHOULDER-GIRDLE MUSCLES

Michele et al (1950), Russek (1952), Long (1956), and Michele & Eisenberg (1968) were amongst

some of the first to draw attention to how commonly TrP activity in muscles in the neck and shoulder girdle is the cause of pain being referred down the arm. Then in 1971, Aronson et al published a report on 16 patients seen by them over an 8-month period with brachial pain emanating from TrPs that had been misdiagnosed as being due to a radiculopathy. They stated that they reported these because they felt it was still not sufficiently well recognized that brachial pain of myofascial origin may readily be mistaken for pain of cervical nerve root origin in those cases where their patterns of referral down the arm are similar. They also stated that prior to these patients being seen by them, because their pain had a cervical nerve root distribution, they had been misdiagnosed by orthopaedic and neurosurgeons as suffering from nerve root entrapment and subjected to prolonged periods of neck traction and the wearing of cervical collars.

They pointed out that what led them to the correct diagnosis was the absence of objective neurological signs and the discovery on careful palpation of exquisitely tender trigger areas with pressure on these causing the pain to be reproduced.

Muscles in the neck and shoulder girdle with TrP pain referral similar to that of radiculopathic pain referral are the supraspinatus, the infraspinatus, the scalenus anterior and the levator scapulae.

## TrP activity in the supraspinatus

As stated in Chapter 13, pain from TrPs in this muscle is referred to the outer side of the shoulder over the area of the deltoid muscle and down the outer side of the upper arm to the lateral epicondyle, where it is often felt particularly strongly. Its pattern of referral, therefore, coincides with the cutaneous area of distribution of the C5 nerve root, and for this reason its clinical presentation is similar to that of pain from entrapment of this nerve (Reynolds 1981).

## TrP activity in the infraspinatus

As stated in Chapter 13, pain from TrPs in this muscle is referred to the front of the shoulder, the anterolateral border of the arm and forearm, and sometimes it extends as far as the radial aspect of the hand. Its pattern of referral, therefore, coincides with the cutaneous area of distribution of the C5, C6 and C7 nerve roots and for this reason its clinical presentation is similar to that of pain from entrapment of these nerve roots (Reynolds 1981).

## TrP activity in the scalenus anterior

As stated in Chapter 12, pain from TrPs in this muscle is referred down both the anterior and posterior aspects of the upper arm, the radial border of the forearm, and terminates in the thumb and index finger, and, therefore, may also simulate a C5–C7 nerve root lesion (Reynolds 1981). Such pain is likely to persist for months or years as TrPs in this muscle, because of its anatomical position, are particularly liable to be overlooked.

A man (52 years of age) was referred to me with an 11-year history of pain down the outer side of the right arm extending from the shoulder to the index finger and thumb. The pain had been intermittent with episodes of it being brought on by bouts of heavy lifting at work. He had had numerous courses of physiotherapy directed to the neck for what he was told was a 'trapped nerve'. Having received no benefit from these he decided to try acupuncture as a last resort!

On examination of the neck there were two exquisitely tender TrPs in the right scalenus anterior muscle, with pressure on one of these causing pain to shoot down the arm to the thumb in the same distribution as the spontaneously occurring pain. The deactivation of these by means of superficial dry needling carried out at these two points quickly brought the pain under control.

## TrP activity in the levator scapulae

As stated in the previous chapter, TrP activity in the levator scapulae muscle is a common cause of pain being referred down the arm. Michele & Eisenberg (1968) estimated that it is responsible for more than 90% of all cases of cervicobrachial pain. The pain from TrPs in this muscle is referred down the inner side of the arm to the ring and little fingers in a similar manner to that of C8 T1 nerve root entrapment pain.

Electromyography may be required to distinguish MTrP pain from cervical nerve root entrapment pain, but in practice this is rarely necessary because when TrP activity is responsible for the pain, pressure on the relevant TrP almost always, in my experience, causes pain to shoot down the arm in the distribution of the spontaneously occurring pain.

A prison officer (54 years of age), 2 years before presentation, developed pain in his neck as a result of falling off his motor bike. At that time he was told that his neck X-ray showed quite marked arthritic changes, but in spite of this, the pain only lasted for 3 weeks. He was then symptom-free until 9 months before being referred to me after suffering a car collision-evoked whiplash injury to his neck. At first the neck felt persistently stiff with pain on turning it to the left side. After some weeks, he also began to get pain down the inner side of the left arm, with pins and needles in the ring and little fingers.

He was given a variety of different forms of treatment in the physiotherapy department, including neck traction, and was told to wear a collar. When after 9 months the pain in the neck and arm had not improved, and he had lost much time off work, he informed his doctor he would like to try acupuncture.

On examination there was quite marked limitation of neck movements on the left side and, in addition, there were several TrPs to be found in the muscles of the neck and shoulder girdle. In the levator scapulae muscle there were two: one at the angle of the neck, and one at the site where the muscle is inserted into the superior angle of the scapula. These were of particular interest because pressure on either of them caused pain to radiate down the medial side of the arm to the ring and little fingers in exactly the same distribution as that of pain from a C8 T1 nerve root lesion.

Following deactivation of these TrPs by the carrying out of superficial dry needling on two occasions the pain was brought sufficiently under control for him to be able to return to work.

## CERVICAL RADICULOPATHIC BRACHIAL PAIN FOLLOWED BY THE DEVELOPMENT OF MTrP BRACHIAL PAIN

From what has already been said, it may be seen that the patterns of pain referral down the arm from either compression of a cervical nerve root or TrP activity in a neck or shoulder girdle muscle may in certain cases be identical. To add to the confusion it has to be remembered that a muscle, such as for example the pectoralis minor or scalene anterior, when shortened as a result of TrP activity, may compress roots of the underlying brachial plexus with, as a consequence, radiculopathic and TrP pain radiating down the arm concomitantly. It should also be remembered that, as Simons et al (1999, p. 81) have pointed out, TrP activity is liable to develop as a secondary event in muscles innervated by an entrapped nerve root due to the effect nerve root compression has on a TrP's dysfunctional motor endplates.

## PAIN REFERRAL DOWN THE ARM FROM THE HEART AND FROM TrPs IN THE CHEST WALL MUSCLES

Pain that radiates down the arm does not of course necessarily stem from either a cervical nerve root lesion or from TrPs in the muscles of the neck or shoulder girdle. It may also, as already stated in Chapter 12, be referred down the arm from TrPs in the muscles of the chest wall or from the heart in coronary artery disease.

Pain down the arm from TrP activity in muscles of the chest wall is usually readily distinguished from pain emanating from the muscles of the neck, because the pain is almost always felt in the chest itself as well as in the arm, as may be seen from the diagrams of the TrP pain patterns of such muscles as the pectoralis major (Fig. 12.7), pectoralis minor (Fig. 12.10), serratus anterior (Fig. 12.11), serratus posterior superior (Fig. 12.13) and the latissimus dorsi (Fig. 12.15).

It is important to remember, however, that whilst anginal pain is usually felt across the front of the chest, as well as at other sites such as the neck and arm, at times it may be predominantly felt in the neck and arm, and occasionally it may be confined entirely to the arm. The latter may be somewhat misleading and is not sufficiently well recognized, despite it having been well known to William Heberden (1818) nearly 200 years ago, as may be seen from reading Chapter 70 entitled 'Pectoris Dolor' in his famous *Commentaries on the History and Cure of Diseases*.

## TRICEPS MUSCLE

This is the only muscle in the upper arm in which TrP activity is likely to give rise to widespread pain affecting both the neck and arm.

## Activation of TrPs

TrPs may become activated in the long, medial or lateral heads of the muscle as a result of it becoming overloaded during the carrying out of sports such as tennis and golf or doing 'press ups'. Also, when this happens as a result of sitting for any length of time with the arm held forwards without the elbow being adequately supported, such as when driving a car for a long distance.

TrPs in the medial and lateral heads give rise to localized pain around the epicondyles of the humerus and will therefore be referred to later in the chapter when discussing lateral and medial epicondylalgia.

## LONG HEAD OF THE TRICEPS

It is TrP activity in the long head of the triceps that cause pain to radiate over a wide area of the neck and arm.

## Specific pattern of pain referral

Pain from these TrPs is referred upwards over the posterior part of the shoulder, occasionally to the base of the neck and sometimes down the back of the forearm to the wrist (Fig. 13.13). It is because of this pattern that the pain is sometimes confused with that of a C7 radiculopathy.

## TrP examination

TrPs in this head are usually to be found deep in the belly of the muscle just below the level of the posterior axillary fold (Fig. 13.13). They are present in taut bands which, when plucked, give local twitch responses.

When TrPs in the long head are the cause of pain it is not possible to press the upraised arm hard against the ear when the elbow is kept straight (Fig. 13.14).

## Deactivation of TrPs

When deactivating TrPs in the triceps muscle by means of the carrying out of superficial dry needling, the patient should lie in the semi-prone position with the affected arm uppermost.

## BRACHIAL PLEXUS INJURIES

The brachial plexus may be damaged by stab wounds, bullets, or iatrogenically by surgical operations on the neck. The nerves in such cases, however, usually remain in continuity and, with present day neurosurgical techniques, repair operations usually result in good functional recovery without any serious residual pain.

When, however, this plexus is damaged during the course of irradiating neoplastic glands in the neck, this may lead many years later to gradual wasting of the muscles of the hand and the development of severe pain. This neuropathic type of pain is not readily controlled by drugs or acupuncture, but transcutaneous electrical nerve stimulation (TENS) sometimes proves helpful.

## Avulsion of brachial plexus cervical nerve roots

By far the commonest type of brachial plexus injury at the present time is the tearing away of its nerve roots from the spinal cord during the course of a motorcycle accident. This type of traction lesion, unfortunately usually affects an otherwise fit young man leaving him with an irreversibly paralyzed and totally anaesthetic arm, and one in which, in almost 90% of cases, there is severe intractable pain that takes the form of a persistent severe burning as if the arm is on fire (causalgia), and superimposed upon this are episodic paroxysms of intense momentary shooting pain through the arm.

As Wynn Parry (1980, 1984) pointed out, the single most helpful method of gaining some relief from the pain is for the patient to distract his mind from it by concentrating on work or hobbies. By this means it is often possible for him to get through a working day quite comfortably but, as soon as he sits down to relax in the evening, the pain builds up and at times becomes almost unbearable.

Analgesic drugs have little effect on it, but Wynn Parry (1984) has found TENS to be helpful.

With respect to this, just as acupuncture does not work if needles, whether they be stimulated manually or electrically, are inserted into a part of the body deprived of feeling, so TENS does not work if the electrodes are applied to skin that is anaesthetic. It is therefore essential in combating the pain of a nerve root avulsion lesion firstly to map out the area of anaesthesia and then to place the electrodes on skin above the upper level of this.

## Compression of the brachial plexus (thoracic outlet syndrome)

Until about 30 years ago, it was widely taught that a common cause of generalized pain spreading down the arm from the neck, with pins and needles in the fingers, was compression of the lower trunk of the brachial plexus, either by it being stretched as it passed over a cervical rib, or compressed as it passed between the scalenus anterior and a normal first rib (the scalenus anterior syndrome).

It is now realized that, although a cervical rib is frequently seen on routine X-rays of the neck, only in about 10% of cases does it cause symptoms, and also that entrapment of the brachial plexus by the scalenus anterior muscle with its very similar clinical picture is also uncommon. Nevertheless, when a patient presents with pain in the arm in the distribution of the C8 T1 nerve roots, such causes of what collectively is known as the thoracic outlet syndrome have to be considered.

In this syndrome there is pain down the inner side of the arm, often from the elbow downwards, associated with paraesthesiae such as numbness or pins and needles affecting the ulnar side of the hand; also some sensory loss on the ulnar side of the hand and forearm, and wasting of the small muscles of the hand supplied by the ulnar nerve, such as the interossei and adductor pollicis.

When these neurological symptoms and signs are due to stretching of the brachial plexus over a cervical rib, there may also be evidence of compression of the subclavian artery, including a bruit to be heard in the neck on auscultation and circulatory changes to be found in the fingers.

The stretching of the brachial plexus over a cervical rib most commonly gives rise to symptoms and signs in middle-aged women when loss of tone in the muscles of the shoulder girdle causes this to droop. Relief from pain may, therefore, often be obtained by exercises designed to strengthen these muscles. However, when vascular changes predominate, or there is progressive wasting of the muscles of the hand, then the rib should be removed. Before embarking upon this, care should be taken to exclude an ulnar nerve lesion at the elbow as this may cause similar neurological signs in the forearm and hand.

When the underlying cause of the syndrome is a taut shortened scalenus anterior, then the neurological changes may be associated with symptoms from pressure on the subclavian vein, and only rarely with those associated with pressure on the artery.

Scalenotomy for the relief of pain in the scalenus anterior syndrome proved to be disappointing and is no longer performed. If the condition occurs because of myofascial TrPs in the scalenus anterior then these should be deactivated by the carrying out of superficial dry needling.

With respect to all this it has to be remembered that when pain arises as a result of the development of TrP activity in this muscle, without shortenening of it due to this giving rise to pressure on the brachial plexus, then the referral of pain is down the radial side of the forearm and hand (Ch. 12).

Finally, it cannot be stressed too strongly that in all cases where there is pain down the inner side of the arm from the neck with pins and needles in the ring and little fingers, in the absence of objective neurological signs and of signs of vascular compression, an active search for TrPs in the levator scapulae should always be made, as this is frequently a cause of pain in this distribution (Ch. 14).

## LATERAL EPICONDYLALGIA (SYNS: LATERAL EPICONDYLITIS, TENNIS ELBOW)

### Terminology

The disorder in which in response to repeated microtrauma severe pain develops in the lateral epicondylar region, with pressure on the lateral epicondyle and resisted dorsiflexion at the wrist making it worse, is best called lateral epicondylalgia. This is because tennis elbow is a misnomer, as the playing of tennis is an aetiological factor in its production in less than 5% of the people affected by it (Coonrad & Hooper 1973), and because epicondylitis is an inappropriate term as there is no inflammation of the epicondyle itself.

## Pathophysiology

### Enthesopathy

This disorder is an enthesopathy affecting the common extensor tendon at its attachment to the lateral epicondyle. Chard & Hazleman (1989), from studying biopsy material taken prior to the carrying out of surgery for this disorder, found that initially there is an inflammatory reaction in and later degenerative tissue damage of this tendon. Potter et al (1995) have since reached the same conclusion as a result of correlating MRI, histopathological and surgical findings.

## Inflammatory reaction and TrP activity

Doubt concerning the type of inflammatory lesion present in this disorder has recently been raised as a result of Ljung et al (1999) investigating it by means of employing immunohistochemistry and antibodies to the neuropeptides Substance P (SP) and calcitonin gene-related peptide. It was shown by this means that nerve fibres distributed in association with a subpopulation of small blood vessels showed SP-like and calcitonin gene-related peptide-like immunoreactivity. Furthermore, contrary to what is generally believed, there were no inflammatory-cell infiltrates and only a few solitary mast cells.

This study therefore provided evidence in support of suggestions previously made that the inflammatory reaction in this disorder is of a neurogenic type with the release of these neuropeptides from sensory afferent nerve endings causing microvascular leakage and local oedema formation. A finding that clearly has important implications with respect to the rationale for the use of corticosteroids in its treatment.

Another important discovery made in recent years is that the pain in this disorder is not only due to the development of an enthesopathy but also to the development of TrP activity in various muscles in the vicinity of the elbow. These include the supinator, brachioradialis, extensor carpi radialis longus and brevis, extensor digitorum and the lower end of the lateral margin of the medial head of the triceps (Simons et al 1999, pp. 734–742).

## Clinical features

In this disorder there is a persistent dull ache with, at times, bouts of acute pain on the outer side of the elbow. The pain is aggravated by putting the wrist extensors on the stretch, such as when the pronated wrist is passively flexed. It is also made worse by any action that causes these muscles to contract, such as when the wrist is extended against resistance. It is possible therefore to lift a chair comfortably when it is gripped with the hand, palm upwards, but there is considerable aggravation of the pain when this is done with the hand palm downwards.

There is, in addition, some weakness of the grip with a tendency to drop objects. Also, any attempt to sustain a grip such as when shaking hands aggravates the pain.

The lateral epicondyle is invariably extremely tender. Also, in some cases the surrounding tissues feel warm and appear to be swollen.

## Differential diagnosis

Other causes for pain in the lateral epicondylar region include arthritis of the elbow joint, and referral of it there either as a result of cervical nerve root entrapment or because of the development of TrP activity in a muscle of the neck, particularly the supraspinatus.

## Factors responsible for development of TrP activity

TrP activity in muscles in the vicinity of the epicondyle develops as a result of trauma. This activity may arise when there is direct injury to the elbow or when the muscles and their attachments at or near to the elbow become suddenly wrenched. It more often arises, however, when the muscles are traumatized as a result of repeated strenuous extensor movements at the wrist.

The supinator, as its name implies, is the principal muscle responsible for supinating the hand and forearm at the radioulnar joint, but the biceps assists with the movement providing the elbow is flexed slightly. It therefore follows that whenever the muscle is liable to be subjected to undue strain, such as when hitting a tennis ball backhanded, both the elbow and wrist should be held in a slightly flexed position. It is when tennis players fail to do this and take backhand shots with the arm straight that the supinator becomes overloaded. This then causes TrP activity to develop in it with, as a consequence, the referral of pain to the lateral epicondyle.

It is not, however, only tennis players who are liable to develop the disorder, but anybody who has to hold the arm straight with the forearm in a position of supination for any length of time, or has to carry a load with the elbows flexed and the hands held in the pronated position. Heavy objects in fact should always be carried with the hand palm upwards, as then much of the strain is taken by the biceps.

Other common activities liable to put an abnormal strain on this muscle include the repeated turning of a stiff door knob, the unscrewing of a tight jar lid, the controlling of a heavy dog straining at the leash, and the raking of leaves.

Similar activities may also sometimes lead to the activation of TrPs in the brachioradialis and the extensor carpi radialis longus. In addition, TrPs may become activated in the extensor digitorum as a result of forceful repetitive movements of the fingers by such people as musicians, craftsmen and gardeners.

## TrP examination at the elbow

TrPs in the supinator are usually to be found at its distal attachment to the anterior surface of the radius just below the insertion of the tendon of the biceps into the radial tuberosity. When searching for them the hand should be fully *supinated*. Also the brachioradialis should be pushed out of the way in a lateral direction. This is most readily done

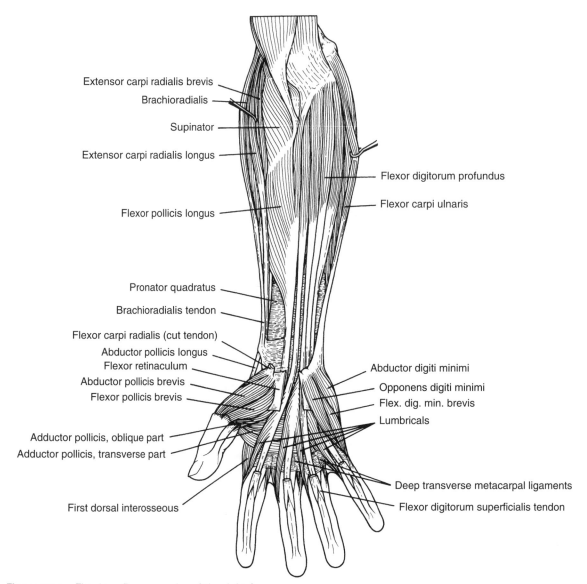

**Figure 15.1** The deep flexor muscles of the right forearm.

if the elbow is slightly flexed. Any TrPs present will then be found to lie just under the skin between the biceps tendon medially and the brachioradialis laterally (Fig. 15.1).

The finding of TrPs in the brachioradialis and extensor carpi radialis longus should be carried out with the elbow slightly flexed and with the foream resting comfortably on a pillow in the prone position (Fig. 15.2). They are located about 3 cm distal to the lateral epicondyle (Figs 15.3 & 15.4).

The locating of TrPs in the extensor digitorum should be carried out with the arm in the same position as for the brachioradialis and extensor carpi radialis longus. TrPs in this muscle lie about 6 cm below the lateral epicondyle (Fig. 15.5).

The anatomical arrangement of the triceps muscle is such that the medial head just above the elbow extends from one side of the arm to the other beneath the muscle's common tendon of attachment to the olecranon process of the ulna.

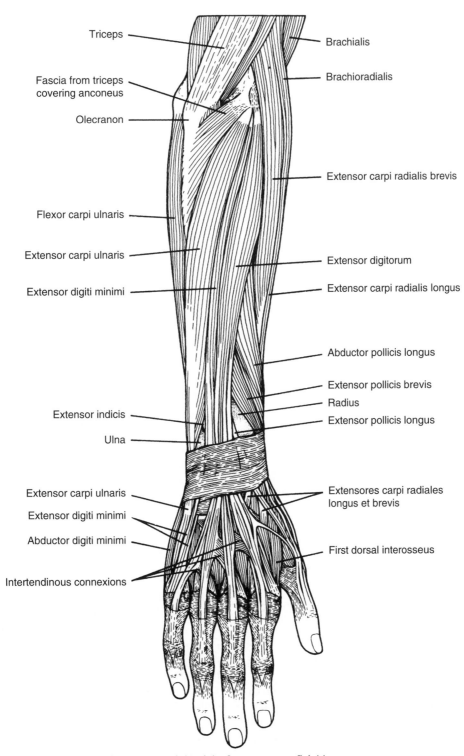

**Figure 15.2**    Muscles of the extensor aspect of the right forearm, superficial layer.

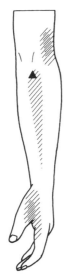

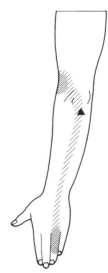

**Figure 15.3**   Pattern of pain referral from a trigger point (▲) in the brachioradialis muscle.

**Figure 15.5**   The pattern of pain referral from a trigger point (▲) in the extensor digitorum muscle (ring finger extensor).

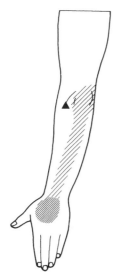

**Figure 15.4**   Pattern of pain referral from a trigger point (▲) in the extensor carpi radialis longus muscle.

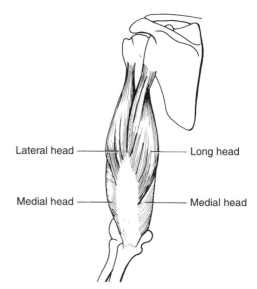

**Figure 15.6**   The medial, lateral and long heads of the triceps muscle. It should be noted that the lower part of the medial head just above the elbow extends from one side of the arm to the other beneath the muscle's common tendon of attachment to the olecranon process of the ulna.

The lower part of the lateral border of the medial head is, therefore, just above the lateral epicondyle, and the lower part of the medial border of this head is just above the medial epicondyle (Fig. 15.6).

A TrP in the medial border refers pain to the medial epicondyle and sometimes down the arm to the ring and little fingers and will be discussed again when considering medial epicondylalgia

and when considering the differential diagnosis of ulnar nerve entrapment (p. 240).

It is a TrP in the lateral border of the medial head just above the elbow which commonly refers

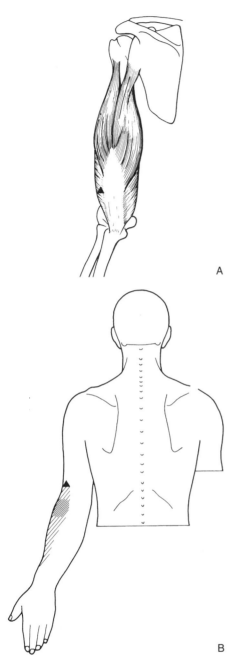

**Figure 15.7**  (A) Trigger point in the lateral border of the medial head of the triceps muscle. (B) Pattern of pain referral from this trigger point.

pain to the lateral epicondyle in 'tennis elbow'. It is found about 4 cm or approximately 1.5 in above the lateral epicondyle near to the attachments of the extensor carpi radialis longus and the brachioradialis (Figs 15.7A & B).

## Treatment

### Non-steroidal anti-inflammatory drug administration

Hay et al (1999), in a randomized controlled trial carried out to compare the relative efficacy of a local corticosteroid and the NSAID naproxen for the treatment of this disorder, concluded that a 2-week course of this NSAID gave no better pain relief than that provided by a placebo.

### Local injection of a corticosteroid

It is a long established practice to inject a steroid at the enthesopathy site. Methods of doing this vary but a widely employed one (Chard 1995) is to inject at the site of maximum tenderness on the lateral epicondyle a hydrocortisone (10–25 mgs)/local anaesthetic mixture with the needle inserted far enough for it to impinge upon the periosteum. A fan-shaped injection procedure is then carried out that involves frequent partial withdrawals and reinsertions of the needle. The main disadvantage of this technique is that it is liable to give rise to much pain during the time it is being carried out.

### Reviews of steroid injection clinical trials

A review carried out by Assendelft et al (1996) of 12 clinical trials led them to conclude that the pain relief following a corticosteroid injection in this disorder is usually relatively short-lasting and often has to be repeated after 4–6 weeks.

A sytematic review of randomized controlled trials identified by a search of six databases carried out by Smidt et al (2002) led them to conclude that it is not possible to draw firm conclusions as to the long-term effectiveness of steroid injections in this disorder due to the lack of high-quality studies; therefore, more better designed, conducted and reported randomized controlled trials with intermediate and long-term follow up are needed.

Altay et al (2002), employing the peppering technique already described have compared the pain-relieving effectiveness of injecting a corticosteroid (triamcinolone)/local anaesthetic mixture with that of injecting a local anaesthetic alone into the lateral epicondyle. That they obtained equally

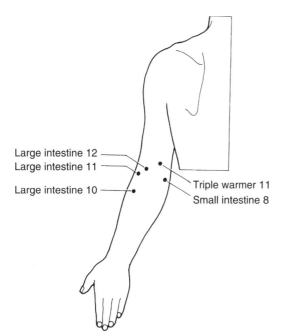

**Figure 15.8** Traditional Chinese acupuncture points at the back of the elbow.

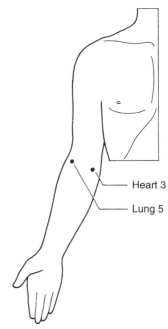

**Figure 15.9** Traditional Chinese acupuncture points on the inner and outer sides of the front of the elbow.

good results raises the possibility that with both types of treatment the pain relief was due to the effect of the one factor common to both – the peppering of the periosteum with a needle (i.e. to the carrying out of acupuncture).

### Acupuncture carried out at traditional Chinese acupuncture points

Haker & Lundeberg (1990) carried out a study in 82 patients with lateral epicondylalgia to compare the pain-alleviating effect of inserting needles deeply into five traditional Chinese acupuncture points (Large intestine 10, 11, 12 [Fig. 15.8], Lung 5 [Fig. 15.9] and Sanjiao 5, a point immediately above the transverse crease of the wrist on its dorsal side) with that of inserting them superficially at those sites. In each of the two groups the needles were left in situ for 20 minutes, 2–3 times a week, for a total of 10 treatments.

The results of this trial showed that deep needling is superior to superficial needling when carried out at these traditional Chinese acupuncture points.

### Acupuncture carried out concomitantly at the lateral epicondyle's point of maximum tenderness, traditional Chinese acupuncture points and TrP sites

In view of differences of opinion concerning the optimum method of employing acupuncture for the treatment of lateral epicondylalgia, Webster-Harrison et al (2002) have carried out an e-mail-collated consensus study. Those taking part in this were 14 medical practitioners who teach on the British Medical Acupuncture Society's training courses.

The consensus of opinion was that the optimum acupuncture treatment and the one that should be used in any future randomized controlled trial is as follows.

At the initial treatment needles should be inserted deeply into the following traditional Chinese acupuncture points – Large intestine 4 (situated in first dorsal interosseous muscle) and Large intestine 11 (situated in the depression at the lateral end of the transverse cubital crease). A needle should also be inserted at the lateral epicondyle's point of maximum tenderness far enough for it to reach the periosteum. In addition, needles should be inserted at three TrP sites. The duration of needling at the traditional Chinese points should be 5 minutes, and at the periosteum site and TrP sites it should be limited to no more than 3 minutes.

On subsequent occasions the strength of stimulation at these sites should be increased or decreased according to an individual patient's responsiveness to the initial treatment.

It was recommended that acupuncture should be carried out weekly for a minimum of 2 weeks and that up to eight treatments should be given if evidence of improvement warrants this.

The main purpose of formulating this standard acupuncture treatment regime is for it to be used in any future large-scale randomized controlled trial. There is certainly a great need for one as Green et al (2002), from a very extensive computer search for trials carried out between 1966 and 2001, found that during that time there had only been four small randomized controlled trials worth considering. And from the results of those they were led to conclude: 'There is insufficient evidence to either support or refute the use of acupuncture (either needle or laser) in the treatment of lateral elbow pain …. Further trials, utilising appropriate methods and adequate sample sizes, are needed before conclusions can be drawn regarding the effect of acupuncture on tennis elbow.'

My personal current practice is to carry out both pecking of the periosteum at the lateral epicondyle's point of maximum tenderness and superficial dry needling at all the TrP sites found to be present in the nearby muscles.

## MEDICAL EPICONDYLALGIA (SYNS: MEDIAL EPICONDYLITIS, GOLFER'S ELBOW)

This is a similar condition to that which affects the lateral epicondyle, but one that occurs far less commonly. It arises when, as a result of the flexor muscles of the wrist and hand becoming strained, TrPs become activated in these muscles near to their common tendon attachment to the medial epicondyle.

It is characteristic of this disorder that resisted flexion of the wrist, when the elbow is extended, aggravates the pain.

The advantages and disadvantages of a local corticosteroid in this condition are similar to those

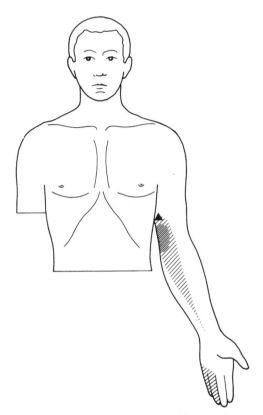

**Figure 15.10**  Pattern of pain referral from a trigger point in the medial border of the medial head of the triceps muscle.

when using this form of treatment in lateral epicondylalgia so they will not be further discussed.

Acupuncture carried out in a similar manner to that used in the treatment of lateral epicondylalgia is a worthwhile alternative, and, with respect to TrPs, there are two of these that usually have to be deactivated. One is to be found in the common flexor tendon near to its attachment to the medial epicondyle not far from the traditional Chinese acupuncture point Heart 3 (Fig. 15.9); the other is to be found along the medial border of the medial head of the triceps immediately above the medial epicondyle (Fig. 15.10), and therefore in the region of the Chinese acupuncture point Small Intestine 8 (Fig. 15.8).

## PAIN IN THE WRIST AND HAND FROM TrPs IN THE FOREARM MUSCLES

Persistent pain confined to the wrist and hand region may occur as a direct result of some local disorder, or it may arise indirectly as a result of it being referred there from TrPs some distance away in the muscles of the forearm. It is particularly essential to bear the possibility of the latter in mind as, otherwise, with there being nothing abnormal to find at the site where the pain is felt, there is always the risk that any patient suffering from this may be considered to be either neurotic or a malingerer.

Although it is now over 40 years since Kelly (1944) first drew attention to the clinical importance of this particular cause of pain in the wrist and hand, too little attention is still being paid to it in current medical teaching, and, therefore, it will be dealt with at some length.

## Forearm extensor muscles

The forearm extensor muscles in which TrP activity is liable to cause pain to be referred to the wrist and hand include the extensor carpi radialis longus, the extensor carpi radialis brevis, the extensor carpi ulnaris, and the extensor digitorum. TrP activity in the anatomically closely related brachioradialis and supinator muscles may also be responsible for this (Fig. 15.2).

### Activation of TrPs in these muscles

TrPs in these muscles are liable to become activated as a result of carrying out forceful twisting movements with some tool such as a screwdriver or trowel whilst holding it with a very firm grip.

### Specific TrP pain patterns

**Supinator muscle** TrPs in the supinator muscle refer pain primarily to the lateral epicondyle, but at times they may also cause it to be felt in the region of the first dorsal interosseous muscle (Fig. 15.11).

**Brachioradialis muscle** TrPs in the brachioradialis muscle, in contradistinction to those in the supinator muscle, refer pain primarily to the region

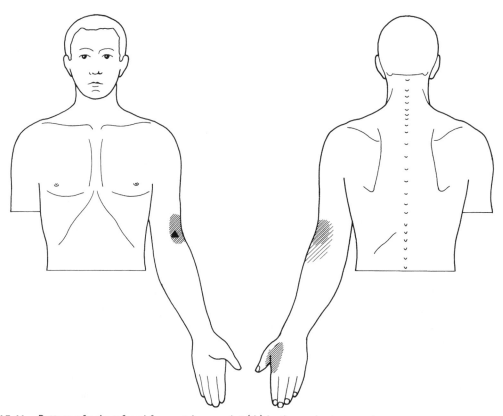

**Figure 15.11**  Pattern of pain referral from a trigger point (▲) in the supinator muscle.

of the 1st dorsal interosseous muscle, and only occasionally to the lateral epicondyle (Fig. 15.3).

**Extensor carpi radialis longus**    TrPs in the extensor carpi radialis longus refer pain to the lateral epicondyle and down the forearm to be felt predominantly on the dorsum of the hand in the region of the anatomical 'snuff box' – the hollow on the outer side of the wrist between the tendons of the extensor pollicis radialis longus and brevis (Fig. 15.4).

It has to be remembered that when TrPs in the above muscles refer pain to the region of the 1st dorsal interosseous muscle or the anatomical 'snuff box', satellite TrPs may develop at these sites, and have to be distinguished from primarily activated ones that, as will be discussed later, may also develop at these sites as a result of trauma to the wrist.

It is also of interest to note in passing that the Chinese in their traditional system of acupuncture have a well-known point, Large Intestine 4 (Ho-Ku or Hegu), in the first dorsal interosseous muscle

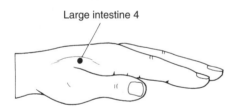

**Figure 15.12**    The traditional Chinese acupuncture point Large Intestine 4 (Hoku or Hegu) in the 1st dorsal interosseous muscle.

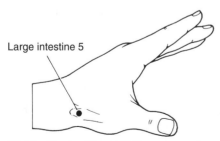

**Figure 15.13**    The traditional Chinese acupunture point Large Intestine 5 (Yang Xi) in the anatomical snuff box – the hollow on the outer side of the wrist between the tendons of the extensor pollicis radialis longus and brevis muscles.

(Fig. 15.12), and another point, Large Intestine 5 (Yang Xi in the anatomical 'snuff box', Fig. 15.13).

**Extensor digitorum**    TrPs in the extensor digitorum cause pain to be referred down the back of the forearm, back of the hand and into individual fingers, depending on which muscle fibres are involved. The middle finger extensor probably is the one most often involved (Fig. 15.14).

TrPs in the ring and little finger extensors are also liable to cause pain to be referred upwards to the lateral epicondyle (Fig. 15.5).

**Extensor carpi radialis brevis**    TrPs in the extensor carpi radialis brevis are found below the level of those occurring in the extensor carpi radialis longus at about 6 cm (or approximately 2 in) below the elbow crease. Pain from these TrPs is referred to the back of the hand and wrist (Fig. 15.15).

**Extensor carpi ulnaris**    TrPs in this muscle occur at about the same level in the forearm as those in the extensor carpi radialis brevis, and as Gutstein (1938) showed, refer pain to a localized area around the ulnar side of the back of the wrist (Fig. 15.16).

The following case illustrates how TrPs in several extensor forearm muscles may be responsible for the development of a composite pain pattern.

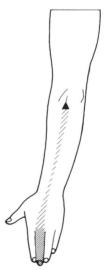

**Figure 15.14**    The pattern of pain referral from a trigger point (▲) in the extensor digitorum muscle (middle finger extensor).

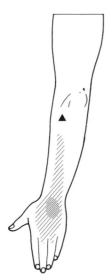

**Figure 15.15**   The pattern of pain referral from a trigger point (▲) in the extensor carpi radialis brevis muscle.

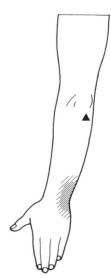

**Figure 15.16**   The pattern of pain referral from a trigger point (▲) in the extensor carpi ulnaris muscle.

A housewife (60 years of age), who was also a keen gardener, and who frequently gripped the handle of a trowel tightly whilst weeding, presented with a 9-month history of pain at the back of the wrist, at the base of the thumb, and in the fingers, together with some discomfort in the outer part of the elbow.

She complained that the fingers felt bloated and as if they were going to burst. She also complained that the grip of her hand was becoming increasingly weak, and that this, together with the pain and swelling of her fingers, and the consequent difficulty with bending them, had led her to become concerned that she might be developing arthritis.

The patient was examined sitting comfortably on a chair with the forearm resting on a pillow, and the elbow slightly bent.

The weak grip was confirmed by getting the patient to squeeze two of my fingers. This action also increased the pain both at the elbow and in the hand.

Flat palpation of the extensor muscles just below the lateral epicondyle revealed TrPs to be present in the extensor carpi radialis longus, and these must have been partly responsible for the lateral epicondyle pain, and pain at the base of the thumb. There were also TrPs in the extensor carpi radialis brevis, which must have been responsible for the pain at the back of the wrist and TrPs in the extensor digitorum that must have been partly responsible for the pain at the elbow, and also in the fingers.

Deactivation of these TrPs by means of the carrying out of superficial dry needling on four occasions at weekly intervals relieved her of the pain, but on going back to gardening she again developed pain in the hand as a result of the reactivation of TrPs in the forearm and eventually she decided it was better to employ someone to do the weeding!

## Forearm flexor muscles

The forearm flexor muscles in which TrP activity is liable to cause pain to be referred to the front of the wrist and hand include the flexor carpi radialis, the flexor carpi ulnaris, and the flexor digitorum (superficialis and profundus), all of which are attached proximally to the medial epicondyle by means of a common tendon; also the flexor pollicis longus which is attached proximally to the radius.

### Anatomical relationships of the muscles

In order to be able to identify in which of these various muscles a particular TrP is located, it is helpful to remember that they are arranged in three layers with the superficial layer consisting of the flexor carpi radialis, and the flexor carpi ulnaris, separated by the palmaris longus; the intermediate layer consists of the flexor digitorum

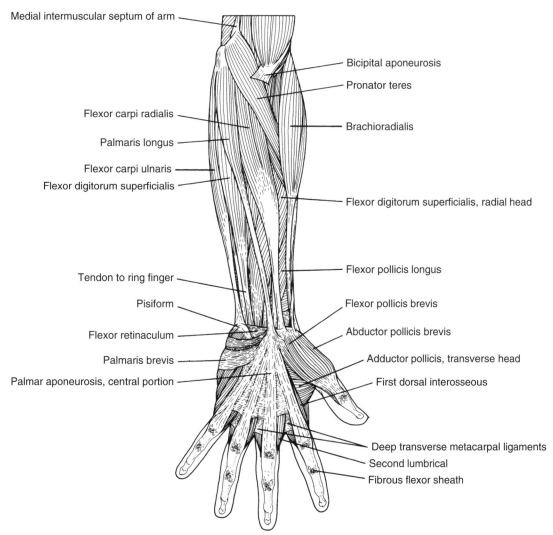

Medial intermuscular septum of arm

Bicipital aponeurosis

Pronator teres

Flexor carpi radialis

Brachioradialis

Palmaris longus

Flexor carpi ulnaris

Flexor digitorum superficialis

Flexor digitorum superficialis, radial head

Flexor pollicis longus

Tendon to ring finger

Pisiform

Flexor pollicis brevis

Flexor retinaculum

Abductor pollicis brevis

Palmaris brevis

Adductor pollicis, transverse head

Palmar aponeurosis, central portion

First dorsal interosseous

Deep transverse metacarpal ligaments

Second lumbrical

Fibrous flexor sheath

**Figure 15.17**   The superficial flexor muscles of the left forearm, the palmar aponeurosis and the digital fibrous flexor sheaths.

superficialis (Fig. 15.17); and the deep layer consists of the flexor digitorum profundus, and the flexor pollicis longus (Fig. 15.1).

### Activation of TrPs

TrPs situated in the hand and finger flexor muscles in the forearm are liable to be activated by prolonged gripping. It commonly occurs, for example, when the steering wheel of a car is gripped tightly during a long journey, particularly when the hands are placed on the top of the steering wheel in the flexed position.

TrPs in the flexor pollicis longus become activated as a result of gripping tightly with the thumb whilst carrying out any twisting pulling movement such as may occur when weeding.

### Specific pain patterns and TrP locations

**Flexor carpi radialis and flexor carpi ulnaris**
TrPs in these two muscles cause pain to be referred either to the radial aspect or the ulnar aspect of the palmar surface of the wrist according to which one is involved (Fig. 15.18). The TrPs in either of these muscles are to be found high up the forearm just

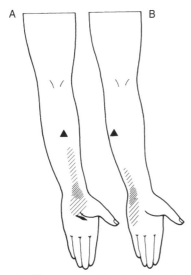

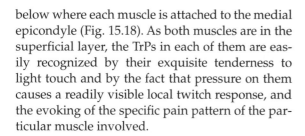

**Figure 15.18**    The patterns of pain referral from trigger points (▲) in (A) the flexor carpi radialis muscle and (B) the flexor carpi ulnaris muscle.

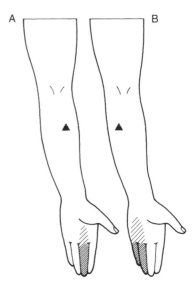

**Figure 15.19**    The patterns of pain referral from trigger points (▲) in the flexor digitorum superficialis (A) radial head (B) humeral head.

below where each muscle is attached to the medial epicondyle (Fig. 15.18). As both muscles are in the superficial layer, the TrPs in each of them are easily recognized by their exquisite tenderness to light touch and by the fact that pressure on them causes a readily visible local twitch response, and the evoking of the specific pain pattern of the particular muscle involved.

**Flexor digitorum superficialis and profundus**
TrPs in various parts of these two muscles refer pain to individual fingers. Such points are to be found at almost the same level in the forearm as those in the flexor carpi radialis and ulnaris (Fig. 15.19). However, as the digital flexors lie deep to the hand flexors, any TrPs in them are more difficult to locate, and require firm pressure to elicit the deep seated tenderness associated with their presence, and even with this, neither a local twitch response nor any of the various specific pain patterns can be evoked.

**Flexor pollicis longus**    TrPs in this muscle cause pain to be felt in the thumb. As this muscle is deep lying, firm pressure is required to elicit any TrP tenderness in it. Such points are usually to be found on the radial side of the forearm about one-quarter way up from the wrist crease (Fig. 15.20).

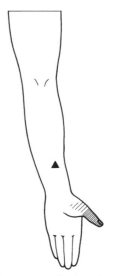

**Figure 15.20**    The pattern of pain referral from a trigger point (▲) in the flexor pollicis longus muscle.

## Ulnar nerve entrapment at the elbow (cubital tunnel syndrome)

The ulnar nerve at the elbow is held in a groove behind the medial epicondyle by a fibrous expansion of the common flexor tendon. It then enters the forearm beneath an arch formed by the humeral and ulnar heads of the flexor carpi ulnaris muscle to occupy a space bounded by the flexor carpi ulnaris superficially and medially, the flexor digitorum superficialis superficially and laterally, and the flexor digitorum profundus behind it.

The ulnar nerve is at risk of being damaged either by external pressure being applied to it where it lies behind the medial epicondyle, or by it becoming constricted in the cubital tunnel by arthritic or other structural changes affecting the elbow joint. Not infrequently, however, this entrapment may occur in the absence of structural pathological changes. In some of these cases there is evidence of TrP activity in the forearm flexor muscles, but exactly how this leads to pressure being exerted on the nerve is far from clear.

The symptoms of ulnar nerve entrapment are gradual in onset with numbness and tingling affecting the fifth finger and the ulnar half of the ring finger, followed at a later stage by weakness and wasting of the small muscles of the hand. If the ulnar nerve becomes damaged where it lies behind the medial epicondyle, then pressure on the nerve at that site will reproduce the symptoms. The only effective treatment when the nerve is bound down by fibrous tissue is a surgical operation to release it from the groove and transpose it to the front of the elbow. If, on the other hand, TrPs are found to be present just below the medial epicondyle in the flexor muscles, then deactivating them may in some cases, presumably by reducing tension in the muscles, be sufficient to relieve the pressure on the nerve.

It should be noted that pain is not an outstanding feature with ulnar nerve entrapment and, therefore, in all cases when pain affects the medial side of the forearm and hand, an alternative diagnosis should be sought. The differential diagnosis including cervical nerve root entrapment (C8 T1 nerve roots), TrP activity in the levator scapulae muscle (Ch. 14) and TrP activity in the medial border of the medial head of the triceps.

### TrP in the medial distal border of the medial head of the triceps

A TrP may be found in the medial border of the medial head of triceps just above the medial malleolus.

### Specific pattern of pain referral

It refers pain to the medial epicondyle (p. 210) and down the inner side of the anterior forearm to terminate in the ring and little fingers (Fig. 15.10).

### TrP location

It is best located and then deactivated with a dry needle, with the patient lying down in the supine position with the arm externally rotated, the forearm supinated, the elbow slightly flexed, and the whole of the arm supported comfortably on a pillow.

The following case illustrates how failure to recognize TrP activity in muscles around the medial epicondyle could have resulted in an unnecessary operation.

A ward sister (36 years of age) complained that for 1 year she had had pain around the left elbow radiating down the inner side of the arm with some discomfort in the little and ring fingers. An orthopaedic surgeon thought it was due to ulnar nerve root entrapment and recommended that the nerve should be transposed from behind the medial epicondyle to the front of the joint. The patient, not liking the thought of having an operation, asked to be referred to me to see whether acupuncture had anything to offer.

On examination there were two exquisitely tender TrPs, one in the medial border of the medial head of the triceps just above the medial epicondyle and another just below it. After deactivating these by means of the carrying out of superficial dry needling on three occasions, she was relieved of her symptoms.

## Palmaris longus and pronator teres muscles

TrP activity in these two forearm muscles may also cause pain to be referred to the hand.

### Palmaris longus

This vestigial muscle is not always present, but when it is, it also is attached proximally to the medial epicondyle and distally to the palmar fascia, and has as its main action the cupping of the hand. It also assists flexion of the hand at the wrist.

It lies, as previously stated, in the superficial layer of the flexor forearm muscles, between the flexor carpi ulnaris and the flexor carpi radialis (Fig. 15.17).

**Location of TrPs**    TrPs in this muscle are found high up in the forearm just below the medial epicondyle (Fig. 15.21).

**Activation of TrPs**    These TrPs may become activated as a result of repeatedly gripping some object such as a tennis racquet or tool excessively tightly. They may also become activated as a secondary event whenever pain is referred to the upper part of the forearm from similar points just above the medial epicondyle in the medial head of the triceps muscle. In addition, Simons et al (1999, p. 746) have observed that patients with Dupuytren's contracture invariably have one or more active TrP(s) in this forearm muscle.

**Specific pattern of pain referral**    There is a persistent unpleasant tingling sensation in the palm of the hand, and the patient complains of discomfort on applying pressure to any object held in the palm. This, therefore, makes the handling of tools difficult.

**Deactivation of TrPs**    Deactivation of these TrPs just below the elbow is carried out with the forearm extended and well supported.

*Pronator teres*

This forearm muscle, whilst not a flexor of the hand or fingers, is conveniently dealt with here in view of its anatomical relationship in the flexor forearm muscles. This muscle is attached above by two heads, the humeral head being attached to the medial epicondyle, and the ulnar head to the coronoid process of the ulna. The median nerve enters the forearm between these two heads. The muscle distally is attached to the lateral surface of the radius (Fig. 15.17).

**Location of the TrP**    A TrP in this muscle may be found just below the crease of the elbow, in the proximal part of the muscle, to the medial side of the biceps tendon (Fig. 15.22). Activity in it is liable to develop as a result of a fracture at either the elbow or wrist.

**Specific pattern of pain referral**    Pain from a TrP in this muscle is referred down the anterior surface on the radial side to be felt in particular around the radial side of the wrist, in much the same area as pain from TrP activity in the flexor carpi radialis (Fig. 15.22).

A patient with an active TrP in this muscle finds it difficult to turn the hand into the fully supinated position and usually is not able to turn it beyond the mid position.

## Pain in the wrist and hand from local TrPs

Any activity that puts a strain on the muscles in the region of the wrist or hand, including the thumb

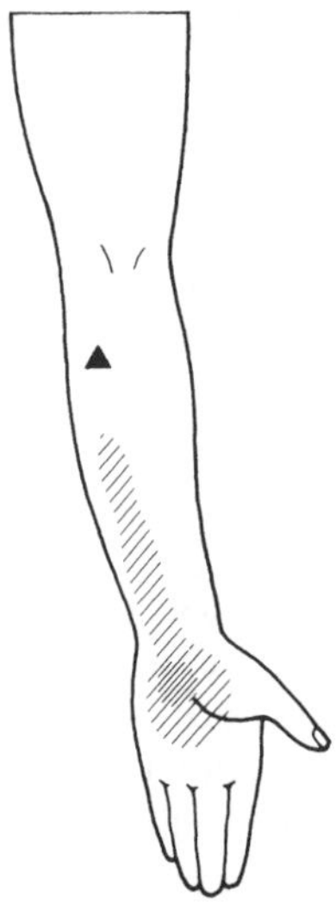

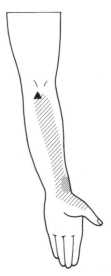

**Figure 15.21**    The pattern of pain referral from a trigger point (▲) in the palmaris longus muscle.

**Figure 15.22**    The pattern of pain referral from a trigger point (▲) in the pronator teres muscle.

and fingers, may lead to the development of persistent pain at these sites as a result of the development of TrP activity in them. However, what is not so well known is that pain in exactly the same distribution may also occur because of TrP activity developing some distance away in the muscles of the forearm.

It, therefore, follows that in every case where pain in the hand develops as a result of TrP activity, it is essential to ascertain whether this is occurring locally in the hand, or high up in the forearm, or both, before any decision can be made as to where acupuncture needles should be inserted.

It is because this is of such fundamental importance that a somewhat lengthy account of myofascial TrPs in the forearm has just been given, and it is hoped that this will help to clarify any confusion concerning the subject prior to turning to the more straightforward concept of wrist and hand pain occurring as a result of local TrP activity.

However, before doing this, consideration must be given to pain at the wrist occurring as a result of median nerve compression in the carpal tunnel, and also as a result of tenosynovitis around the wrist joint.

## Carpal tunnel syndrome

Although this syndrome became recognized as a clinical entity soon after World War II (Brain et al 1947), and there are now good descriptions of it in standard textbooks, a brief account of it must be given here as the pain at the wrist, which often radiates up the arm, sometimes as far as the shoulder, has to be distinguished from other causes of pain in the arm, and particularly from pain ascending up the arm as a result of myofascial TrP activity.

It occurs principally in middle-aged women, but may occur in younger women and is occasionally seen in men. The cause of compression of the median nerve in the carpal tunnel is usually not known but it is sometimes due to a tenosynovitis in rheumatoid arthritis, fluid retention during pregnancy, and soft tissue swelling in either myxoedema or acromegaly.

The essential symptoms are pain in the arm and paraesthesiae in the fingers. The pain is characteristically nocturnal, awaking the patient in the early hours of the morning. It is felt at the wrist, but often ascends up the arm, at times as high as the shoulder. The paraesthesiae usually affect the index, middle and radial side of the ring finger, but surprisingly on occasions may involve the little finger.

These nocturnal symptoms are often relieved by hanging the arm over the side of the bed. On waking in the morning, the hand often feels stiff and swollen.

During the day, the arm is not troublesome but the paraesthesiae persist and are made worse by any activity such as knitting or holding a book.

The condition, as might be expected, most often affects the dominant side but eventually it may become bilateral. The nocturnal pain, and the nocturnal and diurnal paraesthesiae may persist for many months without any objective neurological signs developing, but eventually weakness and wasting of two of the thenar muscles (abductor pollicis brevis and opponens pollicis) cause flattening of the outer half of the thenar eminence.

On examination, the pain and tingling can often be provoked by applying pressure to a point of exquisite tenderness over the anterior carpal ligament. If any doubt as to the diagnosis remains, an electrical conduction test may be carried out, but it has to be remembered that this test may be misleadingly normal in cases with a short history.

**Treatment**   Initially conservative measures should be used including the avoidance of activities that aggravate the symptoms and the wearing of a splint at night. Should symptoms persist, and particularly when there is evidence of muscle wasting, decompression of the median nerve by division of the flexor retinaculum is essential.

## Tenosynovitis in the wrist region

This is a common cause of pain in the region of the wrist. Inflammation of the synovial sheaths surrounding the tendons around the wrist joint is liable to occur whenever the forearm muscles are used excessively or the fingers are worked both hard and rapidly. The condition may therefore occur as a result of recreational pursuits or occupational tasks.

Pain, which can be quite severe, is felt along the line of one or more tendons at the wrist. It is usually associated with swelling, and characteristically crepitus will be detected on moving the tendon. The tenosynovitis affecting the conjoined tendons of the extensor pollicis brevis and abductor pollicis longus as they pass over the styloid process of the radius (de Quervain's disease) is liable to occur as a result of any activity associated with strenuous repetitive movement of the thumb. In this condition there is pain and tenderness over the styloid process and, in particular, crepitus may be elicited on extending the thumb.

**Treatment** For this disorder, rest of the affected part on a splint or in plaster is helpful. Cases that do not respond to this should have an injection of a corticosteroid into the tendon sheath. Extreme care, however, has to be taken not to inject the material into the tendon itself as this may cause it to rupture.

### Pain in the thumb

Pain in the thumb may occur as a result of it being referred there from TrPs in the muscles of the forearm or from TrPs locally in the muscles around the thumb. The muscles around the thumb liable to contain these include the adductor pollicis, and a muscle mass consisting of the opponens pollicis covered by the abductor and flexor pollicis brevis. In practice, it is difficult to differentiate between these three muscles when attempting to locate TrPs in them but it would seem to be the opponens pollicis in which TrP activity most commonly occur.

When TrP activity develops in these muscles it also often takes place in the 1st dorsal interosseous muscle with a point of exquisite tenderness to be found in the anatomical snuff box.

The relative anatomical relationship of the adductor and opponens pollicis, and the approximate position of their TrPs and patterns of pain referral from them are shown in Figures 15.23, 15.24 and 15.25. The action of the adductor pollicis is to bring the thumb adjacent to and parallel with the index finger. The action of the opponens pollicis is to bring the thumb across the palm to touch the pads of the ring and little fingers. TrP activity is liable to arise in these muscles whenever the thumb is strained by some form of sustained gripping action. Writing or sewing therefore may do this when continued for long periods, but perhaps the

commonest activity to cause it is weeding when the ground is dry.

Gardening is therefore a good example of where TrP activity developing locally in the muscles around the thumb or in the forearm is liable to cause pain to arise in it. TrPs some distance above the wrist in the flexor pollicis longus may be activated by twisting and pulling movements associated with pulling out weeds. And TrPs just below the lateral epicondyle, in either the extensor carpi radialis longus or the brachioradialis, are likely to be activated by tightly gripping the handle of a trowel whilst shifting heavy soil.

**Post-traumatic pain in the thumb** When pain following trauma to the thumb persists long after any overt evidence of tissue damage has disappeared, it is usually due to the development of TrP activity. The following case is a good example of this.

A housewife (50 years of age) fractured her left wrist. Soon after the plaster was removed she noticed pain at the base of the left thumb that persisted for about 2 months. It then recurred intermittently, two to three times a year, for about 3–4 weeks at a time. After this had gone on for about 4 years, she was referred to me for assessment.

On getting her to analyze in detail any particular circumstances associated with the onset of the pain, it soon became apparent that this always started when she cooked for more than two people, and used especially large and heavy saucepans, which for some inexplicable reason, considering she was right-handed, she was always in the habit of lifting them off the stove with the left hand.

On examination, the appearances of the thumb were normal, but there were exquisitely tender TrPs in the adductor pollicis, the opponens pollicis, and the 1st dorsal interosseous muscle. Deactivation of these by means of the carrying out of superficial dry needling on two occasions relieved the pain. Following this she made a determined effort to lift the saucepans with her right hand and has had no further trouble.

When post-traumatic pain in a peripheral structure such as the thumb has persisted continuously for some time, it may eventually start to spread up the limb. It would seem that Leriche (1939) must have observed this in what he called 'posttraumatic

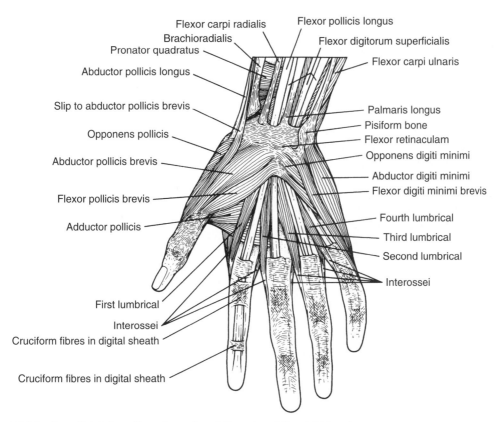

**Figure 15.23**    Superficial dissection of muscles of the palm of the right hand.

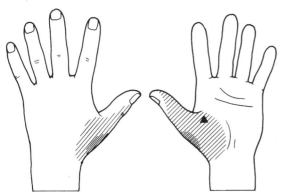

**Figure 15.24**    The pattern of pain referral from a trigger point (▲) in the adductor pollicis muscle.

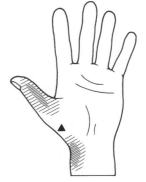

**Figure 15.25**    The pattern of pain referral from a trigger point (▲) in the opponens pollicis muscle.

spreading neuralgia' and also Taylor (1938) in what he called 'ascending neuritis'.

As this type of antidromic referral of pain is not well recognized, other than with median nerve entrapment, two examples of it occurring following trauma will be described.

A 16-year-old schoolgirl tripped and, in falling, wrenched her right thumb backwards by catching it on the edge of a desk.

There was much immediate pain with, according to her, considerable swelling and bruising of the tissues at the base of the thumb. When, after 6 weeks, the latter disappeared but the pain persisted, she was referred to an orthopaedic specialist. An X-ray of the hand showed no abnormality and in particular no evidence of a fractured scaphoid. However, in view of the persistent pain, he immobilized the thumb and wrist in a plaster, but on removing this 6 weeks later, the pain was as bad as ever, and, in addition, the thumb felt stiff and weak. Physiotherapy was, therefore, given and a month later she was discharged from his care. The pain persisted making gripping a pen difficult and interfering with her school work. As the appearances of the thumb and wrist were normal, her doctor began to wonder whether anxiety about forthcoming exams was a factor in the prolongation of her symptoms, but he became concerned when the pain started to spread up the outer side of her arm, at first as far as the elbow, but eventually up to the shoulder.

Eight months after the accident she was referred to me for assessment as to whether acupuncture might be helpful. On examination there was nothing abnormal to be seen but there was some generalized tenderness of the thumb with restriction of its movements, and also there were TrPs to be found on the outer, inner and dorsal aspects of the base of the thumb and in the anatomical 'snuff box'. Three needles were therefore inserted around the base of the thumb and one into the anatomical 'snuff box'. When a needle was put into the latter site, pain immediately shot up the outer side of the arm towards the elbow along the line of distribution of the spontaneously occurring pain.

When seen 1 week later, she reported she had experienced relief from pain but only for 3 days. On re-examining her, it became obvious that satellite TrPs in the extensor muscles just below the lateral epicondyle, in the deltoid, and in the supraspinatus had been overlooked on the first occasion. Needles were, therefore, inserted into the tissues overlying these points as well as the ones around the base of the thumb. Treatment at regular intervals had to be given for another 2 months before lasting relief from the pain was obtained.

The second case is that of a 40-year-old woman whose son, who suffered from a learning disability, attacked her and caught hold of her right thumb, wrenching it backwards. Bruising and swelling around the joint fairly quickly subsided, but it left her with persistent pain, which was not only felt around the thumb but after a time gradually spread up the outer side of the arm.

When seen by me 1 year after the injury, the pain in her thumb at rest and, in particular, on using it, was seriously affecting her life. TrPs were found around the base of the thumb, and satellite ones at the elbow and in the shoulder girdle. These had to be deactivated nine times over the course of the next 3 months before permanent control of the pain was finally obtained.

### Pain in the palm of the hand

It will be remembered from what was said earlier that a persistent prickling type of discomfort in the palm of the hand may develop when TrPs become activated just below the elbow in the palmaris longus muscle. This sometimes occurs in patients with contracture of, and tender nodules in the palm from the development of Dupuytren's contracture. In addition, localized pain in the palm, also in association with the presence of a tender nodule, may occur in the disorder known as trigger finger.

**Trigger finger** Repeated trauma to the hand may lead to the development of a reaction in the sheath of one of the digital flexor tendons in the palm and when this occurs the finger when flexed becomes locked.

In this condition, usually referred to as a trigger finger, there is an exquisitely tender point at the site of a nodule in the palm just proximal to the head of the metacarpal bone.

Traditionally, it is taught that a corticosteroid should be injected locally into the synovial sheath, but this is not necessary and, of course, if by a mistake it should happen to be put into the tendon, it can cause this to rupture. However, there is no need to use this form of treatment as the condition can be relieved equally well simply by inserting a needle into the point of maximum tenderness, and stimulating the nerve endings at that site by rotating the needle a few times.

There are three aspects concerning this that never cease to surprise me. Firstly, that the needle only has to be inserted a short distance into the skin. Secondly, that the response to needle stimulation in this condition is good, with it usually only being necessary to carry it out on one or two occasions, even when the disorder has been present for some considerable time. Thirdly, that with this technique not only is the pain readily controlled, but the finger movement is also quickly restored to normal. The following case is quoted as a typical example.

A 62-year-old company director had had a trigger finger (ring finger on the right hand) for 6 months. It was not so much the locking of the finger on flexion that worried him as the discomfort in the palm when trying to grip a golf club! His doctor, somewhat surprisingly, did not inject hydrocortisone into the tendon sheath, but contented himself with telling the patient that the condition was not bad enough to warrant an operation! Eventually the patient persuaded the doctor to let him try the effects of acupuncture and so he was referred to me.

On examination, there was the usual exquisitely tender point in the palm. A needle was inserted into the skin overlying this and then subjected to a rotary movement until the immediate pain induced by the needle penetrating the skin had been replaced by a feeling of numbness. This occurred after about 20 rotary movements of the needle. On withdrawing the needle, there was no residual tenderness at the site, and not only could he move the finger freely, but, more important, from this particular patient's point of view, he could grip a golf club comfortably! Since having treatment on two occasions he has had no further trouble.

## Pain in the fingers

As has already been said, pain and swelling of the fingers may occur as a result of the activation of TrPs high up in the forearm in either the flexor digitorum (p. 240) or the extensor digitorum (p. 237).

Pain in the fingers with stiffness of their movements may also occur because of the activation of TrPs in the interosseous muscles of the hand. TrPs in these may be activated as a primary event when even a small object has to be held firmly for a long time, such as a needle by a seamstress, or a paintbrush by an artist.

## Heberden's nodes

A Heberden's node is a small nodule that develops on the dorsolateral or dorsomedial aspect of a terminal phalanx at its joint. At first it may be painful and tender but eventually it is symptomless.

The significance of Heberden's nodes is still no more certain than when (Simons et al 1999, p. 788) asked 'What are these little hard knobs, about the size of a small pea, which are frequently seen upon the finger, particularly a little below the top, near the joint?'

In more recent years it has become customary to associate these with the development of osteoarthritis of the finger joints, but (Simons et al 1999, p. 788) state that in addition they are frequently associated with the primary activation of TrPs in the interossei.

### Tender points around arthritic small joints of the hand

Exquisitely tender points are often to be found on palpating the tissues around osteoarthritic small joints of the hands. There are no absolute rules as to their distribution and one has to palpate carefully around a painful joint in order to find them. Deactivation of them with a needle often has a markedly pain-relieving effect.

## SOME MULTIFACTORIAL BRACHIAL PAIN DISORDERS

As stated in the introduction to this chapter these include lateral and medial epicondylalgia, neuralgic amyotrophy, the shoulder–hand syndrome and repetitive strain injury. The elbow pain disorders having already been discussed it now only remains necessary to consider the other three.

## Neuralgic amyotrophy

This disorder, also called cryptogenic brachial plexus neuropathy, is one where for some reason, possibly a viral infection, there is a sudden onset of severe pain in the shoulder and upper arm followed eventually by the development of weakness and wasting of muscles such as the serratus anterior, deltoid, supraspinatus, infraspinatus and trapezius. This initial pain usually spontaneously subsides within a relatively short time but overloading of the wasted muscles eventually causes TrP activity to develop in them with, as a consequence, the production of myofascial TrP pain that requires the carrying out of superficial dry needling for its relief.

## Shoulder–hand syndrome

This sympathetically mediated brachial pain disorder is one that arises secondary to the development of a frozen shoulder (see Ch. 13).

It usually has a gradual onset, with initially there being a severe burning pain in the shoulder region accompanied by vasomotor changes in the hand. Then, after a time, despite the shoulder pain usually starting to become less intense, trophic changes begin to take place with atrophy of brachial muscles, thickening of the palmar fascia and atrophy of the nails. In addition, TrP activity is liable to develop in the atrophied muscles.

The treatment of this disorder, as Sola (1999) has pointed out, is difficult and includes the giving of narcotics for the relief of the very severe pain, sympathetic blocks, the deactivation of TrPs and the carrying out of exercises to maintain function.

## Repetitive strain injury

This injury, which over the years has been known by a number of different names including, occupational cervicobrachial disorder, occupational overuse syndrome, chronic upper limb pain syndrome, refractory cervicobrachial syndrome, localized fibromyalgia and cumulative trauma disorder, first came to be recognized as being a clinical entity when keyboard operators in Australia began to complain of work-related brachial pain in the early 1980s.

In Britain there started to be a dramatic rise in its reported incidence in the 1990s (Reilly 1995). with keyboard operators employed in clearing banks, the newspaper industry and various other large organizations such as the Inland Revenue, the Post Office and British Broadcasting Corporation being amongst those suffering from it.

As the various factors contributing to its development, pathophysiology and clinical manifestations have been discussed by me at some length elsewhere (Baldry 2001), it is only necessary here to reiterate that it is now becoming increasingly widely recognized that much of the pain at an early stage in this disorder emanates from myofascial TrPs (Grange & Littlejohn 1993, Headley 1997, Lin et al 1997).

There is reason to believe that it is the sensory afferent barrage set up as a result of persistent nociceptor activity in these structures that is one of the main causes for nociceptive neurons in the dorsal horn undergoing neuroplastic changes with the development of central sensitisation. This central sensitisation then, in turn, is not only responsible for the persistence of the nociceptive TrP pain, but also for the spread of it. In addition, A-beta-mediated pain starts to develop as a result of these sensitised dorsal horn neurons responding to light-touch-induced stimulation of mechanoreceptors in the skin.

The persistent sensory afferent input to the dorsal horn from peripheral nociceptive pain sources including TrPs also has a stimulating effect on spinal-cord-situated sympathetic preganglionic neurons with, as a consequence, the development of sympathetically maintained pain of a burning character and the production of allodynia. Also, in some cases, this sympathetic overactivity is responsible for coldness of the affected limb and swelling of its tissues.

Deactivation of the myofascial TrPs should be carried out and measures taken to prevent their reactivation as early in the course of the disorder as possible in order to help avoid the development of cental sensitisation and the various pain disorders that arise as a result of this.

## References

Altay T, Gunal I, Ozturk H 2002 Local injections for lateral epicondylitis. Clinical Orthopedics 398: 127–130

Aronson P R, Murray D G, Fitzsimmons R M 1971 Myofascitis: a frequently overlooked cause of pain in cervical root distribution. North Carolina Medical Journal 32: 463–465

Assendelft W J, Hay E M, Adshead R et al 1996 Corticosteroid injections for lateral epicondylitis : a systematic overview. British Journal of General Practice 46(405): 209–216

Baldry P E 2001 Repetitive strain injury. In: Myofascial pain and fibromyalgia syndromes. Churchill Livingstone, Edinburgh, pp. 193–196

Brain W R, Wright A D, Wilkinson M 1947 Spontaneous compression of both median nerves in the carpal tunnel. Lancet 1: 277–282

Chard M D 1995 Injections of periarticular tissues – the elbow region. In: Klippel J H, Dieppe P H (eds) Practical Rheumatology. Times Mirror International Publishers, London, pp. 115–116

Chard M D, Hazleman B L 1989 Tennis elbow – a reappraisal. British Journal of Rheumatology 28(3): 186–189

Coonrad R W, Hooper W R 1973 Tennis elbow: course, natural history, conservative and surgical management. Journal of Bone and Joint Surgery (Am) 55: 1177–1187

Grange G, Littlejohn G O 1993 Prevalence of myofascial pain syndrome in fibromyalgia syndrome and regional pain syndrome: a comparative study. Journal of Musculoskeletal Pain 1(2): 19–35

Green S, Buchbinder R, Barnsley L, Hall S, White M, Smidt N, Assendelft W 2002 Acupuncture for lateral elbow pain. Cochrane Database Systematic Review (1): CD 003527

Gutstein N 1938 Diagnosis and treatment of muscular rheumatism. British Journal of Physical Medicine 1: 302–321

Haker E, Lundeberg T 1990 Acupuncture treatment in epicondylalgia: a comparative study of two acupuncture techniques. Clinical Journal of Pain 6: 221–226

Hay E M, Paterson S M, Lewis M, Hosie G, Croft P 1999 Pragmatic randomised controlled trial of local corticosteroid injection and naproxen for treatment of lateral epicondylitis of elbow in primary care. British Medical Journal 319(7215): 964–968

Headley B J 1997 Physiologic risk factors. In: Sanders M (ed) Management of cumulative trauma disorders. Butterworth-Heinemann, London, pp. 107–127

Heberden W 1818 Pectoris dolor. In: Commentaries on the history and cure of diseases. Wells & Lilly, Boston

Kelly M 1944 Pain in the forearm and hand due to muscular lesions. Medical Journal of Australia 2: 185–188

Leriche R 1939 The surgery of pain. Translated and edited by A. Young Archibald. Baillière Tindall & Cox, London

Lin T Y, Teixeira M J, Fischer A A et al 1997 Work-related musculoskeletal disorders. Physical Medicine and Rehabilitation Clinics of North America, Philidelphia, pp. 113–117

Long C 1956 Myofascial pain syndromes – Part II. Syndromes of the head, neck and shoulder girdle. Henry Ford Hospital Medical Bulletin 4: 22–28

Ljung B O, Forsgren S, Friden J 1999 Substance P and calcitonin gene-related peptide expression: the extensor carpi radialis brevis muscle origin: implication for the etiology of tennis elbow. Journal of Orthopaedic Research 17(4): 554–559

Michele A A, Davies J J, Krueger F J, Lichtor J M 1950 Scapulocostal syndrome (fatigue-postural paradox). New York State Journal of Medicine 50: 1353–1356

Michele A A, Eisenberg J 1968 Scapulocostal syndrome. Archives of Physical Medicine and Rehabilitation 49: 383–387

Potter H G, Hannafin J A, Morwessel R M et al 1995 Lateral epicondylitis: correlation of MR imaging, surgical and histopathological findings. Radiology 196(1): 43–46

Reilly P A 1995 Approaches to RSI in the United Kingdom. Journal of Musculoskeletal Pain 3(2): 123–125

Reynolds M D 1981 Myofascial trigger point syndromes in the practice of rheumatology. Archives of Physical Medicine and Rehabilitation 62: 111–114

Russek A C 1952 Diagnosis and treatment of scapulocostal syndrome. Journal of the American Medical Association 150: 25–27

Simons D G, Travell J G, Simons L S 1999 Myofascial pain and dysfunction. The trigger point manual, Vol. 1, 2nd edn. Williams & Wilkins, Baltimore

Smidt N, Assendelft W J, van der Windt D A, Hay E M, Buchbinder S, Bouter L M 2002 Corticosteroid injections for lateral epicondylitis: a systematic review. Pain 96(1–2): 23–40

Sola A E 1999 Upper extremity pain. In: Wall P D, Melzack R (eds) Textbook of pain, 4th edn. Churchill Livingstone, Edinburgh

Sola A E, Kuitert J H 1955 Myofascial trigger point pain in the neck and shoulder girdle. Northwest Medicine 54: 980–984

Taylor J 1938 Surgical treatment of pain. Lancet II: 1151–1154

Webster – Harrison P, White A, Rae J 2002 Acupuncture for tennis elbow: an e-mail consensus to define a standardised treatment in a GP's surgery. Acupuncture in Medicine 20(4): 181–185

Wynn Parry C B 1980 Pain in avulsion lesions of the brachial plexus. Pain 9: 45–53

Wynn Parry C B 1984 Brachial plexus injuries. British Journal of Hospital Medicine 32(3): 130–139

Chapter **16**

# Pain in the head and face

## INTRODUCTION

In this chapter attention will first be drawn to the pathogenesis, pathophysiology, clinical manifestations and management of migraine and tension-type headaches. Following this, the diagnosis and treatment of myofascial trigger point (MTrP) pain referred to the temperomandibular region, the face and the head will be discussed.

## MIGRAINE

Migraine may conveniently be divided into the classical and common types.

Classical migraine usually takes the form of self-limiting episodes of severe throbbing pain affecting one side of the head, often in association with nausea, vomiting, photophobia and facial pallor. An attack is generally preceded by one or another prodromal symptom including, most commonly, a disturbance of vision, but also at times tingling and numbness down one side of the body, and occasionally a disturbance of speech.

Common migraine, as its name implies, occurs far more often. It is less likely to be unilateral and although it may be associated with nausea and vomiting, there are no prodromal symptoms.

### Aetiology

A striking feature of migraine and one that is of considerable relevance when considering its aetiology is that it is three times commoner in women than men. This female preponderance would seem to be associated with vascular changes that occur as a result of fluctuations in oestrogen and progesterone levels, and there is a tendency for the disorder to occur in association with menstruation, early pregnancy, the menopause and the taking of the contraceptive pill.

An attack may also be brought on in some people by the intake of certain foodstuffs such as chocolate, citrus fruits, tyramine-containing cheeses and alcohol, especially red wine. Alcohol is a non-specific vasodilator, whereas tyramine leads to the release of noradrenaline in migrainous patients that causes a cerebral vasoconstriction followed by a rebound vasodilation.

Attack may also be associated with a fall in the level of blood sugar, either from fasting or as a reactive hypoglycaemia following the ingestion of an excessive amount of carbohydrate. As will be discussed later, when attempting to prevent the recurrence of migraine it is essential to exclude, as far as possible, these various causative factors before turning to the use of acupuncture.

## Pathophysiology

The three factors responsible for its development are vascular, myofascial and emotional.

### Vascular component

Although the ingenious blood flow studies in migraine with the radioisotope xenon, carried out by Olesen & Lauritzen (1982), have shown that the circulatory changes in this condition are not as straightforward as previously thought, it is still generally agreed that in classical migraine the prodromal phase is associated with cerebral vasoconstriction, and that in both common and classical migraine the painful stage is characterized by a significant dilation of extracranial and intracranial blood vessels.

When in this disorder, for some as yet unknown reason, trigeminal unmyelinated C-sensory afferent nociceptors in the walls of blood vessels in the brain, meninges and venous sinuses become activated, vasoactive neuropeptides such as Substance P (SP), calcitonin gene-related peptide and neurokinin A are released with the setting up of a neurogenic inflammatory reaction (Moskowitz & Cutrer 1993). The consequence of this is for noxiously generated information to be conveyed to that part of the trigeminal brain stem's sensory nuclear complex known as the subnucleus caudalis.

The subnucleus caudalis, which because of its morphological and physiological similarities to spinal dorsal horns is also known as the medullary dorsal horn, not only receives this vascular-mediated input, but also, as will later be discussed, myofascial and emotionally evoked (supraspinal) ones.

Following integration of these three inputs at this site, migraine-evoking activity is transmitted up the quinto-thalamic tract to the thalamus. On reaching the latter, this migraine-evoking activity is influenced by a serotenergic input from the midbrain's dorsal raphe nucleus and by a catecholaminergic one from the pontine-situated locus coeruleus before being transmitted to the cerebral cortex.

### Myofascial component

When palpation of the head and neck muscles of patients subject to migraine is carried out, both during and in between attacks of this disorder, it is evident that there is not only widespread tenderness of these muscles, but also small discrete focal points of maximum tenderness.

That these intramuscularly situated points are important sources of pain in this disorder was first confirmed by Hay (1976) when he showed that an injection of a local anaesthetic into them during an attack aborted it and in between attacks reduced the frequency with which they developed. Similarly, when Tfelt-Hansen et al (1981) systematically examined the muscles of the neck and scalp in 50 patients during typical common migraine attacks, they found tender points to be present in these muscles in all cases. Moreover, an injection into these tender points during an attack of either a local anaesthetic or saline, both proving to be equally effective, caused 24 out of 48 of these patients to become symptom-free within 70 min. This was a much shorter time than the average natural duration of an attack.

As the results with saline were found to be as good as those obtained with a local anaesthetic, it is reasonable to conclude that the effectiveness of the latter when injected into tender points in migraine is not, as Hay (1976) suggests, because it blocks the flow of nerve impulses from these points, but because both this and a saline injection bring about a needle-evoked stimulation of nerve endings similar to that obtained by the employment of the acupuncture technique of dry needling.

When Loh et al (1984) compared the effects of acupuncture and drug therapy in patients with migraine and muscle tension headaches, they found tender points in the neck and scalp muscles in 34 out of 41 cases examined in between attacks and, not surprisingly, considering what has just been said, found acupuncture to be a worthwhile prophylactic when these points were present but not when they were absent. As the stimulation of peripheral nerve endings at tender points in the muscles of the neck and scalp, either by injecting a chemical into them or by inserting a dry needle into them during the migraine, is sometimes capable of foreshortening its duration, and considering that if this is carried out between incidences it often prevents recurrence, it seems reasonable to conclude that these tender points must be TrPs. Also in favour of this is the clinical observation that the overzealous stimulation of these points with dry needles in a migrainous subject is liable to bring on an attack of migraine.

These TrPs in the muscles of the neck and scalp will be referred to again when discussing the treatment of migraine with acupuncture, but before turning to this, it is necessary to draw attention to some of the changes observed in the plasma and CSF levels of endogenous opioid substances in simple and migrainous headaches, as these may have some relevance when considering the rationale for using this form of therapy.

Sicuteri et al (1978) found low concentrations of a morphine-like substance in the cerebrospinal fluid of chronic headache patients. Anselmi et al (1980) in a study of idiopathic headache sufferers found similarly low levels both in the cerebrospinal fluid (CSF) and plasma. It also has been shown that during a migraine attack the plasma beta-endorphin levels are significantly lower than in between attacks. It would seem possible, therefore, that the periodicity of migraine may, in part, be related to fluctuations in the levels of these naturally occurring pain suppressors. The discovery by Facchinetti et al (1981) that a group of patients with chronic headache, who reacted poorly to acupuncture, had low levels of plasma beta-endorphin may also be of much significance when one considers the manner in which acupuncture is thought to achieve its analgesic effect (Ch. 10).

### Emotional (supraspinal) component

Henryk-Gutt & Rees (1973) found that up to about 70% of migraineurs consider that emotional upsets play an important part in the development of their headaches. And it is now generally recognized that measures to help reduce stress are an essential part of the prophylactic management of the disorder.

### Vascular-myofascial-supraspinal (emotional) paradigm

Olesen (1991), in the light of what is known concerning the vascular, myofascial and supraspinal (emotional) contributions to migraine has formulated a vascular-supraspinal-myogenic (VSM) model to account for its varying manifestations.

According to this model it is the varying strengths of these three inputs to the trigeminal subnucleus caudalis that determines the character of an attack. Thus, when all three inputs are equally strong migraine with aura develops. When the myofascial and supraspinal components are stronger than the vascular one, migraine without aura develops. And when the vascular input is strong but the other two are weak, only a migraine aura develops.

## Biochemical changes

It has been shown that changes in the serotonin, noradrenaline and oestrogen levels in the body contribute to the development of migraine.

### Serotonin (5-hydroxytryptamine)

As Marcus (1995) has pointed out, support for the belief that alterations in blood and brain serotonin levels influence the development of migraine comes from a number of recently carried out studies.

Goadsby & Lance (1990), showed that migraine may be relieved by increasing the level of serotonin in the blood by means of giving an intravenous infusion of a 0.1% solution of it. Marcus

(1995) has suggested that a possible reason why increasing the peripheral serotonin level by this means may relieve migraine is that it has an auto-inhibitory effect on the brain's serotonin-producing centre in the dorsal raphe nucleus.

Conversely, Bank (1991) has shown that as a result of increasing the production of serotonin in the brain by means of administering the serotonin-releasing agent reserpine, it is possible to precipitate an attack of migraine. And that the effect of giving the serotonin receptor antagonist methysergide is to block this reserpine-induced effect.

### Noradrenaline (norepinephrine)

Curran et al (1965) have shown that during attacks of migraine plasma noradrenaline levels decrease and their metabolites increase. The significance of this finding, however, is not certain. It could be because this catecholamine is primarily involved in the pathogenesis of migraine or, alternatively, it may simply be due to a pain-evoked stress reaction.

### Oestrogen

Marcus (1995), during the course of studying the interrelationship between oestrogen levels and recurring migraine, found that 60% of females who suffer from this type of headache have an increased incidence of it around the time of menstruation, and that 14% of women with this disorder only have it then. There is evidence to show that the onset of menstrual-related migraine coincides with the time that there is an oestrogen deficiency and that in order to counteract this it is necessary for oestrogen to be administered premenstrually (Somerville 1975).

### Use of acupuncture in the treatment of migraine

As already indicated, acupuncture is capable of aborting an attack of migraine, but its main use is in the prevention of attacks. It is, of course, remarkable that it is possible to prevent migraine developing by stimulating nerve endings in between headaches. The only other painful disorder that comes to mind in which acupuncture is used prophylactically in this manner is dysmenorrhoea

when, according to traditional Chinese teaching it is helpful, premenstrually, to stimulate the so-called Spleen 6 point situated in the lower part of the leg about a hand's breadth above the medial malleolus (Fig. 16.1).

When considering the place of acupuncture relative to other forms of therapy in the prophylaxis of migraine, it has to be remembered that it is a time-consuming procedure. Each treatment session lasts for about 20–30 minutes, and in those cases in which the technique proves to be helpful, treatment has to be repeated on a number of occasions at frequent intervals. There is, moreover, no way of predicting which patients will benefit from it, and, for this reason, every patient has to be given a preliminary trial of three treatments at weekly intervals before a decision can be made as to whether or not to continue with it.

My policy, therefore, when presented with a patient whose attacks of migraine are sufficiently frequent as to require prophylactic treatment, is firstly to ascertain whether or not food substances, alcohol, the contraceptive pill or psychogenic

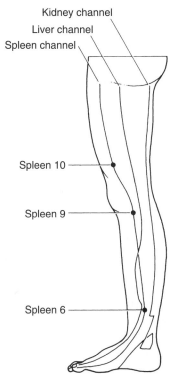

**Figure 16.1** The traditional Chinese acupuncture points Spleen 6, 9 & 10.

factors are contributing to the situation. It has to be admitted that the exercise of excluding a suspect food substance or a particular type of alcoholic drink does not usually seem to be particularly rewarding. The reduction of nervous tension, however, by means of hypnotherapy, and teaching the patient to practise autohypnosis on a daily basis, is, in my experience, often very helpful. Most cases also require prophylactic drug therapy. Some patients find the beta-adrenoceptor blocking drug propranolol effective, others obtain greater benefit from the anti-serotonin agent pizotifen, whilst others prefer the alpha-2 receptor agonist drug clonidine. Plum (1982), however, finds the most effective and the safest agent in migraine prophylaxis to be amitriptyline, thus confirming Lance & Curran's (1964) carefully conducted cross-over trial, which showed this drug to be the best of a number of drugs in the treatment of chronic tension headache. That trial was particularly noteworthy as it showed that the response to amitriptyline could not be correlated with the presence or absence of depressive symptoms. Since then, others have shown that this drug may be an even more effective migraine prophylactic in non-depressed patients than in those overtly depressed (Couch et al 1976, Couch & Hassanein 1976).

It is now recognized that the tricyclic group of drugs have both an antidepressant effect and an entirely separate analgesic effect. The analgesic effect not only comes on more rapidly than any mood change, but is also obtained with a relatively low dosage (average 75 mg each evening). This is mentioned not only because of its importance so far as the treatment of migraine and other types of chronic pain are concerned, but also, in particular, because it is now known that both the analgesic and the antidepressant effects of tricyclic drugs are brought about by their action on the central serotoninergic system. Because of this, they help to potentiate the effectiveness of acupuncture, a technique that, it will be remembered (Ch. 10), depends largely for its action on evoking activity in the serotonin-mediated descending inhibitory system in the central nervous system.

The implications of all this, so far as migraine is concerned, are that this disorder is sometimes responsive to amitriptyline and sometimes to acupuncture, and that there are good grounds for believing that a combination of the two might be even more effective, but statistically controlled trials to confirm this have yet to be carried out.

The situation may therefore be summarized by saying that the place for acupuncture is when for one reason or another the various drugs already mentioned are contraindicated, or when side-effects from them leads to them being discontinued, or when they fail to reduce the frequency and severity of the headaches.

### Location of points to be stimulated

Acupuncture is usually only of value in the treatment of migraine when there are tender points in the muscles of the neck and scalp. For reasons previously given, there are good grounds for referring to these as TrPs, and some people, including myself, believe that the most logical means of carrying out acupuncture in this condition is to insert needles into the tissues overlying them. The identification of these points, therefore, necessitates a systematic search of the muscles down the back of the neck, across the top of the shoulders, and over the scalp, each time a person is treated. However, as will be seen from some of the clinical trials to be discussed later, many physicians with considerable experience in the use of needle stimulation therapy, prefer to use the same set of predetermined traditional Chinese acupuncture points in every case. These include one just medial to the mastoid process (Gall Bladder 20), one over the middle of the upper border of the trapezius (Gall Bladder 21) and points in the temporal region also on the Gall Bladder meridian (Fig. 16.2) together with a point in the first dorsal interosseous muscle of the hand (Large Intestine 4) (Fig. 15.11) and one in the first dorsal interosseous muscle of the foot (Liver 3) (Fig. 16.3).

The muscles in which activated TrPs are to be found in migraine and tension headaches include the paravertebrally situated posterior cervical muscles, the trapezius muscle at the highest point of the shoulder girdle, the sternocleidomastoid muscle and the temporalis muscle. These latter two muscles will be further discussed later in the chapter.

**Posterior cervical muscles**   Sites at which TrPs may become activated in the four layers of the

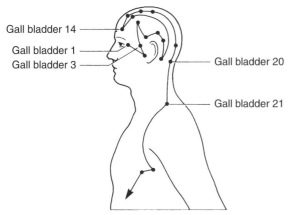

Gall bladder 14
Gall bladder 1
Gall bladder 3
Gall bladder 20
Gall bladder 21

**Figure 16.2** The upper part of the traditional Chinese Gall Bladder meridian. The lower part, not shown, extends down the outside of the trunk, leg and foot to terminate at the base of the 4th toe.

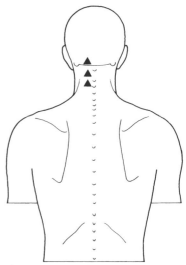

**Figure 16.4** Trigger points (s) in the posterior cervical muscles at the upper part of the back of the neck.

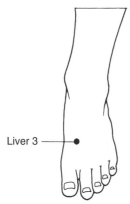

Liver 3

**Figure 16.3** The traditional Chinese acupuncture point Liver 3.

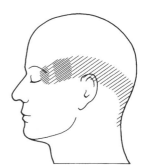

**Figure 16.5** A commonly occurring pattern of pain referral from the posterior cervical muscle trigger points shown in Figure 14.4.

posterior cervical muscles (in descending order of depth – the trapezius, the splenii, the semispinalis muscles, and multifidi together with the rotatores) are shown in Figure 16.4. The referral of pain from these TrPs varies somewhat according to the particular point or points involved and the muscle or muscles in which they are situated, but in general it is to the occiput, and from there along the side of the head to the temporal region, and in some cases, to the eye (Fig. 16.5).

When palpating a TrP in the posterior cervical group of muscles, it is not usually possible to be certain in which particular muscle it lies but this does not matter as the deactivation of any of these points, as with TrPs in general, is best carried out by means of light manual stimulation of a needle

inserted superficially to a depth of approximately 5 mm. This is particularly important when treating migraine as any form of vigorous stimulation may cause an attack of pain to develop.

**Trapezius muscle** There is almost invariably an exquisitely tender TrP in the upper free border of the trapezius muscle about midway between the spine and the acromium, corresponding in position with the traditional Chinese acupuncture point Gall Bladder 21. The referral of pain from this TrP is up the side of the neck, and when particularly severe, it is also referred along the side of the head to the temple and eye (Fig. 16.6D). The deactivation of this point should be carried out in a similar manner.

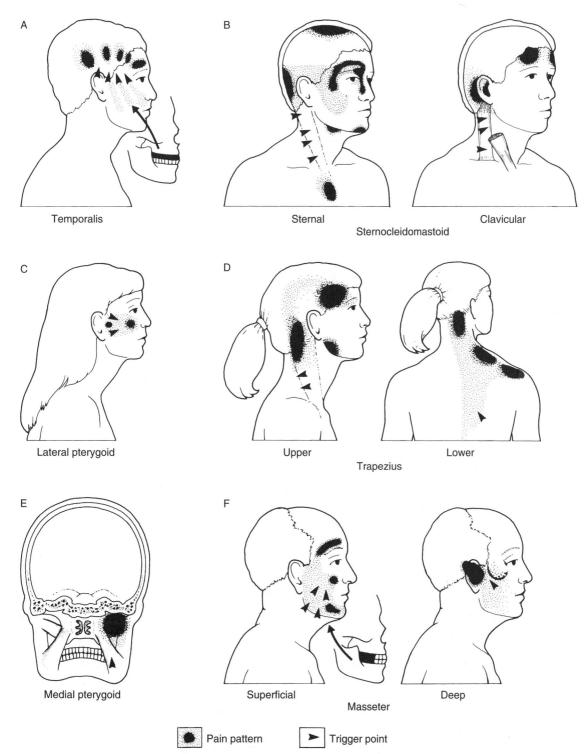

Figure 16.6    Patterns of pain referral from trigger points in masticatory muscles and two neck muscles. (Reproduced with permission of D G Simons and J G Travell from Wall P D and Melzack R (eds) 1984 *Textbook of Pain*.)

There is such a close spatial correlation between Western style TrPs and traditional Chinese acupuncture points around the head and neck involved in the treatment of migraine that it probably makes little difference to the outcome as to which are used. But what does require to be carefully investigated is whether in the treatment of this disorder there is anything to be gained by following the traditional Chinese practice of inserting needles into points some distance away in the hand and foot.

*Distant points* It will be remembered from Chapter 1 that according to the traditional Chinese approach to acupuncture various parts of the body are said to be linked by channels known as acu-tracts or meridians so that pain in one part of the body can be treated either by inserting needles locally at that site, or by inserting them into points some distance away from the area of pain, providing that both the latter and the distant points lie along the same meridian. As discussed in Chapter 2, ever since the Western world first heard about acupuncture 300 years ago, it has always been very sceptical about acu-tracts or meridians, knowing that contrary to the teaching of the ancient Chinese, they are anatomically not demonstrable. It is, therefore, extremely interesting that in recent years neuroanatomical research has shown that certain parts of the body are linked in a manner hitherto not thought possible. For example, studies by Rossi & Brodal (1956) and those by Torvik (1956) show that there are direct projections from the spinal cord to the trigeminal nucleus. Micro-electrode studies carried out in cats by Sessle et al (1981) also demonstrated that the responsiveness evoked in individual neurons in the trigeminal subnucleus caudalis as a result of stimulating the tooth pulp is considerably inhibited by stimulation of the forepaws.

Such observations have considerable relevance to the practice of acupuncture. For example, Mann et al (1973), in discussing some cases of chronic pain treated with acupuncture, stated: 'In the case of pain in the distribution of the trigeminal nerve, acupuncture was applied to the ipsilateral extremities.' And they went on to explain that this was done because 'there is a projection from the spinal cord to the spinal trigeminal nucleus of both sides, and stimulation of limb nerves can bring about primary afferent depolarisation in the spinal trigeminal nucleus'.

Neuroanatomical studies carried out in the Western world during recent years therefore give credence to the ancient belief of the Chinese that by stimulating a point called by them Hoku (The Joining of the Valleys) or Large Intestine 4, in the first dorsal interosseous muscle of the hand (Fig. 15.11), it is possible to control pain occurring in the face and scalp.

It will be remembered, however, from Chapter 9, that several investigators, including Andersson & Holmgren (1975), Jeans (1979), and also Chapman et al (1980), who have compared the relative effectiveness of near and distant points, have concluded that stimulating points near to the site of pain is more effective than stimulating distant ones.

Certainly, when attempting to alleviate musculoskeletal pain by Western-style TrP acupuncture, it is only considered necessary to stimulate the TrPs believed to be the source of pain. It is therefore interesting to note that when it comes to alleviating the pain of migraine, or to preventing it from recurring, many physicians in the Western world with considerable experience in the use of acupuncture employ both proximal and distal points. Loh et al (1984), for example, in their statistically controlled trial of acupuncture versus drug therapy, in cases of migraine and muscle tension headaches of such severity as to warrant referral to the National Hospital for Nervous Diseases in London, used local traditional acupuncture points around the neck and scalp (Gall bladder 20 and 21 in the neck; Gall bladder 3 in the temple and 14 in the forehead [Fig. 16.2]) together with two distant points – one in the first dorsal interosseous muscle in the hand (Large intestine 4 [Fig. 15.11]), and the other in the first dorsal interosseous muscle in the foot (Liver 3 [Fig. 16.3]). And by using this combination of points, they were able to conclude 'that acupuncture is a beneficial treatment for headache and migraine for some patients, and that its more widespread use is justified'.

Vincent (1989) also stimulated local and distant traditional Chinese acupuncture points in a well-designed, carefully conducted, randomized controlled trial in which he was able to show that 'true acupuncture was significantly more effective than the control procedure (see Ch. 11) in reducing the pain of migraine'.

It has to be said, however, that the situation is far from straightforward as Jensen et al (1979), in their placebo versus acupuncture trial using university students in Denmark suffering from repeated headaches, used only the distal point Liver 3 in the foot but, nevertheless, in spite of employing this point alone concluded 'that acupuncture is a relevant therapy for headache with a definite symptomatic effect'.

Felix Mann (1996) has also for many years been recommending the needle-evoked stimulation of nerve endings at the Liver 3 point in patients with migraine. And Campbell (2001) during the course of discussing this states:

> ... One should always look for trigger points in the head and neck and these should generally be treated if they are present. However, Liver 3 alone can also work and if it does it has certain advantages: it is quicker to perform and is something that patients can do for themselves if necessary. Features that suggest trying Liver 3 first are a convincing history of headaches being precipitated by particular foods (chocolate, cheese) or by alcohol and the occurence of a visual or other type of aura before the headaches. In other words I think that Liver 3 is probably the first treatment to try for classic migraine and migraine triggered by food sensitivities. ...

In view of these diverse, but seemingly successful methods of using acupuncture in the prevention of primary headaches, there is, in my opinion, a pressing need for controlled trials to be set up in order to compare the relative efficacy in migraine of stimulating:

1. local and distant points
2. local points only
3. distant points only.

Unfortunately, one of the difficulties in assessing the value of any type of treatment in migraine is that it is a type of disorder that is liable to be readily responsive to a placebo. Matthews (1983) in discussing this matter states:

> ... the placebo effect in migraine is so marked that virtually any form of treatment administered with sufficient aplomb, as for example, acupuncture, will produce a remission in a high proportion of patients.

The results of Dowson et al's trial (1985), in which the effect of traditional Chinese acupuncture and that of a placebo in the treatment of simple and migrainous headache were compared, tend to confirm this view. This was an extremely well conducted, single blind, randomized study with certain particularly commendable features, including the use of pain diaries in which patients conscientiously recorded their treatment responses for 4 weeks prior to treatment, during 6 weeks of treatment and for 24 weeks follow-up; and, the employment of an extremely well-thought-out type of placebo treatment that involved the placing of two electrodes on the skin over the mastoid process connected to a TENS stimulator, the circuitry of which was so adjusted as to allow the red light on the machine to flash whilst preventing any current from reaching the patient. The authors admit that:

> ... the numbers entered into the study are small and we have analysed those suffering from simple headache and migrainous headaches together. It is possible that a larger study with a separate analysis for specific types of headache might reveal that acupuncture is successful in some instances, but not in others.

And they conclude:

> ... it appears that the complaint of headache is very sensitive to placebo therapy, but it is possible that acupuncture has a real therapeutic effect of approximately 20% over placebo. We would, therefore, recommend that future studies should be planned with more patients and on the basis of this assumption.

## TENSION–TYPE HEADACHES

The Headache Classification Committee of the International Headache Society (1988) introduced the term tension-type headache (T-TH) to include a number of other hitherto commonly employed ones. These were tension headaches, muscle contraction headaches, psychogenic headache and stress headache.

## Clinical manifestations

A T-TH characteristically takes the form of a dull aching sensation or vice-like constriction that usually affects the whole of the head, but may in some cases be localized to one or other region of it.

On clinical examination a number of pericranial muscles are found to be tender. Lous & Olesen (1982) found that the muscles most commonly affected in this way were the sternocleidomastoid and masseter (92%), the temporalis (76%), and the lateral pterygoid (70%). Furthermore, systematic palpation of each muscle in turn reveals the presence of well-defined points of maximum tenderness that, as Simons (2001) has persuasively argued, have all the characteristics of active MTrPs.

## The activation of MTrPs

Originally it was thought that compression of small blood vessels in the muscles, brought about as a result of the latter undergoing psychogenic-evoked contraction leads to ischaemia-induced activation of nociceptors at MTrP sites.

This theory, however, had to be discarded once Peterson et al (1995) and Schoenen et al (1991) failed to confirm increased electromyographic (EMG) activity of the head and neck muscles in T-TH. And because, as Olesen & Bonica (1990) have pointed out, any muscle contraction that may be present in this disorder is never of sufficient degree to constrict blood vessels.

EMG studies carried out at MTrP sites by Lewis (1994) and by McNulty et al (1994) have, however, shown that psychological stress is capable of activating MTrPs seemingly as a result of it causing autonomic nervous system hyperactivity. Banks et al (1998), have provided confirmation of this by showing that localized EMG activity found to be present within MTrPs is significantly and dramatically increased by a psychological stressor such as mental arithmetic and decreased by autogenous relaxation training.

## Measures to reduce the frequency and severity of tension–type headaches

Prophylactic measures should be employed whenever the frequency of the headaches is more than two a week and the duration of each episode is for more than 3–4 hours.

### Pharmacotherapy

Amitryptyline is widely employed with a dose of 10–20 mg/day often being all that is required to reduce the frequency of the attacks. Alternatively, a serotonin-specific reuptake inhibitor such as fluoxetine may be employed. Saper et al (1994), have shown in a controlled trial that this is more effective than a placebo.

### Acupuncture

Needle-evoked nerve stimulation at traditional Chinese acupuncture points cannot be recommended on present evidence. Vincent (1990), in a study involving 14 patients, found that it was superior to sham acupuncture in only four of them. And Tavola et al (1992) found it to be no more effective than a placebo.

TrP acupuncture, however, clearly has a sound physiological basis in view of it having been shown that a nociceptive input to the subnucleus caudalis from TrPs in the neck muscles is a primary reason for the disorder developing. Patients with T-TH, like those with migraine, are in general strong reactors and so short duration (approximately 30 seconds) superficial dry needling carried out at MTrP sites is usually all that is required.

## MIGRAINE AND TENSION TYPE HEADACHES – A CONTINUUM

It is now generally recognized that migraine and T-TH are so closely related as to form a continuum (Baldry 2001).

Hopkins (1993) during the course of discussing this has stated:

> … A consensus has developed that patients with chronic recurrent headaches have at different times varying amounts of the features that have, in the past, been called migrainous … and at other times features of headaches that have in the past been called tension headaches or muscle-contraction headaches …

It was for this reason that Loh et al (1984), when comparing the relative effectiveness of acupuncture and standard medical management in the treatment of chronic recurrent headache, stated that they had to include these two types of cephalalgia in the same trial because 'patients commonly have both kinds of headache and frequently do not differentiate them when they report their progress. Although there are clear-cut examples of migraine and of muscle-tension headaches, there are many headaches where it is artificial to assign them to one or other of these two categories.'

Olesen (1991) is of the opinion that what determines whether a patient at any particular time develops a tension-type headache or migraine is the relative strengths of three inputs – vascular, myofascial and emotional (supraspinal). With migraine there are, in descending order of strengths, vascular, supraspinal and myofascial inputs to the subnucleus caudalis. In contrast to this, with T-TH they are myofascial, supraspinal, and vascular ones.

## CLUSTER HEADACHES (MIGRAINOUS NEURALGIA)

This is a relatively rare disorder, but one that has to be distinguished from migraine, particularly as both may occur in the same patient. Also because the management is different and because, so far as my limited experience is concerned in attempting to treat it with acupuncture, it is not relieved by this form of treatment. It is a condition that predominantly affects men in the 40–60 years age group. It is characterized by an excruciating pain around the eye, spreading to the face and temple, with profuse watering and redness of the eye and stuffiness of the nose. Each attack lasts from about 20–120 min once or several times every day in a 'cluster' lasting 3–8 weeks. The symptom-free intervals between the clusters are widely variable.

The patient usually knows what time of day or night to expect an attack and an ergotamine suppository inserted some hours before will often abort it. Other prophylactic agents currently being used are lithium carbonate and nifedipine (Silberstein et al 1998).

## PAIN IN AND AROUND THE TEMPEROMANDIBULAR JOINT

It must be emphasized at the outset that pain in and around this joint is rarely due to arthritis. Admittedly, patients with rheumatoid arthritis sometimes have radiographic evidence of this in the joint, but pain from it is uncommon (Chalmers & Blair 1973). Similarly, osteoarthritic changes shown on an X-ray of this joint are usually no more than a fortuitous radiological finding (Cawson 1984). In the later years of adolescence, pain in the region of this joint is very commonly due to caries in a partially erupted wisdom tooth.

Another important cause of pain in this region is the development of MTrP activity. A disorder that Schwartz (1956) called the temperomandibular joint pain-dysfunction syndrome and others have termed the myofascial pain dysfunction syndrome (Laskin 1969, Mikhail & Rosen 1980). Sharav (1999), when recently discussing it at some length, simply called it temperomandibular myofascial pain. My personal preference, however, is to call it the temperomandibular MTrP pain syndrome as this has the merit of drawing attention to the all important source of the pain.

## The temperomandibular MTrP pain syndrome

This disorder, which mainly affects women, may develop at any age. The patient experiences a dull, continuous, poorly localized ache mostly around the ear, the angle of the mandible and the temporal area but also often in the jaws, teeth and side of the face. The continuous ache is punctuated by momentary jabs of sharp pain (Bell 1977). The patient may also complain of various clicking or popping noises in the joint on opening the mouth, and also of limited mouth opening and dizziness (Sharav et al 1978).

On examination, the limited mouth opening and the abnormal sounds in the joint that sometimes are produced on attempting this may be confirmed. The muscles around the joint are tender and systematic palpation of these reveals the presence of focal points of exquisite tenderness, or TrPs, particularly in the lateral pterygoid, the masseter, and the medial pterygoid muscles (Travell & Simons 1983, pp. 168–182). The exact location of these TrPs will be described later, but first it is necessary to say something about the aetiology of the syndrome and its management in general, for it is certainly no good directing treatment at these points alone without at the same time correcting other disorders.

## Aetiology of the syndrome and its management

There would seem to be a triad of factors responsible for the condition including occlusal disturbances, psychological disorders, and perhaps because of one or other or both of these, the activation of TrPs in the masticatory muscles.

## Occlusal disturbances

There is much controversy concerning the part played by occlusal disturbances in the aetiology of this syndrome. Some authorities, such as Clarke (1982), believe there is no significant difference between those occurring in patients with this syndrome and those found in asymptomatic controls. Others, such as Sharav (1999), consider that such disturbances are a prerequisite for the development of dysfunction and pain. And it should be noted in relationship to this that the American Dental Association (Ayer 1983) has lent its support to the view that the use of dental appliances designed to temporarily modify the occlusion are helpful in the treatment of this condition.

## Psychological disorders

Since Schwartz (1956) first drew attention to the importance of psychological disorders in the aetiology of this condition, it is generally agreed that anxiety, depression, frustration, and resentment may singly or collectively contribute to this syndrome with bruxism – a purposeless grinding or gnashing of the teeth – being an outward manifestation of such disorders of mood.

Treatment must therefore include the prescribing of an antidepressant or tranquillizer according to whichever is most appropriate, or the use of various relaxation techniques such as biofeedback (Stem et al 1979) or hypnotherapy. My preference is for the latter and to teach the patient to practise autohypnosis on a regular basis each day.

## MTrPs

The masticatory muscles in which activated TrPs are likely to be found include the lateral pterygoid, the masseter, the medial pterygoid, and the temporalis muscles. Greene et al (1969) in a study of

277 patients with temperomandibular joint pain dysfunction found that, of those in pain, 84% had tenderness of the lateral pterygoid and 70% had tenderness of the masseter muscle.

Sharav et al (1978) observed much the same in a series of 42 patients, with active TrPs occurring in the lateral pterygoid in 83% and in the masseter in 69%.

As in practice, it is better to deactivate TrPs in the masseter muscle before dealing with those in the more deeply lying lateral pterygoid muscle; the masseter muscle will be considered first.

**Masseter muscle** The masseter muscle consists of a superficial and deep part. The superficial part, which is the larger of the two, arises from the zygomatic process of the maxilla, and the zygomatic arch. Its fibres pass downwards and backwards to be inserted into the angle and lower half of the ramus of the mandible. The deep part, much of which is concealed by the superficial part arises from the zygomatic arch, and its fibres pass vertically downwards to be inserted into the lateral surface of the coronoid process and upper half of the ramus of the mandible (Fig. 16.7).

*Activation of TrPs* TrPs in this muscle may become activated as part of the myofascial pain syndrome, but additionally when there is prolonged overstretching of the muscle as sometimes occurs during a dental operation or as a result of the direct trauma of an accident, and secondarily, when pain is referred to the region of this muscle from TrP activity in the sternocleidomastoid muscle. The TrP activity is the cause of referred pain, restriction of jaw opening and, somewhat surprisingly, tinnitus (Travell 1960).

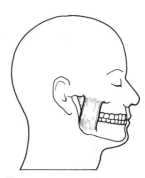

**Figure 16.7** The masseter muscle.

*Specific pattern of pain referral* TrPs in the superficial layer of the muscle are responsible for pain being referred along both the maxilla and mandible, around the molar teeth, and in and around the temperomandibular joint (Fig. 16.6F).

Those in the deep layer refer to the region of the temperomandibular joint and ear (Fig. 16.6F). They may also be responsible for the development of tinnitus. Deafness or giddiness, however, never occur.

**TrP examination**    In locating TrPs, it is necessary to put the muscle on the stretch by propping open the mouth. A cylindrical cardboard air-tube used for respiratory function measurements is very useful for this purpose.

TrPs in the superficial part of the muscle usually occur near to either the upper or lower attachments, where they are best located by flat palpation. On occasions they may be found in its belly and are then best located by gripping the muscle between a finger inserted into the mouth and the thumb pressed against the cheek. TrPs in the deep part are located by palpating it where it overlies the posterior part of the ramus of the mandible, just in front of the external auditory meatus.

*Deactivation of TrPs*    When deactivating a TrP with a dry needle, the point should be either fixed

between two fingers placed side by side extra-orally, or it should be held in a pincer grip, between a finger inside the mouth, and the thumb on the outside pressing against the cheek.

**Lateral (external) pterygoid muscle**    The lateral pterygoid muscle lies deep to, and mainly behind, the coronoid process and zygomatic arch. It is made up of two divisions – the superior and inferior.

*Attachments*    The superior division is attached in front to the sphenoid bone and behind to the capsule of the temperomandibular joint. The inferior division is attached in front to the lateral pterygoid plate and behind to the neck of the mandible (Fig. 16.8).

*Activation of TrPs*    This occurs with malocclusion of the teeth or with overuse of the muscle as a result of anxiety-induced bruxism, or both.

*Specific pattern of pain referral*    TrPs in this muscle are responsible for pain being referred to the temperomandibular joint and around the region of the maxillary sinus (Fig. 16.6C).

*TrP examination*    The locating of TrPs at the anterior attachment of the inferior division is best carried out by intraoral palpation. With the mouth open and the lower jaw drawn towards the side to be examined, a finger is squeezed between the maxilla and the coronoid process of the mandible,

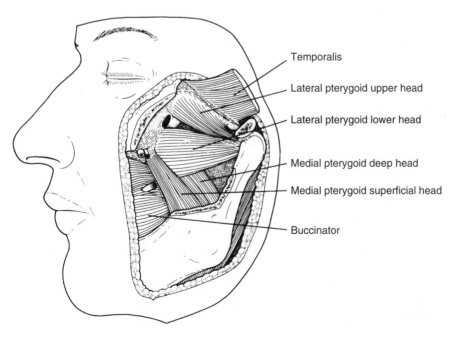

Temporalis

Lateral pterygoid upper head

Lateral pterygoid lower head

Medial pterygoid deep head

Medial pterygoid superficial head

Buccinator

**Figure 16.8**    The left ptyerygoid muscles. The zygomatic arch and part of the ramus of the mandible have been removed.

along the roots of the upper molar teeth. If the space is too narrow to admit a finger, some instrument such as the handle of a dental mirror should be employed. The finger is slid as far along the length of the coronoid process as possible, a manoeuvre facilitated by having the mouth partially closed. Pressure is then applied in an inwards direction towards the lateral pterygoid plate to test for the exquisite tenderness of TrP activation. Similar tenderness from a TrP in the temporalis muscle at its attachment to the coronoid process may be elicited by pressing with the finger, at exactly the same site but in an outwards direction.

TrPs in other parts of the muscle are best located by extraoral examination. It must be remembered, however, that it is impossible to palpate the muscle from the outside with the mouth closed because the superior division is then behind the zygomatic arch, and the inferior division behind the ramus of the mandible. The examination, therefore, must always be carried out with the mouth open. It is then possible to palpate the mid parts of both the superior and inferior division through the bony aperture, bounded above by the zygomatic arch, and below by the coronoid process anteriorly and the condyloid process posteriorly (the mandibular notch). In order to palpate the mid part of the superior division, pressure should be exerted in an upwards and forwards direction, and for the inferior division it should be applied in a downwards and forwards direction. It is only possible to elicit tenderness at these sites, however, if TrPs in the overlying masseter muscle have previously been deactivated.

### Deactivation of TrPs

**INTRAORAL APPROACH** It is possible to deactivate TrPs in the anterior part of the inferior division by inserting a needle intraorally, but this should only be attempted by someone skilled in manipulating needles within the mouth. Otherwise it is better to use an external approach.

**EXTRAORAL APPROACH** In order to deactivate TrPs in the lateral pterygoid muscle extraorally, the patient should be placed in the supine position and the mouth propped open.

For TrPs in the anterior part of the inferior division, the needle is inserted through the masseter muscle, and then through the mandibular notch in the direction of the upper molar teeth.

For TrPs in the anterior part of the superior division, the needle is passed under the zygomatic arch just anterior to the temperomandibular joint in an upwards and forwards direction towards the orbit.

For TrPs further back, in either division of the muscle, the needle is inserted through the mandibular notch perpendicular to the surface and slightly posteriorly. To reach the superior division, the needle is directed upwards beneath the zygomatic arch, and to reach the inferior division the needle is directed downwards towards the angle of the mandible.

**Medial pterygoid muscle** If, after deactivating TrPs in the masseter and lateral pterygoid muscles, opening the mouth is still painful and restricted with, in addition, some difficulty in swallowing, then it is possible that there are active TrPs in the medial pterygoid muscle.

*Attachments* The medial pterygoid muscle is attached below to the angle of the jaw and above to the lateral pterygoid plate (Fig. 16.8).

*TrP examination* The patient should be placed in the supine position, with the mouth propped open. The muscle is first palpated from the outside by pressing a finger against the inner surface of the mandible at its angle. At this site the lower end of the muscle is just within reach of the finger. An intraoral examination is then carried out in order to reach parts of the muscle higher up. With the pad of the finger facing outwards, it is inserted into the mouth and slid behind the lower molar teeth until it encounters the bony edge of the ramus of the mandible, and just behind this, it comes up against the muscle running in a vertical direction (Fig. 16.6E).

*Deactivation of TrPs* Deactivation of TrPs in this muscle is technically difficult but fortunately as Travell & Simons (1983, p. 254) point out, it is usually possible to control the pain by stretching the muscle, and then applying a vapocoolant spray to it. The patient is placed in the supine position and encouraged to stretch the muscle by placing two fingers behind the lower incisor teeth, and the thumb under the chin, and then pulling the mandible forwards and downwards to open the jaws fully. Whilst this is being done, the vapocoolant spray is swept from the neck below upwards towards the temperomandibular joint. It is important to ensure that the spray does not go into the eye by placing a pad over it.

**Temporalis muscle**    The temporalis muscle is the third most commonly involved of the masticatory muscles after the masseter and lateral pterygoid in this myofascial TrP pain syndrome (Greene et al 1969) but as the activation of TrPs in this muscle may also occur for many other reasons, all of the various causes will be considered together later in the chapter.

## TRIGEMINAL NEURALGIA

Trigeminal neuralgia clearly has to be included in the differential diagnosis of pain in and around the face, but as this book is primarily concerned with musculoskeletal pain, only brief reference will be made to its clinical features in order that it may be distinguished from other causes of facial pain. This condition of unknown aetiology may develop at any age, but it is most commonly seen from the age of 50 years onwards. In young people, it occasionally heralds the onset of multiple sclerosis.

The pain usually involves the 2nd or 3rd divisions of the nerve. It commonly takes the form of unilateral, brief, very severe electric-shock like stabs repeated at frequent intervals in short-lasting bouts with intervals of freedom from pain varying in duration from minutes to hours. After several weeks, the pain spontaneously remits but recurs some time later. Unfortunately, there is a tendency over the course of time for the remission periods to get shorter whilst the bouts of pain in an attack get progressively more severe, and the attacks last longer.

Each bout of pain is usually precipitated by some non-noxious stimulus such as shaving, washing, or even just touching or moving the face. Also, in some people, eating, drinking or brushing the teeth may bring on an attack.

It is important to note that with idiopathic trigeminal neuralgia there are no abnormal physical signs including no sensory loss.

## Treatment

Carbamazepine is the drug of choice in the treatment of this condition, but unfortunately, in about 25% of patients it is ineffective and in about 25% of patients it cannot be tolerated. Therefore, only about 50% can be successfully treated with it (Loeser 1984).

Other anticonvulsants currently being used in the treatment of this disorder include lamotrigine and tizanidine (Zakrzewska 1999). A systematic review of the use of them in the treatment of neuropathic pain, including trigeminal neuralgia, has been carried out by McQuay et al (1995). The alternative, when medical management proves to be ineffective, is to carry out one or other of the various surgical procedures now available (Zakrzewska 1999).

## ATYPICAL FACIAL PAIN

Pain in the face, which from its character is clearly not due to trigeminal neuralgia, and which, following careful investigation, is not found to be due to disease of the teeth, bones or sinuses, is often diagnosed as atypical facial pain. The very term signifies how ill-defined the condition is, and regrettably all too often the possibility of the pain being referred from TrPs in muscles in this region is not considered. It must be admitted, however, that there is a group of patients who have pain in the face, which, unlike that of trigeminal neuralgia, is persistent in character, is often associated with an area of sensory loss, and not infrequently is bilateral. Also, on examination, in addition to there being no evidence of disease of any of the structures of the face, there is also no evidence of TrP activity in the neighbouring muscles, and, therefore, by a process of exclusion, the only diagnosis possible is one of atypical facial pain (Weddington & Blazer 1979).

As patients with atypical facial pain often show some evidence of emotional instability, treatment usually consists of giving an antidepressant, sometimes in combination with a phenothiazine. Such drugs, however, are only occasionally helpful in this condition. The anticonvulsants, carbamazepine and diphenylhydantoin, are also sometimes recommended, but there seems to be no scientific basis for this and only a small number of patients are likely to be helped. Side effects from any of these drugs are common and such treatment should never be embarked upon until, by careful examination, the possibility that the pain may be coming from myofascial TrPs has been carefully excluded.

## TRAUMA–INDUCED MYOFASCIAL TrP CEPHALALGIA

This particular type of cephalalgia does not appear as a separate entity in the International Headache Society's Classification (Headache Classification Committee of the International Headache Society 1988), but those who include a search for TrPs as part of their routine physical examination in all cases of persistent head pain have come to realize that it is an extremely common, but poorly recognized disorder. The TrP activity may develop (Baldry 1999) as a result of sudden severe trauma, such as that brought about by a whiplash injury or because of muscle overloading from, for example, the adoption of a faulty posture. This TrP activity is liable to develop in one or more of the following muscles – the trapezius and posterior cervical group (see Ch. 14), the sternocleidomastoid, the temporalis and the occipito-frontalis.

## Sternocleidomastoid muscle

Many errors in diagnosis and, consequently, much inappropriate treatment are due to a lack of awareness that the activation of TrPs in the sternocleidomastoid muscle is an important cause of persistent pain in the head and face, and also, in certain cases, is the cause of a distressing type of postural dizziness.

### Activation of TrPs

TrPs frequently become activated in the upper part of this muscle on one side of the neck in patients with tension headaches, in those with migraine, and in those with both. They may also become activated in any part of this muscle when the neck is kept turned to one side for any length of time, such as, for example, when typing a long report from shorthand notes.

They may become activated in the muscles on both sides of the neck as a result of the head being tilted backwards for some time such as, for example, when painting a ceiling or sitting at the front of the theatre watching a play being performed on a high stage. However, one of the commonest causes of bilateral activation of TrPs in this muscle is when the muscles on both sides of the neck become strained as a result of a whiplash injury occurring as a result of one car running into the back of another. When this happens, TrPs in the levator scapulae, posterior cervical, and the trapezius muscles also become activated with the development of a painful stiff neck (Ch. 14); whilst TrPs in the sternocleidomastoid muscle are liable to give rise to a variety of symptoms including pain in the head and face, and postural dizziness.

### Symptoms from TrP activation in the sternocleidomastoid muscle

TrPs at the upper part of the sternal division of the muscle near to its insertion into the mastoid process are responsible for pain being referred to the occipital region and to the top of the head, often with marked tenderness of the area of the scalp affected (Fig. 16.6B). Those in the mid-part of this division refer pain along the supraorbital ridge, around the eye, and into the cheek (Fig. 16.6B). The activation of TrPs in this part of the muscle sometimes occurs in association with TrP activity in other muscles such as the temporalis, the masseter, the external pterygoid, the orbicularis oculi and the zygomaticus, and unless the presence of TrPs in these muscles is recognized, the composite pain pattern is liable to be misdiagnosed as that of atypical facial neuralgia.

Travell (1981) reported a very interesting case of TrP activity in muscles such as those just mentioned that had been the cause of intractable pain in the face for 13 years before the true cause of the pain was finally established. It is perhaps unfortunate that she referred to this as a case of atypical facial neuralgia for, in my view, such a diagnosis should be reserved for that group of cases in which myofascial TrP activity is not present, and that cases in which pain is due to this are better referred to as examples of the chronic facial myofascial TrP pain syndrome.

TrPs at the lower end of this division near to its attachment to the sternum refer pain in a downwards direction over the upper part of the sternum. The pattern of this is such that it is liable to be mistaken for pain that is myocardial in origin (Fig. 16.6B).

TrPs in the deeper clavicular part of the muscle are likely to refer pain either into the ear and postauricular region, or across the front of the forehead (Fig. 16.6B).

TrP activity in the sternal division also affects the autonomic nervous system and may be the cause of conjunctival redness and watering of the eye and nose similar to that seen with migrainous neuralgia (Travell 1960, 1981). This is liable to be very confusing when this TrP activity is responsible for pain developing around the eye, except of course that in migrainous neuralgia an attack of pain, although very intense, usually only lasts for less than 1 hour. TrP activity in this muscle may also cause disturbed proprioception with the development of postural dizziness.

## Disturbances of proprioception brought about by TrP activity in the sternocleidomastoid muscle

Cohen's investigations (1959, 1961) into body orientation carried out in monkeys have shown that, whilst it is the function of the labyrinths to give information concerning the position of the head in space, information concerning the position of the head in relationship to the body comes from proprioceptive mechanisms in the neck. In humans, the main muscle concerned with this would seem to be the sternocleidomastoid and it is because of this that unilateral TrP activation in it is often the cause of postural dizziness developing.

In my experience, it never takes the form of giddiness or vertigo if, by these terms, one means a sudden disturbance of balance associated with a sensation of rotation either of the person concerned or of their surroundings, but rather it is a sensation of unsteadiness and loss of balance with a tendency to veer to one side when attempting to walk in a certain direction. This disorientation and loss of co-ordination is mainly postural and occurs when movements of the body or head involve a change in tension in the affected sternocleidomastoid muscle. Such symptoms may be associated with nausea, but never with vomiting, tinnitus or nystagmus. In the differential diagnosis, an anxiety state, and also in the elderly, vertebrobasilar ischaemia have to be considered. Postural dizziness due to sternocleidomastoid TrP activity may occur at any age, with

Weeks & Travell (1955) reporting a case of it occurring in an 11-year-old girl.

Travell, who was one of the first to recognize this condition, and who in 1955 published a report of 31 adults suffering from it, maintains that the TrPs responsible for this phenomenon are always situated in the clavicular part of this muscle, and that, therefore, it is associated with frontal headache with either the one or the other dominating the clinical picture (Travell 1967).

Most of the cases of this type of postural imbalance that have come under my care have been in patients who, in addition to having TrP activity in this muscle, also have had painful stiff necks due to similar activity occurring in other muscles of the neck as a result of whiplash injuries. It is always interesting to observe how often in the referral letter this unsteadiness is assumed to be due to 'nerves' brought on by the shock of the accident. It is also remarkable how often the disorder disappears once the appropriate TrPs have been deactivated by inserting dry needles into them.

In considering the mechanism by which postural dizziness occurs as a result of TrP activity in the sternocleidomastoid muscle, it has to be remembered that the sensory innervation of this muscle comes from the anterior primary rami of the 2nd and 3rd cervical nerves, and that Cohen (1961) in experiments on monkeys and baboons produced an exactly similar type of unsteadiness and loss of balance in these animals by artificially cutting off the sensory input from these two nerves.

Furthermore, the clinical implications of this are that when pain in the head, superficial tenderness of the scalp, postural dizziness and nausea occur as a result of some injury in which there has been marked hyperextension of the neck, the two possibilities that have to be considered are that the symptoms may be due either to TrP activation in the sternocleidomastoid muscle, or to direct injury to an upper cervical spinal nerve.

Behrmann (1983) reviewed 17 cases in which these symptoms were due to a traumatic neuropathy of the 2nd cervical spinal nerve, and in 12 of them the injury to the nerve was caused by exactly the same type of acceleration-deceleration road-traffic accident, with a wrenching movement of the head, as that which is liable to cause TrP activation in the sternocleidomastoid muscle.

The main distinguishing feature would seem to be that with the TrP syndrome there is no sensory loss, but with trauma to the second cervical spinal nerve, there is diminished sensation to pin prick over one side of the head or localized to the periorbital, temporal, or suboccipital areas.

## POST–TRAUMATIC HEADACHE

The post-concussional syndrome of headaches, persistent tenderness of the scalp, postural dizziness, irritability, and failure of concentration is a well-recognized entity but one about which there is considerable diversity of opinion concerning its aetiology. Many experienced clinicians, such as Matthews & Miller (1972) incline to the belief that it is psychogenic in origin. In support of this view, Matthews & Miller point out that the condition is commoner after minor head injuries than it is after major ones, and that it rarely occurs in head injuries sustained in the house or during sport. Indeed, it arises most often from trauma incurred during a traffic accident, and even more frequently from trauma associated with an industrial accident, and particularly in those circumstances when there is a claim for compensation – and to quote these authors '"treatment" is fruitless'. From the few cases of post-traumatic headache, either with or without a history of concussion that have come under my care, it is my belief that TrP activation in the muscles of the neck, such as the splenii, trapezius and sternocleidomastoid muscles, is an important cause not only of persistent headache, but also of persistent scalp tenderness and postural dizziness. It is also my belief that in all such cases a systematic search for TrPs is mandatory because, when present, deactivation by means of dry needle stimulation is likely to prove helpful. This is a view also supported by the observations of Rubin (1981). There is, therefore, a pressing need for a large-scale survey of cases of post-traumatic headache and dizziness in order to establish the true incidence of myofascial TrP activity in this condition.

Certainly the post-traumatic headache syndrome not only occurs as a result of head injuries, but may also develop whenever the muscles of the neck are subjected to the trauma of being held persistently in a state of hyperextension, as, for example, in the following case, when this occurred as a result of a meningitis.

A female business executive (41 years of age) developed severe retraction of her neck during the course of what was said to be a viral meningitis. The illness was sufficiently bad for her to be kept in hospital for 6 weeks. Shortly after getting over the acute stage of the illness, she began to develop severe bilateral temporal headaches, a painful stiff neck, and a feeling of unsteadiness on walking. Eighteen months later, because of these symptoms persisting, she was admitted to a neurological unit for investigations including a brain scan. No abnormality was found but she continued to have these symptoms and, by the time she was referred to me 3 years later, she was frequently off work because of the severity of the headaches and was taking 8 Ponstans a day. On examination, there were exquisitely tender TrPs in the posterior cervical muscles, the levator scapulae, the trapezius, and the sternocleidomastoid muscles. Deactivation of these by means of the carrying out of superficial dry needling gradually caused her symptoms to abate but the procedure had to be repeated at regular intervals over the course of the next 3 months before the headaches and postural dizziness were finally brought under control.

## TORTICOLLIS

Torticollis (Latin, *tortus* – twisted; *collum* – neck) is of two distinct types. The one is a spasmodic contraction of the neck muscles due to a lesion in the basal ganglia, and the other a constant pulling over of the neck muscles due to the activation of TrPs in them.

The clinical picture of **spasmodic torticollis** is one in which there is paroxysmal contraction of the neck muscles causing the head to be frequently and involuntarily turned forcibly to one side. This is a very distressing condition and one in which eventually the head may become permanently turned to one side. On examination, there is an obvious severe and painful contraction of the sternocleidomastoid muscle but, on closer inspection, it becomes obvious that all of the muscles of the neck are involved.

Treatment is far from easy, but selective blocking of the muscles identified as being responsible for the abnormal movements using repeated injections of botulinum toxin is sometimes helpful.

The other type of wry neck, and one that it is essential to distinguish from the spasmodic type as it is so far more readily treatable, is the one in which there is persistent contraction of the neck muscles causing the neck to be constantly pulled over to that side, and occurring as a result of the activation of TrPs in various muscles of the neck, including the posterior cervical muscles, the levator scapulae, the trapezius and the sternocleidomastoid muscle.

A man (30 years of age) had, in his early teens, been accidentally shot in the head causing him to have a depressed fracture of the skull and a hemiplegia. Since that time he had had much pain in the neck with restriction of neck movements and recurrent headaches. He was referred to me, because during the previous 18 months he had developed a constant and painful spasm of his neck muscles causing the neck to become increasingly pulled over to the affected side. On examination, there were numerous, obviously very active, TrPs in the muscles of the neck. These were deactivated by means of the carrying out of superficial dry needling initially once a week and after a time at less frequent intervals.

After 4 weeks, the pain in the neck became appreciably less, but treatment had to be continued for another 4 weeks before he could begin to keep his neck upright without discomfort. Eventually, however, with further treatment spread over several months, his long-standing headaches and pain in the neck disappeared. Also, he entirely lost any evidence of a torticollis and regained full movements of the neck. Another interesting aspect of the case that is worth noting is that on the initial examination there was exquisite tenderness of the scalp around the craniotomy scar and, on closer examination, it became apparent that there was one focal point of maximum tenderness in the scar itself. It was considered, therefore, that this must be a TrP, and, although needling it was difficult due to the scar being tough, and also because it was a very painful procedure, the treatment, nevertheless, very quickly brought about a dramatic lessening of the generalized tenderness around the scar; and as a result of repeating it a few further times, the tenderness disappeared altogether.

## TEMPORALIS MUSCLE (Fig. 16.9)

This muscle, which is attached to the temporal bone above and the coronoid process of the mandible below, quite commonly develops TrP activity in it. This may occur in people who are tense, in migrainous subjects, and in those with the temperomandibular myofascial TrP pain syndrome. It is also liable to occur when the muscle is suddenly cooled by being exposed to a draught, or when it is subjected to direct trauma such as may occur with a fall on the head or being hit by a golf ball. In addition, it may develop as a secondary event when pain is referred to the temporal region from TrPs in either the sternocleidomastoid or upper trapezius muscle.

*Location of TrPs and their specific pain patterns* The sites at which TrPs are likely to be found include:

1. the anterior part of the temple at the lateral end of the supraorbital ridge
2. midway between this point and the ear along the line of the zygomatic arch
3. on the same line just in front of the ear
4. just above the ear.

The referral of pain from a TrP at site 1 is along the supraorbital ridge and, on occasions, towards the upper incisors; that from a TrP at sites 2 and 3 is locally in the region of the temple and sometimes

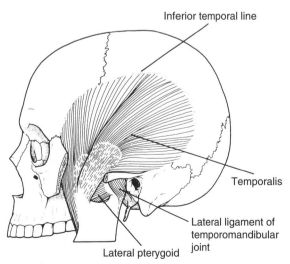

**Figure 16.9** Left temporalis. The zygomatic arch and masseter have been removed.

Inferior temporal line

Temporalis

Lateral ligament of temporomandibular joint

Lateral pterygoid

downwards into the teeth of the upper jaw; and that from a TrP at site 4 is in a backwards and upwards direction from it (Fig. 16.6A).

*Locating TrPs* When examining the temporalis muscle for TrPs, they are more readily found if the muscle is put slightly on the stretch by having the mouth propped partially open.

*TrP deactivation* It is relatively easy to deactivate TrPs in this muscle by means of the carrying out of superficial dry needling but even with this care must be taken not to puncture the temporal artery.

*Differential diagnosis* It has to be said that, although persistent pain in the temporal region is commonly due to TrP activation, when it occurs in the middle-aged and elderly, the possibility that it may be due to giant cell arteritis must always be considered. In this disorder the pain may be in any part of the head but is commonest in the temporal region, and when this is so it is often made worse by mastication – a state of affairs sometimes somewhat ineptly referred to as jaw claudication considering that the jaw is incapable of limping! On examination, the temporal artery is characteristically thickened and pulseless, there is much surrounding tenderness, and, in some cases, the overlying skin is reddened. The physical signs, however, are often by no means obvious and in any case of doubt it is essential to have the ESR measured as

with this condition it is invariably appreciably elevated.

This disorder has been discussed at some length because, unless the possibility of it occurring is taken into consideration, the pain and tenderness associated with it may all too readily be assumed to be due to TrP activation. This is a mistake that could have far-reaching consequences, because, whilst time is being wasted treating the condition with acupuncture rather than with a corticosteroid, there is always the risk of blindness developing.

## TrP ACTIVITY IN SKIN MUSCLES: ORBICULARIS OCULI, ZYGOMATICUS AND OCCIPITOFRONTALIS (Fig. 16.10)

### Orbicularis oculi

TrPs may become activated in this muscle as a primary event in someone who persistently frowns, or as a secondary event when pain is referred to the orbit from TrPs in the sternomastoid muscle.

The TrP lies above the eyelid just beneath the eyebrow against the bone of the orbit. The referral of pain from this is down the side of the nose (Fig. 16.11).

In deactivating this point with a dry needle, superficial needling is particularly necessary

**Figure 16.10** Muscles of the scalp and face. Right lateral aspect.

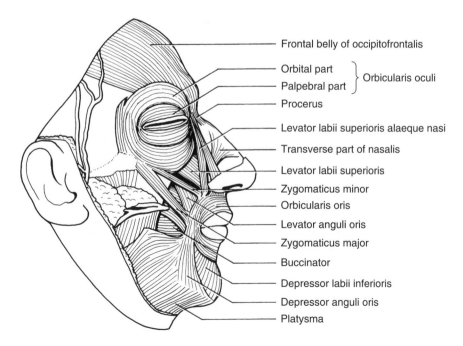

Frontal belly of occipitofrontalis

Orbital part
Palpebral part } Orbicularis oculi

Procerus

Levator labii superioris alaeque nasi

Transverse part of nasalis

Levator labii superioris

Zygomaticus minor

Orbicularis oris

Levator anguli oris

Zygomaticus major

Buccinator

Depressor labii inferioris

Depressor anguli oris

Platysma

because due to the laxity of the tissues at this site there is a risk of a haematoma developing.

## Zygomaticus major

This muscle, which assists in controlling facial expression by drawing the angle of the mouth upwards and backwards, attaches above to the zygomatic bone, and below to the angle of the mouth.

A TrP in it may become activated either as a result of direct trauma to the face or secondary to TrP activation in the masticatory muscles. This point is usually situated just above the corner of the mouth and is best located with the mouth propped wide open and the muscle held in a pincer grip with one digit intraorally and the other extraorally. Pain from it is referred upwards along the side of the nose to the forehead (Fig. 16.12). The TrP is generally to be found in a palpable band of muscle and to deactivate it, a needle should be inserted into the superficial tissues overlying it.

## Occipitofrontalis muscle

This cutaneous muscle of the scalp is in two parts – the frontalis situated anteriorly, and the occipitalis situated posteriorly. The action of both of them acting together is to wrinkle the forehead.

A TrP in the frontalis is liable to become activated in someone who persistently frowns, and also, when TrPs in the sternomastoid muscle refer pain to the frontal region of the head.

The TrP is usually situated above the inner end of the eyebrow. Pain from this is referred locally around the TrP site. In order to deactivate it, a needle should be inserted superficially and obliquely into the skin (Fig. 16.13). A TrP in the occipitalis part of the muscle often becomes activated as a result of TrPs in the posterior cervical muscles referring pain to the occipital region. It refers pain over the side of the head from the occiput to the orbit (Fig. 16.14). It is readily identified by palpating gently over the back of the head and this point also should be deactivated by inserting a needle superficially and obliquely into the skin.

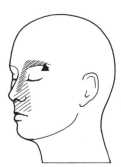

**Figure 16.11** The pattern of pain referral from a trigger point in the orbicularis oculi muscle.

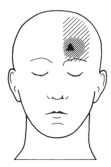

**Figure 16.13** The pattern of pain referral from a trigger point in the frontalis belly of the occipitofrontalis muscle.

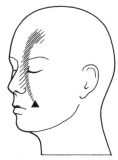

**Figure 16.12** The pattern of pain referral from a trigger point in the zygomaticus muscle.

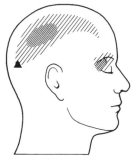

**Figure 16.14** The pattern of pain referral from a trigger point in the occipitalis belly of the occipitofrontalis muscle.

# References

Andersson A, Holmgren E 1975 On acupuncture analgesia and the mechanism of pain. American Journal of Chinese Medicine 3: 311–334

Anselmi B, Baldi E, Casacci F, Salmon S 1980 Endogenous opioids in cerebrospinal fluid and blood in idiopathic headache sufferers. Headache 20: 294–299

Ayer W 1983 Report of the president's conference on the examination, diagnosis and management of temperomandibular disorders. Journal of American Dental Association 106: 75–77

Baldry P E 1999 Aetiology and treatment of some common cephalalgias. Acupuncture in Medicine 17(1): 22–35

Baldry P E 2001 Myofascial pain and fibromyalgia syndrome. Churchill Livingstone, Edinburgh

Bank J 1991 Brainstem auditory evoked potentials in migraine after Rausedyl provocation. Cephalalgia 11: 277–279

Banks S L, Jacobs D W, Gervitz R, Hubbard D R 1998 Effects of autogenic relaxation training on electromyographic activity in active myofascial trigger points. Journal of Musculoskeletal Pain 6(4): 23–32

Behrmann S 1983 Traumatic neuropathy of second cervical spinal nerves. British Medical Journal 286: 1312–1313

Bell W E 1977 Management of masticatory pain. In: Alling C C, Mayhan P E (eds) Facial pain, 2nd edn. Lea & Febiger, Philadelphia

Campbell A 2001 Acupuncture in practice. Beyond points and meridians. Butterworth-Heinemann, Oxford, p. 92

Cawson R A 1984 Pain in the temperomandibular joint. British Medical Journal 288: 1857–1858

Chalmers I M, Blair G S 1973 Rheumatoid arthritis of the temperomandibular joint. Quarterly Journal of Medicine 42: 369–386

Chapman C R, Colpitts Y M, Benedetti C, Kitaeff R, Gehrig J D 1980 Evoked potential assessment of acupuncture analgesia, attempted reversal with naloxone. Pain 9: 183–197

Clarke N G 1982 Occlusion and myofascial pain dysfunction; is there a relationship? Journal of American Dental Association 85: 892

Cohen L A 1959 Body orientation and motor coordination in animals with impaired neck sensation. Federation Proceedings 18: 28

Cohen L A 1961 Role of eye and neck proprioceptive mechanisms in body orientation and motor co-ordination. Journal of Neurophysiology 24: 1–11

Couch J R, Hassanein R S 1976 Amitriptyline in migraine prophylaxis. Archives of Neurology (Chicago) 36: 695–699

Couch J R, Ziegler D K, Hassanein R S 1976 Amitriptyline in the prophylaxis of migraine. Effectiveness and relationship of antimigraine and antidepressant effect. Neurology (Minneapolis) 26: 121–127

Curran D A, Hinterberger H, Lance J W 1965 Total plasma serotonin, 5-hydroxyindolacetic acid and p-hydroxy-m-methoxymandelic acid excretion in normal and migrainous subjects. Brain 88: 997–1009

Dowson D I, Lewith G T, Machin D 1985 The effects of acupuncture versus placebo in the treatment of headache. Pain 21: 35–42

Facchinetti F, Nappi G, Savoldi F, Genazzi A R 1981 Primary headaches: reduced circulating beta-lipoprotein and beta-endorphin levels with impaired reactivity to acupuncture. Cephalgia 1: 95–203

Goadsby P J, Lance J W 1990 Physiopathology of migraine. Revue du Practicien 40: 389–394

Greene C S, Lerman M D, Sutcher H D, Leskin D M 1969 The TMJ pain-dysfunction syndrome: heterogeneity of the patient population. Journal of American Dental Association 79: 1168–1172

Hay K M 1976 The treatment of pain in trigger areas in migraine. The Journal of the Royal College of General Practitioners 26: 372–376

Headache Classification Committee of the International Headache Society 1988 Classification and diagnostic criteria for headache disorders, cranial neuralgias and facial pain. Cephalalgia (suppl)7: 1–96

Henryk-Gutt R, Rees W L 1973 Psychological aspects of migraine. Journal of Psychomatic Research 17: 141–153

Hopkins A 1993 Clinical neurology. A modern approach. Oxford University Press, Oxford, p. 117

Jeans M E 1979 Relief of chronic pain by brief, intense transcutaneous electrical stimulation – a double blind study. In: Bonica J J, Liebeskind J C, Albe-Fessard D G (eds) Advances in pain research and therapy 3. Raven Press, New York, p. 601–606

Jensen L B, Melsen B, Jensen S B 1979 Effect of acupuncture on headache measured by reduction in number of attacks and use of drugs. Scandinavian Journal of Dental Research 87: 373–380

Lance J W, Curran D A 1964 Treatment of chronic tension headache. Lancet 1: 1236–1239

Laskin D M 1969 Etiology of the pain dysfunction syndrome. Journal of American Dental Association 79: 147–153

Lewis C 1994 Needle trigger point and surface frontal EMG measurements of psychophysiological responses in tension-type headache patients. Biofeedback and Self-regulation 3: 274–275

Loeser J D 1984 Tic douloureux and atypical facial pain. In: Wall P, Melzack R (eds) Textbook of pain. Churchill Livingstone, Edinburgh, p. 430

Loh L, Nathan P W, Schott G D, Siekha K J 1984 Acupuncture versus medical treatment for migraine and muscle tension headaches. Journal of Neurology, Neurosurgery and Psychiatry 47: 333–337

Lous I, Olesen J 1982 Evaluation of pericranial tenderness and oral function in patients with common migraine, muscle contraction headache and 'combination headache'. Pain 12: 385–393

Marcus P 1995 Interrelationships of neurochemicals, estrogen and recurring headache. Pain 62: 129–139

Mann F 1996 Reinventing acupuncture. A new concept of ancient medicine. Butterworth-Heinmann, Oxford, p. 6

Mann F, Bowsher D, Mumford J, Lipton S, Miles J 1973 Treatment of intractable pain by acupuncture. Lancet II: 57–60

Matthews W B, 1983 Headache. In: Weatherall D A, Ledingham J G G, Warrell D A (eds) Oxford textbook of medicine. Oxford University Press, Oxford, p. 145–149

Matthews W B, Miller H 1972 Diseases of the nervous system. Blackwell Scientific Publications, Oxford, p. 122–123

McNulty W H, Gervitz R N, Hubbard D R et al 1994 Needle electromyographic evaluation of trigger point response to a psychological stressor. Psychophysiology 31(3): 313–316

McQuay H, Carroll D, Jadad A R , Wiffen P, Moore A 1995 Anticonvulsant drugs for management of pain: a systematic review. British Medical Journal 311(7012): 1047–1052

Mikhail M, Rosen H 1980 History and etiology of myofascial pain-dysfunction syndrome. Journal of Prosthetic Dentistry 44: 438–444

Moskowitz M A, Cutrer F M 1993 Sumatriptan: a receptor – targeted treatment for migraine. Annual Review of Medicine 44: 145–154

Olesen J 1991 Clinical and pathophysiolgical observations in migrane and tension-type headache explained by integration of vascular, supraspinal, and myofascial inputs. Pain 46: 125–132

Olesen J, Bonica J 1990 Headache. In: Bonica J J (ed) The management of pain, 2nd edn. Lea & Febiger, Philidelphia, Vol 1, pp. 687–726

Olesen J, Lauritzen M 1982 Spreading cerebral oligaemia in classical and normal cerebral blood flow in migraine. Headache 22: 242–248

Peterson A L, Talcott G W, Kelleher W J et al 1995 Site specificity of pain and tension in tension-type headaches. Headache 35(2): 89–92

Plum F 1982 Headache. In: Wyngaarden J B, Smith L (Jnr) (eds) Cecil's textbook of medicine, 16th edn. Saunders, Philadelphia, pp. 1948–1951

Rossi G F, Brodal A 1956 Spinal afferents to the trigeminal sensory nuclei and to the nucleus of the solitary tract. Confinia Neurologica 16: 321–322

Rubin D 1981 Myofascial trigger point syndromes. An approach to management. Archives of Physical Medicine and Rehabilitation 62: 107–110

Saper J R, Silberstein S D, Lake A E, Winters M E 1994 Double-blind trial of fluoxetine: chronic daily headache and migraine. Headache 34: 497–502

Schoenen J, Gerard P, De Pasqua V et al 1991 EMG activity in pericranial muscles during postural variation and mental activity in healthy volunteers and patients with chronic tension headache. Headache 31: 321–324

Schwartz L L 1956 A temperomandibular joint pain-dysfunction syndrome. Journal of Chronic Diseases 3: 284–293

Sessle B J, Hu J W, Dubner R, Lucier G E 1981 Functional properties of neurons in cat trigeminal subnucleus caudalis (medullary dorsal horn) II. Modulation of responses to noxious and non-noxious stimuli by periaqueductal grey, nucleus raphe magnus, cerebral cortex, and afferent influences, and effect of naloxone. Journal of Neurophysiology 45: 211–255

Sharav Y 1999 Orofacial pain. In: Wall P D, Melzack R (eds) Textbook of pain, 4th edn. Churchill Livingstone, Edinburgh

Sharav Y, Tzukert A, Refaeli B 1978 Muscle pain index in relation to pain dysfunction and dizziness associated with the myofascial pain-dysfunction syndrome. Oral Surgery 46: 742–747

Sicuteri F, Anselmi B, Curradi C, Michelacci S, Sassi A 1978 Morphine-like factors in CSF of headache patients. In: Costa E, Trabucci M (eds) Advances in biochemical psychopharmacology 18. Raven Press, New York, pp. 363–370

Silberstein S D, Lipton R B, Goadsby P J 1998 Headache in clinical practice. Isis Medical Media, Oxford

Simons D 2001 Tension-type headaches. In: Mense S, Simons D (eds) Muscle pain. Lippincott, Williams & Wilkins, Philadelphia, pp. 113–115

Somerville B W 1975 Estrogen – withdrawal migraine. Duration of exposure required and attempted prophylaxis by premenstrual estrogen administration. Neurology 25: 239–244

Stem P G, Mothersill K J, Brooke R I 1979 Biofeedback and a cognitive behavioral approach to treatment of myofascial pain-dysfunction syndrome. Behavior Therapy 10: 29–34

Tavola T, Gala C, Conte G, Invenizzi G 1992 Traditional Chinese acupuncture in tension-type headache: a controlled study. Pain 48: 325–329

Tfelt-Hansen P, Lous I, Oleson J 1981 Prevalence and significance of muscle tenderness during common migraine attacks. Headache 21: 49–54

Torvik A 1956 Afferent connections to the sensory trigeminal nuclei, the nucleus of the solitary tract and adjacent structures. Journal of Comparative Neurology 106: 51–132

Travell J 1955 Referred pain from skeletal muscle. I. Pectoralis major syndrome of breast pain and soreness II. Sternomastoid syndrome of headache and dizziness. New York State Journal of Medicine 55: 331–339

Travell J 1960 Temperomandibular joint pain referred from muscles of the head and neck. Journal of Prosthetic Dentistry 10: 745–763

Travell J 1967 Mechanical headache. Headache 7: 23–29

Travell J 1981 Identification of myofascial trigger point syndromes: a case of atypical facial neuralgia. Archives of Physical Medicine and Rehabilitation 62: 100–106

Travell J G, Simons D G 1983 Myofascial pain and dysfunction – the trigger point manual. Williams & Wilkins, Baltimore, pp. 168–182

Vincent C A 1989 A controlled trial of the treatment of migraine by acupuncture. The Clinical Journal of Pain 5(4): 305–312

Vincent C A 1990 The treatment of tension headache by acupuncture: a controlled single case design with time series analysis. Journal of Psychosomatic Research 34(5): 553–561

Weddington W N, Blazer D 1979 Atypical facial pain and trigeminal neuralgia: a comparison study. Psychosomatics 20: 348–356

Weeks V D, Travell J 1955 Postural vertigo due to trigger areas in the sternocleidomastoid muscle. Journal of Pediatrics 47: 315–327

Zakrzewska J A 1999 Trigeminal, eye and ear pain. In: Wall P D, Melzack R (eds) Textbook of pain, 4th edn, Ch. 32. Churchill Livingstone, Edinburgh

# Chapter 17

# Low-back pain

## CHAPTER CONTENTS

## INTRODUCTION

The main indication for acupuncture in the alleviation of low-back pain is when such pain is mechanical in its relationship to activity, and in particular when it emanates from myofascial trigger points (MTrPs). These may have become activated as a primary event when the muscles containing them have become either overloaded or subjected to direct trauma. Alternatively, but less commonly as a secondary event following the development of nerve root entrapment from, for example, disc prolapse or spondylitic changes in the spine.

It therefore follows that before contemplating the use of such treatment it is necessary to exclude other causes of low-back pain of a non-mechanical nature including inflammatory, metabolic, and neoplastic disorders of the spine; also referred pain from abdominal or pelvic organs; and the pain of peripheral vascular disease.

It is only possible to do this by taking a careful history, by carrying out a detailed physical examination including in particular a systematic search of the musculature of the lower back for trigger points, and by carrying out certain investigations. With respect to the latter, it is essential in all cases to measure the erythrocyte sedimentation rate (ESR) and to have radiographs (PA, oblique and lateral views) of the spine. In certain circumstances it may also be necessary to carry out more highly specialized investigations such as magnetic resonance imaging (MRI) and, on occasions, certain specific biochemical blood tests.

## DIFFERENTIAL DIAGNOSIS BETWEEN MECHANICAL AND NON-MECHANICAL LOW-BACK PAIN

Although it would clearly be inappropriate in a book of this type to enter into a detailed discussion of all the various diagnostic features that help to separate mechanical from non-mechanical low-back pain; it, nevertheless, may help to ensure that acupuncture is not used inappropriately if brief reference is made to a few of the more important ones.

### Mechanical low-back pain

The history given by a patient with low-back pain of mechanical type is quite different from that when the pain is due to some non-mechanical cause, and therefore simply by listening to the patient carefully one can often obtain considerable help in distinguishing between these two fundamentally different types of pain.

The commonest form of low-back pain is that which occurs as a result of some structural dysfunction and, because of the direct relationship it has with activity, it may be said to be of the mechanical type. It tends to be more noticeable in carrying out movements after sitting or lying down for some time. Also, twisting, lifting, bending, and coughing often make it worse. It is relieved by resting and, therefore, as might be expected, there is often a history of it being most troublesome during the course of daytime activities. It may, nevertheless, come on in bed at night as a result of turning or lying awkwardly, but when this occurs it is quickly eased once a comfortable position is found.

There is sometimes a complaint that the pain becomes worse on sitting down. This may seem surprising, but the reason for this will be explained later when discussing the location of TrPs.

It has to be remembered that a history of pain in the buttocks and thighs, brought on by walking and relieved by resting, may be vascular in origin, and develop as a result of aorto-iliac occlusion (Leriche's syndrome). In addition, it is possible for sciatica to occur as a result of atheromatous obstruction in the internal iliac artery causing ischaemia of the sciatic nerve (Lamerton et al 1983). This is why history-taking must be supplemented with a careful physical examination including palpation of the femoral pulses.

Further, when a patient with low-back pain complains that the legs become painful, weak, and affected by paraesthesiae on walking, and that this is relieved by resting, and, in particular, by adopting a squatting position, the possibility of stenosis of the spinal canal, either congenital or acquired, has to be considered (Porter 1987). This should be investigated accordingly by tomography, or by ultrasonic measurements (Porter et al 1978), or, preferably, by computerized axial tomography (Schumaker et al 1978).

### Non-mechanical low-back pain

Non-mechanical low-back pain occurs far less commonly than that of the mechanical type. It occurs as a result of neoplastic, infective, inflammatory, or metabolic disease of the spine, and for several reasons, including the fact that its intensity bears no relationship to physical activity, the history tends to be different.

The onset is usually insidious, with the pain gradually increasing in intensity, and being as severe when resting at night as it is during the day. It may, in fact, seem to be worse at night because there is nothing to distract the mind from it, and unlike mechanical type pain, it cannot be eased by a change of position.

Ankylosing spondylitis, the principal inflammatory disease affecting the lower back, will be singled out for special mention because of certain distinctive features in the history (Calin et al 1977), and because it is the one non-mechanical disorder in which acupuncture may be of much help in relieving pain. The disease, which affects men five times more commonly than women, declares itself in early adult life by the insidious onset of pain affecting both sides of the lower back and spreading to the buttocks. This pain characteristically causes early morning waking and on rising there is considerable stiffness, but this is relieved by activity. In addition, there may be a history of iritis, and a family history of the disease. Careful attention to the history is essential because, although once the disease has become established the ESR is elevated and there are diagnostic radiographic changes in the sacroiliac joints and lumbar spine, in the early stages both the ESR and the X-ray appearances may be normal. In such circumstances it may sometimes be necessary to carry out technetium scanning of the sacroiliac joints in order to demonstrate the presence of sacroiliitis. When the clinical picture is not straightforward, the HLA-B27 test may also be helpful, as a positive test is strongly suggestive of this disease being the cause of the pain. At the same time, it has to be remembered that it may only be a reflection of a carrier state, with the pain being due to some other cause.

## PAIN REFERRED TO THE BACK FROM ABDOMINAL AND PELVIC ORGANS

When pain in the lower part of the back occurs as a result of it being referred to that site from some abdominal or pelvic disorder, it is usually accompanied by other symptoms that direct attention to the organ involved. This, however, is not invariable, particularly in the initial stages, and one has to be particularly wary when there is a history of recent trauma to the back as this may be diagnostically misleading.

A woman (54 years of age) developed persistent pain across the lower back shortly after being involved in a car accident. The pain was unremitting and in spite of it being present day and night, and not relieved by rest, the trauma was assumed to be responsible, and in view of this she spent several months having physiotherapy. By the time she was referred to me for an opinion as to whether acupuncture might be helpful, the character of the pain together with the fact that she was losing weight and feeling generally unwell, led to further investigations that ultimately revealed the presence of a carcinoma of the body of the pancreas.

## DUAL PATHOLOGY

When taking the history it has to be remembered that in spite of the philosophical maxim of the 14th-century Franciscan, William of Occam, that 'Entities are not to be multiplied without necessity' (Occam's razor), symptoms indicative of abdominal or pelvic disease, and low-back pain may not necessarily be due to the same cause.

Several cases have been referred to me by a gastroenterological colleague for acupuncture because, although there have been symptoms of an abdominal disorder, such as the irritable bowel syndrome, or diverticulitis, there has in addition been low-back pain that, from its relationship to posture and movement, has clearly been of a mechanical type and, therefore, eminently suitable for this form of treatment.

## CLINICAL EXAMINATION

As a detailed account of the proper manner in which to examine the back is to be found in any standard textbook, only some of the more salient features will be mentioned here with special reference to those of particular importance in coming to a decision as to whether or not acupuncture might be helpful in the symptomatic relief of lumbosacral pain.

The examination really begins as soon as the patient enters the room, and particularly whilst taking the history, as observations at that stage concerning the patient's appearance, expression, and manner of describing symptoms often give a good indication as to whether or not there is likely to be an underlying debilitating disease. In this way an idea as to the degree to which the pain is affecting the patient and the psychological make-up of the individual can also be obtained. As will be explained later, there is often a complex inter-relationship between psyche and soma in the pathogenesis of mechanical type low-back pain, which often influences the response to any form of treatment, including acupuncture, and which often makes it necessary to treat both the mind and the body.

The first part of the formal examination of the back should be carried out with the patient standing and with sufficient clothes removed to give an uninterrupted view of the whole length of the spine and legs.

On inspection, the trained eye will readily note the café-au-lait patch possibly indicative of a neurofibroma, the midline dimple or tufts of hair over a spina bifida occulta, the patch of erythema ab igne from prolonged usage of a hot water bottle, and the lower lumbar hump characteristics of spondylolisthesis. However, from an everyday practical point of view, and particularly when acupuncture is likely to be used, the most important observations at this stage are those concerning whether or not there is inequality of the length of the two legs.

## Short–leg syndrome

A short leg, either when this is of congenital origin, or when it is acquired, usually as a result of a fracture, puts a considerable strain on the muscles of the lower back, so that when TrPs in these muscles become activated for one reason or another, the effect of this strain is to nullify any attempt to deactivate these points. It is therefore a waste of time employing any technique such as acupuncture for this purpose without at the same time correcting the deformity.

The physical findings associated with relative shortness of one leg include the pelvis being seen to be titled in association with a compensatory scoliosis; also, on the side of the short leg, the shoulder is held lower, the hip is less prominent, there is a loss of the hollow of the flank, and the gluteal fold is lower than the one on the opposite side (Nichols 1960).

Travell & Simons (1983, pp. 105–109) consider that a discrepancy in leg length of 1.3 cm (1/2") may cause no symptoms throughout a lifetime if MTrPs do not become activated, but if, for one reason or another, this occurs, then it only needs a discrepancy of 0.5 cm (3/16") to perpetuate this TrP activity.

Travell (1976) believes that the quadratus lumborum is the one muscle in particular in which TrP activity is most likely to persist in the presence of a short leg.

It is important to realize that an uncorrected short leg has far-ranging consequences because it may not only cause low-back pain to become chronic, but it may also, by putting a strain on the ipsilateral muscles of the neck, cause TrPs to become activated in those mucles with the consequent development of persistent neck pain and headaches.

Two commonly used techniques for assessing differences in leg length, carried out with the patient lying down, are unreliable because the patient is non-weight bearing. These include one where a tape measurement is made from the anterior superior iliac spine to the tip of the medial malleolus; and the other where, with the knees straight, the distance is measured between comparable points on the medial malleoli. A better method is to have the undressed patient in the standing position with the feet together. An approximate estimate of the comparative length of two legs can then be made by palpating the iliac crests, or posterior superior iliac spines. Pages of a journal should then be placed under the foot of the short leg, and the number of these gradually increased until the pelvis and shoulder are level. This gives a measure as to how much the shoe on the affected side should be raised, a task that in my experience is best done by a cobbler with a special interest in and experience of this type of work.

## Curves of the lumbar spine

On inspection of the back with the patient standing, the curves of the lumbar spine should also be observed. Loss of its normal lordosis may occur with certain inflammatory conditions but it may also result from pregnancy and obesity. Any scoliosis also should be noted. This may develop in painful conditions as a result of muscle spasm, or as discussed above, it may occur together with a pelvic tilt, when the legs are of unequal length. When due to the former, it is sometimes only seen on forward flexion, whereas with the latter this movement usually causes it to disappear.

## Wasting of the muscles

It should also be noted whether there is any wasting of the muscles. Wasting of the paraspinal muscles, for example, often occurs with chronic inflammatory conditions of the spine.

## Movement of the spine

The movements of the spine should next be tested, including forward flexion, lateral flexion, extension and rotation. In the case of non-mechanical pain due to inflammatory or neoplastic conditions there is often a generalized restriction of all lumbar movements. When pain is of a mechanical type and, therefore, likely to be suitable for treatment with acupuncture, only certain movements are likely to be limited, and observing which these are gives helpful guidance as to where TrPs are likely to be found. TrPs are also often more readily palpable when muscles are put on the stretch. And following treatment with acupuncture, it is wise to re-test the spine's range of movements as in this way attention may be drawn to TrPs that have been overlooked.

## Examination of the patient lying down

For the second part of the examination the patient lies face upwards on the examination couch in order that the abdomen may be examined for evidence of visceral disease. The femoral pulses should also be palpated at this stage.

This should be followed by an assessment of hip and knee movements, a neurological examination, and the carrying out of the straight-leg raising test (Lasègue's sign). A vaginal or rectal examination should then be performed when indicated.

## Search for TrPs

The final part of the examination and one that should be carried out especially carefully is a search for TrPs. This is of particular importance when the pain is found to be of the mechanical type and due to some relatively benign structural disorder because it would seem that it is from activated TrPs that much of this pain emanates. The reason for saying this is that pressure applied to these points aggravates the pain and relief from it may often be obtained simply by deactivating these points by means of the acupuncture technique of inserting dry needles into the tissues overlying them. This search has to be conducted in an unhurried and systematic manner because, unlike the TrPs responsible for similar pain in the neck, which tend to be found at identical sites in everyone, the distribution of TrPs in the lower

back has no fixed pattern and is in fact widely variable from person to person.

The patient should first be placed in the prone position, and the muscles of the back from the lower thoracic region downwards should be palpated by placing the examining hand flat on the back and rolling the skin and subcutaneous tissue over the underlying muscle by means of flexing fingers in a manner similar to that used in kneading dough.

TrPs in the lower back occur as focal areas of exquisite tenderness either in muscle which otherwise feels normal, or in elongated fibrous bands of muscle (palpable bands) or in so-called 'fibrositic' nodules.

It is a good rule to start the search by palpating along the length of the spine in the midline from the level of the 10th dorsal vertebra above, to the coccyx below, and then systematically to examine every part of the musculature on each side of the back in turn, by palpating along lines about 1 cm apart and parallel to the spine, from a similar level above, to the upper border of the buttocks below. The muscles of the buttocks should next be palpated, first using light pressure, and then deep pressure, and this should be followed by palpation of the muscles along the back of the leg.

The patient should then roll on to each side in turn so that the muscles of the flank can be palpated from the iliac crest above to the greater trochanter below, with special attention being paid to the area around the latter structure as it is surprising how often there is a crop of TrPs in muscles near to their sites of attachment to it. The outer side of the thigh should then be palpated because it is common to find TrPs along the length of the tensor fasciae latae and iliotibial tract.

The examination should be completed by getting the patient to lie in the supine position and the search for TrPs continued by palpating the muscles of the anterior abdominal wall and the inner side of the thigh, with special attention being paid to sites where the adductor muscles of the leg become attached to the pelvis and the iliopsoas muscle attaches to the lesser trochanter.

Back pain referred from TrPs in the abdominal wall musculature is discussed in Chapter 20. It is important to remember that TrPs in and around the pubic region and the upper inner part of the thigh, at or near to the site of the attachment of the adductor muscles to the pelvis, may not only be associated with low-back pain, but on occasions are responsible for pain being referred to the hip region, to the scrotum, or to the vagina. It should also be noted that it is activation of these TrPs that sometimes makes a person with low-back pain complain that the pain is worse on sitting down. The following case is a typical example.

A housewife (62 years of age) was referred to me with persistent pain in the lower back and buttocks that was made worse both by certain movements and on sitting down. Dry-needle deactivation of many TrPs in the lower back relieved her of much of the pain but the pain on sitting persisted. There was no TrP in the region of the ischial tuberosity to account for this but there were some exquisitely tender ones at the sites of insertion of the adductor muscles into the pubis, and once these were deactivated the sitting position became comfortable.

An account of some of the commoner sites where TrPs are to be found in the muscles of the lower back, and their specific patterns of pain referral, will be given towards the end of this chapter. It is remarkable how often they coincide in position with traditional Chinese acupuncture points (see Fig. 17.1).

## INVESTIGATIONS OF ASSISTANCE IN DISTINGUISHING BETWEEN THE MECHANICAL AND NON-MECHANICAL TYPES OF LOW-BACK PAIN

### Erythrocyte sedimentation rate (ESR)

The erythrocyte sedimentation rate, using the standard Westergren technique, is one of the most reliable means of distinguishing between these two types of low-back pain in view of the fact that with mechanical type low-back pain the rate is usually not above the upper limit of normal of 25 mm in the first hour, whereas with disorders responsible for non-mechanical type pain the rate is in general well above this. One important exception is early ankylosing spondylitis when the rate in about 20% of cases may for a time remain normal.

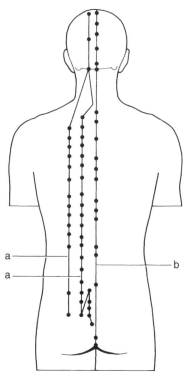

Figure 17.1 The traditional Chinese (a) Urinary bladder and (b) Du acu-tracts.

## Plain radiographs

As will be seen when chronic low-back pain is considered in detail later, there is no clearly defined relationship between its development and the radiographic changes of disc or facet joint degeneration. Also, with acute disc prolapse, the plain X-ray appearances are normal. In the assessment of low-back pain of the mechanical type, therefore, there is little to be learnt from plain radiographs of the spine. The main importance of having them is to exclude non-mechanical causes of low-back pain including infective, inflammatory, and neoplastic lesions. It is essential to bear in mind, however, that in the early stages of such disorders the radiographic appearances may be normal, and, therefore, at times it is wise to have a technetium scan. It is believed that an increased uptake of this radioisotope is dependent on an increased bone blood flow and metabolism, and as this is common to all these various diseases, it necessarily follows that a positive result does not distinguish between them, but does serve to rule out the possibility of the pain being only mechanical in type (McKillop & McDougal 1980).

## Magnetic resonance imaging

MRI, which was introduced in 1982 has proved to be of considerable help in the investigation of low-back pain disorders (Kleefield & O'Reilly 1992).

## SOME CAUSES OF MECHANICAL TYPE LOW-BACK PAIN AND THEIR MANAGEMENT

There are many potential causes of low-back pain of the mechanical type, both psychological and physical, and frequently, several of them contribute to the condition simultaneously. The situation is further complicated by the fact that the exact manner in which some of the factors operate remains obscure. There can be no doubt that it is because of such difficulties that the management of this type of pain remains far from satisfactory, and why the effects of most forms of treatment for it, including acupuncture, are notoriously unpredictable.

It was because of this that Nachemson (1979) was prompted to say:

> Having been engaged in research in this field for nearly 25 years and having been clinically engaged in back problems for nearly the same period of time and as a member and scientific adviser to several international back associations, I can only state that for the majority of our patients, the true cause of low-back pain is unknown … since the cause is unknown there is only symptomatic treatment available.

This undoubtedly is true, so the remainder of this chapter will be devoted to reviewing the clinical characteristics of the various structural disorders in the lower back considered to be capable of giving rise to pain of the mechanical type, and examining the various neurological mechanisms thought to be responsible for this. An attempt will also be made to evaluate the various forms of symptomatic treatment available, in order to assess which of them in the light of our present knowledge seem to be based on sound physiological principles.

The purpose of this is to show that acupuncture may be included amongst these, and that there is much to be gained by using it, either in conjunction with, or at times instead of, some of these other so-called more orthodox forms of treatment.

During the course of this review it will be observed how often with many of these structural disorders, MTrPs are an important source of pain. The activation of points is sometimes a primary event and at other times a secondary one. There is a need for wider recognition of this phenomenon now that it has been shown that deactivation of these points by the acupuncture technique of dry needle stimulation is not only frequently effective in alleviating low-back pain, but also is both simple to apply and safe to use, this being more than can be said for some of the more complex forms of treatment in current use.

## ACUTE LOW-BACK PAIN

The description of Mixter & Barr in 1934 of the symptoms and signs of a prolapsed intervertebral disc (PID) and how the pain from this condition can often be relieved by a laminectomy was undoubtedly of considerable importance. However, since the chemistry of the intervertebral disc has become better understood (Urban & Maroudas 1980), it is now recognized that PID as a cause of acute low-back pain must be a comparatively rare event. The reason for this is that the central nucleus pulposus of a disc, over the years, becomes increasingly inspissated, and it is only possible for it to bulge through a ruptured annulus fibrosus and impinge on a nerve root, whilst it still remains in a relatively fluid state. This is approximately up to the age of 50 years, and during this earlier part of adult life rupture of an annulus fibrosus is uncommon because the degenerative changes are still at an early stage.

As Dixon (1980) rightly points out, disc prolapse is probably the most overdiagnosed cause of low-back pain, and goes on to state that 'indeed the whole myth of the "slipped disc" is one of the deep rooted weeds that have sprung up in this area. Discs do not "slip" in the way in which laymen and not a few doctors imagine'. He believes that this over-diagnosis may be due to the fact that most patients with proved prolapse give a history of past episodes of acute low-back pain without nerve root compression, and that the diagnosis is often one of convenience. Wyke (1980) in support of this view estimates that 'contrary to popular impression … less than 5% of patients with backache have prolapsed intervertebral discs', but at the same time agrees that 70% of those with PID have backache as the initial symptom.

It is now generally accepted that acute mechanical type low-back pain is most commonly due to some primary disorder of muscle, for example, such as when the tendinous attachments of muscles become avulsed, or muscle fibres and their fascial sheaths become torn as a result of the lower back muscles being suddenly overloaded as a result of a heavy object being lifted in the stooping position or, for example, when the muscles become strained by being overloaded for some considerable time. Alternatively, it may occur when the back is exposed to draughts or damp, or, at times, for no obvious reason. Formerly, its development under such circumstances led to a diagnosis of fibrositis or myositis, or more recently to one of myofasciitis. As previously explained (Ch. 5) all such terms are no longer acceptable as inflammatory changes in the muscle have never been demonstrated.

Acute low-back pain also commonly occurs when the nociceptive receptor systems in either the fibrous capsules of the facet joints or the lumbosacral ligaments become stimulated as a result of the spine being subjected to persistent postural stress. The clinical picture, irrespective of the structure or structures involved, is one of acute localized pain with reflex spasm of the paravertebral muscles, and the presence of exquisitely tender TrPs. This picture is identical to that seen with the much rarer acute disc prolapse at a stage before pain extends down the leg. With regard to the activation of TrPs, the only difference is that with disorders of the muscle or ligaments the activation is a primary event, but with facet joint strain or disc prolapse it is a secondary one.

It therefore follows that with the development of acute low-back pain, because of the difficulty in distinguishing clinically between these various causes, it is impossible to make a precise diagnosis, and it is better, in my opinion, to refer to all such cases as being examples of the acute lumbar myofascial TrP pain syndrome. This at least helps

to guard against the all too frequent error of assuming that acute low-back pain must be due to a 'slipped disc', and for this reason alone, automatically subjecting the person concerned to a period of strict bed rest without first of all carrying out a detailed examination. Admittedly acute low-back pain may require bed rest, but it is essentially the severity of the pain that dictates when this is necessary. Bed rest should certainly never be prescribed without there first being a systematic search for TrPs, because, when present, the deactivation of these by acupuncture by alleviating the pain may obviate the need for bed rest, or it may shorten the period for which it is required, as is illustrated by the following case.

A housewife (38 years of age) suddenly developed severe pain in the left lower back after bending for some time doing some strenuous gardening. She therefore took to her bed and called the doctor. After listening to the story, he told her she must have 'slipped a disc', and that she would have to lie flat on her back for 2–3 weeks. This immediately created a domestic crisis as she and her family had planned to drive to Switzerland 2 days later. The husband therefore persuaded the general practitioner to let me see her.

On examination she was lying very still and reluctant to move because of the pain it caused. When, after a certain amount of persuasion, she rolled over sufficiently for her back to be examined, one focal area of exquisite tenderness in the left flank was found, with pressure on this considerably aggravating the pain. After deactivating this TrP with a dry needle, the patient was more comfortable. When seen the next day, she reported that the pain relief had only lasted for about 2 hours, and on re-examination the TrP was as tender as before. It was, therefore, once again deactivated with a dry needle, and this time the pain relief was longer lasting, so that 24 hours later she was able to set off on the journey to Europe without any discomfort.

## Spontaneous resolution of acute low–back pain

It could be argued that in the case just quoted the pain might have resolved spontaneously within a few days, but from its severity and the degree of muscle spasm present, this would seem to have been unlikely.

Nevertheless, it is important to remember in assessing the effects of any form of treatment for acute low-back pain that most of those who suffer from it become symptom-free in 4–6 weeks irrespective of treatment (White 1966, Rowe 1969) and as Waddell (1982) says in discussing the subject 'frequently treatment simply takes the credit for natural history and the passage of time'.

This no doubt is true but acute low-back pain that persists for 4–6 weeks can often seriously interfere with a person's ability to work or to carry out sporting activities, and if it can be shown, as my everyday clinical experience would lead me to believe, that acupuncture by its direct action on TrPs is capable of alleviating the pain more quickly than might be expected if left to resolve spontaneously, then such treatment is obviously well worth using. The difficulties of proving this statistically, however, are formidable as with a condition with such a relatively short natural history, the numbers of cases required both for the treatment and control groups would be extremely large, and in order that such a trial could be completed in a reasonable time, many centres would have to participate.

## ACUTE SCIATICA

Following Mixter & Barr's important contribution to the subject of acute disc prolapse in 1934, it became generally assumed that the diagnosis of this condition, and that of acute sciatica were synonymous and, moreover, it was also widely believed that the sciatic pain was invariably due to the disc exerting pressure on a nerve root.

In recent years it has been found necessary to modify these concepts because, although it is undoubtedly true that acute sciatica may occur when a disc is sufficiently badly prolapsed as to exert pressure on a nerve root, it is now realized that acute pain along the course of the sciatic nerve is more often due to it being referred down the back of the leg from TrPs in the muscles of the lower back. These TrPs become activated either as a result of a partially prolapsed disc causing the back muscles to go into spasm, but even more

frequently as a result of the muscles being subjected to strain during the course of some physical activity.

Firstly, therefore, a description will be given of the clinical picture that arises when acute sciatica is caused by a badly prolapsed disc pressing on a nerve root, and following this, acute sciatica of the referred type will be discussed.

## Acute prolapse of a disc with 'sciatica' due to pressure on a nerve root

There is often a history of recurrent episodes of low-back pain before the eventual sudden onset of sciatica with a severe shooting type of pain that radiates from the lower back, down the leg to the foot.

The discs most likely to prolapse include the one between the 4th and 5th lumbar vertebrae with involvement of the 5th lumbar nerve root, and the one between the 5th lumbar vertebra and the sacrum with involvement of the 1st sacral nerve root. Much less commonly, the disc between the 3rd and 4th vertebrae prolapses with involvement of the 4th lumbar nerve root.

With involvement of the 5th lumbar nerve root, pain is felt in the buttock, down the posterolateral aspect of the thigh and leg, and over the inner half of the foot; dorsi flexion of the toes is weak; and the tendon reflexes are normal.

With involvement of the 1st sacral nerve root, pain is felt in the buttock, down the back of the thigh and leg and along the outer side of the foot; plantar flexion of the foot is weak and the ankle jerk diminished.

With the less common involvement of the 4th lumbar nerve root there is pain down the outer side of the thigh, and the inner side of the leg. There is weakness of knee extension and a diminished knee jerk. The pain in the buttock and thigh, no matter which root is involved, is associated with widespread muscle tenderness and the spasm of paravertebral muscles leads to the spine becoming rigid with a loss of the normal lumbar lordosis and the development of a scoliosis.

In addition to nerve root pain, there is at an early stage of the disorder pain in the back brought about as a result of an inflammatory reaction caused by the liberation of phospholipase A-2 and other enzymes from the nucleus pulposus following its extrusion (Saal et al 1990). This particular type of pain is always worst during the first 3 weeks due to the extruded disc absorbing water and, because of this, temporarily increasing in size.

Eventually, the prolapsed disc becomes smaller partly because of a gradual decrease in its fluid content, but also because of enzymatic resorption and phagocytosis together with resolution of the inflammatory process. It is because of all this that, after a period of time, discogenic pain tends to disappear spontaneously, and this is also why conservative treatment in some cases is all that is required.

### Factors that aggravate the pain

Disc pain is aggravated by sitting, lifting and movements that twist the torso. Relief is usually obtained by lying down. It is also invariably made worse by coughing, sneezing and straining to open the bowels.

### Influence of the vertebral canal's size on the pain

Porter (1993), from carrying out MRI studies, has found that the factor that determines whether or not pain is felt with a disc lesion is the size and shape of the vertebral canal. He compared the vertebral canal measurements in 173 patients with disc protrusion with 671 healthy controls, and found that it is those with disc lesions who have particularly small canal measurements and, therefore who are particularly likely to suffer pain. However, it is not only the size of the canal, but also its shape that matters, with a small trefoil-shaped canal being particularly disadvantageous.

### Straight leg-raising test (Lasègue's sign)

This test involves the passive flexion of the leg at the hip with the knee straight. The test is said to be positive when there is a restriction of movement to 45° or less.

This test is positive with compression of the 5th lumbar or 1st sacral nerve roots, and for many years subsequent to Mixter & Barr's original paper in 1934 it was thought that limitation of straight leg-raising only occurs when there is pressure on a nerve root by a prolapsed intervertebral disc. Therefore, nobody was surprised when Edgar & Park (1974) found the straight leg-raising test to be positive in 94% of patients with a surgically confirmed prolapse pressing on a nerve root, or that in 95% of such cases, pain could be induced in the affected leg by raising the opposite leg (the well leg-raising test). Such teaching, however, has had to be revised since King & Lagger (1976) have shown that a positive Lasègue's sign also occurs with acute sciatica of the referred type, and that in such cases it can be reversed by interrupting the arc between the posterior primary division, the cord, and the anterior primary division of a root segment. This no doubt explains why Spangfort (1972), in a computer-aided analysis of 2504 operations, found that of those patients with acute sciatica shown not to have a prolapsed disc at operation, 88.8% of them had a positive Lasègue's sign pre-operatively.

It therefore now has to be accepted that the restricted straight leg-raising that occurs with acute sciatica is not necessarily indicative of nerve root entrapment as it also occurs when the pain is of the referred type.

### TrPs

Activation of TrPs in the muscles of the back and leg is a prominent feature in all cases of acute disc prolapse. Chu (1995), during the course of carrying out electromyographic studies, has shown that TrPs in the paraspinal muscles commonly become activated as a secondary event following the development of nerve root entrapment. Simons et al (1999) attribute this to compression of motor nerves activating and perpetuating primary TrP dysfunction at the motor endplate.

### Radiographic examination

A plain X-ray of the spine is never of help in the diagnosis of acute disc prolapse because, as explained earlier, it always takes place at a time of life when disc degeneration is at an early stage and, therefore, before there has been time for narrowing of the intervertebral space to take place.

The best means of confirming the presence of a disc prolapse is by the carrying out of MRI. With respect to this, however, it has to be remembered that it is not uncommon for disc protrusion to develop without it giving rise to nerve root entrapment. Jensen et al (1994) showed this when they carried out a MRI study of the lumbar spine in people without back pain and found an appreciable incidence of disc prolapse.

It, therefore, follows that evidence of such a lesion on MRI cannot be assumed to be the cause of any pain that may be present unless there are clinical signs of nerve root entrapment at the same segmental level as that indicated on the scan.

## Acute sciatica of the referred type

From what has been said it is clear that a confident diagnosis of disc prolapse with acute sciatica due to the entrapment of a nerve root can only be made with any degree of confidence when there are objective neurological signs, including motor weakness followed later by muscle wasting, sensory impairment, suppression of tendon reflexes, and, particularly, if it is possible to obtain confirmatory evidence of nerve root compression by the carrying out of MRI.

With most cases of acute sciatica, however, there is no neurological deficit and the pain is referred from TrPs in the muscles and ligaments of the lower back. King & Lagger (1976) believe that this occurs when a partially prolapsed disc impinges on the sinu-vertebral nerve causing the paravertebral muscles and adjacent ligaments innervated by posterior rami to go into acute spasm, with this, in turn, causing TrPs in these structures to become activated. The consequence of this, to quote King & Lagger, is that 'pain impulses initiated in these posterior rami areas are referred to areas innervated by the anterior rami of the same and juxtaposed spinal roots'. In support of their hypothesis is their ability to alleviate this type of pain and, at the same time, to render negative the Lasègue's sign by interrupting this arc between the posterior rami, the cord, and the anterior rami, by deactivating these TrPs. It is only a pity that the methods they chose to use in order to achieve this were somewhat unnecessarily complicated and included radio-frequency percutaneous rhizotomy (Shealy et al 1974) and multiple bilateral percutaneous rhizolysis (Rees & Slade 1974).

The concept, however, that radiation of pain down the leg, in patients with low-back pain, is not necessarily due to nerve root entrapment and that sometimes it may occur as a result of it being referred down the leg from TrPs in the muscles and ligaments of the back, is not a recent one. It was first put forward by Steindler & Luck (1938), when they showed that it is possible to alleviate not only the pain in the back, but also the pain down the leg simply by injecting procaine into a TrP in the lumbar region. It was their observations concerning this that led them to develop their procaine hydrochloride test for use in patients with both low-back and leg pain. The test consists of injecting procaine into a TrP situated in a lumbar muscle or ligament in order to prove whether or not it is from that point that both the low-back and leg pain emanates. Such proof, according to them, required the following five postulates to be fulfilled:

1. The insertion of the needle into the TrP must aggravate the local pain in the back.
2. The insertion of the needle into the TrP must elicit or aggravate the pain referred down the leg.
3. The injection must suppress the referred pain.
4. The injection must suppress local tenderness.
5. Limited lumbar flexion or straight leg-raising must return to normal following the injection.

It is of course now recognized that with referred leg pain from TrPs in the back it is possible to fulfil these criteria of Steindler & Luck even more simply just by inserting an acupuncture needle into the tissues overlying them. This, however, in no way detracts from the importance of their work, and it is only very much to be regretted that until recent years such little attention has been paid to the basic principles propounded by them.

It is clear from what Steindler & Luck had to say on the subject that they believed that with most cases of sciatica of the referred type, the pain stemmed from TrPs activated by what they termed deep ligamentous injuries and myofasciitis. However, the possibility, as suggested by King & Lagger, that such activation may also develop as a result of partial prolapse of a disc does not seem to have occurred to them.

There is no doubt that this type of referred pain may be produced by either of these means but, because, for reasons already given, a prolapsed disc is somewhat of a rarity, the commonest cause would seem to be an acute primary strain of the muscles and ligaments.

## Management of disc prolapse

Surveys, such as those carried out by Friedenberger & Shoemaker in 1954 and by Weber in 1983 have shown that immediate surgery is only required for those with a midline disc rupture causing dysfunction of the bowel or bladder. All other patients with this disorder should initially be treated conservatively, as only a minority of them will ultimately be shown to need surgery.

### Conservative treatment

*Short-term bed rest followed by mobilization* Complete bed rest may be required for the first 1–2 weeks. This should be followed by increasing mobilization and the eventual carrying out of a progressive exercise programme (Manniche et al 1991, Saal & Saal (1989), Wynn Parry 1994).

*Analgesics and corticosteroids* Pain control requires the use of analgesics. In addition, because it is now recognized that much of the initial pain is due to an inflammatory reaction brought about by enzyme release and the consequent liberation of prostaglandins and leukotrienes, corticosteroids are being increasingly used. A drug of this type may be administered either orally (Johnson & Fletcher 1981), or intramuscularly (Green 1975), or, even more commonly, intrathecally. Bogduk (1995), however, during the course of questioning the value of using the latter route has stated, 'there is no compelling data from double-blind trials that vindicate the use of lumbar or caudal epidural steroids'. Despite this, an injection of this type continues to be widely used for the suppression of nerve root inflammation. Currently it is invariably given under fluoroscopic control (Dreyfuss 1993).

### Indications for surgical intervention
The general consensus of opinion is that a discetomy should be carried out in those cases where there is a worsening of the symptoms over the months, together with a progressively increased restriction of straight leg raising and deviation of the lumbar spine to one side. Other indications include pain evoked by contralateral straight-leg raising and a loss of diurnal changes in straight leg raising on the affected side. With a partial disc rupture the diurnal change with this test may be as much as 30°, but once the rupture is complete this is no longer observed and the prognosis without surgery is poor (Porter & Trailescu 1990).

*Post-laminectomy pain* One of the commonest reasons for the persistence of pain following a laminectomy is overlooked TrP activity in the lumbar muscles (Gerwin 1991). These TrPs may have become active either pre-operatively or as a result of the traumatisation of muscles during the operation. They may also develop in incisional scars. It therefore follows that in all cases where pain persists following a laminectomy a search for TrPs is essential and when found to be present deactivated by means of the carrying out of superficial dry needling. The one exception to this is when TrPs in the paravertebral musles have become activated as a secondary event following the development of nerve root compression pain when deep dry needling should be employed (Chu 1995).

There are two other much less common reasons for the pesistence of pain post-operatively. These are: (1) infection in the disc space (Fouquet et al 1992), and (2) the development of arachnoiditis (Ransford & Harries 1972, Symposium 1978).

With respect to all this, it has to be said that, even when strict criteria for surgery are adhered to, there is no certainty that removal of the disc will alleviate the pain. Spangfort (1972), in a review of the results of 2504 laminectomies selected for surgery because of clear-cut neurological signs of nerve root entrapment, found that complete relief of both leg and back pain occurred in only 60% of cases.

Failure to relieve pain in those with nerve root entrapment is usually attributed to one or other of the following causes:

- The exploration being carried out at the wrong site.
- A second disc prolapse being overlooked.
- The nerve root continuing to be compressed by the posterior intervertebral joints.
- Spinal stenosis causing pressure on the nerve root.

- An extraforaminal lateral disc herniation, though this is rare (Nelson 1980).

It may also be due to chronic irreversible nerve damage having developed prior to the operation being carried out (Wynn Parry 1989).

*Spinal fusion*  When pain due to a prolapsed disc is not relieved by laminectomy it is not uncommon to attempt to provide structural support for the spine by means of fusing together several vertebrae. The results of this operation in such circumstances have, however, been very disappointing leading Loeser (1980), somewhat tersely, to remark:

> … the greatest folly of all in the management of low-back pain is the use of fusion of the vertebrae in the absence of demonstrated instability due to a congenital or acquired lesion. There simply is no good evidence that fusion is ever beneficial to the patient with only a herniated lumbar disc; there is considerable evidence that it may be deleterious. Why patients are subjected to a major operative procedure with no evidence of efficacy is beyond my comprehension.

There can be no doubt that one of the major disadvantages of the operation is that by rendering the spine rigid it seriously interferes with the low-threshold mechanoreceptor pain-inhibiting mechanism (Ch. 6), as the action of the latter is entirely dependent on an ability to carry out normal movements. Also, the rigidity of the back seems to put an abnormal strain on the paravertebral muscles, and this in itself must encourage the activation of MTrPs. In addition, it is not uncommon to find iatrogenically induced TrPs in the midline surgical scar.

Patients who have come under my care with persistent pain in spite of having had a spinal fusion following failed laminectomy have, not unnaturally, been very depressed, particularly as most of them have been told that, other than the long-term use of analgesics, there is nothing more that can be done. Each one without exception, however, has been found on examination to have readily demonstrable TrPs and it has been possible to improve the quality of life by repeatedly deactivating these points with a dry needle. Unfortunately, and probably mainly because of the mechanical

disadvantage to which the operation puts the spine, the pain relief from acupuncture is seldom long-lasting and the necessity of having to continue with treatment on a long-term basis has to be explained to the patient at the outset in order to avoid any undue disappointment.

In conclusion, it has to be said that when pain persists following a laminectomy, it is firstly essential to ascertain that it is not due to residual nerve root compression, but once this has been excluded, it is better to attempt to alleviate the pain by the acupuncture technique of deactivating TrPs rather than to embark on a spinal fusion that leaves the spine permanently rigid and rarely relieves the pain.

## CHRONIC MECHANICAL TYPE LOW–BACK PAIN

The pathogenesis of chronic mechanical type low-back pain is poorly understood, and as a consequence of this both the manner in which the condition is investigated, and its treatment are far from satisfactory (Flor & Turk 1984, Turk & Flor 1984). The greatest obstacle to the rational treatment of chronic low-back pain is the difficulty of deciding in any particular case the primary source of the pain. The main possibilities are that the pain comes either from degenerative changes in the intervertebral discs and facet joints, or from MTrPs.

### Pain arising from degenerative changes in the intervertebral discs and facet joints

There can be no doubt that degenerative changes in the spine are potentially capable of causing low-back pain for, as Wyke (1987, p. 59) has pointed out, the structures in the vicinity of the spine in which nociceptive receptor systems are present include the spinal ligaments, the periosteum, the duramater, the walls of the blood vessels, and also the fibrous capsules of the facet joints.

It is generally believed that the degenerative changes in the spine start first in the discs, and that it is the reduction in the vertical height of the lumbar spine occurring as a result of this that encourages the development of arthritic changes in the facet joints (Vernon-Roberts & Pirie 1977).

Hirsch et al (1963) were among the first to show that the facet joint is a potential source of chronic back pain by showing that pain in the back and leg can be artifically induced by injecting 11% hypertonic saline around it.

Mooney & Robertson (1975) studied the matter more specifically by injecting 5% hypertonic saline into a facet joint in five normal individuals and 15 patients with chronic pain in the back and leg. They first ensured that the needle was directly in the joint by means of inserting it under fluoroscopic control and then injected sufficient contrast medium into the joint to outline its capsule. In each case, within about 5 s of injecting the hypertonic saline, pain was felt in the lower back, and within 20 s, this had increased in intensity and had spread to the greater trochanter and down the posterolateral part of the thigh. Such pain patterns, however, are in no way specific. Similar ones have been produced, as discussed in Chapter 4, by Kellgren, and also by Inman & Saunders, by injecting hypertonic saline into muscles and ligaments, and the possibility cannot be excluded that Mooney & Robertson's hypertonic saline did not remain confined to the facet joints, and, by diffusing into the tissues, it may have also stimulated other structures in the vicinity.

Fairbank et al (1981) have also studied the effects of injecting a local anaesthetic into facet joints for the purpose of ascertaining whether or not this procedure might act as a diagnostic aid. In their study, 25 adults suffering for the first time from severe low-back pain, were given an injection into a facet joint under X-ray control. The facet joints selected for injection were situated at points of maximum tenderness. Their results were that 14 obtained immediate relief (the responders) and 11 did not (the non-responders). They concluded that this might suggest that the responders had pain of mechanical origin possibly arising in the facet joint, and that the non-responders' pain may have originated from one of the many other possible sources in the back.

The reason for their conclusions being so tentative was that they were aware that the anaesthetic may not have remained confined to the facet joint, but may have diffused out into the tissues to involve the nerve root or the posterior primary ramus, and that this, in turn, may have affected other structures with a common innervation. It is of course possible that by using points of maximum tenderness for their injection that the anaesthetic was acting on nerve endings at TrPs because, as they admitted, Lewit (1979) had alleviated pain of this type simply by inserting dry needles into such points.

It may therefore be seen that various experimental studies aimed at showing whether or not facet joints are an important source of low-back pain have been somewhat inconclusive, and certainly observations by pathologists and above all by radiologists, would seem to suggest that the widely-held view that chronic mechanical type low-back pain, from middle age onwards, is mainly due to degenerative changes in the lumbar discs and facet joints, is almost certainly erroneous.

It was in 1932 that Schmorl & Junghanns, from their classic autopsy studies of over 4000 spines, established that degenerative changes in the lumbar spine are present in 50% of the population by the end of the 4th decade, in 70% at the end of the 5th decade, and in 90% at the age of 70. And since then, numerous comparative studies by radiologists have shown that the radiographic features of disc degeneration, including the narrowing of intervertebral spaces, osteophyte formation, disc calcification, and Schmorl's nodes, as well as those of facet joint arthrosis, are found as commonly in asymptomatic controls as they are in those with low-back pain (Splithoff 1952, Hult 1954, Hussar & Guller 1956, Horal 1969, Magora & Schwartz 1976).

Furthermore, there is also no evidence to suggest that the intensity of lumbar pain is in direct proportion to the amount of degenerative changes seen on a radiograph. It is not uncommon for a person with only slight changes to have severe pain, and conversely, for a person with advanced changes to be symptomless.

It would therefore seem that, whilst degenerative changes in the spine may make some contribution towards the development of chronic low-back pain, there is no direct correlation between the two, and in everyday clinical practice it would seem important not to assume just because there is radiographic evidence of disc and facet joint degeneration that this is necessarily the cause of the pain, as often this is not more than a chance investigatory finding in someone whose pain can be shown to be primarily muscular in origin. Waddell (1982), with considerable wisdom, comments:

> … the case for degenerative disc disease as the explanation of backache must still be regarded as not proven. It is important to treat patients and not X-rays of spines.

### Lumbar facet joint syndrome

All this not withstanding the lumbar facet joint syndrome is still currently considered by many to be a clinical entity, despite it having no generally accepted pathognomonic symptoms or physical signs (Jackson et al 1988, Schwarzer et al 1994a). It is for this reason that the diagnosis has to be made by determining whether or not the pain is alleviated by injecting, under fluoroscopic control, a local anaesthetic into any joint that on deep palpation is found to be markedly tender or one that, when put through movements, is found to be painful.

**Diagnostic facet joint block procedure**  Originally only one local anaesthetic was employed but this gave such an unacceptably high false-positive responder rate that it is now recommended that the test should be carried out using firstly a short-acting one (lidocaine [lignocaine]) and following this a longer acting one (bupivacaine). Analgesia has to be obtained with both for a patient to be considered a true responder. Unfortunately, however, even with this Schwarzer et al (1994a) had a false-positive rate of 38% and they also found (Schwarzer et al 1994b) that the prevalence of chronic low-back facet joint pain was only 15%.

**Treatment**  The treatment of this disorder is to inject a cortocosteroid/local anaesthetic into the suspected painful joint. There have been two controlled trials to assess the efficacy of this. In the first carried out by Lillius et al (1989) patients judged from a facet joint diagnostic block to have facet joint pain were randomly divided into three groups. Two of these were given either an intra-articular injection of a steroid/local anaesthetic mixture or a pericapsular injection of it. The third group was given an injection of saline into the affected joint. It was found that these three types

of treatment gave similar results with only 36% of the patients overall achieving pain relief lasting for 3 months.

The second trial was carried out by Carette et al (1991), in which the treatment group received an intraarticular injection of prednisolone and the control group an intraarticular injection of saline. Only 42% in the treatment group and 33% in the control group had significant pain relief lasting 3 months.

It may therefore be seen from the results of these two trials that any pain relief provided by a steroid injection was only obtained in a disappointingly small number of patients, and that a saline injection proved to be equally pain relieving. One possibility is that any pain relief obtained with either of these was simply due to the one factor common to both, i.e. the stimulating effect of the needle used for the injection on nerve endings.

Deyo (1991), during the course of commenting on what was found in both these trials, offered another explanation when he said:

> The poor results of these two studies may have occured because, despite careful diagnostic efforts, many patients had a source of pain other than the facet joints, or because a corticosteroid injection is inefficacious even when a facet joint is the source of the pain. In either event, the form of treatment appears to be over-used and minimally effective.

Jackson (1992), 1 year later, with commendable perspicacity posed the question: 'the facet syndrome, myth or reality?' and concluded that his provocative question could only be answered by the carrying out of further clinical trials.

## Chronic lumbar myofascial TrP pain syndrome

Those currently responsible for teaching medicine, when considering the causes of mechanical-type low-back pain, tend to dismiss pain of muscular origin as being of little or no consequence, and hardly worthy of their attention. This is no doubt, in part, not only because the pathology of the underlying condition continues to remain so singularly elusive, but also because it is now generally agreed that the condition is not of an inflammatory nature and, therefore, diagnoses such as fibrositis and myofasciitis are no longer acceptable, so there is even difficulty in knowing what to call the condition!

Everyday clinical experience, however, leads me to agree with Wyke (1987, p. 74) that irritation of the nociceptive receptor system in the lumbar muscles, their fascial sheaths, their tendinous insertions, and in the ligaments of the spine is a common cause of chronic low-back pain. This occurs either directly as a result of various factors to be discussed acting locally on the muscle or ligaments, or indirectly, as a result of anxiety causing them to be held in a state of persistent tension. There can be no doubt that mechanical type low-back pain that is primarily muscular in origin is frequently both severe and incapacitating; and it may affect not only adults, but also children (Bates & Grunwald 1958, Grantham 1977).

Careful examination of the lumbar muscles and the supraspinous ligament in someone with chronic mechanical type low-back pain frequently reveals the presence of focal points of exquisite tenderness. In the lower back these points may be found in muscle that otherwise feels normal, but often they are present in palpable bands or fibrositic nodules that develop in the substance of the muscles. Of particular significance is the fact that pressure applied to these points exacerbates any pain felt locally in the back, and at times causes pain to radiate down the leg in the same distribution as that occurring spontaneously. This of course is no recent observation for, as explained in Chapter 4, Kellgren first drew attention to the significance of 'tender spots' in muscles as progenitors of musculoskeletal pain nearly half a century ago, and once Janet Travell shortly after this, for obvious reasons, called them TrPs, she and others have written extensively about them.

Unfortunately, when the idea that TrPs might be an important source of low-back pain was first put forward, the climate of opinion was against it due to the medical profession in the Western world at that time being firmly wedded to the belief that acute 'lumbago' and sciatica are principally caused by the prolapse of an intervertebral disc, and that chronic 'lumbago' and sciatica occur

as a result of degenerative changes in the discs and facet joints.

This for many years was to remain one of the deeply entrenched beliefs of medical orthodoxy. It is, therefore, very much to the credit of St Claire Strange, that in his Presidential address to the section of orthopaedics of the Royal Society of Medicine, London, in 1966, he had the boldness to question the validity of this view by stating that, whilst he had no doubt that such lesions may at times be the cause of low-back pain, he was certain from his everyday clinical experience that they were not the only ones, and that, in investigating such pain, more attention should be paid to examining the muscles for points of maximum tenderness in what he termed 'muscle bundles in spasm' that are, 'sometimes "as slender as the shaft of a pin" and at other times "as thick as a pencil"', or in other words to look for what today would be called TrPs in palpable bands. His insistence on the importance of such an examination stemmed from his belief that it is from these structures that much of the pain emanates, for, as he said, when you press on one of these tender spots 'the patient knows you have "found the spot", found the site of the pain from which he is complaining. And you can see it in his face'.

Since the 1930s, therefore, a succession of people have drawn attention to the importance of TrPs in the aetiology of musculoskeletal pain, including that which affects the lower back, and yet those currently engaged in research into the problems of low-back pain still pay scant attention to them.

However, now that such leading authorities on the neurophysiology of pain as Melzack & Wall (1982) have come to recognize the importance of TrPs in the genesis of musculoskeletal pain in general, those engaged in investigating and managing chronic mechanical type low-back pain can no longer afford to ignore the part played by these structures in its development.

There is, as yet, no adequate explanation as to why some people more than others are prone to activate TrPs in their lumbar muscles, and for this reason to be particularly liable to suffer from chronic low-back pain. Certainly there is no definite evidence that structural disorders of the spine make any significant contribution to this. Admittedly, it is theoretically possible for MTrPs to become acti-vated as a result of structural disorders of the spine causing the lumbar muscles to go into spasm, but, as has already been discussed, so far as degenera-tive changes are concerned, a number of well-controlled studies have failed to show any direct relationship between the presence of radiograph-ically observable degenerative changes in the discs and facet joints, and the development of inter-mittently recurrent low-back pain.

There is, in addition, no definite evidence that other structural disorders such as sacralization of the spine, spondylolisthesis, or various abnormal curvatures of the spine are associated with the activation of TrPs. It has, for example, been gener-ally assumed that the abnormal fusion that some-times occurs between the 5th lumbar vertebra and the sacrum – so-called sacralization of the spine – is a cause of chronic low-back pain, but Magora & Schwartz (1978), from their extensive survey, were unable to confirm this.

Similarly, although the forward shift of one vertebra or another – so-called spondylolisthesis – has been said to contribute to the development of chronic low-back pain, the evidence for this is con-flicting with some observers such as Hult (1954), Horal (1969), and Torgerson & Dotter (1976) sup-porting this belief, but with others, including Splithoff (1952) and Rowe (1965), being unable to demonstrate such a relationship.

Furthermore, although congenital or acquired abnormalities such as scoliosis, kyphosis, exagger-ated lordosis, and spina bifida occulta have all been assumed to cause chronic low-back pain, sev-eral studies including those of Hult (1954), Horal (1969), Torgerson & Dotter (1976), and Magora & Schwartz (1978) have failed to confirm this.

Before leaving the subject of the possible activ-ation of TrPs in response to structural disorders in the spine, the following observations will be made concerning the most common of these, namely degenerative changes in the discs and facet joints.

Although myofascial TrPs are frequently found to be present in cases of mechanical type low-back pain, where degenerative changes are demonstrable radiographically, there is no correlation between the number of TrPs present and the amount of degenerative change in the spine; furthermore,

distribution of the TrPs in the back often bears no relationship to the part of the spine affected by degenerative changes, and when one comes to consider the treatment of low-back pain by the acupuncture technique of dry needling TrPs, experi-ence shows that it is wrong to assume that the chances of a good response diminish in proportion to the amount of degenerative disease present. On the contrary, a patient with little or no degenerative changes in the spine may, for reasons to be dis-cussed later, have a poor response to this type of treatment, whereas, conversely, a patient with advanced degenerative disease may respond well.

A woman (89 years of age), who had had episodes of low-back pain since the age of 35 years, and had experienced severe pain in the left buttock for 1 year, asked her doctor if she might try acupuncture, only to be told that this would be a waste of time as the X-ray of her lumbar spine showed that the pain was due to severe arthritis. However, she finally got her own way! And, on examination, there were only two TrPs to be found, which were in muscles situated in the postero-inferior part of the chest wall at the level of the 10th and 11th ribs. The pain in the buttock must clearly have been referred from these (Fig. 15.3) as it disappeared after deactivating them with a dry needle on only two occasions. Following this she remained free from pain for 18 months in spite of the advanced 'arthritic changes' in the spine.

It is from having had a similarly good response to acupuncture in a large number of cases of chronic low-back pain with equally advanced degenera-tive changes on X-rays of the spine, that leads me to believe that such changes in the discs and facet joints are often no more than a chance radiographic finding in someone whose pain is primarily due to the activation of TrPs by factors acting directly on the muscles themselves.

Those who treat chronic low-back pain by manipulating the spine might not agree with this but, nevertheless, it would seem reasonable to postulate that any success they may have with this form of treatment may be due more to their manipulative procedures exerting traction on muscles than to any effect these procedures may have on the spine itself. This would certainly be in keeping with Travell's observation (1968) that it is possible to inactivate myofascial TrPs by passively stretching affected muscles.

### Physical and psychological factors capable of activating myofascial TrPs

Some of the physical factors capable of activating myofascial TrPs in the lumbar muscles include, as Travell & Simons (1983, p. 644) point out, the sudden overloading of the muscles as when lifting objects whilst in an awkward position such as with the back twisted and flexed; or when they are subjected to sustained overloading, as may occur during the pursuit of athletic activities, or at work, particularly when this involves much heavy lifting, stooping, or the adoption of awkward standing or sitting postures.

Surgeons should also note that the putting of patients into unusual postures such as the Trendelenburg or lithotomy positions for prolonged periods, particularly when the muscles are particularly relaxed due to the effects of a general anaesthetic, is liable to cause the activation of MTrPs with the development of chronic postoperative low-back pain.

Magora (1970), who has extensively investigated the relationship between low-back pain and occupational factors has found that this type of pain is more frequent in those whose work forces them to sit for prolonged periods, than in those who constantly move about. And that heavy lifting, particularly when this is only occasional, is a frequent cause of this type of pain. He also found that low-back pain occurs with about the same frequency in those with sedentary occupations as in those doing heavy labour, but the sedentary worker's symptoms come on more after weekend athletic activities.

It is interesting to note, too, that, although he found a high incidence of absence from work amongst manual workers because of the pain preventing them from carrying out their duties, the incidence of back pain correlated best with how physically demanding workers perceived their work to be, rather than how objectively demanding it was. As he pointed out, its incidence is also more closely related to whether there are psychological problems at the workplace or at home rather than to objective physical factors. When Westrin (1973) studied low-back pain, he concluded that its incidence is especially high in those not happy with their job situation, those who are divorced, or those who have problems with alcohol.

This therefore leads to a consideration of psychological factors that so far as chronic low-back pain is concerned, seem to be of particular importance as TrP activators. Turk & Flor (1984) state that 'chronic back pain is increasingly viewed as a psychophysiological and psychosocial problem stemming from the interaction of physical, psychological and social factors'. It has, in fact, to be accepted that the condition is often multifactorial and this reflects itself in its treatment, which not infrequently has to include therapeutic procedures directed both to the mind and the body.

There is a large group of patients who hold the muscles of their scalp, neck, or lower back in a state of persistent tension in response to nervous strain, and as already discussed in Chapter 7 this leads to the activation of TrPs in these muscles with, as a result, of this, the development of either persistent headaches, or chronic pain in the neck, or chronic low-back pain, or a combination of these.

Some people come to recognize that their attacks of pain coincide with times of particular stress. One young executive, for example, told me that public speaking terrified him, and that his low-back pain always came on about 2 weeks before having to address a business conference. Others can date the onset of recurrent low-back pain to some specific time when they were subjected to some particularly distressing experience. One housewife, for example, told me that her attacks of neck and low-back pain started the year that both her husband and only daughter died within 6 months of each other.

It obviously cannot be assumed that either an anxiety state or an agitated depressive one (reactive depression), occurring in association with chronic low-back pain, has necessarily contributed to the development of this, because often such mood changes develop some months after the onset of the pain, and in such circumstances have to be considered to have arisen as a result of it.

It is important to realize that so-called psychological low-back pain is, in reality, psychosomatic because, as has already been explained, there are almost invariably TrPs to be found in the muscles usually in the form of foci of maximum tenderness in palpable bands or 'fibrositic' nodules. This has considerable diagnostic and therapuetic implications because when an overtly anxious person with low-back pain is found to have no abnormality of the spine on X-rays, no evidence of disease in the pelvis, and as all too often happens, the TrPs in the muscles are overlooked, there is a tendency for it to be assumed that the pain must be entirely psychological in origin, and for the patient concerned to be referred to a psychiatrist. This, in my experience, is rarely helpful, not because of any lack of expertise on the part of the latter, but because in such a case it does not matter how much psychotherapy is given, it will in no way influence the course of the pain unless at the same time the TrPs are deactivated. The converse, however, is also true, that when psychological factors contribute to low-back pain no amount of TrP deactivation by acupuncture or by any other means will give any lasting relief from the pain, unless at the same time some form of therapy is given to reduce the nervous tension.

It is my belief that, whenever possible, it is preferable for the patient to receive both these forms of treatment from the same physician, and it is for this reason that the patients with psychosomatic low-back pain under my care receive from me a combination of hypnotherapy and acupuncture.

An even more serious error, and one which not infrequently occurs because of a general lack of understanding concerning the significance of TrPs, and, therefore, a failure to look for them, is to conclude that a patient with normal X-ray appearances of the lumbar spine is in need of psychological help, or, even, is frankly malingering, when in fact the pain is entirely of organic origin. An example of this is given here.

A housewife, at the age of 35 years was referred to an orthopaedic surgeon because of persistent low-back pain, only to be told that the pain could not be coming from her back because the X-ray of her spine was normal. She was then referred to a gynaecologist, who finding no abnormality on physical examination, carried out a dilatation and curettage. This operation

was complicated 10 days later by a near-fatal pulmonary infarct. The patient then continued to be quite markedly incapacitated by persistent pain for another 2–3 years, and, as during this time certain marital difficulties had arisen, it was assumed that the pain must be of psychological origin and she was referred to a psychiatrist. It was very much to his credit that he frankly admitted he could find no psychiatric cause for the pain, and the patient in desperation then asked her doctor whether she could try acupuncture.

On examination, there were some TrPs in quite enormous, exquisitely tender fibrositic nodules and palpable bands. Once these TrPs had been deactivated with a dry needle at weekly intervals on four occasions, she obtained lasting relief from pain for the first time for many years.

It has to be admitted that some people whose low-back pain has occurred as a result of injury at work or in a traffic accident, and who are claiming compensation for this, do exaggerate their symptoms. Unfortunately, however, a litigant is sometimes unjustifiably assumed to be doing this, often for no better reason than that the X-ray of the spine is normal, when a careful examination of the back would show a sound physical basis for the pain in the form of activated TrPs in the muscles.

A self-employed heating engineer, very anxious to keep his business going but unable to do so because of persistent low-back pain following a car accident, very much resented being told by an orthopaedic surgeon that his symptoms would not improve until his claim for compensation had been settled, particularly as when he eventually decided to try acupuncture, it only required dry needle stimulation of TrPs to be carried out on three occasions before his pain was sufficiently alleviated for him to return to quite hard physical work.

Finally, before leaving the subject of the influence of psychological factors on chronic low-back pain, it has to be said that, in my experience, acupuncture often fails to relieve this type of pain in those who, because of long-standing neuroticism, persistently hold their lumbar muscles in a state of tension, and similarly is rarely helpful in those who develop low-back pain as a manifestation of conversion hysteria in order to escape from seemingly intolerable domestic, marital or occupational obligations.

A prison officer, who had complained of low-back pain for many years, was finally persuaded by his general practitioner to come to me for treatment with acupuncture. During the course of taking the history it seemed obvious that for some time he had found the pain to be extremely useful to him in so much that it enabled him to avoid some of the more arduous duties associated with his job. It, therefore, came as no surprise to me when, after two sessions, he failed to attend for any further treatment. He told his doctor that this was because the treatment had made him worse, but almost certainly it was because, perhaps unknowingly, he was afraid it might eventually make him better!

## IMPORTANCE OF DISTINGUISHING BETWEEN NOCICEPTIVE AND RADICULOPATHIC CHRONIC LOW-BACK AND LEG PAIN

It is important to realize that the insidious development of combined low-back and 'sciatic-type' leg pain may be either nociceptive, radiculopathic, or a mixture of both. For all too long there has been a belief that pain in this distribution, particularly when it is accompanied by restricted straight leg raising, must be due to nerve root entrapment. However, from what has already been said, and as will be seen when TrP pain referral patterns from individual muscles in the lower back are considered, it is evident that chronic 'sciatica', even when it is associated with restricted straight leg raising, may be entirely due to the primary activation of MTrPs. At the same time, it has to be clearly understood that MTrPs may become activated as a secondary event in areas affected by pain from nerve root entrapment.

It therefore follows that in all cases a systematic search for TrPs is essential. Also, in those cases where the history or physical signs suggest that the pain might be radiculopathic, further investigations, such as computerized axial tomography (CAT scanning) or MRI should be carried out.

Pain in this distribution occurring as the result of the primary activation of MTrPs is readily relieved by acupuncture. If, however, there is any suggestion that the pain might be due to nerve root entrapment, then it is better not to embark upon acupuncture until this has been fully investigated. The reasons for this are that, should nerve root entrapment be present, not only will the deactivation of TrPs with dry needles do no more than temporarily alleviate the pain, but also the longer the nerve root remains compressed, the more likely it is to become irreversibly damaged, so that, even if surgical decompression is eventually carried out, the operation may not relieve the pain.

Wynn Parry (1989), from reviewing experimental studies carried out by various people over the past years has concluded that compression of a nerve ultimately leads to the development of irreversible pain-producing degenerative changes both in the nerve itself and in the central nervous system. As he points out, it is this peripheral and central damage that is the main reason for surgery failing to relieve symptoms from nerve root compression and why, when this happens, further operations are also doomed to failure.

As therefore it is essential to be able to recognize the clinical manifestations of the various causes of chronic nerve root entrapment in the lower back these will now be considered.

### Spondylolisthesis

Spondylolisthesis, the forward displacement of a vertebra relative to the one below it, may either be congenital or acquired. Nelson (1987) reviewed the diagnosis and management of five separate types, but only the degenerative type that affects adults from the age of 40 years onwards will be discussed.

#### Symptoms and signs

Degenerative spondylolisthesis affects mainly females and occurs predominately at the L 4/5 level. The back pain is aggravated by activity, relieved by resting and is commonly made worse by standing. The pain in the leg is in the distribution of a nerve root with physical examination revealing the presence of a motor and sensory deficit. In addition, bilateral paraesthesiae and muscle weakness may be present in those cases in which degenerative changes have led to the development of spinal stenosis.

## Investigations

Plain radiography, and either CAT scanning or MRI are necessary in order to confirm the diagnosis.

## Treatment

Conservative treatment may be all that is necessary in mild cases, but surgery is required for the relief of severe pain with evidence of nerve root compression.

# Spinal stenosis

Eisenstein (1977), from a comparison of African and Caucasoid skeletons, showed that it is when a congenitally narrowed spinal canal becomes further narrowed as a result of the development of degenerative changes in the posterior facet joints that symptoms develop. The clinical manifestations depend on whether the stenosis is of the central canal, or of the lateral root canal.

## Central canal stenosis (neurogenic claudication)

The patient, usually a middle-aged male, gives a long history of low-back pain and a more recent one of a vice-like claudication type pain with feelings of numbness, tingling and heaviness affecting one or both legs. The pain, as when due to vascular disease, is brought on by walking and relieved by resting. Characteristically, relief from the pain is obtained by bending forwards. It is for this reason that patients with this disorder adopt an ape-like posture with both hips and knees flexed – the so-called simian stance (Simkin 1982). It is also because bending forwards relieves the pain that patients have less pain walking up a hill than down a hill and continue to be able to cycle long distances even when it is too painful to walk more than short distances on the flat (Figs 17.2 & 17.3).

## Clinical examination

Physical signs are widely variable. In some cases there is some limitation of straight leg raising and evidence of a lower motor neurone lesion, but with others their straight leg raising is normal and there are no abnormal neurological signs.

Peripheral pulses may or may not be palpable depending on whether arterial occlusion is or is not also present. The provisional diagnosis therefore mainly comes from the history.

## Investigations

Plain radiographs of the lumbar spine frequently show diffuse degenerative changes; a myelogram shows segmental filling defects or a total block and ultrasound measurements confirm the reduced diameter of the vertebral canal.

## Treatment

When symptoms are relatively mild, conservative measures may be helpful, but in those cases where there is severe pain and walking is restricted to

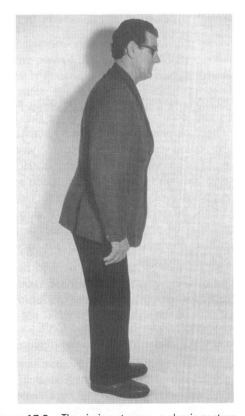

**Figure 17.2**    The simian stance – a classic posture adopted by patients with neurogenic claudication, with flexed hips and knees. Reproduced with Professor Porter's permission from *The Lumbar Spine and Back Pain*, *Churchill Livingstone* 1987.

(a)

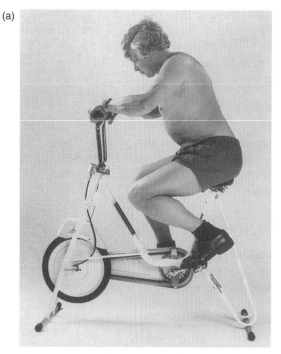

(b)

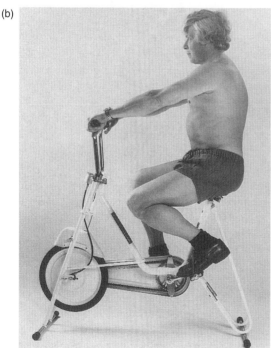

**Figure 17.3** The cycle test. The cycling distance is the same in vascular intermittent claudication whether the spine is flexed (a) or upright (b). The extended spine in (b) limits the cycling distance in neurogenic claudication. Reproduced with Professor Porter's permission from *The Lumbar Spine and Back Pain*, Churchill Livingstone 1987.

short distances in association with a progressive neurological deficit, it is essential to carry out some form of surgical decompression.

## Lateral root canal stenosis

In this condition pain in the back with radiation down one leg occurs as a result of stenosis at this site causing entrapment of a nerve root – usually the 5th lumbar or 1st sacral. The stenosis may occur as the result of bony encroachment from osteophytes or ossified spinal ligaments, or from soft tissue changes including facet joint capsule hypertrophy, posterior longitudinal ligament thickening and scar tissue developing around a ruptured annulus fibrosus or extruded nucleus pulposus.

### Symptoms

The sciatic pain is in the same distribution as with a disc lesion but, unlike the latter, it is not relieved by lying down and remains severe and unremitting both day and night. Fortunately, however, unlike with disc pain, coughing and sneezing does not make it worse. In a series of 78 cases reported by Getty et al (1981), 58% also had numbness and paraesthesiae in the leg and 17% had claudication.

### Physical signs

These are widely variable. In the series of patients reported by Getty et al (1981), only 49% showed evidence of a motor deficit and only 38% had impairment of sensation to light touch and pinprick. Perhaps most surprising of all, most had a normal straight leg raising test.

It is probably because patients with lateral canal stenosis are liable to have bizarre sensory symptoms together with a paucity of physical signs, and frequently have unrestricted straight leg raising despite complaining of severe sciatica that the diagnosis in the past was frequently overlooked and patients suffering from it ran the risk of being considered to be neurotic.

### Investigations

Plain radiographs may show a reduction of the L5/S1 disc space. A CAT scan will usually reveal the presence of degenerative changes in the facet joints, but similar changes may also be evident in patients who do not suffer from back pain.

It is not possible to demonstrate the presence of nerve root entrapment in a stenosed lateral canal on a myelogram. Leyshon et al (1981), however, have shown that the diagnosis may be confirmed by electromyographic studies.

### Management

Porter et al (1984) have shown that the root pain not infrequently gradually subsides spontaneously. However, as Wynn Parry (1989) points out, the difficulty is that whilst waiting for this to happen a proportion of patients develop irreversible pain-producing changes both in the entrapped nerve and in the central nervous system. It is obvious, therefore, that any decision concerning if and when surgical decompression should be carried out requires considerable clinical experience.

### Indications for acupuncture and TENS

There is an important place for acupuncture and TENS as part of the conservative treatment of lumbar chronic nerve-root entrapment pain and also post-operatively in those cases where surgery has failed to relieve this.

Acupuncture is of particular value in those cases where the nerve root is not severely compressed and much of the pain is coming from secondarily activated MTrPs.

TENS is likely to be more helpful in cases where the pain is predominately neurogenic, but it must be remembered that the electrodes should never be placed on anaesthetic skin, but always on skin where the sensation is normal in order that the high-frequency low-intensity stimulus provided by this form of therapy may be enabled to recruit A-beta nerve fibres.

## MANAGEMENT OF CHRONIC LOW-BACK PAIN

It is a measure of the general public's disillusionment with all the various conventional methods of treating chronic low-back pain that it is ever increasingly turning to alternative forms of therapy including acupuncture.

It is not possible, however, to come to any conclusions concerning the possible place of acupuncture in the treatment of chronic low-back pain without first of all critically appraising some of the other more widely used forms of treatment, including drugs, physiotherapy, spinal supports, and steroid injections.

## Drugs

### Analgesics

Various non-narcotic pain-killing drugs such as aspirin, phenacetin, paracetomol and pentazocine, together with a number of non-steroidal antiinflammatory drugs, and even, at times, narcotic ones such as pethidine, are prescribed for chronic back pain. Although they are all capable of relieving pain for short periods, this is more than offset by the disadvantages of using them on a long-term basis including tolerance, habituation and side effects, many of which are liable to be of a serious nature.

### Antidepressants

Patients with chronic low-back pain are sometimes sufficiently depressed as to require a tricyclic antidepressant, but in addition a drug of this type may also be used for its analgesic effect.

The evidence that tricyclic antidepressants have an analgesic action independent of their antidepressive properties includes Monks' (1981) having found that the onset of analgesia in chronic pain conditions with this group of drugs is more rapid (3–7 days) than that of their antidepressant effect (14–21 days). Couch & Hassanein (1976) having shown that they are capable of producing chronic pain relief in the absence of an antidepressant response, and Couch et al (1976) having reported that this may also occur in patients in whom there is no detectable evidence of depression.

It would seem that the analgesic and antidepressant effects of this group of drugs are due to their ability to increase the concentration in the brain and spinal cord of amine transmitters such as serotonin (Sternbach et al 1976). Controlled trials comparing a tricyclic antidepressant with a placebo in chronic low-back pain have given somewhat equivocal results with Sternbach et al (1976) showing that amitriptyline, and Jenkins et al (1976) showing that imipramine, are no better than a placebo, but with Sternbach et al (1976) showing that clomipramine (Anafranil) is more effective than a placebo.

### Muscle relaxants

As nervously holding muscles tense aggravates musculoskeletal pain, it might be thought that diazepam would be helpful in the management of chronic low-back pain, but Hingorani (1966), from the results of a double-blind controlled trial, was unable to confirm this.

## Physiotherapy

### Ultrasound

Sclapbach (1991) has pointed out that despite the fact that ultrasound is probably one of the most frequently used physiotherapeutic modalities for the relief of musculoskeletal pain, there have been remarkably few controlled studies to assess its effectiveness for this purpose.

During the past 35 years there have only been nine such trials and, of these, only one has been in patients with low-back pain. This was a study carried out by Nwuga (1983) who compared bed rest and ultrasound, bed rest and sham ultrasound, and bed rest alone for the relief of acute low-back pain from intervertebral disc prolapse. Unfortunately, as bed rest was used in all three groups and is known to be effective itself in relieving acute low-back pain (Deyo et al 1986, Wiesel et al 1980), the results of the trial are difficult to interpret.

Sclapbach (1991), from a review of these nine studies, is of the opinion that, 'based on the results of the few available controlled trials, it must be concluded that we are far from being able to judge either the efficacy or inefficacy of therapeutic ultrasound'.

### Exercises

Exercises are sometimes advocated, but there is no good evidence that increasing the strength of the lumbar muscles reduces the frequency with which low-back pain recurs, and, indeed, Nachemson

(1980) warns against them in view of the fact that they may increase the load on the lumbar spine to unacceptable levels.

### Manipulation

This highly specialized form of physical therapy has many advocates and is widely practised by doctors and others but, having no personal experience of its use, it would be wrong for me to express any opinion concerning its efficacy, other than to say that, from a study of the literature it would seem that, whilst it is of undoubted value in the treatment of acute low-back pain (Berquist-Ullman & Larsson 1977), its place in the management of chronic low-back pain is far less certain (Doran & Newell 1975, Glover et al 1974, Evans et al 1978, Sims-Williams et al 1982).

### Spinal supports

Corsets are widely prescribed, but in spite of the fact that, at times, they are incredibly elaborate there is little or no evidence that they are of any benefit. A corset may, in fact, do harm, because by limiting the movements of the back it may lead to wasting of the muscles and, in addition, it is liable to suppress the action of the low-threshold mechanoreceptor large diameter fibre pain-modulating mechanism (Ch. 6). Furthermore, a corset sometimes aggravates low-back pain by exerting pressure on TrPs. Quinet & Hadler (1979) in referring to these devices remark:

> The widespread use of these gimmicks ought to be curtailed until we have data suggesting that our patients are more likely to profit from their continued use than are orthopaedic supply houses.

## Injections of a corticosteroid and/or local anaesthetic into points of maximum tenderness

Since Kellgren, nearly 50 years ago, started injecting novocain into 'tender spots' in order to alleviate musculoskeletal pain, this type of treatment has been commonly employed in the treatment of low-back pain. Then once corticosteroids became available, the injection of a steroid/local anaesthetic mixture has been used (Bourne 1979). And in order to decide whether there was any advantage in using a steroid, Bourne (1984) decided to compare the effects of injecting, on repeated occasions, either, a corticosteroid/lidocaine (lignocaine) mixture, or lidocaine (lignocaine) by itself, into points of maximum tenderness in the lower back, in the treatment of chronic back pain. He concluded that the mixture gave better results.

It should be noted that the injection was sometimes given under the deep fascia but at other times into the periosteum, and, also, that amongst the transient side effects were menstrual irregularities, flushing of the face and glycosuria. Bourne ascribed the good results obtained with a steroid to certain softening and stretching effects on the collagen, together with the growing of new fibrocytes, and a consequent reduction in tissue tension described by Ketchum et al (1968) and Ketchum (1971). If, indeed, this type of tissue reaction does contribute to pain relief, it is bound to take time and hardly accounts for the immediate relief from pain so often observed when tender 'spots' are needled.

The alternative explanation is that a corticosteroid, when introduced into the tissues, and particularly when injected around the periosteum, has a powerful irritant effect on peripheral nerve endings, and in a similar manner to stimulating nerve endings with a dry needle, evokes activity in pain-modulating mechanisms in the central nervous system.

## TrP acupuncture

From what has just been said in reviewing some of the present methods of treating chronic low-back pain, it is clear that none of them are particularly effective, some are associated with undesirable side effects, and some can only be carried out in specially equipped centres. Few would disagree with Waddell (1982) when he says:

> Future improvements in treatment for backache and the creation of a truly scientific basis for treatment depend on better biochemical understanding, more accurate identification and localization of the source of pain, recognition of specific clinical syndromes within mechanical

backache, and critical evaluation of the effectiveness of treatment. While awaiting such developments it is best to use the simplest, safest, and cheapest treatment possible.

Acupuncture certainly fulfils these criteria, and there is therefore much to be said for exploring its use in everyday clinical practice and, above all, by the setting up of statistically controlled clinical trials. In my view, because of its simplicity, it is best to employ it as a first line of treatment, and then to turn to other more complex therapeutic procedures in those cases not helped by it.

The TrPs from which chronic neck pain is referred are situated in much the same muscles in everyone, but this certainly is not so with the TrPs responsible for chronic low-back and leg pain, and for this reason the task of finding them is that much more difficult. However, the task is facilitated by having a knowledge of specific patterns of pain referral from TrPs in individual muscles.

### Paraspinal musculature

TrPs in the paraspinal musculature may occur either in the superficial group of muscles known collectively as the erector spinae, or in muscles deep to this such as the multifidus and rotatores.

The two muscles in the superficial group (the erector spinae) most likely to develop TrPs are the longissimus thoracis and lateral to this, the iliocostalis lumborum muscle (Fig. 17.4).

Referred pain from TrPs in these muscles is mainly felt locally in areas immediately adjacent to these points, but sometimes it is felt at a distance. As King & Lagger (1976) have shown, TrPs in the erector spinae muscles may cause pain to be referred down the course of the sciatic nerve. And, as Travell & Simons (1983, p. 637) have stated, TrPs in the iliocostalis lumborum muscle at the upper lumbar level, and in the longissimus thoracis at the lower thoracic level, cause pain to be referred to the buttock (Figs 17.5 & 17.6). It is because of this that, earlier in this chapter, it was stressed that the search for TrPs must always start some distance above the 12th rib.

The two muscles in the deep group likely to develop TrPs are the multifidi and rotatores. Pain from these TrPs is referred to the midline with the development of exquisite tenderness on palpating

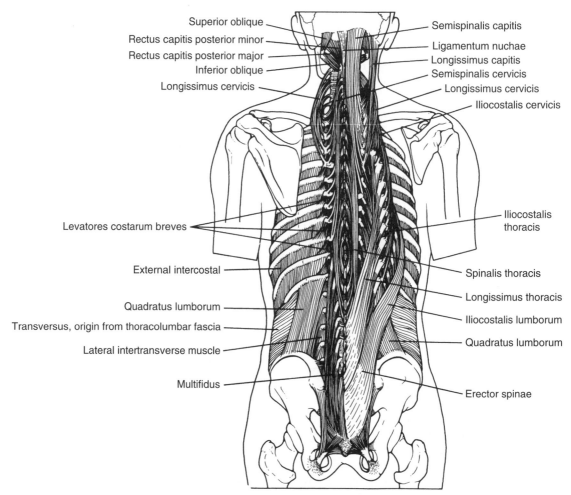

**Figure 17.4** The deep muscles of the back. On the left side the erector spinae and its upward continuations (with the exception of the longissimus cervicis, which has been displaced laterally) and the semispinalis capitis have been removed.

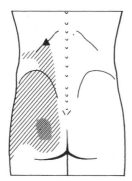

**Figure 17.5** The pattern of pain referral from a trigger point (▲) in the ilicostalis lumborum muscle.

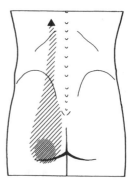

**Figure 17.6** The pattern of pain referral from a trigger point (▲) in the longissimus thoracis muscle.

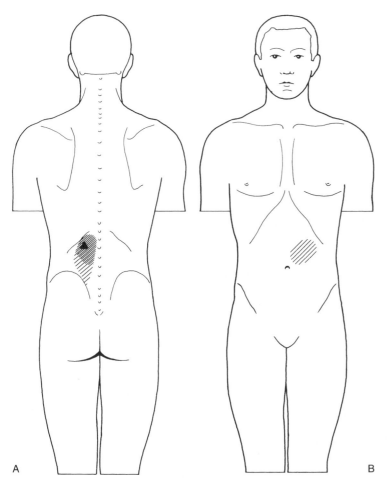

**Figure 17.7A&B**   The pattern of pain referral from a trigger point (▲) in the deep group of paraspinal muscles (multifidi and rotatores) in the upper lumbar region.

A

B

the spinous processes (Fig. 17.7A). Deep TrPs low down in the sacral region may also refer pain in a downwards direction to the coccyx and cause it to become very tender (Fig. 17.8).

It should also be noted, as stated by Travell & Simons (1983, p. 637), that TrPs in the iliocostalis muscle in the lower part of the thorax and in the multifidus muscle anywhere along the length of the lumbar spine may refer pain anteriorly to the abdomen, and that such pain may readily be misinterpreted as being visceral in origin (Fig. 17.7B).

**Examination to locate TrPs in these muscles**   The examination to locate TrPs in the paraspinal muscles should be conducted either with the patient seated and leaning forwards to flex the spine or with the patient in the semiprone position with the painful side uppermost, and the knees

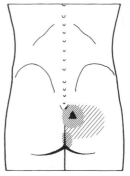

**Figure 17.8**   The pattern of pain referral from a trigger point (▲) in the deep group of paraspinal muscles (multifidi and rotatores) in the sacral region.

brought up towards the chest. The full prone position should be avoided because, if the muscles are allowed to become too relaxed, it is difficult to identify palpable bands.

TrPs in the superficial erector spinae muscles are readily felt by palpating down the length of the paravertebral gutter.

In order to identify a TrP in one of the deeper muscles it is necessary to apply firm pressure immediately lateral to the spine in a posteromedial direction towards the body of a vertebra at the level of a tender spinous process.

**Deactivation of TrPs**    TrPs in the superficial paraspinal muscles should be deactivated with needles inserted at right angles to the skin, except in the lower thoracic region where, to avoid any chance of penetrating the pleura, it is wiser to insert them tangentially.

In deactivating TrPs in the more deeply situated paraspinal muscles, the needles have to be inserted lateral to the midline and in a diagonal direction towards the vertebral bodies.

### Supraspinous ligament connecting the apices of the lumbar vertebral spines

TrPs in the paraspinal muscles are often accompanied by TrPs in the midline supraspinous ligament, and when present these should also be deactivated.

**Traditional Chinese acupuncture points**    As will be seen from Figure 17.1, traditional Chinese acupuncture points are located down the midline in the so-called 'Du' channel, and in the paravertebral region in the so-called 'Urinary Bladder' channel. There is, therefore, a close spatial correlation between points in the Chinese system and the TrPs just described.

### Quadratus lumborum muscle (Fig. 17.9)

It is relatively common for TrPs to become activated in this muscle but because it lies deep to the paraspinal muscles they tend to get overlooked (Travell 1976). Sola & Williams in 1956 reported it to be a frequent cause of unilateral low-back pain amongst young adults in the American Air Force.

**Activation of TrPs**    TrPs in this muscle become activated either when, because of a sudden twisting or stooping movement, an acute strain is put on the muscle, or when because of bending for long periods the muscle is subjected to sustained or

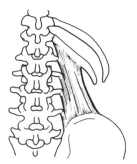

Figure 17.9    The quadratus lumborum muscle.

repeated overload. The patient may then complain of pain on walking, but particularly on stooping or twisting, such as when turning over in the bed, also on rising from a chair, and with sharp respiratory movements such as coughing or sneezing.

**Specific patterns of pain referral**    The pattern of pain referral depends on whether the TrPs are in the superficial lateral part or the deeper medial part of the muscle. When TrPs are located in the lateral part, the pain is referred down to the outer side of the iliac crest and over the greater trochanter (Fig. 17.10). It may also extend anteriorly towards the groin. When they are located in the medial part, the pain is referred to the region of the sacroiliac joint and buttock (Fig. 17.11). According to Sola & Williams (1956) TrP activity in this muscle is also a frequent cause of anterior abdominal pain.

**TrP examination**    TrPs in this muscle, particularly in its deeper medial part, are liable to be overlooked unless care is taken to put the muscle on the stretch. The patient whilst lying on the unaffected side, as during the examination of the paraspinal muscles, should separate the 12th rib from the iliac crest, by reaching upwards with the free arm whilst at the same time drawing down the pelvis by dropping the uppermost thigh backwards on to the couch. This manoeuvre brings the muscle nearer to the surface whilst at the same time tensing it.

TrPs in the superficial lateral part of the muscle tend to be found, either where it inserts into the 12th rib, or into the iliac crest.

TrPs in the medial deeper part of the muscle may be located by exerting firm pressure directed

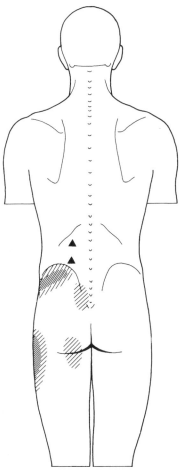

**Figure 17.10** The pattern of pain referral from trigger points (▲) in the lateral part of the quadratus lumborum muscle.

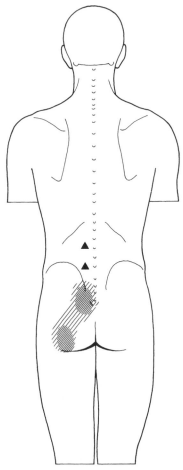

**Figure 17.11** The pattern of pain referral from trigger points (▲) in the medial part of the quadratus lumborum muscle.

medially towards the transverse processes of the vertebrae. Again TrPs in this part of the muscle tend to cluster in the upper part around the 12th rib or in the lower part at the level of the 4th lumbar vertebra.

### Glutei muscles (see Fig. 18.6)

TrPs in the gluteus maximus may occur at any of a variety of sites in the belly of this muscle. They become activated as a primary event or secondarily when pain is referred to the buttock from TrPs in muscles situated in the postero-inferior part of the chest wall.

Pain from TrPs in this muscle is referred locally to the buttock itself and the coccyx (Fig. 17.12).

TrPs in the gluteus medius and minimus are often found near to their insertions into the greater trochanter. The referral of pain from these is into the buttock, and also sometimes down the outer side of the thigh along the length of the iliotibial tract, and when this happens it is often associated with the secondary activation of TrPs in this structure (Fig. 17.13).

With TrPs situated more posteriorly in one or other of these muscles, the pain is referred down the back of the thigh when it may be misdiagnosed as sciatica (Fig. 17.14).

Deactivation of TrPs in the glutei and iliotibial tract with a dry needle usually presents no difficulties, providing it is carried out systematically and no TrPs are overlooked.

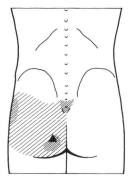

**Figure 17.12**   The pattern of pain referral from a trigger point (▲) in the gluteus maximus muscle.

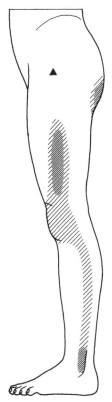

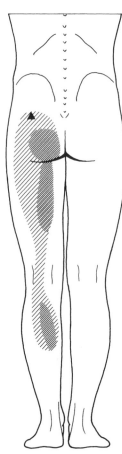

**Figure 17.14**   The pattern of pain referral from a trigger point (▲) in the posterior part of either the gluteus medius or minimum muscles.

**Figure 17.13**   The pattern of pain referral from a trigger point (▲) in either the gluteus medius or minimus near to the attachment of these muscles to the greater trochanter.

## Piriformis muscle (Fig. 17.15)

TrP activation in the piriformis muscle may also cause pain to be referred to the buttock, to the hip, and down the back of the leg in the distribution of the sciatic nerve (Fig. 17.16).

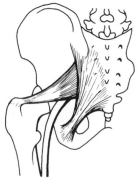

**Figure 17.15**   The outer part of the piriformis muscle with its attachment to the greater trochanter. The sciatic nerve is shown in its normal position behind this muscle.

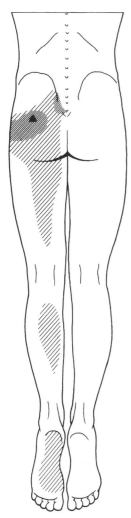

result of the development of trauma-induced TrP activity may cause entrapment of the nerve and the development of 'sciatica' – the so-called piriformis syndrome.

**Piriformis syndrome**   The type of trauma responsible for TrP activity developing in this syndrome includes the overloading of the muscle, such as when twisting the trunk sideways during the course of bending to pick up a heavy object. Also, direct trauma to the muscle such as, for example, in a road traffic accident. And when the muscle is held in a shortened position for any length of time such as may happen when lying with the hips flexed and legs widely abducted during the course of a surgical operation.

The syndrome occurs six times more often in women than in men (Cailliet 1977). On examination there is marked tenderness over the sciatic notch, and the pain is made worse by attempting to abduct and externally rotate the thigh against resistance. This test is most readily carried out by applying resistance to the outside of the thigh whilst the patient in the sitting position attempts to abduct the leg (Pace & Nagle 1976).

TrP tenderness may be elicited by exerting deep pressure on the lateral part of the muscle through the overlying gluteal muscles. Active TrPs near to its medial attachment, however, can only be located when pressure is applied to the region of the greater sciatic notch during the course of carrying out a rectal or vaginal examination.

Cummings (2000) has recently provided a comprehensive, well-referenced review concerning the diagnostic features, the clinical examination and the various procedures available for the treatment of this syndrome. These include stretching of the muscle with or without the application of a vapocoolant spray, the application of external pressure, rectal massage and acupuncture. With respect to the latter he recommends:

… brief dry needling of TrPs with a 75 mm acupuncture needle in piriformis. The position adopted for needling is that which puts piriformis on stretch. The needle is inserted over the site of maximum tenderness and advanced until the increased resistance of the stretched muscle is reached or the patient recognises their pain … When aiming for the most medial portion of

**Figure 17.16**   The pattern of pain referral from a trigger point (▲) in the piriformis muscle.

This muscle, an external rotator of the hip, arises from the internal surface of the sacrum, and then passes outwards and downwards through the sciatic notch to become inserted into the greater trochanter of the femur (Fig. 18.6).

The sciatic nerve on leaving the pelvis is normally situated behind the muscle (Fig. 17.15) but in more than 10% of people the peroneal part of the nerve passes through the belly of the muscle (Grant 1978), and in less than 1% of people the entire sciatic nerve passes through the muscle (Beaton & Anson 1937). In those patients in whom part or the whole of the sciatic nerve takes this course, shortening of the muscle as a

piriformis accessible externally an additional needle can be inserted as a guide of depth on to the
sacrum at the medial border of the sciatic notch …

## Pain in and around the sacroiliac joint

Pain in the region of the sacroiliac joint in a young
man may herald the onset of ankylosing spondylitis
and appropriate investigations should be carried
out to exclude this. Pain from sacroiliac strain may
also occur during the last few months of pregnancy
and in the postpartum period, but it is doubtful
whether it is possible to subject this joint to strain
at any other time of life.

During the later stages of pregnancy, hormonally-
induced laxity of the ligaments of the joint takes
place, and this is sometimes associated with pain
both in the region of this joint and the hip, and, on
occasions, down the front of the thigh. On examination, there is often quite marked tenderness over
one or both sacroiliac joints, but the temptation
to attempt to relieve this pain by inserting dry
needles into points of maximum tenderness should,
in my opinion, be resisted. This is because now
that it has been shown that it is possible to induce
labour at full term by stimulating nerve endings in
the pelvic region, it might be difficult to defend
oneself in a court of law if acupuncture carried out
near to term for the treatment of low-back pain
appeared to be responsible for labour starting
prematurely. It was as well that my policy of not
carrying out acupuncture during pregnancy was
adhered to in the case of the 8-months pregnant
woman who was particularly anxious for me to
alleviate some persistent sacroiliac pain by means
of this technique, because 2 days after advising her
against having acupuncture in view of her being
pregnant, she spontaneously went into labour!

Pain in the region of the sacroiliac joint may also
occur following pregnancy when the joint, having
opened during delivery, fails to close properly.
Radiographic investigation may also show evidence
of misalignment of the pubic rami. The sacroiliac
pain may be relieved by inserting a dry needle into
a point of maximum tenderness along the line of
the joint but, in my experience, this usually, even
when repeated, only gives temporary relief, and
if the pain becomes chronic, there is a case for
strengthening the ligaments by injecting a sclerosing
agent into them.

## Sacroiliac strain unrelated to pregnancy

Low-back pain occuring without any relationship
to pregnancy is often diagnosed as being due to
sacroiliac strain, particularly by osteopaths, but
the joint normally has such little movement, due
to it being held in position by particularly strong
ligaments, that other than during pregnancy it
seems very unlikely to be subjected to strain, and
also it seems equally unlikely that it is amenable
to manipulative procedures. However, it has to
be admitted that in cases of chronic low-back pain
there is often exquisite tenderness on applying
pressure to the 'dimple' overlying the joint, and
the insertion of an acupuncture needle into the
point of maximum tenderness is often very helpful.

## Iliopsoas muscle (Fig. 17.17A)

In the investigation of chronic low-back pain no
examination for TrPs is complete without finally
turning the patient into the supine position to
check for TrPs in the anterior abdominal wall and
in the groin.

The activation of a TrP immediately below the
inguinal ligament, in the tendon of the iliopsoas
muscle where it lies in close relationship to the
femoral artery, just before it becomes inserted into
the lesser trochanter of the femur, is a cause of pain
being referred up a line immediately lateral to the
spine in the paravertebral gutter, and also in some
cases down the front of the thigh (Figs 17.17A,B).
Deactivation of the TrP with a dry needle is best
carried out with the thigh abducted and externally
rotated, and with care being taken not to damage
the femoral nerve.

TrP activity in the iliopsoas muscle may be associated with similar activity in muscles in the lower
back such as the quadratus lumborum, but occasionally it is present on its own. It is important
to examine the groin routinely for TrPs in all cases
of low-back pain as otherwise they can easily be
overlooked.

A physical training instructor (34 years of age), whilst
playing football, twisted his left leg and shortly after
developed pain in the left lower back, and down the
back of the leg a far as the calf; any stretching
movement of the trunk made the pain worse. An
osteopath manipulated his spine on several occasions
but without any improvement in the pain, and after

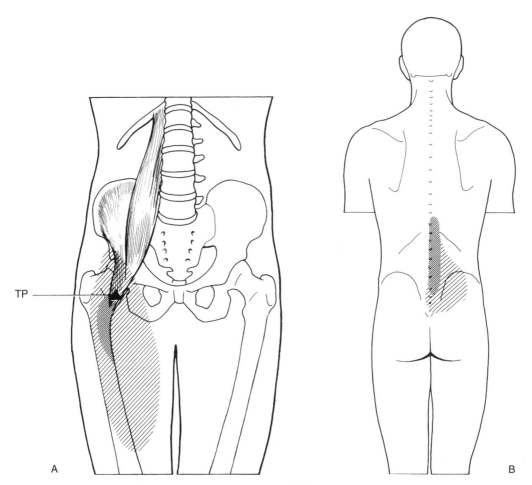

**Figure 17.17A&B**    Patterns of pain referral from a trigger point (▲) in the iliopsoas muscle near to its insertion into the lesser trochanter.

this had persisted for 12 months, he was sent to me for possible treatment with acupuncture. In view of the history there was no doubt in my mind that TrPs would be readily demonstrable in the muscles of the lower back, and it came as a great surprise to me when this proved not to be so. However, on getting him to lie on his back, TrPs were found in the groin, in the iliopsoas and adductor tendons. It is interesting to note that, as so often happens, in spite of them being exquisitely tender, he was quite unaware of their presence until pressure was put on them at the time of the examination. Also of particular interest was the fact that the insertion of a needle into one of them evoked a transient sensation of pain in the back and down the leg in exactly the same distribution as that occurring spontaneously. Furthermore, the importance of the part played by these TrPs in provoking the pain

was further confirmed by the latter being alleviated quite dramatically once they were deactivated with dry needles. The first time that this was done he was pain-free for 3 days, and, although the pain had been present for over a year, it was only necessary to repeat the procedure on two further occasions at weekly intervals before he obtained lasting relief.

### Clinical trials to assess the effectiveness of acupuncture in the treatment of chronic low-back pain

The general consensus of opinion among those with much experience of using acupuncture in the treatment of chronic low-back pain is that it provides worthwhile symptomatic relief in about 70% of cases. This, however, can be considered to be no more than a clinical impression, as the number of statistically controlled trials so far conducted has been small, and of those that have been carried out, most have been poorly designed and have lacked sufficient numbers of patients in them.

It has to be admitted that the objective assessment of the effectiveness of acupuncture, or any other type of treatment, in relieving chronic low-back pain is particularly difficult because the considerable uncertainty concerning the aetiological factors responsible for this type of pain in any particular individual, makes it virtually impossible to divide cases into clearly definable sub-groups. It is because of this that the Working Group on Back Pain (1979), set up by the Minister of Health, considered that in order to be certain that randomization ensured that all the various factors likely to influence the outcome of treatment are equally distributed amongst the actively treated group and the control group in any such trial, it might well be necessary to study up to 500 pairs or more. The Working Group, however, being well aware of the very considerable practical problems associated with conducting trials of such magnitude, suggested that initially it might be more expedient to settle for less than that which might be considered to be ideal.

Some of the problems related to statistically controlled trials designed to assess the effectiveness of acupuncture in relieving musculoskeletal pain including that which affects the lower back have already been considered in Chapter 11, and so at this stage nothing more need be said other than to draw attention to some personal observations made during the course of using this form of treatment in a large number of cases of chronic low-back pain that seem to me to be of relevance when planning, carrying out, and assessing the results of such trials.

Firstly, it is my belief that the response to acupuncture seems to bear little or no relationship to the amount of degenerative changes a person has in the lumbar discs or facet joints, but it does seem to be very much influenced by his or her psychological state. By this it is meant that at one end of the spectrum psychologically stable people with low-back pain often respond well to acupuncture, in spite of having advanced degenerative changes in their spine, whereas at the other end of the spectrum, the response to this form of treatment in people who hold their lumbar muscles in a state of persistent tension because of chronic anxiety is liable to be poor, even when the X-rays of their spines are normal. The implication of this, with respect to clinical trials, might seem to be that, so far as psychosocial factors and degenerative changes in the spine are concerned, that of the two, it is particularly important that randomization ensures that neuroticism is evenly spread between the treatment and control groups. It was no doubt considerations such as these that led Mendelson et al (1983), in their statistically controlled study of the use of acupuncture in low-back pain, to carry out a detailed pre-trial psychological assessment in all their patients. And there are many who now believe that psychosocial factors are of such importance both in the aetiology of chronic low-back pain, and in causing it to persist, as to make it essential with some patients to employ various psychological forms of relaxation therapy, such as hypnosis (Crasilneck 1979) or biofeedback (Keefe et al 1981), in addition to physical measures applied locally to the back, such as acupuncture. Trials in anxious low-back pain patients to assess whether or not the use of acupuncture and a relaxation technique give better results than those obtained by the use of one of these treatments on its own have not as yet been carried out.

Before leaving the subject, it must be admitted that the belief that unrelieved chronic anxiety tends to nullify the effects of acupuncture is not held by everyone, with, for example, Levine et al (1976) finding that a high score on psychometric indicators of anxiety and depression is a significant predictor of successful needle puncture analgesia in patients with chronic pain. It is clear, therefore, that with such diversity of views on this subject there is much scope for clinical trials specifically designed to resolve this issue.

The other matter that has to be considered when discussing the design of clinical trials to assess the efficacy of acupuncture in relieving chronic low-back pain, and, for that matter, all other forms of musculoskeletal pain, is that responders to acupuncture may be divided into a group consisting of those who obtain long-lasting relief from chronic pain after a comparatively few treatment sessions, and another group consisting of those who benefit from acupuncture but require ongoing treatment over a long period in order to keep chronic pain adequately suppressed.

These differences in people's reaction to acupuncture so far as low-back pain is concerned, again seem to bear little or no relationship to the type or extent of any pathological changes that may happen to be present in their spines, but, as with musculoskeletal pain anywhere in the body, it does seem to depend on the varying manner in which individuals' endogenous pain-modulating mechanism respond to peripheral nociceptive stimulation.

The ability of acupuncture in some people at times not only to give symptomatic relief, but to cut short a long-standing episode of pain is well recognized, and a possible explanation for this phenomenon is given in Chapter 10. However, it has to be realized that such a response may, on occasions, be more apparent than real and be due to the acupuncture treatment being given coincidentally with the onset of a natural remission. If by chance this should happen to occur with a number of patients in a clinical trial, then of course it might seriously interfere with the results. And it was in an attempt to safeguard against this as much as is possible that Macdonald et al (1983), in their statistically controlled trial of acupuncture in the relief of chronic low-back pain, only included patients whose pain had persisted for at least 1 year. Their reasoning behind this was, of course, that the longer chronic pain persists, the less likely it is to undergo a spontaneous remission.

Many chronic low-back pain sufferers only obtain relatively short periods of symptomatic relief from acupuncture and because of this have to be given it at fairly frequent intervals on a long-term basis. Such relief, however, is clearly of great benefit to them, and repeated treatment with a procedure so free of side effects as acupuncture is, of course, a small price to pay for it. Fox & Melzack (1976) clearly had this in mind when, during the course of commenting on the results of their comparative trial of transcutaneous electrical stimulation and acupuncture in the treatment of chronic low-back pain, they stated:

> ... transcutaneous stimulation and acupuncture, however, are not 'cures' and repeated treatments are usually necessary to provide continuing

periods of relief. When it is recalled that many of the patients in this study had suffered pain for years, and several had undergone major surgery without relief, the value of a technique which brings partial relief for a few hours or days at a time is especially evident. It makes the difference between unbearable and bearable pain, between a sedentary, sometimes bed-ridden life and one that, for at least several hours or days a week, allows a normal social, family, or business life. Even a few hours or days of pain at tolerable levels permits some of these patients to live with more dignity and self-assurance, so that life in general becomes more bearable.

These differing effects of acupuncture on chronic low-back pain, with at times it being capable of giving long-lasting relief, and at other times giving short-term, but nevertheless much appreciated, relief, have to be taken into account when evaluating the results of clinical trials.

Furthermore, when planning such trials it has to be remembered that individuals vary widely as to how much peripheral nerve stimulation they require in order to obtain optimum response, and also as to how many times treatment has to be given in order to bring the pain under control. It would therefore seem expedient, when drawing up protocols for these trials, to allow for these varying treatment requirements, by permitting the rules governing the administration of the acupuncture and the control type of therapy to be more flexible than those governing the prescribing of pharmacological substances in drug trials.

Such considerations of course apply to acupuncture trials in general and have already been referred to in Chapter 11, but it is appropriate to draw attention to them again here because it would seem that up to now only Macdonald et al (1983) have realistically taken them into account when drawing up the protocol for their trial in patients with chronic low-back pain. In that trial the effect of inserting needles superficially through the skin to an approximate depth of 4 mm at TrP sites was compared with that obtained by a placebo treatment consisting of the placing of electrodes on the skin at similar points and then attaching them to a non-functioning TENS machine. The protocol for this trial laid down that treatment both in the acupuncture group and in the placebo control group should be given once a week. For the acupuncture group, it was decided that each treatment should take the form of needles being left in situ, without any form of rotation, for 5 min, and that if, on any occasion, such treatment failed to produce beneficial results, then at the next treatment the needle insertion time had to be doubled, and if necessary on a further occasion doubled again up to a maximum of 20 min. If there was still no response, electroacupuncture had to be used. It was laid down that, initially, impulses of $700\,\mu s$ duration should be obtained at a frequency of $2\,Hz$, with the amplitude being increased approximately every 2 min to maintain the stimulation just above the pain threshold. Again if 5 min of this treatment produced no effect, the duration had to be doubled at each treatment up to a maximum of 20 min. The number of treatments given could be varied according to an individual's response with an arbitrarily defined upper limit of 10. The number of treatments was reduced, however, if further improvement failed to occur, or, indeed, if the pain continued to progress.

The rules governing the application of electrodes to the skin over the TrPs in the control group were exactly similar, including that if the patient reported a worsening of the pain immediately following 'treatment', as happened in three cases, then in exactly the same way as with the needle insertion time in the acupuncture group, the electrode application time was reduced.

The trial was small, but nevertheless, largely due to its design, it was possible to show a statistically significant superiority of superficial dry needling over placebo in the alleviation of chronic low-back pain.

Ernst & White (1998), have recently carried out a meta-analysis of all the various randomized controlled trials conducted to date to assess the value of acupuncture in the treatment of back pain. During the course of discussing their findings Ernst (1999) has concluded that reasonably good evidence supports the use of acupuncture in the treatment of this disorder but goes on to say that 'unfortunately numerous caveats prevent firmer conclusions'.

One of my criticisms is that in the majority of trials the effects of needling carried out at traditional Chinese acupuncture points and sham points have been compared. This is of dubious value because, as emphasized by van Tulder et al (1999), in their systematic review of the effectiveness of acupuncture in the management of acute and chronic low-back pain, the needling of so-called sham points must invariably afford a certain amount of pain relief for reasons discussed at some length in Chapter 11, so as to make it difficult to compare the relative effectiveness of the two types of treatment.

Another shortcoming is that low-back pain is a symptom not a specific entity, so that patients admitted to such trials are likely to be suffering from a variety of different disorders with the pain in some of them being nociceptive and in others neuropathic. This makes the interpretation of results virtually impossible as the responsiveness to acupuncture of these two types of pain is likely to be very different. It is for this reason that Thomas & Lundberg (1994) are to be commended for specifically discussing the importance of modes of acupuncture in the treatment of chronic nociceptive low-back pain.

Two recent trials are worthy of special mention, as in both, care was taken to include only patients suffering from the MTrP pain syndrome.

Kovacs et al (1997) carried out a randomized, double-blind, multi-centre trial to assess the value of treatment called by them neuroreflexotherapy directed at TrPs in low-back muscles. This form of therapy consisted of the implantation of staples inserted 2 mm below the surface of the skin at TrP sites in the lumbar muscles for up to 90 days and epidermal burins (metal studs) inserted into tender points in the ear for up to 20 days. A control group was treated in a similar manner, but with the devices implanted 5 cm away from the TrPs in the back and the tender areas in the ear. From the results they concluded that:

> … neuroreflexotherapy intervention seems to be a simple and effective treatment for rapid amelioration of pain episodes in patients with chronic low back pain … but further studies are essential to confirm the present results on a larger sample.

Ceccherelli et al (2002) carried out a double-blind, randomized controlled study in patients with lumbar myofascial pain to compare shallow needling (insertion of the needle to a depth of 2 mm) in one group and deep needling (insertion of the needle to a depth of 1.5 cm) in another group carried out at eight traditional Chinese acupuncture sites and four TrP sites. From their results they concluded that deeply applied stimulation has a better therapeutic effect than shallow needling.

As most people who treat the myofascial pain syndrome do so by directing treatment at all of the TrPs present in each individual case, there is clearly a need for large scale trials to be carried out to compare the effectiveness of doing this in three groups of patients. One group treated with shallow needling (2 mm insertion at the TrP sites), a second treated with superficial needling (5–10 mm insertion at the TrP sites) and a third with needles inserted deeply into the TrPs themselves.

# References

Bates T, Grunwald E 1958 Myofascial pain in childhood. Journal of Pediatrics 53: 148–209

Beaton L E, Anson B J 1937 The relation of the sciatic nerve and of its subdivision to the piriformis muscle. Anatomical Record 70(suppl 1): 1–5

Berquist-Ullman M, Larsson U 1977 Acute low-back pain in industry. A controlled prospective study with special reference to therapy and confounding factors. Acta Orthopaedica Scandinavica 170(suppl)

Bogduk N 1995 Spine update, epidural steroids. Spine 20(7): 845–848

Bourne I H J 1979 Treatment of backache with local injections. The Practitioner 222: 708–711

Bourne I H J 1984 Treatment of chronic back pain comparing corticosteroid-lignocaine injections with lignocaine alone. The Practitioner 228: 333–338

Cailliet R 1977 Soft tissue pain and disability. F A Davies, Philadelphia, p. 99

Calin A, Porta J, Fries J F F 1977 The clinical history as a screening test for ankylosing spondylitis. Journal of the American Medical Association 273: 2613–2615

Carette S, Marcoux S, Truchon R et al 1991 A controlled trial of corticosteroid injections into facet joints for chronic low back pain. New England Journal of Medicine 325(14): 1002–1007

Ceccherelli F, Rigoni M T, Gagliardi G, Ruzzante L 2002 Comparison of superficial and deep acupuncture in the treatment of lumbar myofascial pain: a double-blind randomized controlled study. The Clinical Journal of Pain 18: 149–153

Chu J 1995 Dry needling (intramuscular stimulation) in myofascial pain related to lumbosacral radiculopathy. European Journal of Physical Medicine and Rehabilitation 5(4): 106–121

Couch J R, Hassanein R S 1976 Migraine and depression: effect of amitriptyline prophylaxis. Transactions of the American Neurological Association 101: 1–4

Couch J R, Ziegler D K, Hassanein R S 1976 Amitriptyline in the prophylaxis of migraine. Effectiveness and relationship of anti-migraine and anti-depressant effects. Neurology 26: 121–127

Crasilneck H B 1979 Hypnosis in the control of chronic low-back pain. American Journal of Clinical Hypnosis 22: 71–78

Cummings M 2000 Piriformis syndrome. Acupuncture in Medicine 18(2): 108–121

Deyo R A 1991 Fads in the treatment of low back pain. New England Journal of Medicine 325: 1039–1040

Deyo R A, Diehl A K, Rosenthal M 1986 How many days of bed rest for acute low-back pain? A randomized clinical trial. New England Journal of Medicine 315: 1064–1070

Dixon J St J 1980 Introduction. In: Jayson M I V (ed) The lumbar spine and back pain, 2nd edn. Pitman, London, p. XI & 147

Doran D M L, Newell D J 1975 Manipulation in the treatment of low-back pain, a multicentre study. British Medical Journal 2: 161–164

Dreyfuss 1993 Epidural steroid injections. A procedure ideally performed with fluoroscopic control and contrast media. International Spinal Injection Society Newsletter 1: 34–40

Edgar M A, Park W M 1974 Induced pain patterns in passive straight-leg raising in lower lumbar disc protrusion. Journal of Bone and Joint Surgery 56B: 658–667

Eisenstein S 1977 The morphometry and pathological anatomy of the lumbar spine in South African negroes and caucasoids with special reference to spinal stenosis. Journal of Bone and Joint Surgery 59B: 173–180

Ernst E 1999 Clinical effectiveness of acupuncture: an overview of systematic reviews. In: Ernst E, White A (eds) Acupuncture, a scientific appraisal. Butterworth-Heinemann, Oxford

Ernst E , White A R 1998 Acupuncture for back pain: a meta-analysis of randomized controlled trials. Archives of Internal Medicine 158: 2235–2241

Evans D P, Burke M S, Lloyd K N, Roberts G M 1978 Lumbar spinal manipulation on trial. Part I Clinical assessment. Rheumatology and Rehabilitation 17: 46–53

Fairbank J C T, Park W M, McCall I W, O'Brien J P 1981 Apophyseal injection of local anaesthetic as a diagnostic aid in primary low-back pain syndromes. Spine 6: 598–605

Flor H, Turk D C 1984 Etiological theories and treatments for chronic back pain. Part I Somatic models and interventions. Pain 19: 105–121

Fouquet B, Goupille P, Jattiot F et al 1992 Discitis after disc surgery. Features of 'aseptic' and 'septic' forms. Spine 17: 356–358

Fox E, Melzack R 1976 Transcutaneous electrical stimulation and acupuncture – a comparison of treatment for low-back pain. Pain 2: 141–148

Friedenberg Z B, Shoemaker R C 1954 The results of non-operative treatment of ruptured lumbar discs. American Journal of Surgery 86: 933–935

Gerwin R 1991 Myofascial aspects of low back pain. Neurosurgery Clinics of North America 2(4): 761–784

Getty C J M, Johnson J R, Kirwan E O'G et al 1981 Partial undercutting facetectomy for bony entrapment of the lumbar nerve root. Journal of Bone and Joint Surgery 63B: 330–335

Glover J R, Morris J G, Khosla T 1974 Back pain – a randomized clinical trial of rotational manipulation of the trunk. British Journal of Industrial Medicine 31: 59–64

Grant J C 1978 An atlas of human anatomy, 7th edn. Williams & Wilkins, Baltimore

Grantham V A 1977 Backache in boys – a new problem? The Practitioner 218: 226–229

Green L N 1975 Dexamethasone in the management of symptoms due to herniated lumbar disc. Journal of Neurology Neurosurgery and Psychiatry 38: 1211–1217

Hingorani K 1966 Diazepam in backache. A double blind controlled trial. Annals of Physical Medicine 8: 303–306

Hirsch C, Ingelmark B, Miller M 1963 The anatomical basis for low-back pain. Acta Orthopaedica Scandinavica 33: 1–17

Horal J 1969 The clinical appearance of low-back pain disorders in the city of Gothenberg, Sweden. Acta Orthopaedica Scandinavica 118(suppl): 8–73

Hult L 1954 Cervical dorsal and lumbar spinal syndromes. A field investigation of a non-selected material of 1200 workers in different occupations with special reference to disc degeneration and so-called muscular rheumatism. Acta Orthopaedica Scandinavica 17(suppl): 1–102

Hussar A E, Guller E J 1956 Correlation of pain and the roentgenographic findings of spondylosis of the cervical and lumbar spine. American Journal of Medical Science 232: 518–527

Jackson R P 1992 The facet syndrome, myth or reality? Clinical Orthopaedics and Related Research 279: 110–120

Jackson R P, Jacobs R R Montesano P X 1988 Facet joint injection in low back pain. A prospective stastistical study. Spine 13: 966–971

Jenkins D G, Ebbutt A F, Evans C D 1976 Imipramine in treatment of low-back pain. Journal of International Medical Research 4(suppl 2): 28–40

Jensen M C, Brant-Zawadzki M N, Obouchowski N et al 1994 Magnetic resonance imaging of the lumbar spine in people without back pain. New England Journal of Medicine 331: 69–73

Johnson E W, Fletcher E R 1981 Lumbosacral radiculopathy. Review of 100 consecutive cases. Archives of Physical Medicine and Rehabilitation 62: 321–323

Keefe F J, Schapira B, Williams R B, Brown C, Surwet R S 1981 EMG assisted relaxation training in the management of chronic low-back pain. American Journal of Clinical Biofeedback 4: 93–103

Ketchum L D 1971 Effects of triamcinolone on tendon healing and function. A laboratory study. Plastic and Reconstructive Surgery 47: 471–482

Ketchum L D, Robinson D W, Masters F W 1968 The degradiation of mature collagen. A laboratory study. Plastic and Reconstructive Surgery 40: 89–91

King J S, Lagger R 1976 Sciatica viewed as a referred pain syndrome. Surgical Neurology 5: 46–50

Kleefield J, O'Reilly G V 1992 Magnetic resonance and radiological imaging in the evaluation of back pain. In: Aronoff G M (ed) Evaluation and treatment of chronic pain, 2nd edn. Williams & Wilkins, Baltimore

Kovacs F M, Abraira V, Pozo F, Kleinbaum D G et al 1997 Local and remote sustained trigger point therapy for exacerbations of chronic low back pain. A randomized, double-blind, controlled, multicenter trial. Spine 22(7): 786–797

Lamerton A J, Banninster R, Wittington R, Seifert M H, Eastcott H H G 1983 'Claudication' of the sciatic nerve. British Medical Journal 286: 1785–1786

Levine J, Gormley J, Fields H L 1976 Observation on the analgesic effects of needle puncture (acupuncture). Pain 2: 149–159

Leyshon A, Kirwan E O, Wynn Parry C B 1981 Electrical studies in the diagnosis of compression of the lumbar root. Journal of Bone and Joint Surgery 63B: 51–75

Lewit K 1979 The needle effect in the relief of myofascial pain. Pain 6: 83–90

Lillius G, Laasonen E M, Myllynen P, Harilainen A, Gronlund G 1989 Lumbar facet joint syndrome. A randomised clinical trial. Journal of Bone and Joint Surgery (British) 71: 681–684

Loeser J D 1980 Low-back pain. In: Bonica J J (ed) Pain. Raven Press, New York, pp. 363–377

Macdonald A J R, Macrae K D, Master B R, Rubin A P 1983 Superficial acupuncture in the relief of chronic low-back pain. Annals of the Royal College of Surgeons of England 65: 44–46

McKillop J H, McDougal I R 1980 The role of skeletal scanning in clinical oncology. British Medical Journal 281: 407–410

Magora A 1970 Investigation of the relation between low-back pain and occupation to age, sex, community, education and other factors. Industrial Medicine and Surgery 39: 465–471

Magora A, Schwartz A 1976 Relation between the low-back pain syndrome and X-ray findings. 1. Degenerative osteoarthritis. Scandinavian Journal of Rehabilitation Medicine 8: 115–175

Magora A, Schwartz A 1978 Relation between the low-back pain syndrome and X-ray findings. 2. Transitional vertebra (mainly sacralization). Scandinavian Journal of Rehabilitation Medicine 10: 135–145

Manniche C, Lundberg E, Christensen I, Bentzen L , Hasselsoe G 1991 Intensive dynamic back exercises for chronic low-back pain. A clinical trial. Pain 47: 53–63

Melzack R, Wall P D 1982 The challenge of pain. Penguin Books, Harmondsworth, pp. 249–254

Mendelson G, Selwood T S, Kranz H, Loh T S, Kidson M A, Scott D S 1983 Acupuncture treatment of chronic back pain: a double blind placebo controlled trial. American Journal of Medicine 74: 49–55

Mixter W J, Barr J S 1934 Rupture of the intervertebral disc with involvement of the spinal canal. New England Journal of Medicine 211: 210–215

Monks R C 1981 The use of psychotropic drugs in human chronic pain. A review. 6th World Congress of the International College of Psychosomatic Medicine, Montreal, Canada, Sept 15

Mooney V, Robertson J 1975 The facet syndrome. Clinical Orthopaedics and Related Research 115: 149–156

Nachemson A 1979 A critical look at the treatment for low-back pain. Scandinavian Journal of Rehabilitation Medicine 11: 143–149

Nachemson A 1980 A critical look at conservative treatment for low-back pain. In: Jayson M I V (ed) The Lumbar spine and back pain, 2nd edn. Pitman, London, p. 459

Nelson M A 1980 Surgery of the spine. In: Jayson M I V (ed) The lumbar spine and back pain, 2nd edn. Pitman, London, p. 477

Nelson M A 1987 Indications for spinal surgery in low back pain. In: Jayson M I V (ed) The lumbar spine and back pain, 3rd edn. Churchill Livingstone, Edinburgh, pp. 321–352

Nichols P J R 1960 Short-leg syndrome. British Medical Journal 1: 1863–1865

Nwuga V C B 1983 Ultrasound in treatment of back pain arising from prolapsed intervertebral disc. Archives of Physical Medicine and Rehabilitation 64: 88–89

Pace J B, Nagle D 1976 Piriform syndrome. The Western Journal of Medicine 124: 435–439

Porter R W 1987 Spinal stenosis in the central and root canal. In: Jayson M I V (ed) The lumbar spine and back pain, 3rd edn. Churchill Livingstone, Edinburgh, pp. 383–400

Porter R W 1993 Management of back pain, 2nd edn. Churchill Livingstone, Edinburgh, p. 168

Porter R W, Hibbert C, Evans C 1984 The natural history of root entrapment syndrome. Spine 9: 418–422

Porter R W, Wicks M, Ottewell D 1978 Measurement of the spinal canal by diagnostic ultrasound. Journal of Bone and Joint Surgery 60B: 481–487

Porter R W, Trailescu I F 1990 Diurnal changes in straight leg raising. Spine 15: 103–106

Quinet R J, Hadler N M 1979 Diagnosis and treatment of backache. Seminars in Arthritis and Rheumatics 8: 261–287

Ransford A O, Harries B J 1972 Localised arachnoiditis complicating lumbar disc lesions. Journal of Bone and Joint Surgery 54B: 656–665

Rees W S, Slade H W 1974 Multiple bilateral percutaneous rhizolysis in the treatment of the slipped disc syndrome. Paper delivered before the American Association of Neurological Surgeons meeting in St Louis Missouri, April 22–25, 1974

Rowe M L 1965 Disc surgery and chronic low-back pain. Journal of Occupational Medicine 7: 196–202

Rowe M L 1969 Low back pain in industry. A position paper. Journal of Occupational Medicine 11: 161–169

Saal J S, Franson R C, Dobrow R et al 1990 High levels of inflammatory phospholipase A2 activity in lumbar disc herniations. Spine 15: 674–678

Saal J A, Saal J S 1989 Non-operative treatment of herniated lumbar intervertebral disc with radiculopathy. An outcome study. Spine 14: 431–437

Schmorl G, Junghanns H 1932 Die gesunde und kranke Wirbelseule im Roentgenbild. Thieme, Leipzig

Schumaker T M, Genant H K, Korobkin M, Bovill T R 1978 Computerized tomography – its use in space-occupying lesions of the musculoskeletal system. Journal of Bone and Joint Surgery 60A: 600–607

Schwarzer A C, Aprill C N, Derby R, Fortin J, Kine G, Bogduk N 1994a Clinical features of patients with pain stemming from lumbar zygapophysial joints. Is the lumbar facet syndrome a clinical entity? Spine 19: 1132–1137

Schwarzer A C, Aprill C N, Derby R, Fortin J, Kine G, Bogduk N 1994b The relative contributions of the disc and zygapophysial joint in chronic low back pain. Spine 19: 801–806

Sclapbach P 1991 Ultrasound. In: Schlapbach P, Gerber N J (eds) Physiotherapy: controlled trials and facts, rheumatology. Karger, Basel, Vol. 14, pp. 163–170

Shealy C N, Prieto A Jnr, Burton C, Long D M 1974 Radiofrequency percutaneous rhizotomy of the articular nerve of Luschka – an alternative approach to chronic low-back pain and sciatica. Paper delivered before the American Association of Neurological Surgeons' meeting, Los Angeles, California, April 9th 1974

Simons D, Travell J G, Simons L S 1999 Myofascial pain and dysfunction. The trigger point manual, Vol. 1, 2nd edn, Williams & Wilkins, Baltimore, p. 81

Simkin P A 1982 Simian stance: a sign of spinal stenosis. Lancet 2: 652–653

Sims-Williams H, Jayson M I, Young S M, Baddeley H, Collins E 1982 Controlled trial of mobilization and manipulation for patients with low-back pain in general practice. British Medical Journal 2: 1338–1340

Sola A E, Williams R L 1956 Myofascial pain syndromes. Neurology (Minneapolis) 6: 91–95

Spangfort E V 1972 The lumbar disc herniation. A computer-aided analysis of 2504 operations. Acta Orthopaedica Scandinavica supplement 142: 1–95

Splithoff C A 1952 Lumbosacral junction. Roentgenographic comparison of patients with and without backaches. Journal of the American Medical Association 152: 1610–1613

Steindler A, Luck J V 1938 Differential diagnosis of pain low in the back. Journal of the American Medical Association 110: 106–112

Sternbach R A, Janowsky D S, Huey I Y, Segal D S 1976 Effects of altering brain serotonin activity on human chronic pain. In: Bonica J J, Albe Fessard D (eds) Advances in pain research and therapy 1. Raven Press, New York, pp. 601–606

Strange F G St Clair 1966 Debunking the disc. Proceedings of the Royal Society of Medicine 59: 952–956

Symposium 1978 Lumbar arachnoiditis: nomenclature, etiology and pathology. Spine 3: 21–92

Thomas M, Lundberg T 1994 Importance of modes of acupuncture in the treatment of chronic nociceptive low back pain. Acta Anaesthesiologica Scandivacica 38: 63–69

Torgerson W R, Dotter W E 1976 Comparative roentgenographic study of the asymptomatic and symptomatic lumbar spine. Journal of Bone and Joint Surgery 58A: 850–853

Travell J 1968 Office hours: day and night. The World Publishing Company, New York

Travell J G 1976 The quadratus lumborum muscle, an overlooked cause of low-back pain. Archives of Physical Medicine and Rehabilitation 57: 566

Travell J G, Simons D G 1983 Myofascial pain and dysfunction. The trigger point manual. Williams & Wilkins, Baltimore, pp. 105–109, 644, 637

Turk D C, Flor H 1984 Etiological theories and treatments for chronic back pain II. Psychological models and interactions. Pain 19: 209–233

Urban T, Maroudas A 1980 In: Graham R (ed) Clinics in rheumatic diseases, Vol. 6, no 1. Saunders, Philadelphia, p. 51

van Tulder M W, Cherkin D C, Berman B, Lao L, Koes B W 1999 The effectiveness of acupuncture in the management of acute and chronic low back pain. A systematic review within the framework of the Cochrane Collaboration Back Review Group. Spine 24: 1113–1123

Vernon-Roberts B, Pirie C J 1977 Degenerative changes in the intervertebral discs and their sequelae. Rheumatology and Rehabilitation 16: 13–21

Waddell G 1982 An approach to backache. British Journal of Hospital Medicine 28(3): 187–219

Weber B 1983 Lumbar disc herniation: a controlled prospective study with ten years' observation. Spine 8: 131–140

Westrin C G 1973 Low back sick-listing. A sociological and medical insurance investigation. Scandinavian Journal of Social Medicine, Supplement 7

White A W M 1966 Low-back pain in men receiving workmen's compensation. Canadian Medical Journal 95: 50–56

Wiesel S W, Cuckler J M, De Luca F et al 1980 Acute low back pain: an objective analysis of conservative therapy. Spine 5: 324–330

Working Group on Back Pain 1979 Department of Health and Social Security. Her Majesty's Stationery Office, London

Wyke B 1980 The neurology of low-back pain. In: Jayson M I V (ed) The lumbar spine and back pain, 2nd edn. Pitman, London, p. 307

Wyke B 1987 The neurology of low-back pain. In: Jayson M I V (ed) The lumbar spine and back pain, 3rd edn. Churchill Livingstone, Edinburgh, pp. 59, 74

Wynn Parry C B 1989 The failed back. In: Wall P D, Melzack R (eds) Textbook of pain, 2nd edn. Churchill Livingstone, Edinburgh, pp. 341–353

Wynn Parry C B 1994 The failed back. In: Wall P D, Melzack R (eds) Textbook of pain, 3rd edn. Churchill Livingstone, Edinburgh, p. 1082

Chapter **18**

# Pain in the lower limb

## CHAPTER CONTENTS

## INTRODUCTION

As pain in the leg from entrapment of lumbar nerve roots and from trigger points (TrPs) in the muscles of the lower back and buttocks has been dealt with in the previous chapter, and as pain in and around the hip, knee, and ankle joints will be discussed in Chapter 19, this chapter will be restricted to a consideration of pain in the lower limb occurring as a result of the activation of TrPs in muscles of the lower limb itself.

Investigations to ascertain the cause of persistent pain in the leg are usually directed at excluding diseases of the bones or joints, circulatory disorders, and neuropathies, but the possibility that such pain might occur as a result of the activation of TrPs in the muscles is all too frequently passed over, with the result that it is often allowed to continue for much longer than it need.

A man (75 years of age) began to get pain in the calves, ankles, and the soles of the feet on climbing stairs, together with troublesome cramps in the calves at night disturbing his sleep. After the symptoms had been present for 4 weeks, he sought medical advice. As investigations at that time showed no evidence of arthritis, no circulatory disturbance, and no evidence of a diabetic neuropathy, he was treated symptomatically with paracetamol for the pain on exertion, and quinine sulphate for the nocturnal cramps. These, however, had little or no effect and after a further 3 months he was referred to me as a case of persistent pain in the legs of unknown cause.

On taking this history, it became apparent that the patient spent much time cruising on the river. This involved frequently opening heavy lock gates, and to assist with this he was in the habit of pressing hard with his legs against concrete blocks. It would seem that this must have strained the muscles of his calves for, on examination, there were numerous exquisitely tender TrPs in the gastrocnemius and soleus muscles. Deactivation of these with dry needles on only one occasion gave him relief from the symptoms for 3 days, and after repeating the procedure a further three times at weekly intervals they disappeared altogether. A state of affairs of course that could have been achieved both more quickly and at an earlier stage if only the diagnosis had been made more promptly.

The muscles in the leg which, in my experience, most often develop active TrPs are the adductor longus, the quadriceps femoris group of muscles, the hamstrings, the tibialis anterior, the gastrocnemius, the soleus, the peronei and the dorsal interossei.

## ADDUCTOR LONGUS MUSCLES (Fig. 18.1)

TrPs in the adductor longus commonly develop near to its insertion into the pubis, and as referral of pain from these is predominantly into the groin, as well as down the inner side of the thigh, consideration will be given to pain from TrPs in this muscle when discussing pelvic pain in Chapter 20.

## QUADRICEPS FEMORIS GROUP OF MUSCLES (Fig. 18.1)

TrPs may become activated in any of the quadriceps group of muscles (the rectus femoris, the vastus medialis, the vastus intermedius and the vastus lateralis), when these muscles become strained either as a primary event, or secondarily to walking badly because of some painful disorder in the foot, ankle or knee.

With arthritis of the knee it is the vastus medialis that most commonly develops TrPs. The vastus medialis is the main muscular support of the knee, and as pointed out by Travell (1952), the development of TrP activity in it, whether this be due to a primary muscle strain, or to arthritis in the knee, is liable to cause the knee to become unstable and for

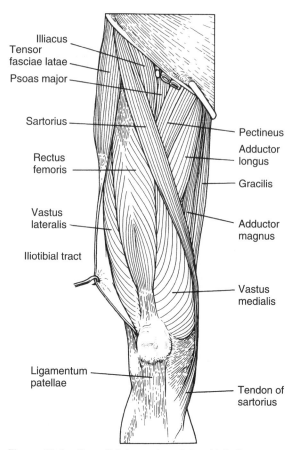

**Figure 18.1** Superficial muscles of the thigh. Extensor aspect.

it suddenly to give way. This often occurs before this TrP activity is a cause of pain. It therefore follows that a history of painless buckling of the knee is an indication for examining this muscle for a TrP and, if present, for it to be deactivated by means of inserting a dry needle into the tissues overlying it.

For those interested in comparing positions of TrPs with those of traditional Chinese acupuncture points, it should be noted that the TrP in the vastus medialis just above the knee is in close relationship to the traditional Chinese point Spleen 10 (Fig. 16.1) and one in the vastus lateralis, just above the knee, occurs close to the Chinese point Gall bladder 33 (Fig. 18.2).

Pain from a TrP just above the knee in the vastus medialis, is felt around the inner side of the knee (Fig. 18.3).

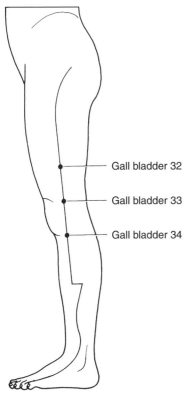

Figure 18.2    Some traditional Chinese acupuncture points along the Gall Bladder meridian in the region of the knee joint.

Gall bladder 32

Gall bladder 33

Gall bladder 34

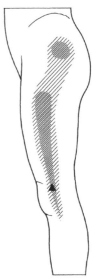

**Figure 18.4**    The pattern of pain referral from a trigger point (▲) in the vastus lateralis muscle.

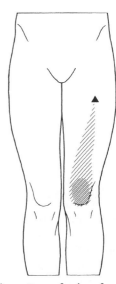

**Figure 18.5**    The pattern of pain referral from a trigger point (▲) in the rectus femoris muscle.

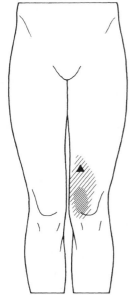

**Figure 18.3**    The pattern of pain referral from a trigger point (▲) in the vastus medialis muscle.

Pain from a TrP just above the knee, in the vastus lateralis, is referred up the side of the thigh, from the TrP below, up as far as the greater trochanter above (Fig. 18.4).

TrPs in the vastus intermedius and rectus femoris are usually to be found in the upper third of the thigh, and pain from these is referred down the anterior surface of the thigh (Fig. 18.5).

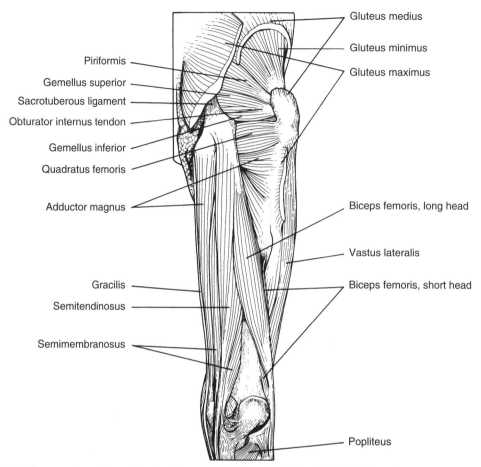

Piriformis
Gemellus superior
Sacrotuberous ligament
Obturator internus tendon
Gemellus inferior
Quadratus femoris

Adductor magnus

Gracilis
Semitendinosus

Semimembranosus

Gluteus medius
Gluteus minimus
Gluteus maximus

Biceps femoris, long head

Vastus lateralis

Biceps femoris, short head

Popliteus

**Figure 18.6** The muscles of the gluteal region and flexor aspect of the right thigh. Posterior aspect.

## HAMSTRINGS (Fig. 18.6)

TrPs in the hamstring muscles – the biceps femoris, the semimembranosus and the semitendinosus – are liable to become activated either in the bellies of these muscles high up on the posterior surface of the thigh or in their tendons at their sites of attachment just below the knee. It will be remembered that the lower attachment of the biceps femoris, the lateral hamstring, is by a tendon inserted into the fibula; the semimembranosus is inserted into the medial condyle of the tibia; and the semitendinosus, together with the gracilis and sartorius muscles, are inserted by a conjoined tendon – the pes anserinus (the goose's foot) – into the upper part of the medial surface of the tibia (Fig. 18.7).

Pain from TrPs in the bellies of these muscles is referred mainly to the region of the popliteal fossa (Fig. 18.8).

## Pain from TrPs

When TrPs are widespread throughout the bellies of the hamstrings, they cause these muscles to become shortened with, as a consequence of this, restricted flexion of the hip and a positive straight-leg raising test (Simons & Travell 1984).

## TIBIALIS ANTERIOR MUSCLE (Fig. 18.9)

The tibialis anterior muscle, which arises mainly from the upper two-thirds of the lateral surface of the tibia, is a thick fleshy muscle that ends in a tendon attached on the medial side of the foot to the medial cuneiform bone and the first metatarsal bone.

Active TrPs usually occur in the belly of the muscle, with pain from this being referred down the front of the shin, the medial side of the ankle

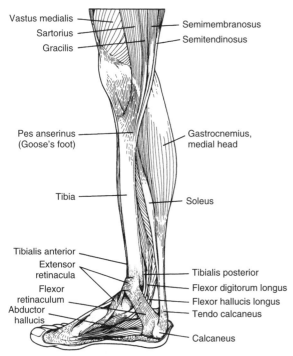

Figure 18.7    The muscles of the right leg, medial aspect.

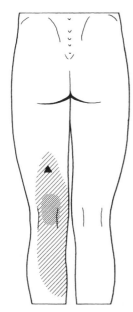

Figure 18.8    The pattern of pain referral from a trigger point (▲) in the belly of the biceps femoris muscle.

and foot, and sometimes extending as far as the big toe (Fig. 18.10).

TrP activity in this muscle is liable to develop in athletes and, as Sola & Williams (1956) have

pointed out, in members of the armed services who do much marching. The pain is quickly brought under control by deactivating the TrP with a dry needle, but is liable to recur if any activity responsible for the TrP activation is persisted with.

## GASTROCNEMIUS MUSCLE (Fig. 18.11)

TrPs become activated in the belly of the muscle in the centre of the calf as a result of the muscle becoming strained either, as a primary event, or when a limp develops as a result of a painful disorder occurring in the heel or foot, and also when, because of a circulatory disorder, the muscle becomes ischaemic (Fig. 18.12).

The pain from TrPs in this muscle is felt in the calf and the sole of the foot. It is often worse on walking uphill, and may be associated with the development of nocturnal cramps. As may be seen from the case quoted at the beginning of the chapter, nocturnal cramps should not be treated with quinine sulphate until a search for TrPs in this muscle has been carried out, because, if these are present, the cramps will not be brought under control until they have been deactivated.

## SOLEUS MUSCLE (Figs 18.9 & 18.11)

The soleus, a broad flat muscle situated immediately anterior to the gastrocnemius, and which, together with the latter, is inserted into the calcaneus by means of the Achilles tendon, is liable to develop TrPs in its distal third for the same reasons as they do in the gastrocnemius.

Pain from these TrPs is referred distally along the Achilles tendon to the heel (Fig. 18.13). Simons & Travell (1983) state that the pain may also be referred upwards to the sacroiliac joint. No case with this particular pattern of referral has, as yet, come under my care. They also point out that the ankle jerk may be decreased or absent in patients with TrP activity in the soleus. And that the deactivation of the TrPs restores this reflex to normal.

## Activation of TrPs in the gastrocnemius and soleus as a consequence of lower leg ischaemia

Intermittent claudication (L. *claudicatio*, limping or lameness), a condition characterized by calf pain

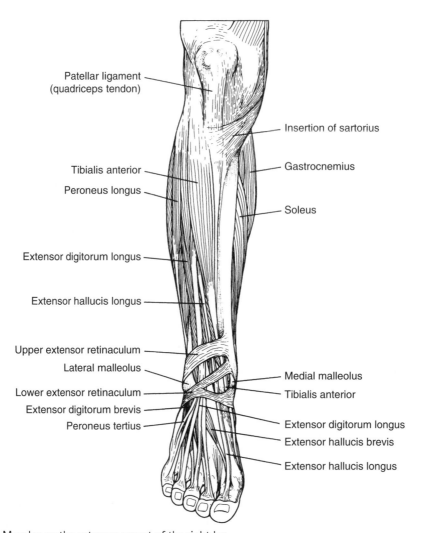

**Figure 18.9** Muscles on the extensor aspect of the right leg.

brought on by exertion and relieved by resting (angina cruris), is primarily due to femoropopliteal artery occulusion. However, Dorigo et al (1979) have shown that another factor contributing to the pain is the activation of TrPs in the gastrocnemius and soleus when these muscles become ischaemic as a result of an impaired arterial blood supply to the leg. They further showed that deactivating these TrPs, by injecting procaine into them, increases the exercise capacity of the limb in spite of the blood flow to the limb remaining the same. Deactivation of TrPs in these two muscles is therefore a worthwhile symptomatic therapeutic procedure in this condition and one that can be carried out even

more readily and just as effectively by inserting dry needles into the tissues overlying these TrPs.

## PAINFUL HEEL

Persistent pain may develop in the heel, either by being referred from TrPs in the soleus muscle, or from an inflammatory reaction occurring in either the Achilles tendon, or the plantar fascia. This inflammatory reaction in both Achilles tendinitis and plantar fasciitis may develop as a result of some underlying disease such as ankylosing spondylitis, psoriatic arthropathy, or Reiter's disease. More commonly, however, it occurs as a result of an injury to

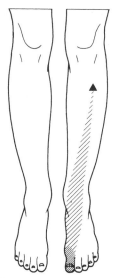

**Figure 18.10** The pattern of pain referral from a trigger point (▲) in the tibialis anterior muscle.

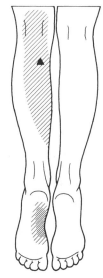

**Figure 18.12** The pattern of pain referral from a trigger point (▲) in the gastrocnemius muscle.

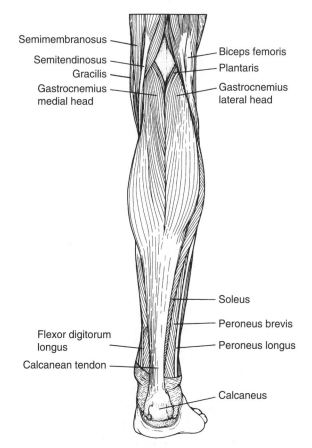

Semimembranosus

Semitendinosus

Gracilis

Gastrocnemius medial head

Biceps femoris

Plantaris

Gastrocnemius lateral head

Soleus

Peroneus brevis

Flexor digitorum longus

Calcanean tendon

Peroneus longus

Calcaneus

**Figure 18.11** Muscles of the right calf; superficial layer.

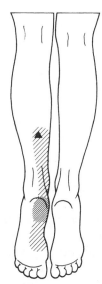

**Figure 18.13** The pattern of pain referral from a trigger point (▲) in the soleus muscle.

the heel or pressure from an ill-fitting shoe. At times it seems to occur for no apparent cause.

## Achilles tendinitis

It is particularly important to distinguish between pain developing in the base of the heel as a result of an inflammatory lesion in the tendon and pain referred to that site from TrPs in the soleus muscle. In Achilles tendinitis, the tendon is liable to be slightly swollen and there may be crepitus over it when the foot is moved. Also, on examination, exquisitely tender TrPs are to be found in the tissues around the tendon.

The pain may be relieved by inserting dry needles into the tissues overlying these TrPs. Admittedly, this usually has to be repeated three or more times at weekly intervals in order to obtain any lasting benefit but it is certainly preferable to injecting hydrocortisone into them. Not only is hydrocortisone associated with the development of much post-injection pain, but also, should it inadvertently be injected into the tendon itself, this structure may rupture and then need to be repaired surgically.

## Plantar fasciitis

The plantar fascia is attached by a tendon inserted into the periosteum of the calcaneus. Trauma, with tearing or stretching of the plantar tendon fibres, causes the periosteum to become detached from the calcaneus, with, as a consequence of this, the development of subperiosteal inflammation, the laying down of fibrous tissue, the deposition of calcium and the formation of a calcaneal spur. It is thought that the initial pain and discomfort is probably due to the soft-tissue inflammation and that at a later stage it is due to the spur (Cailliet 1977). However, not infrequently, there is radiographic evidence of a calcaneal spur in people who are asymptomatic. Furthermore, plantar fasciitis may occur without the development of a spur. Radiographically a calcaneal spur in traumatic fasciitis has smooth borders in contrast to one occurring in association with a seronegative arthropathy when they are fuzzy.

Plantar fasciitis leads to the development of severe pain under the heel, and also, in some cases, in the sole of the foot. It is a condition that most often occurs in those whose work requires much standing. On examination, there is a point of maximum tenderness close to where the plantar tendon attaches to the calcaneus. It is standard practice to inject hydrocortisone plus a local anaesthetic into this point. It is often necessary to carry out this procedure more than once. It is also possible to control the pain simply by inserting into the point of maximum tenderness a dry needle and then leaving it in situ for 3–5 minutes. There is no need to carry out any twirling movements, particularly as at this particular site, it is liable to cause considerable pain. If the needle is left in place for a sufficient length of time, with this varying according to the needs of the individual patient, it will be found on withdrawing it, that the original exquisite tenderness has disappeared, and that weight bearing can be carried out far more comfortably. For long-term pain relief, however, it is usually necessary to repeat this procedure on several occasions. In addition, strain should be taken off the plantar fascia by the wearing of a sorbo rubber heel pad with the centre cut out.

## METATARSALGIA

Metatarsalgia, a condition characterized by the development of pain and tenderness in the region of the metatarsal heads, may be either congenital or acquired.

### Congenital metatarsalgia (Morton's syndrome)

The underlying abnormality consists of a congenitally short first metatarsal bone and a relatively long second one (Morton 1952, 1955). This makes the foot unstable with a tendency for the ankle to rock inwards on standing. It is because of this that the ankle often becomes recurrently sprained. Calluses are liable to form under the prominent second metatarsal head. Also, on examination, the second toe is seen to protrude. The diagnosis is readily confirmed by an X-ray of the foot taken with the patient standing. The structural instability of the foot, and the pain in the sole occurring as a result, causes the patient to hobble. This, in turn, puts a strain on muscles throughout the whole of the leg and because of this pain, frequently becomes widespread due to the activation of TrPs in various muscles.

The instability of the foot is liable to result in the hip being held in an adducted and internally rotated position, the knee being internally rotated, and the ankle pronated. As a consequence of this, TrPs become activated in the glutei muscles, particularly the gluteus medius (p. 304), the vastus medialis (p. 332), and the peroneus longus and brevis (Travell 1975).

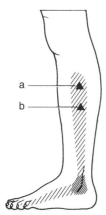

**Figure 18.14**  The pattern of pain referral from a trigger point (▲) in (a) the peroneus longus muscle (b) the peroneus brevis muscle.

TrPs in the peroneus longus are to be found on the lateral surface of the leg about a hand's breadth below the head of the fibula. TrPs in the peroneus brevis occur lower down the outside of the leg about two hand breadths above the external malleolus. Pain from TrPs in both these muscles is referred down the outer side of the leg and foot often as far as the little toe, with it being felt particularly strongly on the outer side of the ankle (Fig. 18.14).

The pain in the foot is best combated by placing a pad in the shoe under the head of the first metatarsal bone. Widespread pain throughout the leg necessitates careful examination of the muscles from the hip downwards for TrPs and any that are exquisitely tender should then be deactivated by means of inserting needles into them.

## Acquired metatarsalgia

An anatomical abnormality such as claw-toes or an equinus deformity of the foot leads to stretching of the interosseous ligament and depression of the transverse arch so that instead of, as normally, most of the weight being placed on the 1st and 5th metatarsal heads, it is transferred to the 2nd, 3rd and 4th heads causing them to become painful and tender.

Treatment is directed at elevating the arch by inserting a pad inside the shoe under the 2nd and 3rd metatarsal bones *proximal* to the heads. It should not be placed under the heads themselves as this aggravates the pain.

Another cause for pain developing in the sole of the foot is a neuroma on the digital nerve between the 3rd and 4th toes, or, occasionally, between the 2nd and 3rd ones (Morton's neuroma). This condition, for some reason, most often occurs in middle-aged women who characteristically find when affected by it that taking off their shoes and massaging the soles of their feet gives them comfort.

On examination, the pain is aggravated by pressing between the metatarsal heads rather than over them. The pain is relieved by wearing broader shoes and by elevating the transverse arch by suitably padding the inside of the shoe. It is also sometimes necessary to attempt to suppress the pain by inserting a dry needle into a point of maximum tenderness. If this fails to give relief, a hydrocortisone-local anaesthetic mixture should be injected into it. In particularly stubborn cases the neuroma may have to be excised. It also has to be remembered that metatarsalgia may also herald the onset of rheumatoid arthritis, long before the disease manifests itself by the development of a polyarthritis.

Finally, it is important to bear in mind that metatarsalgia, no matter how it is caused, may, by placing a strain on the muscles of the leg, lead to TrPs becoming activated in them, with, as a result of this, pain developing over a wide area. Such widespread pain is best brought under control by deactivating these TrPs by means of the acupuncture technique of inserting dry needles into the tissues overlying them.

## PAIN IN A TOE

Pain in a toe is clearly most often due to some obvious local pathology, but occasionally the pain persists in spite of the tissues in and around the toe having a normal appearance. In such a case it is likely that the pain is being referred to that site from a TrP some distance away.

Trauma may cause TrPs to become activated in a dorsal interosseous muscle. When this occurs, pain is referred to the side of the toe to which the muscle is attached. In relation to this it will be remembered that the 1st dorsal interosseous muscle is attached to the medial side of the 2nd toe. The 2nd, 3rd and 4th dorsal interosseous muscles are attached to the lateral side of the 2nd, 3rd and 4th toes.

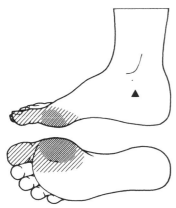

**Figure 18.15** The referral of pain to the big toe from a trigger point near to the medial malleolus.

A schoolgirl (14 years of age) complained bitterly of pain in the big toe. Her doctor was at a loss to account for this as the appearances of the toe were normal and an X-ray of the foot showed no abnormality.

When, 6 months later, she was seen by me, the only abnormality to be found was an exquisitely tender point on the inside of the foot just in front of the medial malleolus. Long-term relief from the pain was obtained by deactivating this TrP with a dry needle on two occasions. On going back over the history it seems likely that she had activated the TrP some months previously at a time when she wrenched her ankle in the gymnasium.

Pain in the big toe may be referred from a TrP high up on the outer aspect of the leg in the tibialis anterior muscle, or from a TrP in the region of the medial malleolus (Fig. 18.15).

## References

Cailliet R 1977 Soft tissue pain and disability. F A Davis, Philadelphia, p. 288–290

Dorigo B, Bartoli V, Gristillo D, Beconi D 1979 Fibrositic myofascial pain in intermittent claudication. Effect of anaesthetic block of trigger points on exercise tolerance. Pain 6: 183–190

Morton D J 1952 Human locomotion and body form. A study of gravity and man. Williams & Wilkins, Baltimore

Morton D J 1955 Foot disorders in women. Journal of the American Medical Women's Association Feb 10: 41–46

Simons D G, Travell J G 1983 Myofascial origins of low back pain. Postgraduate Medicine 73: 66–108

Simons D G, Travell J G 1984 Myofascial pain syndromes. In: Wall P D, Melzack R (eds) Textbook of Pain. Churchill Livingstone, Edinburgh, p. 271

Sola A E, Williams R L 1956 Myofascial pain syndromes. Neurology (Minneapolis) 6: 91–95

Travell J 1952 Pain mechanisms in connective tissue. In: Ragan C (ed) Connective Tissues, Transactions of the Second Conference, 1951, Josiah Macy Jnr Foundation, New York, p. 86–125

Travell J 1975 Pain and the Dudley J Morton foot (long second toe). Archives of Physical Medicine and Rehabilitation 56: 566

## INTRODUCTION

In this chapter pain in and around various joints that have not already been considered in previous chapters will be discussed. A detailed account will be given as to how acupuncture may be used to alleviate the pain of osteoarthritis, and also the pain in and around a non-arthritic joint that occurs as a result of its referral there from distant myofascial trigger points (MTrPs). Brief reference will also be made to its limited application in the treatment of rheumatoid arthritis.

## OSTEOARTHRITIS

In order to be able to give a rational explanation as to how acupuncture may be used, either alone, or in conjunction with other forms of treatment, in the alleviation of osteoarthritic pain, it is first necessary to give a short summary of present-day knowledge concerning the aetiology and pathology of the disorder. In particular it is important to consider the various mechanisms thought to be responsible for the development of its characteristic type of pain.

### Modes of presentation

The manner in which this condition presents and the course it takes are widely variable depending on whether it affects one joint alone or many, and in the case of the latter, depending on which joints in particular are involved. Its presentation and natural history are also influenced by whether it occurs as a separate entity or as part of some systemic disease.

## Joints involved

The joints most commonly affected by this disorder are the knee, hip and small joints of the hands and feet, including the carpo-metacarpal joint of the thumb, the terminal interphalangeal joints of the fingers (sometimes in association with Heberden's nodes), the proximal interphalangeal joints (sometimes in association with Bouchard's nodes), and the metatarsophalangeal joint of the big toe.

The disorder may be monarticular but it is not uncommon, particularly in women, for it to be generalized and affect the knees and small joints of the hands and feet concomitantly (Huskisson et al 1979).

Other joints that may occasionally become osteoarthritic are the shoulder and elbow. The cervical and lumbar facet joints are also usually included amongst those liable to be affected but, as already discussed in Chapters 14 and 17, degenerative changes both in these joints and the intervertebral discs in the disorder known as spondylitis only cause chronic cervical and lumbar pain to develop when they give rise to nerve root entrapment.

## Predisposing factors

It is generally agreed that genetic factors play a major role in the development of osteoarthritis (Stecher 1955, Kellgren et al 1963) but, as Harper & Nuki (1980) have pointed out, there is still much to be learnt about these.

This genetic predisposition is of particular importance because for a long time the disorder was considered to be more likely to occur in joints repeatedly subjected to trauma. It was said, for example, to be more common in miners working underground, particularly in confined spaces. Huskisson (1985), however, points out that this apparent, somewhat simplistic link between osteoarthritis and trauma is not confirmed by recent studies that show, for example, that osteoarthritis of the knee is no commoner in parachute jumpers or footballers, except in those who have had a meniscectomy, and then there would seem to be some genetically determined underlying biochemical predilection in addition to the mechanical insult to the joint.

Other predisposing factors include age, gender, obesity and race (Creamer 1999).

## Monarticular hip disease

Osteoarthritis of the hip joint sometimes occurs alone, and would then seem to be a separate entity if for no other reason than, unlike generalized osteoarthritis, it is commoner in men (Wood 1976). The clinical course is also different. Pain in generalized osteoarthritis tends to be episodic but the pain in monarticular hip disease is usually persistent with a slow or, at times, rapid increase in intensity. This is a distinction of some importance considering how essential it is to take into account the natural history of pain from any particular joint when attempting to assess the effectiveness of some treatment, such as acupuncture, in relieving it.

## Primary and secondary osteoarthritis

Osteoarthritis is traditionally divided into two groups, a primary one, and one in which it occurs secondary to some underlying disorder. This, however, is far from satisfactory because although, admittedly, examples of the latter include congenital, traumatic and inflammatory conditions acting locally and various metabolic diseases such as alkaptonuria and haemochromatosis affecting the body in general, it is often by no means clear why so-called secondary osteoarthritis should develop as a result of, for example, some relatively minor congenital disorder of a joint. The term primary is also somewhat of a misnomer. Idiopathic or cryptogenic would be far more appropriate, for there is no doubt that the more that becomes known about the condition, the smaller this group will become.

## Biochemical and mechanical factors in the aetiology of the disease

As stated earlier, the long-held concept that primary osteoarthritis is entirely mechanical in origin and due to 'wear and tear' of the cartilage is no longer tenable. It is true that a mechanical factor plays a part in its development, but there are now good reasons for believing that biochemical factors, yet to be identified, must also contribute.

## Inflammation of the synovium

In recent years it has become apparent that chronic inflammation of the synovium is an important feature in the pathology of the disease. This is a finding of considerable significance as it has led to a better understanding of the mechanisms responsible for the pain, and as a direct result of this to a more rational approach to methods of alleviating it.

The disease in fact was originally known as osteoarthritis, but in order to emphasize what was considered to be its mechanistic nature, it became fashionable, not so long ago, to call it osteoarthrosis. However, with recent recognition (Dieppe 1978) that inflammation of the synovium is an important part of the pathological process, it is clearly preferable to revert to the original terminology. The tissue first to be affected and ultimately destroyed in osteoarthritis is cartilage, and fragments of this floating in the joint space are known to cause an inflammatory reaction in the synovium (George & Chrisman 1968). In addition, various chemical substances, such as pyrophosphates (McCarty 1976) and hydroxyapatite (Dieppe et al 1976, Schumacher et al 1977), found on occasions in crystal form in osteoarthritic joints, may also contribute to this inflammatory response in some patients.

The realization that an inflammation of the synovium similar to that seen in rheumatoid arthritis occurs in osteoarthritis has come from observations made both by clinicians and pathologists.

Clinically, it has now become widely recognized that an osteoarthritic joint may not only be painful but may also show evidence of warmth, swelling, redness, and stiffness on waking and after prolonged sitting. These are, as Ehrlich (1975) has pointed out, all classical symptoms and signs of inflammation. It is interesting to note with respect to this that Huskisson et al (1979), in comparing and contrasting the clinical features of 100 consecutive cases of rheumatoid arthritis and 100 consecutive cases of osteoarthritis, frequently found evidence of inflammation in those with osteoarthritis. Such evidence included morning stiffness, redness of distal interphalangeal joints, warmth, and effusion in the knees. And as they said:

> ... the absence of morning stiffness has often been suggested as a helpful diagnostic feature of osteoarthritis, but it was noted by almost as

many of our patients with osteoarthritis as those with rheumatoid arthritis. Synovial fluid also provided evidence for a low-grade inflammation with greater than normal number of cells.

Evidence for an inflammatory reaction being present has also been obtained by thermography confirming that osteoarthritic joints are warm (Collins et al 1976), although not to the same degree as in rheumatoid arthritis, thus confirming the clinical impression that the reaction is less severe.

Pathological evidence of an inflammatory reaction in the synovium includes Cooper et al's (1981) finding of this to be present in synovial tissue taken from patients with osteoarthritis as commonly as in tissue taken from patients with rheumatoid arthritis. Schumacher et al (1981) observed synovial inflammation to be present in a large proportion of osteoarthritic knees examined at autopsy, and Goldenberg et al (1982) noted its presence in the majority of synovial specimens taken from osteoarthritic patients during the course of surgical operations.

Much space has been devoted to discussing this inflammatory change, because, as Fassbender (1975) has said, and as will be seen from the following discussion, it is in general only when synovitis occurs in an osteoarthritic joint that it becomes painful.

## Pathological changes in an osteoarthritic joint, and the relationship of these to the production of pain

As has already been stated, the primary change in osteoarthritis is the destruction of the articular cartilage, and with the narrowing of the joint space that occurs as a result of this, changes take place fairly quickly in the underlying bone (Radin et al 1976). These include microfractures, sclerosis, and remodelling of the bone with the formation of osteophytes and the development of cysts.

When attempting to understand how pain may arise in an osteoarthritic joint, it is important to appreciate that there are no receptor nerve endings in the articular cartilage, synovium, or the menisci (Wyke 1981). Pain therefore cannot arise directly from the cartilage itself.

Subchondral bone, however, is well supplied with nerves and therefore it would not be unreasonable to assume that the various changes just described that take place in it and that start to develop at an early stage in the disease, are likely to generate pain. It is therefore somewhat surprising to find that there is no good evidence for this. For example, Lawrence et al (1966), in studying the relationship between symptoms and X-ray changes in an extensive population survey, found that bone cysts in the metacarpophalangeal joints and hip joints were seen no more frequently in those with pain than in those without pain. And Danielsson's (1964) 10 years' prospective study of patients with osteophytes in the region of the hip showed that they contributed little to the evolution of the osteoarthritic process or to the development of pain.

This therefore explains the seeming paradox that it is possible to have extensive osteoarthritic changes in a joint, including a well-marked loss of joint space, sclerosis, cysts and osteophytes demonstrable radiographically, and yet for the joint not to be painful. And, as a corollary to this, it can never be assumed just because an X-ray shows changes of the disease in a joint that any pain from which a person may be suffering necessarily comes from this source. It is only possible to make a decision about this following a careful clinical examination.

Although it is true that at rest pain in the knee or hip may occur as a result of intramedullary venous stasis and hypertension both in patients with osteoarthritis of these joints and in those without (Arnoldi et al 1980), most of the various forms of pain that often occur episodically in osteoarthritis, including the morning stiffness and the aching type of discomfort that initially comes on with movements but subsequently occurs at rest and also at night, would seem to develop only if and when there is inflammation of the synovium.

The synovium itself, as stated earlier, is devoid of nociceptive receptors but when it becomes inflamed, and because of the effect this has on other tissues, pain occurs as a result of stimulation of nerve endings in the synovial blood vessels, the joint capsule, the fat pads, the collateral ligaments, and the adjacent muscles. There are various ways in which this occurs.

Firstly, there are nociceptive receptors in the adventitial sheaths of the vessels in the wall of the synovial sac, and when the latter becomes inflamed, stretching of these receptors leads to the production of pain.

Secondly, pain occurs because chemical substances such as 5-hydroxytryptamine, prostaglandins, histamine, and polypeptide kinins released from inflamed synovial cells get carried in the synovial fluid to the adjacent articular fat pads and joint capsule, where they have an irritant effect on the nociceptive receptors in these structures.

Thirdly, the fibrosis that ultimately develops in the capsule, and even at times in the adjacent muscles, in cases in which the inflammatory process becomes chronic, causes the tissues to contract, and this again leads to stimulation of their sensory receptors, particularly with movements of the joint.

Fourthly, pain develops because the changes that take place in an osteoarthritic joint lead to strain developing in various periarticular structures including the adjacent collateral ligaments, the muscle tendons, particularly at their sites of attachment to bone, the muscles around the joint, and in cases where a faulty posture develops, in muscles some distance from it. As a result exquisitely tender 'spots' (points of maximum tenderness) develop in periarticular structures. The exquisite tenderness of these points is due to them being sites where nociceptive nerve endings are in an activated and sensitized state, and it is because of this that they are particularly important sources of osteoarthritic pain so that, as will later be discussed, treatment directed at conteracting this increased nociceptive activity by means of the carrying out of superficial dry needling is often all that is necessary to abolish the arthralgia. These points of maximum tenderness when present in muscles and ligaments in the vicinity of the joint have the characteristics of TrPs, with pressure applied to them causing pain to be referred to the joint region. Others, however, such as those to be found in the tissues around arthritic small joints of the hand and in articular fat pads of knees have the characteristics of tender points, with pressure applied to them causing pain to be felt locally at these sites.

## Pain and its correlation with X-ray changes

It can therefore be seen from what has just been said that the reason for pain developing in an osteoarthritic joint is not because of cartilage damage, or of structural alterations in the subchondrial bone's architecture, but mainly because of changes in the soft tissues of the joint and periarticular structures causing nociceptive nerve ending activity to develop at trigger and tender point sites. As previously mentioned, this explains why pain in osteoarthritis does not necessarily correlate with the extent of the radiological changes. The one exception to this is osteoarthritis of the hip where generally the pain is proportional to the extent of the joint damage seen on a radiograph (Kellgren 1961).

## Management of osteoarthritis

As there is, as yet, no means of arresting osteoarthritis, its management in the main is directed towards the symptomatic relief of pain up to the time when replacement of the joint proves to be necessary.

It is my belief that a TrP approach to acupuncture has an important place in this but it should not be looked upon as a technique necessarily to be used on its own but rather one that at times should be used in conjunction with other forms of therapy. It is therefore necessary to say something about the advantages and disadvantages of these in order that their place relative to that of acupuncture can be seen in a proper perspective.

### Dieting

Many studies have shown a relationship between obesity and osteoarthritis, particularly when this affects the knee joint in women (Felson et al 1988, Schouten et al 1992).

Martin et al (1996), in a study of post-menopausal obese women with knee osteoarthritis have shown that dieting and exercise carried out over a 6-month period led to the alleviation of the pain and improved function.

### Analgesics

Simple analgesics may be helpful, but the discovery that the occurrence of pain in this disorder is closely associated with the development of an inflammatory process has led to an increased use of nonsteroidal anti-inflammatory drugs (NSAIDs).

When considering the use of an analgesic or a NSAID, it is as well to remember that aspirin has the properties of both.

**Non-steroidal anti-inflammatory drugs**    It has to be kept in mind when contemplating the use of NSAIDs in osteoarthritis that most of the patients suffering from this are elderly, and that because of this their metabolism and excretion of drugs are often impaired. Moreover, because those in later life frequently need a variety of drugs for many different complaints, there is always the risk of drugs interacting. NSAIDs, for example, often increase the effects of anticoagulants, and decrease those of diuretics.

NSAIDs, too, by inhibiting the synthesis of prostaglandins, are liable to aggravate late-onset asthma, and in conditions such as the nephrotic syndrome, hepatocellular failure, and cardiac failure, in which glomerular filtration is prostaglandin-dependent, their use is liable to precipitate uraemia and increase oedema. Also, because of their effect on prostaglandins they are liable to cause gastrointestinal bleeding, either from an erosive gastritis or peptic ulcer, which is a particularly serious event in an elderly arteriosclerotic person.

Although it is generally agreed that all NSAIDs have potentially dangerous side effects, their advantages must be weighed against their disadvantages, and there is no doubt that when used judiciously this group of drugs often gives dramatic relief.

It is important to bear in mind that they should never be prescribed on a long-term basis, but always intermittently and even then in the lowest possible dosage. Also, there are times when the presence of other conditions or individual intolerance precludes their use, and since adverse reports concerning them have reached the popular press, an increasing number of the public are refusing to take them. Furthermore, as Creamer (1999) has said 'evidence for the superiority of NSAIDS over paracetamol is largely lacking and, at least under trial conditions, many patients on chronic NSAID therapy for knee osteoarthritis can cease medication without apparent deterioration in symptoms'.

### Physiotherapy

Controlled trials of different forms of physiotherapy including immersing the hands in warm wax, short-wave diathermy, infra-red irradiation, and faradism show that all of them give a certain amount of temporary relief, but none are of any lasting value (Hamilton et al 1959). There are certain physical measures, however, that are of considerable help. For those with osteoarthritis of the hip or knee, it is useful to carry a walking stick held in the contralateral hand. Warm baths and swimming are of benefit for those with hip disease. It has also been shown (Fisher et al 1993) that quadriceps strengthening exercises reduce pain and improve function in patients with knee osteoarthritis.

### Intra-articular injections of corticosteroids

As the pain in osteoarthritis would seem to be directly related to the development of an inflammatory reaction in the synovium it might be thought that it would be helpful to inject a corticosteroid into the joint. In general, however, the results have been disappointing. Miller et al (1958) and Wright et al (1960) showed that such injections give no better results than can be obtained from injections of a placebo. Admittedly, Dieppe et al (1980), using a long-acting preparation, triamcinolone hexacetonide, found that the relief from pain with this was greater than with a placebo, but even so the benefit was so slight and short lasting as to lead them to conclude that this form of treatment could not be recommended for use in everyday clinical practice.

This notwithstanding, controlled trials of the use of intra-articular steroids in the treatment of knee osteoarthritis provide some evidence of their efficacy, but only for up to 4 weeks (Creamer 1997).

### Aspiration of a synovial effusion

The effusion developing as a result of synovitis is sometimes so large that the volume of fluid itself causes pain. In such a case simply aspirating it often affords considerable relief.

### Treatment directed at periarticular points of maximum tenderness

There is no doubt that when attempting to alleviate osteoarthritic pain by some method applied locally to the joint, by far the best is to employ some technique directed specifically at the TrPs and tender points that, as stated earlier, are to be found in various structures in and around the joint. There are essentially three ways of doing this: either

to inject hydrocortisone or a local anaesthetic into them as advocated by Dixon (1965) for the relief of osteoarthritic knee joint pain, or to deactivate them by means of the acupuncture technique of stimulating A-delta nerve fibres in the overlying tissues with dry needles.

When deciding which of these methods to adopt, it has to be remembered that a local anaesthetic, when injected into either a TrP or a tender point, does not depend for its pain-suppressing effect on its ability to anaesthetize nerve endings. In the same way a corticosteroid does not achieve this effect solely because of its local anti-inflammatory action. What these methods have in common, as with the injection of many other substances, including saline, is that of having a non-specific irritant effect on A-delta nerve fibres that in turn activates centrally placed pain-modulating mechanisms, in exactly the same manner as the carrying out of superficial dry needling at such points achieves this. Furthermore, there is reason to believe that this latter form of treatment increases plasma cortisol levels. Roth et al (1997), in experiments on 20 healthy male students, showed that manual stimulation of acupuncture points brings about a significant increase in cortisol levels 5, 25 and 45 min after cessation of the stimulation. It is findings such as this that may explain, as Pomeranz (2001) has said, why acupuncture is helpful in suppressing the inflammation of arthritis.

The clinical observation that not infrequently following manual acupuncture for the relief of pain in an osteoarthritic small joint of the hand there is a significant decrease in the periarticular soft-tissue swelling may presumably be because of this. The following case is a particularly striking example:

A housewife (62 years of age) was referred to me with a 6-month history of severe pain from an osteoarthritic first carpometacarpal joint. On examination, the tissues around the joint were noted to be considerably swollen. Nevertheless, within 3 days of deactivating TrPs with dry needles for the first time, the swelling totally disappeared, and after a further three treatment sessions there was long-term relief from pain.

## PAIN FROM A SPRAINED JOINT

When a joint becomes sprained much of the pain is likely to arise as a result of TrPs in the soft tissues around it becoming activated and may, consequently, be alleviated by the carrying out of superficial dry needling at these points.

## KNEE JOINT

### Pain in and around a normal knee joint

Pain in and around a normal knee joint may be referred there from an arthritic hip joint. Also from TrPs in one or more muscles some distance from the joint. These include (Baldry 2001) the anteriorly situated adductor longus, rectus femoris, vastus medialis, vastus lateralis and the posteriorly situated semimembranosus, semitendinosus, biceps femoris and popliteus.

### Osteoarthritis of the knee joint

Osteoarthritis commonly involves the knee joint and when it does so it affects either the patellofemoral compartment, or the medial or lateral tibiofemoral compartments, or any combination of these.

#### Patellofemoral compartment

Involvement of the patellofemoral compartment is occasionally the predominant feature and has to be distinguished from chondromalacia patellae, a disorder of adolescents and young adults. This particular disorder often starts between the ages of 15 and 30 years, and usually begins on the medial aspect of the patella. The reason for this, as Wiberg (1941) has shown, is that whereas contact between the lateral facet of the patella and the femur is good at all stages of flexion, contact between the medial facet and its corresponding condyle on the femur is poor at about 90° of flexion with, as a consequence of this, undue wear of the cartilage taking place at this site. The condition, somewhat surprisingly, sometimes gradually remits, but at other times slowly progresses over the years and becomes indistinguishable from osteoarthritis.

The symptoms of the condition are pain behind the patella on walking and, in particular, on descending stairs. On examination of the joint, there is patella crepitation. A good diagnostic test is

the eliciting of pain by getting the patient to contract the quadriceps whilst the patella is held firmly against the femoral condyles. Also, in favour of the diagnosis is the eliciting of pain by sliding the patella to one side or the other, with the leg extended. On palpation of the soft tissues TrPs are to be found along the sides of the patella. The commonest site for these is its upper lateral edge (Dixon 1965).

The pain in this condition, which typically is intermittent in nature, is readily alleviated by deactivating these TrPs by means of inserting dry needles into the tissues overlying them. It is a procedure, however, because of the nature of the disease, that usually has to be repeated from time to time. Occasionally the pain is so persistent as to necessitate some form of surgery being carried out.

#### Tibiofemoral compartments

With osteoarthritis of the tibiofemoral compartments, changes usually occur in both the medial and lateral ones but they are commonly most marked on the medial side.

Pain arises as a result of TrP activity developing in the collateral ligaments, in tendons adjacent to them, in the articular fat pads, and in muscles near to and, at times, some distance from the joint. Also, in muscles in and around the popliteal fossa.

**TrPs in the collateral ligaments**    TrPs are usually to be found in these ligaments at their upper and lower attachments (Fig. 19.1). One of the commonest sites is the anteromedial aspect of the upper part of the tibia in the area somewhat fancifully known as the pes anserinus or goose's foot (Fig. 18.7). The pes anserinus is where the lower part of the medial collateral ligament, and superficial to this, the tendons of the sartorius, gracilis, and semitendinosus muscles become attached to the tibia. A bursa is present between the ligament and tendons.

Careful inspection will often reveal several TrPs in this area, and for the best results, it is necessary to deactivate each one of them with a dry needle. It is interesting to note, however, that in the traditional Chinese system, there is only one acupuncture point in this area – the so-called Spleen 9 (Fig. 16.3).

**Tender points in the medial and lateral articular fat pads**    The fat pads are extrasynovial, but

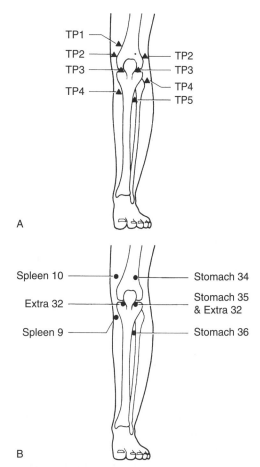

**Figure 19.1A and B** (A) Trigger points (▲) on the anterior aspect of the knee. (1) in the vastus medialis muscle. (2) & (4) at the upper and lower insertions of the collateral ligaments. (3) in fat pads (Both these trigger points corresponding in position with traditional Chinese acupuncture points Extra 32 and, on the lateral side also with Stomach 35). (5) Trigger point corresponding in position with traditional Chinese acupuncture point Stomach 36. (B) Traditional Chinese acupuncture points (•).

occasions without pain developing, they are the cause of the knee suddenly buckling. As Travell (1951) has pointed out, this structure is the main muscular support of the knee and when, as sometimes happens, TrP activity in it occurs in isolation, the contraction of the muscle is in some way inhibited before pain develops, with, in consequence, the knee suddenly giving way without warning, and causing what is tantamount to a 'drop' attack.

**TrPs in the iliotibial tract** The strain imposed on the lower limb by an osteoarthritic knee joint sometimes leads to TrPs developing along the outer side of the thigh in the iliotibial tract, and below the knee between the tibia and fibula, with one often coinciding in position with the well-known Chinese acupuncture point, Stomach 36 (Fig. 19.1).

**TrPs in the popliteal fossa** The main sites where TrPs are sometimes to be found in the popliteal fossa are in the midline and along its outer borders (Fig. 19.2). The point, at the centre of the fossa in the midline, situated in the popliteus muscle, corresponds in position with the traditional Chinese acupuncture point, Urinary Bladder 40. On the outer side points may be found, above, in the biceps femoris, and below, in the lateral head of the gastrocnemius. And, on the inner side, points may be found, above, in the vicinity of the semimembranosus and semitendinosus tendons, and below, in the medial head of the gastrocnemius. It is interesting to note that there are two Chinese acupuncture points on the outer sides of the popliteal fossa namely, Urinary Bladder 39 on the lateral side, and Kidney 10 on the medial side (Fig. 19.2).

*Factors influencing response to treatment*

Whilst bearing in mind that osteoarthritic pain in the knee, certainly in the earlier stages of the disease, tends to be episodic with natural remissions, it would seem that with treatment directed at TrPs in and around the joint, it is possible to obtain, often in a quite dramatic manner, long-lasting relief from pain of many months' duration.

Factors, however, that may influence the response include joint instability, obesity and unequal leg length.

intracapsular, and change their shape with every movement of the knee. Tender points in these structures are to be found on either side of the quadriceps tendon. The medial fat pad is the one most commonly affected (Fig. 19.1).

**TrPs in the vastus medialis muscle** TrPs are often found in the vastus medialis muscle just above the knee (Fig. 19.1). In conjunction with TrPs at other sites they may be a source of pain, but on

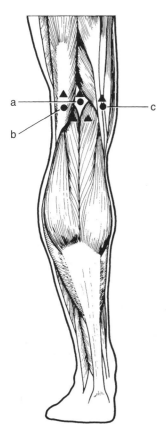

**Figure 19.2**   Trigger points (▲) and traditional Chinese acupuncture points (•) in the region of the popliteal fossa. The central trigger point corresponds in position with the traditional Chinese acupuncture point Urinary Bladder 40(a). Acupuncture points b & c are Urinary Bladder 39 and Kidney 10 respectively.

### Joint instability

Progressive degenerative changes in the cartilage and subchondrial bone may ultimately lead to development of considerable joint instability. When this occurs, the strain imposed upon the surrounding ligaments and muscles causes TrPs in these structures to remain in a state of persistent activity. It is because of this that any relief from pain obtained by deactivating these TrPs with dry needles tends to be only short lived. However, in spite of this, it is often possible by repeating treatment at frequent intervals to considerably improve the quality of a person's life.

A housewife (62 years of age) was referred to me for acupuncture with a 5-year history of severe pain in the right knee, which for the past year had become so bad that she could do nothing more than hobble around the house with the aid of a stick.

On examination there was evidence of marked joint instability; also, the scar of a patellectomy carried out for osteoarthritis of the patellofemoral compartment. The current X-ray showed extensive changes of this disease, affecting particularly the medial tibiofemoral compartment.

Exquisitely tender TrPs were found in and around the medial collateral ligament, with deactivation of these by dry needle stimulation giving immediate relief from pain. But, in spite of repeating this procedure on several occasions, the relief never lasted for more than 2–3 weeks. The patient would not contemplate undergoing any further surgery. However, by repeating acupuncture every 3 weeks for over 4 years now, the pain has been kept under such good control as to allow her to lead a reasonably active life, including doing her own shopping and gardening. The object lesson here is that with acupuncture, provided a patient has sufficient tenacity of purpose to persevere with treatment, it is often possible to obtain long-term benefit from the cumulative effects of short-term pain relief.

### Obesity

It is not uncommon for a person suffering from obesity to develop osteoarthritis of the knee joint. The relationship between the two, however, is far from clear. The rarity of the disease developing in the ankle joint, except when it has been subjected to some form of trauma, shows that excessive weight bearing is not an important aetiological factor. There is no doubt, however, that obesity aggravates the condition and this is probably because of the fact that it impedes the body's normal movements. Dixon (1965) considers the 'Fat lady's knee' to be a distinct clinical syndrome that includes medial ligament strain, excessive tenderness over the medial ligament, and tender hypertrophy of fat pads medial and posterior to the knee. In his series of cases with this syndrome, infiltration of the medial ligament and tender fat pads with a local anaesthetic produced no lasting benefit.

He found that the pain was relieved in the minority who could be persuaded to lose weight, but concluded that the full syndrome of 'Fat lady's knee' is hard to help. This has not always been my experience when treating osteoarthritis of the knee in obese women with acupuncture, although for any lasting benefit to be obtained this has to be repeated several times. Unfortunately, Dixon does not state how often injections of a local anaesthetic were given. If only once, as the report seems to imply, then it is no wonder that the results were disappointing. Many fat middle-aged females that have been under my care with this condition have obtained relatively long remissions from pain that has been present for several months or years after deactivating TrPs by means of the carrying out of superficial dry needling firstly weekly and then, if necessary, depending on each patient's individual responsiveness, at gradually increasing intervals. The following case is one of the more impressive examples:

A 22 stone (139.7 kg) lady hobbled into my consulting room on a stick having persuaded her general practitioner to let her try acupuncture for severe pain of 8 years' duration in osteoarthritic knees. He told her that in view of her considerable obesity she was wasting her time. This was an opinion that, at that time, was shared by me, especially as on examination there was considerable swelling of the joints with a well-marked genu varus deformity. However, not to disappoint her, needles were inserted into the tissues overlying TrPs in the medial ligament and the vastus medialis muscle. After two treatments the pain was sufficiently alleviated as to allow her to give up using a stick, and after two more treatments, i.e. 1 month from starting treatment, she became virtually free from pain. In addition, in spite of only managing to lose about 2 stone, she remained like this for 12 months. At that stage further treatment had to be given, but once again her response was similarly gratifying.

## Short leg syndrome

It is important in examining the knee joint to take account of the length of the two legs (see Ch. 17), as when there is real or apparent shortening of one leg, the knee on the *contralateral* side is liable to become osteoarthritic. This occurs because the compensatory position of flexion and external rotation in which the 'longer' leg is held on walking, causes abnormal stretching of the medial ligament, and the excessive lateral mobility of the knee joint occurring as a result of this, leads to the development of destructive changes in the joint and particularly its lateral femoropatellar compartment.

Any relief from pain obtained by deactivating TrPs that develop in the soft tissues is liable to be short lived unless the shortness of the contralateral leg is corrected by the wearing of a raised shoe.

## Pain referred to the knee from some distant site

As Kellgren pointed out over 40 years ago (Ch. 4), pain in the region of the knee may occur as a result of being referred there either from the hip joint, or from tissues around the lumbar spine, or from the muscles of the thigh. Any examination of a painful knee should, therefore, always include an examination for TrPs in muscles or tendons at these sites. Radiographic evidence of arthritis in the knee joint is no reason for omitting this search because, as already stated, no matter how extensive the cartilage and bone changes from this may be, they are not in themselves a cause of pain.

A schoolmistress (56 years of age) was sent to me with a 5-month history of severe pain in the knees, due, according to the referral letter, to radiographically confirmed osteoarthritis in these joints.

On examination, the contours and movements of the joints were normal and, most important of all, there were no TrPs in the soft tissues around them. There were, however, exquisitely tender ones in the region of both sacroiliac joints, also down the outer sides of the legs in the upper parts of the iliotibial tracts, and in muscles in the upper inner parts of the thighs.

In order to alleviate the knee pain, it was necessary to deactivate all of these TrPs by inserting dry needles into the tissues overlying them and, in order to obtain lasting benefit, to repeat this procedure on five occasions at weekly intervals.

## Persistent pain from a 'strained' non-osteoarthritic knee

The activation of TrPs in the soft tissues around the knee joint, in exactly the same sites as in osteoarthritis, may occur as a result of trauma. As anywhere else in the body, failure to recognize their presence and to deal with them appropriately may lead to many months of unnecessary disability.

A builder's labourer (43 years of age) fell off some scaffolding, and shortly after this the left knee became swollen and painful. The swelling quickly subsided but the pain persisted and 3 months after the accident, he was seen by an orthopaedic surgeon. He detected no abnormality either on clinical examination or on arthroscopy, and, more to placate the patient than for any other reason, arranged for him to have a course of physiotherapy. When, after a further 2 months, the pain was no better, the surgeon concluded that there could be no organic cause for it.

After the patient had been off work for 9 months, and in imminent danger of losing his job, his doctor referred him to me for assessment as to whether acupuncture might be of help.

The patient, a sensible, placid and, quite obviously, normally a very hard working type of person, told me that he was in a state of despair because, although he had full movements of the knee, it ached persistently and this was so bad at nights as to prevent him from getting any sleep.

On examination, there were two exquisitely tender TrPs immediately adjacent to the upper medial and lateral edges of the patella, and another one on the medial aspect of the tibia just below the knee. After deactivating these TrPs with dry needles on only two occasions, he lost his pain and within a very short time was able to get back to work.

## Hip osteoarthritis

Osteoarthritis of the hip may develop in adults under the age of 40 years, if the joint has been damaged by some inflammatory arthritis, or subjected to strain from some congenital or acquired deformity. Far more commonly, however, it affects people from middle age onwards.

The pain in osteoarthritis of this joint takes the form of a severe dull ache that, over the course of time, gets progressively worse. It is, therefore, unlike the episodic type of pain that so commonly occurs when other joints are affected by this disorder. It is felt especially in the groin, the inguinal region, over the greater trochanter, and outer side of the buttock.

The pain may also be referred to the knee joint due to both this and the hip joint being innervated by the obturator nerve. The strain imposed on the muscles of the back may cause pain to develop in the lumbar region and it may also radiate down the thigh, particularly on the outer side.

The pain, which initially is aggravated by walking and relieved by resting, is at a later stage present the whole time. On clinical examination, there is pain on movement of the joint, and limitation of its movements with those particularly affected being internal rotation and extension. Atrophy of the gluteal and quadriceps muscles may be observed. On palpation periarticular TrPs are found to be present.

The pain, which in the case of this particular hip joint, is in direct proportion to the extent of joint damage seen on a radiograph (De Ceulaer & Watson Buchanan 1979) would seem to be due to several different causes.

As stated previously, the cartilage does not have a nerve supply and, surprisingly, neither osteophytes (Danielsson 1964) nor bone cysts (Lawrence et al 1966) in themselves would seem to give rise to pain. However, large cysts in the femoral head may cause the latter to collapse with the production of sudden intense pain.

Pain in the hip, as in the knee, both when osteoarthritis is present and when it is not, is occasionally due to intraosseous venous stasis and intraosseous hypertension – the so-called 'intraosseous engorgement pain syndrome' (Lemperg & Arnoldi 1978). This pain, which is worse towards the end of the day's activities, and persists at rest, may be alleviated by lowering the intraosseous pressure by some surgical procedure such as an osteotomy (Arnoldi et al 1971).

The pain that acupuncture is able to influence is that which develops as a result of TrPs that have become activated in the periarticular tissues for the same reasons as those that appear in osteoarthritis of the knee joint.

### Examination for TrPs

No examination to establish the cause of pain in and around the hip joint is complete without a systematic search for TrPs. There are three main sites where these are usually to be found, irrespective of whether the pain is due to osteoarthritis of the hip or is primarily muscular in origin. In distinguishing between these two causes of pain in the region it should be remembered that with osteoarthritis there is often considerable limitation of movements of the joint and usually, but not always, by the time that pain from this condition develops there are characteristic abnormalities to be seen on a radiograph. There are occasions, however, in the early stages of the disease when the pain of a restrictive capsulitis develops before X-ray changes become apparent.

### Location of TrPs in arthritis of the hip joint and non-arthritic painful disorders around it

TrPs are mainly to be found at one or more of the following three sites: the groin, the upper part of the thigh close to where the femoral artery passes behind the inguinal ligament, and in the vicinity of the greater trochanter.

TrPs in the groin usually develop in the adductor longus muscle near to its insertion into the pubic bone (Travell 1950) (Fig. 18.1).

In addition, there is sometimes a TrP to be found immediately below the inguinal ligament, anterior to the capsule of the joint, in the iliopsoas muscle (Fig. 17.15).

TrPs also frequently occur in muscles in the region of the greater trochanter, and in particular in the gluteus medius and minimus close to where these muscles become attached to it. In order not to overlook any of the TrPs in this region it is necessary to palpate the tissues overlying and adjacent to the greater trochanter in a systematic manner, with special attention being paid to the gluteal muscles as they converge towards it from behind, to the various muscles immediately overlying it, and as Sola & Williams (1956) pointed out, to that part of the tensor fasciae latae situated immediately below it (Fig. 19.3).

It should be noted that a TrP in the gluteus medius or minimus close to the greater trochanter may not only give rise to pain in the hip region but may also cause it to be referred down the outer side of the thigh and leg (Fig. 17.13). Also, a TrP immediately below the iliac crest in one or other of these muscles may not only give rise to pain in the hip region, but also cause it to be referred down the back of the thigh and leg (Fig. 17.14).

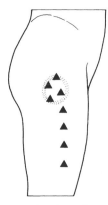

**Figure 19.3**  Trigger points in and around the greater trochanter and along the tensor fasciae latae.

### Deactivation of TrPs

Superficial dry needling carried out at TrP sites in mild-to-moderate osteoarthritis of the hip gives a certain amount of relief from pain but the effect is never as dramatic or as long lasting as it is with osteoarthritis of the knee. There is therefore much to be said for combining the effects of acupuncture and drug therapy including the use of either a NSAIDs, or a simple analgesic, or both.

Treatment to relieve the pain of an osteoarthritic hip usually has to be given over a long period of time and, therefore, one of the great advantages of using both acupuncture and a drug together is that the pain-relieving effect of the former makes it possible to keep the dose of the latter to a minimum, and thereby helps to reduce the risks of any potential side effects from it.

### Non-osteoarthritic hip pain

Dry needling carried out at TrP sites when pain around the hip is primarily of muscular origin is on the other hand very rewarding and often, in my experience, it is possible to bring even quite long-standing pain fairly rapidly under control.

A racehorse breeder (51 years of age) was referred to me by a gastroenterologist because of long-standing epigastric pain emanating from a MTrP just below the xiphisternum (see Ch. 20). The patient, finding that this was quite quickly relieved by acupuncture, then enquired whether similar treatment might help alleviate persistent pain in his right hip! It transpired that 18 years previously he had had a car accident, since when he had had considerable pain in the right groin and hip region causing him to have a pronounced limp.

After having had this limp for about 10 years it got so bad that he was referred to an orthopaedic specialist who encased the lower back and hip in plaster. Apart from making his back muscles weak, this had had no effect, and he was told that, although the X-ray, as yet, showed only a slight abnormality, he would eventually require an operation on his hip, but that, in the meantime, he should keep the pain under control with analgesics.

On examination, there were good movements of the hip joint and the only abnormal finding was the discovery of two TrPs in the adductor longus muscle: one just below the inguinal ligament and the other at the insertion of the tendon into the pubic bone. Quite remarkably, after deactivating these TrPs with dry needles on only two occasions, the pain of 18-years' standing disappeared, and when seen 2 years later it had not recurred.

This is yet another striking example of how TrP activation as a result of trauma may at times cause pain to persist virtually indefinitely, but provided the tissues are otherwise healthy, deactivation of the TrPs, no matter how long this is delayed, quickly alleviates the pain.

### Periosteal pecking

It should be noted that for pain in the hip region Mann (1974) advocates pecking the periosteum of the greater trochanter with a dry needle, and for pain in the knee region, pecking the upper medial aspect of the tibia. Stimulating periosteal nerve endings in this manner is undoubtedly a powerful form of acupuncture, but a somewhat painful one, and in order to assess whether the results obtained by it are any better than those achieved by systematic deactivation of MTrPs around the knee and hip as just described, it would be necessary to carry out a carefully conducted statistically controlled clinical trial.

## Pain in and around the small joints of the hands

The pain from generalized osteoarthritis of the small joints of the hands is usually best controlled by the use of a NSAID, but occasionally one finger joint in particular is especially painful, and in such a case it is helpful to palpate around the joint in order to locate tender points and then to carry out superficial dry needling at these sites. Pain in the first carpometacarpal joint of the thumb is usually more troublesome than in the finger joints presumably because of the important part played by the thumb in grasping objects. For this reason deactivation of tender points around this joint and of TrPs in nearby muscles when it is affected by osteoarthritis is only helpful in the earlier stages of the disease. It is, however, extremely effective in alleviating pain that sometimes persists following a sprain of the joint. Case histories illustrating this have already been given in Chapter 15.

## Pain in the wrist

When a wrist is sprained, TrPs become activated in the periarticular tissues, and the deactivation of these by means of the carrying out of superficial dry needling is very helpful in relieving the pain associated with this condition.

## Pain in the elbow

Osteoarthritis of this joint is rare unless the joint has previously been damaged by trauma or inflammation. However, when, occasionally, it does occur, the acupuncture technique of deactivating TrPs in the periarticular tissue overlying the medial and lateral epicondyles, and in the cubital fossa, is certainly helpful in relieving the pain. Much more commonly, persistent pain develops in the region of the elbow joint due to TrP activation occurring as a result of trauma to the soft tissues. 'Tennis' elbow and 'golf' elbow with pain localized to one or other sides of the joint have already been discussed (Ch. 15). At times, however, this post-traumatic pain around the elbow is more generalized and the movements of the elbow joint, because of this, become restricted.

A man (40 years of age) was ostensibly referred to me because of persistent pain in the neck of 6 months duration. During the course of examination, however, it was noted that the left elbow was supported in a specially constructed leather splint. On enquiring about this it transpired that he had been fitted with this 10 years previously because of persistent pain in the region of the elbow joint following an injury sustained whilst serving in the S.A.S. He said he religiously wore the splint as advised, but it had done little to control the pain and he had learnt to live with it believing that nothing further could be done. All the splint seemed to have done was to make the elbow extremely stiff. An X-ray showed no significant abnormality in the joint itself. However, examination of the surrounding muscles showed there were some exquisitely tender TrPs that clearly had originally been overlooked, and after these had been deactivated with dry needles on four occasions at weekly intervals, the pain was brought under control and full movements of the joint restored.

## Pain in the feet

The only joint in the foot commonly affected by osteoarthritis is the metatarsophalangeal joint of the big toe, and when this occurs as part of the generalized form of the disease is usually mild and rarely requires any special form of treatment.

## Pain in the ankle

It is remarkable that considering that this joint has to bear all the weight of the body that it is rarely affected by osteoarthritis, even when subjected to repeated trauma as, for example, with footballers. When, occasionally, there is persistent pain from osteoarthritis of this joint, activated TrPs are to be found clustered around the malleoli and on the dorsum of the foot midway between these two structures. Deactivation of these by dry needle stimulation, provided this is repeated on several occasions at weekly intervals, will often cause the pain to remit for an appreciable period of time.

TrPs at these sites also become activated when the joint is sprained (Travell & Rinzler 1952, Bonica 1953). As Bonica points out, rather than immobilizing the joint as is standard practice, it is better to get rid of the pain by deactivating the TrPs, and then encourage active movements. He advocated injecting the TrPs with a local anaesthetic, but deactivating them with a dry needle is simpler and just as effective.

## CLINICAL TRIALS TO ASSESS THE VALUE OF ACUPUNCTURE IN RELIEVING OSTEOARTHRITIC PAIN

It is impossible to assess adequately the value of acupuncture in a disorder such as osteoarthritis in which, somewhat paradoxically, progressive and irreversible damage to a joint is often associated with self-limiting episodes of pain, without recourse to carefully conducted large scale clinical trials. Unfortunately, up to now there has been a dearth of these.

The difficulties associated with the carrying out of acupuncture trials in general, and in particular, the problems posed in attempting to compare its effectiveness with that of a placebo were discussed in Chapter 11. It is, however, essential to realize that such difficulties are particulary great when comparing the effectiveness of acupuncture or, for that matter, any other form of treatment with that of a placebo, in alleviating the pain of osteoarthritis, due to the placebo treatment response in this condition often being much in excess of the normally attained 30% level. Traut & Passarelli (1956), for example, found that 59% of 182 patients with osteoarthritic pain obtained relief from this when given lactose tablets!

It is, therefore, not possible to dissent from Evans's (1974) opinion that in order to ascertain whether any form of treatment gives better results than a placebo in the alleviation of osteoarthritic pain, carefully conducted comparative trials are mandatory. This having been said, it is of course essential when carrying out such trials to ensure that the procedure used in the control group is a true placebo!

With respect to this it would, for example, appear to have been unwise for Gaw et al (1975), in their otherwise carefully conducted trial, to assess the efficacy of traditional Chinese acupuncture (TCA) in relieving osteoarthritic pain, to have a control group in which needles were inserted into sites, 'outside of, but contiguous to, traditional acupuncture points', on the assumption that treatment of such a type had only a placebo effect. Patients in both groups responded to their respective treatments equally well, but it would be wrong to conclude from this that acupuncture in the treatment of this condition is no better than a placebo treatment for, as Mann et al (1973) so rightly observed, when discussing the subject of acupuncture in general, 'because of the lack of precise localization of acupuncture points it is difficult to conceive of nearby placebo points'. The implication of this is that the two groups in Gaw et al's study were in reality both treated with acupuncture.

It is clearly for this same reason that Takeda & Wessel (1994) found that both TCA and sham acupuncture significantly reduced pain, disability and stiffness in patients with osteoarthritis of the knee because, although the needles in the so-called sham group were inserted very superficially into the skin, as discussed in Chapters 10 and 11, this is sufficient to stimulate A-delta nerve fibres and by so doing to have a significant pain-blocking effect.

Confirmation of the efficacy of TCA in the treatment of knee osteoarthritis, however, does come from well-planned randomized controlled trials carried out by Berman et al (1999), Christensen et al (1992) and Petrou et al (1988).

TCA points commonly used for the treatment of knee osteoarthritis include Spleen 9 and 10, and Stomach 34 and 36 ( Fig 19.1).

Tillu et al (2001), in a prospective randomized trial to compare the relative efficacy of unilateral and bilateral TCA in the treatment of knee osteoarthritis, used not only these points, but also a distant point – Large intestine 4 in the first dorsal interosseous muscle of the hand (Fig 15.11). They found that unilateral acupuncture is as effective as bilateral acupuncture in increasing function and reducing pain in the affected joint, but whether adding this distant point appreciably improved the effectiveness of the treatment is open to conjecture.

There have been two well-planned trials to assess the efficacy of TCA in alleviating the pain of hip osteoarthritis. One of these was carried out by McIndoe et al (1995) and the other by Haslam (2001).

In McIndoe et al's trial, the relative effectiveness of TCA and intra-articular steroid injections was compared. In Haslam's trial, the effect of acupuncture in one group was compared with that of the giving of advice and the carrying out of exercises in a second group.

Both trials confirmed the efficacy of acupuncture, but what is of particular interest with regard to the one carried out by, Haslam is that six TCA points (GB 29, 30, 34, 43, St 44 & LI4) and 4 'ah shih' points (i.e. TrPs) were needled. The necessity for using both these two neurophysiologically different types of points concomitantly is open to question and can only be determined by carrying out a trial to compare the relative effectiveness of employing TCA in one group of patients, and TrP acupuncture in another group. In view of the close spatial relationship between periarticular TCA points and TrPs (see Figs 19.1 & 19.2) it would seem reasonable to predict that both types of acupuncture will prove to be equally efficacious in relieving osteoarthritic pain. If so, then deciding which one to use routinely in everyday clinical practice will have to depend on each individual therapist's personal proclivity.

## RHEUMATOID ARTHRITIS

In considering whether or not acupuncture has a place in the management of rheumatoid arthritis, it is necessary to bear in mind that the disease goes through two main stages, an early active severe inflammatory phase and a late destructive one.

### Early active acute inflammatory phase

The disease has either a sudden onset with the rapid involvement of many joints or a more insidious one with a gradual spread of the pathological process until ultimately many joints are affected in a roughly symmetrical manner.

In the early active phase of the disease, irrespective of the type of onset, there is an acute inflammatory reaction affecting the synovium of the joints and tendon sheaths. In addition to synovial hypertrophy and effusions, there is also considerable swelling of soft tissues as a result of the development of periarticular inflammatory oedema.

Treatment at this stage of the disease must, of necessity, be directed at combating the acute inflammatory reaction by means of rest, both general and local, physiotherapy and the administration of anti-inflammatory drugs. The severity of the inflammatory reaction and the large number of joints involved precludes considering the use of acupuncture for pain relief at this stage.

## Late destructive phase

The later stages of the disease are characterized by destructive changes in and around the joints with relatively little inflammatory reaction, although with, at times, some secondary osteoarthritic changes.

At this phase of the disease one particular joint may remain persistently painful (Camp 1998) and in such a case superficial dry needling at periarticular tender point sites should be carried out.

## References

Arnoldi C C, Lemperg R K, Linderholm H 1971 Immediate effect of osteotomy on the intramedullary pressure of the femoral head and neck in patients with degenerative osteoarthritis. Acta Orthopaedica Scandinavica 42: 357–365

Arnoldi C C, Djurhuus J C, Heerfordt J, Karte A 1980 Intraosseous phlebography, intraosseous pressure measurements and Tc-polyphosphate scintigraphy in patients with various painful conditions in the hip and knee. Acta Orthopaedica Scandinavica 51: 19–28

Baldry P E 2001 Myofascial pain and fibromyalgia syndromes. Churchill Livingstone, Edinburgh, pp. 266–273

Berman B M, Singh B B, Lao L, Langenberg P, Li H, Hadhazy V et al 1999 A randomized trial of acupuncture as an adjunctive therapy in osteoarthritis of the knee. Rheumatology (Oxford) 38(4): 346–354

Bonica J J 1953 The management of pain. Lea & Febiger, Philadelphia

Camp A V 1998 Acupuncture for rheumatological problems. In: Filshie J, White A (eds) Medical acupuncture – a Western scientific approach. Churchill Livingstone, Edinburgh

Christensen B V, Iuhl I U, Vibek H, Bulow H H, Dreijer N C, Rasmussen H F 1992 Acupuncture treatment of severe knee osteoarthritis. A long-term study. Acta Anaesthesiologica Scandinavica 36(6): 519–525

Collins A J, Ring F, Bacon P A, Brookshaw J D 1976 Thermography and radiology: Complementary methods for the study of inflammatory diseases. Clinical Radiology 27: 237–243

Cooper N S, Soren A, McEwen C, Rosenberger J L 1981 Diagnostic specificity of synovial lesions. Human Pathology 12: 314–328

Creamer P 1997 Intra-articular steroid injections in osteoarthritis: do they work and if so how? (Editorial). Annals of the Rheumatic Diseases 56: 634–635

Creamer P 1999 Osteoarthritis. In: Wall P D , Melzack R (eds) Textbook of pain, 4th edn. Churchill Livingstone, Edinburgh, pp. 493–504

Danielsson L G 1964 Incidence and prognosis of osteo-arthrosis. Acta Orthopaedica Scandinavica 66 (suppl):

De Ceulaer K, Watson Buchanan W 1979 Osteoarthrosis. Medicine 14: 693–699

Dieppe R A, Huskisson E G, Crocker P, Willoughby D A 1976 Apatite deposition disease. A new arthropathy. Lancet 1: 266–268

Dieppe P A 1978 Inflammation in osteoarthritis. Rheumatology and Rehabilitation (suppl): 59–63

Dieppe P A, Sathapatayavongs B, Jones H E, Bacon P A, Ring E F J 1980 Intra-articular steroids in osteoarthritis. Rheumatology and Rehabilitation 19: 212–217

Dixon A St. J 1965 Progress in clinical rheumatology. J A Churchill, London, pp. 313–329

Ehrlich G E 1975 Osteoarthritis beginning with inflammation. Journal of the American Medical Association 232: 157–159

Evans F J 1974 The placebo response in pain reduction. In: Bonica J J (ed) Advances in neurology. International Symposium on Pain. Raven Press, New York

Fassbender H G 1975 Pathology of rheumatic diseases. Springer-Verlag, Berlin (Trans. G Loewi)

Felson D T, Anderson J, Naimark A et al 1988 Obesity and knee osteoarthritis. Annals of Internal Medicine 109: 18–24

Fisher N M, Gresham G E, Abrams M et al 1993 Quantitative effects of physical therapy on muscular and functional performance in subjects with osteoarthritis of the knees. Archives of Physical Medicine and Rehabilitation 74: 840–847

Gaw A C, Chang L W, Shaw L C 1975 Efficacy of acupuncture on osteoarthritic pain. A controlled double-blind study. New England Journal of Medicine 293: 375–378

George R C, Chrisman O D 1968 The role of cartilage polysaccharides in osteoarthritis. Clinical Orthopaedics 57: 259

Goldenberg D L, Egan M S, Cohen A S 1982 Inflammatory synovitis in degenerative joint disease. Journal of Rheumatology 9: 204–209

Hamilton D E, Bywaters E G C, Please N W 1959 A controlled trial of various forms of physiotherapy in arthritis. British Medical Journal 1: 542–544

Harper P, Nuki G 1980 Genetic factors in osteoarthrosis. In: The aetiopathogenesis of osteoarthrosis. Pitman Press, Bath, pp. 184–201

Haslam R 2001 A comparison of acupuncture with advice and exercises on the symptomatic treatment of osteoarthritis of the hip – A randomised controlled trial. Acupuncture in Medicine 19(1): 19–26

Huskisson E C, Dieppe P A, Tucker A K, Cannell L B 1979 Another look at osteoarthritis. Annals of Rheumatic Diseases 38: 423–428

Huskisson E C 1985 Osteoarthritis: Pathogenesis and management. Update Postgraduate Centre series. Update Group, London

Kellgren J H 1961 Osteoarthrosis in patients and populations. British Medical Journal ii: 1–6

Kellgren J H, Lawrence J S, Bier F 1963 Genetic factors in generalized osteoarthritis. Annals of Rheumatic Diseases 22: 237–255

Lawrence J S, Bremner J M, Bier F 1966 Osteoarthrosis. Prevalence in the population and relationship between symptoms and X-ray changes. Annals of Rheumatic Diseases 25: 1–22

Lemperg R K, Arnoldi C C 1978 The significance of intraosseous pressure in normal and diseased states with special reference to the intraosseous engorgement pain syndrome. Clinical Orthopaedics and Related Research 136: 143–156

Mann F 1974 Periosteal acupuncture. In: The treatment of disease by acupuncture, 3rd edn. Heinemann Medical, London, pp. 193–204

Mann F, Bowsher D, Mumford J, Lipton S, Miles J 1973 Treatment of intractable pain by acupuncture. Lancet ii: 57–60

Martin K, Nicklas B J, Bunyard I B et al 1996 Weight loss and walking improve symptoms of knee osteoarthritis. Arthritis and Rheumatism 39(suppl): S225

McCarty D J 1976 Calcium pyrophosphate dihydrate crystal deposition disease. Arthritis and Rheumatism 19: 295

McIndoe A K, Young K, Bone M E 1995 A comparison of acupuncture with intra-articular steroid injection as analgesia for osteoarthritis of the hip. Acupuncture in Medicine 13(2): 67–70

Miller J H, White J, Norton T H 1958 The value of intraarticular injections in osteoarthritis of the knee. Journal of Bone and Joint Surgery 40B: 636–643

Petrou P, Winkler V, Genti G, Balint G 1988 Double-blind trial to evaluate the effect of acupuncture treatment on knee osteoarthrosis. Scandinavian Journal of Acupuncture 3: 112–115

Pomeranz B 2001 Acupuncture analgesia – basic research. In: Stux G, Hammerschlag R (eds) Clinical acupuncture, scientific basis. Springer, Berlin, pp. 1–28

Radin E L, Ehrlich M M, Weiss C A, Parker H G 1976 Osteoarthritis as a state of altered pathology. In: Buchanan W W, Dick C (eds) Recent advances in rheumatology I. Churchill Livingstone, Edinburgh, pp. 1–18

Roth L U, Maret-Maric A, Adler R H, Neuenschwander B E 1997 Acupuncture points have subjective (needling

sensation) and objective (serum cortisol increase) specificity. Acupuncture in Medicine 15(1): 2–5

Schouten J S, van den Ouweland, Valkengurg H A 1992 A 12 year follow up study in the general population on prognostic factors of cartilage loss in OA of the knee. Annals of the Rheumatic Diseases 51: 932–937

Schumacher H R, Smolyo A P, Rose R C, Maurer K 1977 Arthritis associated with apatite crystals. Annals of Internal Medicine 87: 411–416

Schumacher H R, Gordon G, Paul H, Reginato A, Villaneuva T, Cherian V, Gibilisco P 1981 Osteoarthritis, crystal deposition and inflammation. Seminars in Arthritis and Rheumatism 11: 116–119

Sola A E, Williams R L 1956 Myofascial pain syndromes. Neurology 6: 91–95

Stecher R M 1955 Heberden's nodes. A clinical description of osteoarthritis of the finger joints. Annals of Rheumatic Diseases 14: 1–10

Takeda W, Wessel J 1994 Acupuncture for the treatment of pain of osteoarthritic knees. Arthritis Care Research 7(3): 118–122

Tillu A, Roberts C, Tillu S 2001 Unilateral versus bilateral acupuncture on knee function in advanced osteoarthritis of the knee – a prospective randomised trial. Acupuncture in Medicine 19(1): 15–18

Traut E F, Passarelli E W 1956 Study in the controlled therapy of degenerative arthritis. Archives of Internal Medicine 98: 181–186

Travell J 1950 The adductor longus syndrome. A case of groin pain. Its treatment by local block of trigger areas. Bulletin of the New York Academy of Medicine 26: 284–285

Travell J 1951 Pain mechanisms in connective tissues. In: Ragan C, ed. Connective issues. Transactions of the second conference. Josiah Macey Jnr Foundation, New York, pp. 86–125

Travell J, Rinzler S H 1952 The myofascial genesis of pain. Post-graduate Medicine 11: 425–434

Wiberg G 1941 Roentgenographic and anatomic studies of the femoropatellar joint. Acta Orthopaedica Scandinavica 12: 319

Wood P H N 1976 Osteoarthritis in the community. Clinics in Rheumatic Diseases 2: 495–507

Wright V, Chandler G N, Monson R A U, Hartfall S J 1960 Intra-articular therapy in osteoarthritis. Annals of Rheumatic Diseases 19: 257–261

Wyke B 1981 The neurology of joints. A review of general principles. Clinics in Rheumatic Diseases 7: 233–239

Chapter **20**

# Abdominal and pelvic pain

## INTRODUCTION

The type of abdominal and pelvic pain most likely to be helped by acupuncture is that which occurs as a result of the activation of trigger points (TrPs) in the muscles, fasciae, tendons and ligaments of the anterior and lateral abdominal wall, the lower back, the floor of the pelvis, and the upper anterior part of the thigh (Baldry 2001).

Such pain, however, is all too often erroneously assumed to be due to some intra-abdominal lesion and, as a consequence of being inappropriately treated, is often allowed to persist for much longer than is necessary. As Renaer (1984) so rightly says:

> … when confronted with abdominal pain complaints, most doctors will automatically think of pain originating in the abdominal viscera. Yet it would appear strange if tissues so abundantly innervated as the skin and the fasciae of the abdominal wall hardly ever caused pain.

An important reason why doctors tend to overlook the possibility of abdominal pain arising from structures encasing the internal organs is because the majority of present-day textbooks on gastroenterology, together with most sections on the subject in undergraduate textbooks of medicine, whilst giving detailed descriptions of diseases of the viscera and the characteristics of pain associated with these, make little or no reference to the diagnosis and treatment of pain emanating from the abdominal wall itself. This failure on the part of most authors of textbooks to emphasize the importance of distinguishing between visceral and somatic pain is not only surprising, but much to be regretted, as there can be no doubt that pain occurring as the result of activation of TrPs in the abdominal wall is relatively common. One gastroenterologist, who invariably includes this possibility in his differential diagnosis whenever presented with a case of persistent abdominal pain, regularly refers to me an appreciable number of such patients for treatment with acupuncture. It, therefore, came as no surprise to me to find that Ranger et al (1971), working in a large district general hospital, were able to collect a series of 100 patients with abdominal wall pain over a period of 2 years.

Despite this paucity of information concerning abdominal wall TrP pain in most current textbooks, there have been many important contributions to the subject in various journals over the past 50 years or more. One of the earliest was contained in an address entitled 'Myofibrositis as a Simulator of other Maladies', delivered by Murray in 1929 to the Newcastle upon Tyne and Northern Counties Medical Society.

The fact that, because of the time in which Murray lived, he attributed the pain to fibrositis in no way detracts from the importance of his observations concerning what clearly today would be called myofascial trigger point (MTrP) pain. In the part of his address dealing with abdominal wall pain, he says 'such pain is of a dull aching character generally felt at one spot from which it tends to radiate'. He then goes on to state that pain of this type is often made worse by stretching and twisting movements of the trunk, and he stresses the importance of palpating the abdomen with the muscles both in a state of relaxation and of contraction when attempting to distinguish between visceral and somatic pain.

He describes how, by the use of this examination technique, he was able in three cases of persistent abdominal pain to demonstrate that the pain was arising from circumscribed tender areas in the muscles and that pain in the right iliac fossa previously ascribed to chronic appendicitis, pain in the right hypochondrium said to be due to biliary colic, and pain in the epigastrium attributed to a gastritis, was in each case due to what he called 'fibrositis' of the abdominal wall. He concludes by reporting that he was able to relieve this persistent pain, which in two cases had been present for several months, and in one case for 4 years, by applying an iodine and belladonna ointment to the areas of tenderness.

Other physicians who stressed the importance of distinguishing abdominal wall pain from visceral pain during the 1930s were Hunter (1933) and Telling (1935). In addition, Lewis & Kellgren (1939) carried out extremely important experimental work, in both human healthy volunteers and animals, on musculoskeletal pain that arises from the abdominal wall itself, and also that which is referred to the abdomen from muscles in the lower back (see Ch. 4).

From the 1940s onwards, several clinicians have published reports concerning the diagnosis and treatment of abdominal wall MTrP pain based on their own personal series of cases, including Kelly (1942), Young (1943), Gutstein (1944), Theobald (1949), Good (1950a, b), Melnick (1954, 1957a), Long (1956), Mehta & Ranger (1971), Applegate (1972) and Bourne (1980). In addition, Simons et al (1999) have provided an extensive review of the whole subject in their TrP manual.

## ABDOMINAL WALL MTrP PAIN

### Examination of the patient

In order to diagnose MTrP abdominal wall pain and to distinguish it from visceral pain, it is essential to palpate the abdomen with the muscles of the anterior wall both in a relaxed and contracted state, because abdominal wall pain emanates from focal areas of exquisite tenderness, or TrPs, and the tenderness at these points is increased when the muscles are held taut and decreased when they are relaxed.

The procedure and the reason for carrying it out cannot be explained better than by quoting Long (1956) who states:

The painful area is compressed rather firmly beneath a single finger or thumb, with sufficient pressure barely to pass the threshold of pain. The patient is then asked to raise both legs straight, causing both heels to leave the examining surface by a distance of a few inches only. The resultant contraction of the anterior abdominal wall will push the examining finger away from the viscera and simultaneously increasingly compress the abdominal wall beneath the finger. If, on this manouver, the pain increases it is of abdominal wall origin; if it decreases it is of visceral origin.

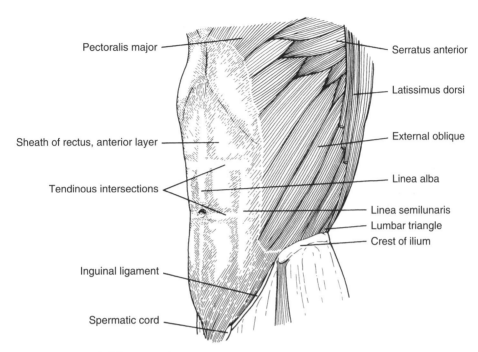

**Figure 20.1**   The left external oblique muscle.

Murray (1929) advocated producing tension in the abdominal muscles by getting the patient to raise the head and upper part of the body from the recumbent position. De Valera & Raftery (1976) recommend getting the patient to elevate both the feet and head. Travell & Simons (1983) advise getting the supine patient to hold a deep breath. There is little to choose between any of these methods and it is my personal practice to adopt whichever one seems to be the most suitable for a particular individual.

## Muscles involved

The principal anterior abdominal wall muscles in which TrPs are liable to become activated include the two rectus abdominis muscles on either side of the midline, and the external and internal oblique muscles in the flanks (Figs 20.1 & 20.2).

## Location of the TrPs

### Rectus abdominis

Common sites for TrP activation in this muscle include the epigastric region near to its insertion into

the lower ribs; in its belly, half-way between the xiphisternum & the umbilicus and half-way between the umbilicus & the pubis; also at or near to its insertion into the pubic bone (Fig. 20.3).

### External and internal obliques

Common sites for TrP activation in these muscles include the hypochondrium, the iliac crest and close to the inguinal ligament. It may also occur anywhere along a line joining the tip of the twelfth rib above and the iliac crest below (Fig. 20.4).

## Symptomatology

Activated TrPs in the anterior abdominal wall may, as with TrPs anywhere else in the body, be responsible for the development of pain but, in addition, because of a somatovisceral reflex in the abdomen, they are also capable of causing other symptoms including anorexia, flatulence, nausea, vomiting, diarrhoea, colic, dysmenorrhoea and dysuria.

Melnick (1954), in a series of 56 patients with abdominal wall TrPs, found the latter to be the cause of flatulence and bloating in 25% of the cases, vomiting in 11%, heartburn in 11% and diarrhoea

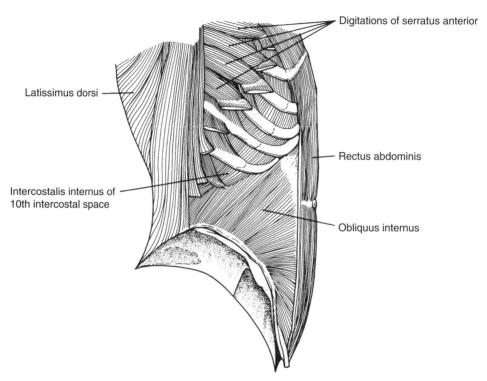

**Figure 20.2** Muscles of the right side of the trunk. The external oblique has been removed to show the internal oblique, but its digitations from the ribs have been preserved. The sheath of the rectus abdominis has been opened and its anterior lamina removed.

in 4%. Theobald (1949) has reported relieving dysmenorrhoea by deactivating TrPs in the lower part of the rectus abdominis about half-way between the umbilicus and pubis, and Hoyt (1953) has reported relieving dysuria by deactivating TrPs in the lower abdominal muscles.

The pain itself often takes the form of a dull ache. Alternatively, it may, as pointed out by Ranger et al (1971) be sharp and burning in character. It tends to be aggravated by twisting or stretching movements of the trunk. Patients sometimes complain more of discomfort than of actual pain (Kelly 1942). This is because, as Travell & Simons (1983) state, 'TrPs in the anterior abdominal wall, and particularly those in the rectus abdominis, are liable to cause the abdomen to become lax and distended with flatus'.

It is also noticeable how often patients with upper abdominal TrP pain complain of this being made worse by the pressure of their clothes. In addition, as pointed out by Murray (1929), epigastric TrP pain may be aggravated by post-prandial distension of the stomach.

A farm labourer (50 years of age) had an 18-month history of epigastric pain that was always worse whenever his abdomen became distended following a meal. After he had been found to have a normal barium meal, gastroscopy, and ultrasound scan, he was referred to me as a possible case of abdominal wall TrP pain. On examination, he had two well-defined exquisitely tender TrPs in the linea alba 3 inches below the xiphisternum and after these had been deactivated with dry needles on two occasions, he had no further trouble.

In addition, pain from TrPs in muscles in the upper part of the abdomen may be brought on by flexing the trunk.

A market gardener (62 years of age), whose work involved much heavy lifting, suffered from attacks of severe pain in the right upper quadrant of the abdomen about 3–4 times a week, with each attack lasting about 15–20 min and coming on whenever his work necessitated him bending over for any length of time. At one stage it was thought he might have some type of diaphragmatic hernia. However, all investigations were negative and after he had had recurrent bouts of pain for 4 years, he was referred to me for an opinion as to whether acupuncture might help to relieve it. On examination, a single TrP was located in the lateral border of the right rectus muscle just below the ribs that had presumably become activated by the strain of heavy lifting. The point was so exquisitely tender to touch that the patient visibly jumped when pressure was applied to it. Somewhat to my surprise in view of the long history, there were no further attacks of pain following deactivation of the TrP with a dry needle on only one occasion.

## Differential diagnosis

Pain and flatulence occurring as a result of TrPs in the right upper quadrant in either, one of the oblique muscles, or in the lateral border of the rectus muscle, is liable to be erroneously ascribed to gall bladder disease, particularly if, by chance, ultrasound scanning reveals the presence of gall stones.

Pain and tenderness in the right lower quadrant occurring as a result of TrP activity in the lateral border of the rectus muscle is apt to be diagnosed as being due to appendicitis, particularly as the TrP frequently occurs in the region of McBurney's point, approximately 1–2 inches from the anterior superior iliac spine along the line joining this spine and the umbilicus. Persistent right iliac fossa pain is rarely, if ever, due to chronic appendicitis but frequently occurs as a result of the activation of a TrP.

Epigastric pain, particularly when accompanied by dyspeptic symptoms and occurring as a result of TrP activity in the rectus abdominis, is liable to be attributed to a hiatus hernia if, by chance, the latter happens to be found on radiographic examination.

Finally, there is a risk of pain in the left lower quadrant from TrPs in the outer border of the rectus or the obliques being considered to be due to diverticulitis if, by chance, a barium enema reveals the presence of diverticulae in the lower part of the colon.

## Factors responsible for the primary activation of anterior abdominal wall TrPs

The various factors responsible for the primary activation of abdominal wall MTrPs include: acute

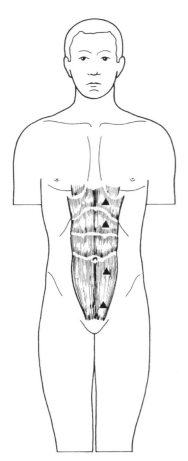

**Figure 20.3** Some common trigger point sites (▲) in the rectus abdominis muscle.

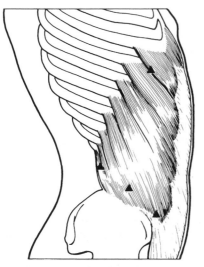

**Figure 20.4** Some commonly occurring trigger point sites (▲) in the external oblique muscle.

trauma to the muscles, as a result, for example, of an accident or surgical operation; repeated minor trauma to, or chronic overloading of them, such as may occur during the course of certain occupational tasks and sporting activities; muscle strain occurring as a result of a faulty posture; viral infections; chronic anxiety, causing the muscles to be held persistently tense; and exposure of them to the cold or damp.

The following abstracts of case notes have been selected from my own series of patients with persistent abdominal wall TrP pain in order to illustrate some of the commoner ways in which TrPs in the abdominal wall undergo primary activation.

## Trauma

A company director (56 years of age) developed severe discomfort and tenderness of the muscles in the right hypochondrium. A cholecystogram was normal. However, the pain persisted and after it had been present for 4 months, he was referred to me. It was significant that the pressure of a tight belt and also flexing his trunk made the pain worse, as on examination there were three well-defined exquisitely tender TrPs in the right external oblique muscle. These must have been activated as a result of trauma, as it transpired that the onset of the symptoms coincided with him being knocked over by a dog. It was only necessary to deactivate these TrPs with dry needles on one occasion to relieve him of his symptoms.

A farrier (37 years of age) suffered bouts of pain in the left upper part of the abdomen. All investigations, including an ultrasound scan of the abdomen, were negative. When seen by me 14 months after the onset of the pain, it had become so incapacitating as to prevent him from working. There were several TrPs in the muscles behind the left lower ribs and these must have become activated by repeated occupational trauma, as he gave a history that the pain always came on after he had spent 2–3 hours shoeing horses, during which time he pressed the legs of the animals tightly against the left upper part of his abdomen. He had no further pain once the TrPs had been deactivated with dry needles on two occasions, and he made adjustments to the manner in which he worked.

A farmer (49 years of age) with a 5-year history of intermittent epigastric pain and with no abnormality on a barium meal or gastroscopy gave a history that he was always worse on the days when he strained himself closing a particularly stiff tailboard of a lorry. He also observed that his upper abdomen often felt quite sore after cattle had knocked against it on market days. Three TrPs were found in the upper part of the rectus muscle and his pain disappeared following the deactivation of these with dry needles on four occasions.

## Faulty posture

A schoolboy (15 years of age) was referred to me with a 4-year history of pain in the right upper part of the abdomen. It was particularly troublesome whenever he put any weight on his right leg in the gymnasium or while playing rugby. He had been fully investigated at a pain clinic with the only abnormality discovered being a minor defect in the 8th dorsal vertebra. Because of this it was considered that the pain might be due to nerve root entrapment but an intercostal nerve block and an epidural injection had proved to be valueless.

On examination he had several exquisitely tender TrPs in the external oblique just below the costal margin and also a number in muscles around the greater trochanter. With hindsight, there can be no doubt that the TrPs in the leg were the first to become activated following a fall when aged 11, and that pain from these caused him to adopt a faulty posture, with the result that, as a secondary event, the TrPs in the abdominal wall became activated. After deactivating these TrPs with dry needles on three occasions, he had no further trouble.

A laboratory technician (31 years of age) with a 4-month history of pain in the right loin radiating anteriorly towards the groin, on being found to have no abnormality in the urogenital tract was referred to me as a possible case of musculoskeletal pain. There were numerous TrPs in muscles both posteriorly and anteriorly. It transpired that the pain always came on after she had been sitting for any length of time at a work bench and she felt herself that she had strained her muscles by sitting on a stool that was too low. The TrPs were readily deactivated and she has had no further pain since insisting on being given a higher stool.

## Exposure to cold or damp

Pain in the muscles of the anterior abdominal wall not infrequently occurs as part of a condition, which, because of the nebulous nature of its underlying pathology, has over the years come to be known by a variety of names including fibrositis, myalgia and, in more recent years, myofascitis. Although there can now be no doubt that the condition is associated with the activation of TrPs in the abdominal wall muscles, the reason for this activation is far from certain. Exposure to cold or damp has traditionaly been considered to be an important aetiological factor but there is of course no absolute proof of this.

## Postoperative pain

Many patients referred to me with abdominal pain that has come on postoperatively have been found to have active TrPs either in the muscles of the lower back or the anterior abdominal wall or both. There is no doubt that the activation has occurred as a result of the muscles having been traumatized or strained during the course of some surgical procedure. In addition, postoperative pain is sometimes due to TrPs developing in surgical scars.

In all such cases the pain continues to be troublesome for a long time unless the TrPs are satisfactorily deactivated.

## Secondary activation of abdominal wall TrPs

TrPs in the anterior abdominal wall can become activated as a secondary event in response to the pain of visceral disease. It is then possible for pain from the abdominal wall TrPs to continue to be troublesome long after the visceral disease has been successfully treated. Melnick (1957b) describes a patient in whom epigastric pain, originally due to a duodenal ulcer, persisted for a long time after the ulcer had healed as a result of the activation of TrPs in the rectus muscle.

The reasons for TrP activity occurring in association with the irritable bowel syndrome would seem to be more complex and, therefore, will be considered separately.

## Irritable bowel syndrome

The irritable bowel syndrome has been defined as, 'syndromes of abdominal pain and disturbance of bowel action of more than 3 months duration without any organic cause' (Blendis 1984). It is a disease that affects not only adults but also children (Apley & Naish 1958). The pain in children is predominantly periumbilical (Stone & Barbero 1970), whereas in adults it is more often over the colon, with the commonest site being the left iliac fossa (Waller & Misiewiez 1969).

Holdstock et al (1969), from manometric studies using radiotelemetering capsules in the small intestine and proximal colon, and air-filled balloons in the sigmoid colon, have shown that attacks of pain in various chronic pain syndromes, including the irritable bowel syndrome, seem to be related to changes in intraluminal pressures in either the small or large intestine.

On clinical examination, there are areas of localized tenderness over one or other parts of the colon with this most often being over the descending part, but sometimes over the transverse part, and occasionally over the whole colon. On palpating the abdomen with the muscles relaxed it seems as if it is the colon that is tender, but, on getting the patient to tense the abdominal wall, it becomes obvious that often much of this tenderness is in localized areas of the abdominal wall muscles.

Kendall et al (1986) and also Hall (1986) consider that these focal areas of tenderness in the muscle occur as a result of a viscerosomatic reflex (Procacci & Zoppi 1983). This may be true, but nevertheless it has to be remembered that Lewis & Kellgren (1939) showed that an injection of a 6% salt solution into the belly of the rectus muscle just below and 1 inch outside the navel gave rise to 'a continuous pain lasting 3 to 5 minutes of unpleasant severity and having a character not to be distinguished from that of colic'. In other words, Lewis & Kellgren, by artificially creating a trigger zone in an abdominal wall muscle, were able, by means of a somatovisceral reflex, to produce a pain not dissimilar to that which occurs with the irritable bowel syndrome.

Furthermore, it has to be remembered that such symptoms as dyspepsia (Watson et al 1976), dysuria (Fielding 1977), and dysmenorrhoea (Waller & Misiewicz 1969) are frequently present in irritable bowel syndrome, and that, as discussed earlier, these are all symptoms that anterior abdominal wall TrPs, by virtue of a somatovisceral reflex, are capable of producing.

The question, therefore, that has to be asked is whether the pain and other symptoms in this condition are primarily due to a disorder of the gut with the focal areas of tenderness in the anterior abdominal wall musculature developing as a secondary event, or whether these tender points are actually TrPs and the prime cause of all these various symptoms? If it is the latter, then it would be reasonable to expect that deactivation of these points by one means or another would relieve the symptoms. Kendall et al, however, state that they have not been able to alleviate the pain by infiltrating them with local anaesthetic agents with or without the addition of steroids. They also have observed that these anterior abdominal wall tender points, unlike TrPs, do not seem to be constant in position but move from place to place.

These observations notwithstanding, what is certain is that many cases of irritable bowel syndrome have been referred to me for treatment with acupuncture because, in addition to having visceral pain, they have also had pain made worse by twisting and stretching movements of the trunk, that was clearly muscular in origin. In all these cases, TrPs have invariably been found to be present at constant sites in the muscles of either the lower back or the anterior abdominal wall. In some instances, this particular type of pain appears to have developed as a result of the skeletal muscles being held tense during bouts of intra-abdominal pain. In other cases it seems as if the irritable bowel syndrome and the TrP pain have arisen independently of each other, which is hardly surprising considering that both this particular disorder of the gut (Esler & Goulston 1973) and musculoskeletal pain disorders (Crown 1978) frequently occur in people of an anxious disposition.

MTrP pain occurring either coincidentally with, or developing as a result of irritable bowel syndrome is well worth treating with acupuncture, because once the TrPs have been deactivated with dry needles any residual visceral pain is so much more readily coped with.

## Deactivation of abdominal wall TrPs

It is obviously possible to deactivate TrPs in the abdominal wall, as elsewhere in the body, by a variety of different methods. Murray (1929) clearly achieved this by applying an iodine and belladonna ointment to the skin overlying them. Many clinicians including Travell & Simons (1983) advocate injecting a local anaesthetic into them. Bourne (1980) favours the use of a corticosteroid local anaesthetic mixture.

Mehta & Ranger (1971), Ranger et al (1971), and also Applegate (1972), presumably because they considered the pain to be due to the entrapment of a cutaneous nerve as it passes through an anterior abdominal wall muscle, felt obliged to inject phenol into a point of maximum tenderness.

There can be no doubt that the reason why all of these methods are capable of alleviating this type of pain is because they all have one property in common, namely an irritant action on A-delta nerve fibres, with this in turn activating pain-modulating mechanisms in the central nervous system. This effect of course can be achieved far more straightforwardly simply by deactivat-ing TrPs with acupuncture needles (Ch. 8). In addition, with regard to this, it has been my experience that anterior abdominal wall TrPs are particularly easy to deactivate with dry needles, so that even with pain of long duration it is rarely necessary to carry out this procedure more than two to three times. This is in marked contrast to TrP pain in either the cervical or lumbar region, where it is often necessary to continue with the treatment for far longer. This may be because during the course of everyday life a much greater mechanical strain is imposed on muscles in the neck and back.

## Pain in the abdomen from TrPs in the lower back

Lewis & Kellgren (1939) were able to show that an injection of hypertonic saline into the supraspinous ligament at the level of the 9th thoracic vertebra gave rise to pain posteriorly in the region of the first lumbar vertebra, and anteriorly over the 9th costal cartilage and down towards the umbilicus. They also observed rigidity of the upper abdominal muscles on the side of the injection when this experimentally induced pain was at its height.

The following year, Kellgren (1940) published an account of several cases in which somatic pain simulated visceral pain. These included the case of a housewife who had a 1-year history of epigastric pain and nausea coming on 1 h after meals, together with epigastric tenderness, but with no abnormality demonstrable on a barium meal. Examination of the back, however, revealed the presence of a mid-dorsal kyphosis of the spine and any attempt to straighten the latter caused the epigastric pain to be reproduced. In addition, there were focal areas of marked tenderness in the region of the 8th and 9th thoracic vertebrae and an injection of novocain into these abolished the epigastric pain and tenderness. Also presented was the case of another housewife with a 6-month history of continuous pain in the right hypochondrium and lower angle of the scapula, together with episodes of more severe pain, nausea, and flatulence. There was tenderness and rigidity of the upper abdominal muscles, but a cholecystogram was normal. She also had a mid-dorsal kyphosis and it was possible to reproduce her pain by forcibly flexing and extending this part of the spine. There were tender areas in the region of the 6th and 7th thoracic interspinous ligaments and, as in the previous case, an injection of Novocaine into these abolished the abdominal pain and rigidity.

These cases, reported by Kellgren nearly 50 years ago, have been quoted in order to show that it has for long been known that abdominal pain may, on occasions, occur as a result of being referred there from TrPs in the lower back, and that in all cases of abdominal pain not obviously due to some visceral disease, it is important to search for TrPs, not only in the anterior abdominal wall musculature, but also in the muscles and ligaments of the lower back.

## Pain in the lower back owing to TrPs in anterior abdominal wall muscles

In my experience whenever a patient with low-back pain finds it is uncomfortable to stand up straight and also when any attempt passively to extend the spine makes the pain worse, it is often because of the activity of TrPs in the lower part of the rectus muscle at or near to its insertion into the

pubic bone, or in the lower border of the external oblique muscle along its insertion into the inguinal ligament. It is, therefore, important in all such cases not only to look for TrPs in the lumbar muscles but also in the anterior abdominal wall.

## PELVIC PAIN

The type of pelvic pain most likely to be amenable to treatment with acupuncture is that which occurs as a result of the activation of TrPs in muscles and ligaments in the pelvic floor and in the adductor longus tendon near or at its attachment to the pubic bone.

### Chronic pelvic floor MTrP pain syndrome

TrP activation in this condition occurs in various muscles and ligaments in the pelvic floor with the principal muscles involved being the levator ani, the coccygeus, the piriformis and the medial fibres of the gluteus maximus (Figs 20.5 & 20.6).

Thiele (1937) was one of the first to draw attention to this condition when he described what he called coccygodynia (pain around the coccyx) from spasm of the levator ani and coccygeus muscles occurring in conjunction with pain around the buttock and down the back of the thigh from spasm of the piriformis.

During the 1940s and 1950s, Thiele and others published papers on coccygodynia, with one of the most interesting being that of Dittrich (1951), as he appears to have been the first person to recognize that pain in this condition occurs as a result of it being referred from TrPs. In his paper he described two cases of coccygeal pain occurring as a result of it being referred to the coccyx from TrPs in adipose tissue in the sacral region. His contribution to the subject is, however, otherwise limited because he seems to have believed that TrPs in this condition only occur at this site and makes no mention of the possibility of them occurring in the muscles of the pelvic floor.

During the course of reviewing the clinical features of coccygodynia, Thiele (1963) pointed out that it is only in the 20% of cases in which coccygeal pain is due to direct trauma that the coccyx is tender, and that in the other 80% of cases not due to trauma this lack of tenderness of the bone means

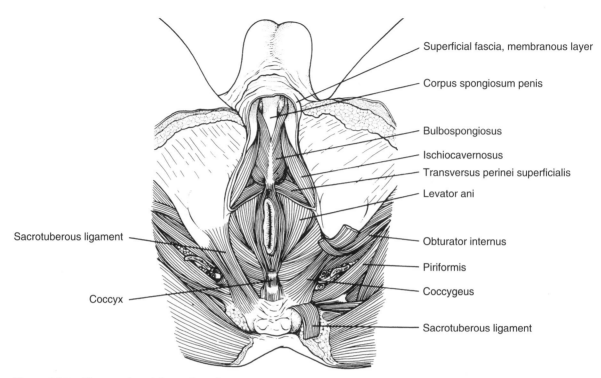

**Figure 20.5**   The muscles of the male perineum.

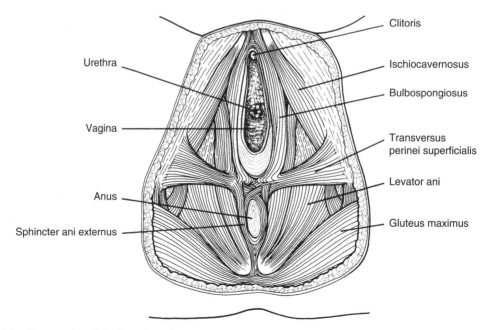

**Figure 20.6**   The muscles of the female perineum.

that the pain cannot be due to disease of this structure itself or to arthritis of the sacrococcygeal joint, but rather that it must be referred to the coccyx from pelvic muscles which, for one reason or another, have gone into spasm.

Coccygodynia is not really a particularly apt name for this disorder because, as Thiele himself recognized when he first introduced the term in the 1930s, the pain is rarely confined to the coccyx. On the other hand, as he originally pointed out, it is a condition that is always associated with spasm of the pelvic floor muscles, and for this reason other physicians have given it a variety of other names including the levator spasm syndrome (Smith 1959), the levator syndrome (McGivney & Cleveland 1965) and the levator ani spasm syndrome (Lilius & Valtonen 1973).

However, none of these terms are entirely satisfactory, as the levator ani muscle is usually only one of the muscles involved and, therefore, much to be preferred is tension myalgia of the pelvic floor, a term introduced by Sinaki et al (1977) at the Mayo Clinic. Nevertheless, even this can be improved upon for there are now good grounds for believing that the pain is referred over a fairly wide area from points of maximum tenderness or TrPs in muscles of the pelvic floor, and for this reason a more appropriate term for it is the chronic pelvic floor MTrP pain syndrome.

## Clinical manifestations

The condition occurs predominantly in females. It is now generally agreed that the commonest and most striking feature is pain coming on when seated. It may also be felt during the acts of sitting down and standing up. There is usually no pain on lying down or on walking about, except that sometimes sudden twisting movements of the trunk are painful. One of my patients found sitting in a chair so distressing that he was reduced to watching television or reading a book kneeling on the floor. Straining at stool may also aggravate the pain, but not as often as might be thought. Sinaki et al (1977) reported it in 33% of their patients. It is also surprising that dyspareunia is rarely a problem. The pain usually takes the form of a somewhat ill-defined aching or throbbing sensation in either the anterior or posterior parts of the perineum or

throughout that region. In addition, the pain may spread to the buttocks, hips and backs of the thighs.

It is generally agreed that this condition mainly occurs in those of an anxious disposition, and from what some of my patients with this condition have told me, it clearly tends to occur in those who tense up the muscles of their pelvic floor at times of stress. There is usually, however, in addition some local cause for the condition developing.

On examination, exquisitely tender TrPs may be found on external examination of the perineum, in some cases, however, they can only be located by the carrying out of a rectal examination.

Patients with this condition seem to be particularly prone to TrP activation and often give a history of TrP pain in other parts of the body such as the neck or lower part of the back. Unfortunately, this syndrome is still not as widely recognized as its importance deserves, the pain all too frequently being attributed to some mechanical disorder of the spine or to some inflammatory condition such as proctitis, prostatitis, cervicitis, urethritis, or vaginitis and, as a consequence of this, treated inappropriately. Alternatively, after the patient has been seen by a series of consultants specializing in orthopaedics, urology, gynaecology and neurology, and they each in turn having found nothing to account for the pain, it is not uncommon for the opinion of a psychiatrist to be sought.

## Aetiology

Many of the physicians who over the years have published reports drawing attention to the pain being due to pelvic floor muscle spasm have considered that in many cases the spasm is secondary to some inflammatory lesion in the pelvis and have emphasized that the pain is not directly due to the latter itself. They have also stated that with many patients there is no inflammatory lesion present. The situation would seem to be that in all cases the spasm of the pelvic floor muscles is due to the activation of TrPs in them, and that in those patients where this is not secondary to some pelvic inflammatory lesion, it is due to the muscles being subjected either to acute trauma or to repeated minor trauma or to chronic strain. The following cases exemplify how one or other of these three factors may lead to the development of this syndrome.

## Acute trauma

A housewife (65 years of age) was referred to me with a 6-month history of persistent posteriorly situated perineal pain. On examination, there was a single exquisitely tender TrP situated half-way between the coccyx and the posterior margin of the anus. The pain quickly subsided once this TrP had been deactivated with dry needles on two occasions. There can be little doubt that this TrP had been activated as a result of surgical trauma as the onset of the pain coincided with an operation for a rectal prolapse.

## Repeated minor trauma

A businessman (58 years of age) with pain in the testicles that came on as soon as he sat down on a chair, and which was relieved by standing or walking about, was investigated by a general surgeon, a urologist, a neurologist, and an orthopaedic specialist. When none of these specialists could account for his pain, it was suggested to him that he should be seen by a psychiatrist. This he refused to do and after the condition had caused him considerable distress for 4 years, his general practitioner, as an act of desperation, referred him to me to see whether acupuncture might help.

On examination there were many exquisitely tender TrPs in the anterior perineal muscles and muscles on the inner side of the thigh near to their attachment to the pubic bone. Deactivation of these TrPs with dry needles gave immediate, but very temporary relief and the procedure had to be repeated 12 times over the course of 5 months before the pain finally disappeared. This man had a long history of low-back pain and it would seem that the reason for him activating TrPs in the pelvic floor was because he had traumatized his perineum by sitting on the hard saddle of a rowing machine for 20 min twice a day for 12 years carrying out exercises designed to strengthen the muscles of his back!

## Recurrent muscle strain

A housewife (48 years of age) developed a throbbing pain mainly around the rectum, but spreading forwards to the anterior perineum and down the thighs. This only came on when she sat down and was relieved by standing. It was made worse when, on sitting, she crossed her legs but was eased by opening them. Two gynaecologists and a neurologist failed to find the cause and after the pain had been present for 3 years she was referred to me to see whether acupuncture might help.

On external examination, there were many TrPs throughout the muscles of the perineum and deactivation of these with dry needles was carried out on several occasions. There was, in addition, much tenderness on rectal examination and she was, therefore, also given rectal massage. These measures, however, only gave her partial relief. She was a very tense person and there is no doubt this aggravated the situation, as there was still further improvement once she had been taught autohypnosis.

The reason for her developing the condition was that she had become obsessed about completely emptying her rectum and for many years had regularly spent up to 20 min each day straining at stool.

## Treatment

Some cases, like those quoted above, have TrPs that can readily be identified on external examination of the pelvic floor, and it is a relatively straight-forward procedure to deactivate these by means of inserting dry needles into them. Response to this, however, is generally slow and in order to obtain any long-term relief it usually has to be repeated many times.

Most cases also have TrPs that are only discernible on rectal examination and with these, rectal massage, similar to that used for massaging the prostate, is said to be helpful (Thiele 1937, 1963). Cummings (2000), however, during the course of discussing this particular form of treatment, has shrewdly commented that it does not appear to have become as popular in the UK as possibly in some other European countries.

Deep heat, by means of diathermy, applied either per rectum or externally, is also useful in helping to relax the muscles (Sinaki et al 1977). In addition, because this condition usually develops in highly anxious people and is aggravated by them nervously holding the pelvic muscles in a state of tension, relaxation techniques such as biofeedback or hypnosis should also be employed.

## Gynaecological MTrP pain

Slocumb (1984, 1990), an American gynaecologist, must be given the credit for being the first to recognize this syndrome. He specifically looked for MTrPs in 177 women referred to his clinic with chronic pelvic pain, and found this to have emanated from TrPs in the anterior abdominal wall (89%), in the vaginal fornices (71%) and in the sacral region (25%). He stressed that when searching for MTrPs in this disorder, the conventional bimanual vaginal examination should not be employed. Instead, he advocated firstly palpating the lower anterior abdominal wall muscles. Then palpating the tissues around the vaginal introitus. Following this, the tissues high up in the paracervical region.

### Pathogenesis

This disorder is due to trauma-evoked MTrP activity occuring either during childbirth or pelvic surgery.

### Character of the pain

The pain is of a diffuse poorly localised aching type. When emanating from TrPs in the lower abdominal wall muscles it is exacerbated when these are stretched either by a distended bladder or twisting of the torso. Pain from TrPs in the vaginal wall is exacerbated by coitus. In addition, TrP activity higher up in the paracervical region is liable to give rise to dysmenorrhoea.

### Treatment

Slocumb deactivated the TrPs by injecting a local anaesthetic into them. However, in view of what is now known about the subject (Ch. 10), it is clear that superficial dry needling is not only simpler but equally effective.

## Adductor longus syndrome

Pain in the groin and down the inner side of the thigh to the knee is liable to be due to a TrP becoming activated in the adductor longus muscle (Travell 1950, Long 1956). In my experience the TrP is most often located in the tendon of this muscle near to or at its insertion into the pubic bone (Fig. 18.1).

This activation may occur secondary to some chronic painful condition such as osteoarthritis of the hip or it may develop as the result of the muscle being subjected to trauma.

In the female this may be the cause of seemingly inexplicable vaginal pain.

A young woman developed a distressing throbbing pain in her vagina and around the urethral orifice when aged 20 years. It was worse after any physical activity such as dancing and sexual intercourse aggravated it. She also noticed that it was more noticeable whenever she was emotionally upset. Over the years she saw several gynaecologists but no cause for it was found and eventually she was sent to a psychiatrist. He, however, was unable to help and after it had been present for 14 years, her general practitioner referred her to me in what he described as a faint hope that acupuncture might help!

On examination, there was an exquisitely tender TrP in the right adductor longus tendon near to its insertion into the pubis. Pressure on this point aggravated the pain and on inserting a needle into it, she exclaimed 'that is my pain' as an electric shock-like sensation shot up into the vagina and down the inner side of her thigh.

Deactivation of the TrP with a dry needle gave temporary relief and after the procedure had been repeated eight times during the course of 12 weeks, the pain no longer returned.

On seeking a reason for the activation of the TrP, it transpired that for some months prior to the onset of the pain she had been in the habit of frequently travelling very long distances seated on the pillion of a motor cycle whilst gripping tightly with her thighs for support.

In the male, TrP activation in this muscle may be the cause of seemingly inexplicable scrotal pain. Several men referred to me with pain in this region have been found to have TrPs in this muscle; but, at the same time, it has to be remembered that TrPs at other sites may also be responsible for this pattern of pain referral.

## Anterior pelvic floor MTrP pain

Muscles in the anterior half of the pelvic floor in which TrP activity may develop include the bulbospongiosus and the ischiocavernosus (Figs 20.5 & 20.6).

### Bulbospongiosus muscle

This muscle is attached posteriorly to the perineal body situated in the centre of the pelvic floor. From there in the female it divides into two parts that anteriorly attach to the clitoris. In the male from its posterior attachment to the perineal body it divides into two parts that wrap around the corpus spongiosum on the posterior aspect of the penis and around the corpus cavernosum on its anterior aspect.

### Ischiocavernosus muscles

These two muscles form the lateral boundaries of the perineum. Posteriorly, in both sexes, the muscle is attached to the ischial tuberosity. Anteriorly, in the male it inserts into the base of the penis and in the female into the base of the clitoris.

**Development of TrP activity in these muscles** TrP activity is liable to develop in these muscles when they are subjected to direct trauma such as when falling astride a hard surface or when strained during the course of carrying out some sporting activity. One of my patients, a keen footballer, damaged them employing a device to strengthen his upper thigh muscles!

**Locating of TrPs in these muscles** In the female TrPs present in the bulbospongiosus may be found by applying firm pressure to the lateral wall of the introitus, and in the ischiocavernosus by applying firm pressure in the region of the clitoris.

In the male TrPs in the bulbospongiosus are located by palpating over the mid-line bulb at the root of the penis and TrPs in the ischiocavernosus muscle by palpating along the lateral aspect of the root of the penis.

Travell & Simons (1992) recommend deactivating these TrPs by injecting a local anaesthetic into them. It is, however, in my experience easier and just as effective to carry out superficial dry needling.

## Scrotal pain

Whenever scrotal pain develops for no obvious reason, the possibility of it being referred to the scrotum from TrPs elsewhere has to be consid-ered.

These TrPs may be either in the external oblique muscle just above the inguinal ligament; or in the adductor longus muscle near to its insertion into the pubic bone; or in the muscles of the pelvic floor; or, as Kellgren (1940) showed, in muscles and ligaments in the upper lumbar region in the vicinity of the 1st lumbar vertebra. The referral of pain to the scrotum from such a distant site presumably is associated with the fact that the genital branch of the genito-femoral nerve arises from the 1st and 2nd lumbar nerves (Yeates 1985).

A man (74 years of age), shortly after having undergone a prostatectomy, developed scrotal pain, which was made worse by various physical activities such as gardening and was aggravated by sitting for long periods in his car. There was no obvious cause for this pain in the testicles or neighbouring pelvic organs. He was, therefore, told that with time it would disappear! However, after it had been troubling him for 3 years he expressed a wish to try the effects of acupuncture.

On examination, physical signs were confined to the lower back where there were several TrPs in various parts of the musculature, including two in exquisitely tender fibrositic nodules immediately to the right of the 1st lumbar vertebra. For anatomical reasons just discussed, it would seen likely that it was from these that the pain was being referred to the scrotum.

As so often happens with TrPs, the patient was unaware of their presence, but on direct questioning he did admit that for about the same period of time he had had some aching in the lower back, but had not thought it worth mentioning as the scrotal pain was so much more distressing.

Deactivation of these TrPs on five occasions over the course of 7 weeks brought the low–back and scrotal pain under control.

The close temporal relationship between the prostatectomy and the onset of aching in the lower back and pain in the scrotum would make it reasonable to assume that the activation of the TrPs was due to the low-back muscles having been strained during the course of the patient being lifted on or off the operating table, or to them being traumatized as a result of the patient lying for some appreciable time on the table.

# References

Apley J, Naish N 1958 Recurrent abdominal pains – a field survey of 1000 school children. Archives of Diseases in Childhood 33: 165–167

Applegate W V 1972 Abdominal cutaneous nerve entrapment syndrome. Surgery 71: 118–124

Baldry P E 2001 Myofascial pain and fibromyalgia syndromes. Churchill Livingstone, Edinburgh

Blendis L M 1984 Abdominal pain. In: Wall P D, Melzack R (eds) Textbook of pain. Churchill Livingstone, Edinburgh, p. 356

Bourne I H J 1980 Treatment of painful conditions of the abdominal wall with local injections. Practitioner 224: 921–925

Crown S 1978 Psychological aspects of low back pain. Rheumatology and Rehabilitation 17: 114–124

Cummings M 2000 Piriformis syndrome. Acupuncture in Medicine 18(2): 108–121

de Valera E, Raftery H 1976 Lower abdominal and pelvic pain in women. In: Bonica J J, Albe-Fessard D (eds) Advances in pain research and therapy, Vol 1. Raven Press, New York, pp. 933–937

Dittrich R J 1951 Coccygodynia as referred pain. Journal of Bone and Joint Surgery 44A: 715–718

Esler M D, Goulston K 1973 Levels of anxiety in colonic disorders. New England Journal of Medicine 288: 16–20

Fielding J F 1977 The irritable bowel syndrome. Clinics in Gastroenterology 6: 607–622

Good M G 1950a The role of skeletal muscles in the pathogenesis of disease. Acta Medica Scandinavica 138: 285–292

Good M G 1950b Pseudo-appendicitis. Acta Medica Scandinavica 138: 348–353

Gutstein R R 1944 The role of abdominal fibrositis in functional indigestion. Mississipi Valley Medical Journal 66: 114–124

Hall M W 1986 Treatment of functional abdominal pain by transcutaneous nerve stimulation (correspondence). British Medical Journal 293: 954–955

Holdstock D J, Misiewicz J J, Waller S L 1969 Observations on the mechanism of abdominal pain. Gut 10: 19–31

Hoyt H S 1953 Segmental nerve lesions as a cause of the trigonitis syndrome. Stanford Medical Bulletin 11: 61–64

Hunter C 1933 Myalgia of the abdominal wall. Canadian Medical Journal 28: 157–161

Kellgren J H 1940 Somatic simulating visceral pain. Clinical Science 4: 303–309

Kelly M 1942 Lumbago and abdominal pain. Medical Journal of Australia 1: 311–317

Kendall G, Sylvester K, Lennard-Jones J E 1986 Treatment of functional abdominal pain by transcutaneous nerve stimulation (correspondence). British Medical Journal 293: 954–955

Lewis T, Kellgren J H 1939 Observations relating to referred pain, viscero-motor reflexes and other associated phenomena. Clinical Science 4: 47–71

Lilius H G, Valtonen E J 1973 The levator ani spasm syndrome: a clinical analysis of 31 cases. Annales Chirurgiae et al Gynaecologiae 62: 93–97

Long C 1956 Myofascial pain syndromes. Part III. Some syndromes of the trunk and thigh. Henry Ford Hospital Medical Bulletin 4: 102–106

McGivney J Q, Cleveland B R 1965 The levator syndrome and its treatment. Southern Medical Journal 58: 505–510

Mehta M, Ranger I 1971 Persistent abdominal pain. Anaesthesia 26(3): 330–333

Melnick J 1954 Treatment of trigger mechanisms in gastrointestinal disease. New York State Journal of Medicine 54: 1324–1330

Melnick J 1957a Symposium on mechanism and management of pain syndromes. Proceedings of the Rudolf Virchow Medical Society, City of New York 16: 135–142

Melnick J 1957b Trigger areas and refractory pain in duodenal ulcer. New York State Journal of Medicine 57: 1037–1076

Murray G R 1929 Myofibrositis as a simulator of other maladies. Lancet 1: 113–116

Procacci P, Zoppi M 1983 Pathophysiology and clinical aspects of visceral and referred pain. In: Bonica J (ed) Advances in pain research and therapy, Vol 5. Raven Press, New York, pp. 643–656

Ranger I, Mehta M, Pennington M 1971 Abdominal wall pain due to nerve entrapment. Practitioner 206: 791–792

Renaer M 1984 Gynaecological pain. In: Wall P D, Melzack R (eds) Textbook of pain. Churchill Livingstone, Edinburgh, p. 373

Simons D, Travell J, Simons L 1998 Myofascial pain and dysfunction. The trigger point manual, Vol 1, Ch. 49. Williams and Wilkins, Baltimore

Slocumb J C 1984 Neurological factors in chronic pelvic pain: trigger points and the abdominal pelvic pain syndrome. American Journal of Obstetrics and Gynaecology 149: 536–543

Slocumb J C 1990 Chronic, somatic, myofascial and neurogenic abdominal pelvic pain. Clinical Obstetrics and Gynaecology 33(91): 143–153

Sinaki M, Merritt J L, Stillwell G K 1977 Tension myalgia of the pelvic floor. Mayo Clinic Proceedings 52: 717–722

Smith W T 1959 Levator spasm syndrome. Minnesota Medicine 42: 1076–1079

Stone R T, Barbero G J 1970 Recurrent abdominal pain in childhood. Pediatrics 45: 732–738

Telling W H 1935 The clinical importance of fibrositis in general practice. British Medical Journal 1: 689–692

Theobald G H 1949 The relief and prevention of referred pain. Journal of Obstetrics and Gynecology of the British Commonwealth 56: 447–460

Thiele G H 1937 Coccygodynia and pain in the superior gluteal region and down the back of the thigh: causation by tonic spasm of the levator ani, coccygeus and piriformis muscles and relief by massage of these muscles. Journal of the American Medical Association 109: 1271–1275

Thiele G H 1963 Coccygodynia: cause and treatment. Diseases of the Colon and Rectum 6: 422–436

Travell J 1950 The adductor longus syndrome: a cause of groin pain. Bulletin of the New York Academy of Medicine 26: 284–285

Travell J G, Simons D G 1983 Myofascial pain and dysfunction. The trigger point manual. Williams & Wilkins, Baltimore, pp. 660–683

Travell J G, Simons D G 1992 Myofascial pain and dysfunction. The trigger point manual, Vol. 2. Williams and Wilkins, Baltimore

Waller S L, Misiewicz J J 1969 Prognosis in the irritable bowel syndrome. Lancet II: 753–756

Watson W C, Sullivan S N, Corke M, Rush D 1976 Incidence of esophageal symptoms in patients with irritable bowel syndrome. Gut 17: 827 (abstract)

Yeates W K 1985 Pain in the scrotum. British Journal of Hospital Medicine 33(2): 101–104

Young D 1943 The effects of Novocaine injections on simulated visceral pain. Annals of Internal Medicine 19: 749–756

# Index

Note: Page references in *italics* indicate illustrations